ISBN 978-0-428-97131-1
PIBN 10786765

This book is a reproduction of an important historical work. Forgotten Books uses state-of-the-art technology to digitally reconstruct the work, preserving the original format whilst repairing imperfections present in the aged copy. In rare cases, an imperfection in the original, such as a blemish or missing page, may be replicated in our edition. We do, however, repair the vast majority of imperfections successfully; any imperfections that remain are intentionally left to preserve the state of such historical works.

THE

AMERICAN

JOURNAL OF OBSTETRICS

AND

DISEASES OF WOMEN AND CHILDREN

EDITED BY

BROOKS H. WELLS, M.D.,

Professor of Gynecology at the New York Polyclinic; Fellow of the American Gynecological Society, the New York Academy of Medicine, the New York Obstetrical Society, the Society of the Alumni of the City Hospital, etc.

VOLUME XLVI.

JULY–DECEMBER, 1902

NEW YORK
WILLIAM WOOD & COMPANY
1902

LIST OF CONTRIBUTORS.

ACKER, GEORGE N., Washington, D. C.
ALDRICH, CHARLES J., Cleveland, O.
ALDRICH, N. B., Fall River, Mass.
ATLEE, L. W., Philadelphia, Pa.
BALDWIN, J. F., Columbus, O.
BANDLER, SAMUEL WYLLYS, New York City.
BONIFIELD, CHARLES L., Cincinnati, O.
BOWEN, W. SINCLAIR, Washington, D. C.
BOYD, GEORGE M., Philadelphia, Pa.
BRANHAM, J. H., Baltimore, Md.
BROMWELL, J. R., Washington, D. C.
BROWN, ADELAIDE, San Francisco, Cal.
CARR, W. P., Washington, D. C.
CLARKE, AUGUSTUS P., Cambridge, Mass.
COOK, GEORGE WYTHE, Washington, D. C.
CROUSE, H. W., Victoria, Tex.
DEAVER, JOHN B., Philadelphia, Pa.
DORSETT, WALTER B., St. Louis, Mo.
DRENNAN, JENNIE G., St. Thomas, Ontario, Can.
DUNNING, L. H., Indianapolis, Ind.
GALLANT, A. ERNEST, New York City.
GILMAN, WARREN R., Worcester, Mass.
GOLDSPOHN, ALBERT, Chicago, Ill.
HALL, RUFUS B., Cincinnati, O.
HAMILTON, CHARLES S., Columbus, O.
HAYD, HERMAN E., Buffalo, N. Y.
HIRST, BARTON COOKE, Philadelphia, Pa.
HUMISTON, WILLIAM H., Cleveland, O.
JENKS, EDWARD W., Detroit, Mich.
KELLY, HOWARD A., Baltimore, Md.
KOLISCHER, G., Chicago, Ill.

McMurtry, Lewis S., Louisville, Ky.
McReynolds, R. P., Philadelphia, Pa.
Manton, W. P., Detroit, Mich.
Morris, Robert T., New York City.
Murphy, John B., Chicago, Ill.
Nairne, J. Stewart, Glasgow, Scotland.
Neff, J. M., Chicago, Ill.
Newman, Henry P., Chicago, Ill.
Noble, Charles P., Philadelphia, Pa.
Porter, Miles F., Fort Wayne, Ind.
Porter, William D., Cincinnati, O.
Price, Joseph, Philadelphia, Pa.
Reich, A., New York City.
Ricketts, Edwin, Cincinnati, O.
Ross, James F. W., Toronto, Can.
Russell, W. W., Baltimore, Md.
Schenck, B. R., Baltimore, Md.
Seymour, William Wotkyns, Troy, N. Y.
Shands, A. R., Washington, D. C.
Simpson, F. F., Pittsburg, Pa.
Smith, A. Lapthorn, Montreal, Can.
Smith, W. S., Baltimore, Md.
Stahl, Frank A., Chicago, Ill.
Stinson, J. Coplin, San Francisco, Cal.
Stone, I. S., Washington, D. C.
Stowe, Herbert Marion, Chicago, Ill.
Tate, Magnus A., Cincinnati, O.
Vander Veer, Albert, Albany, N. Y.
Watkins, Thomas J., Chicago, Ill.
Weber, Samuel L., Chicago, Ill.
Williams, J. J. Gurney, Philadelphia, Pa.
The American Association of Obstetricians and Gynecologists.
The American Gynecological Society.
The Chicago Gynecological Society.
The New York Obstetrical Society.
The Obstetrical Society of London.
The Section on Gynecology, College of Physicians of Philadelphia.
The Washington Obstetrical and Gynecological Society.
The Woman's Hospital Society.

THE AMERICAN

JOURNAL OF OBSTETRICS

AND

DISEASES OF WOMEN AND CHILDREN.

Vol. XLVI. JULY, 1902. No. 1.

ORIGINAL COMMUNICATIONS.

ECTOPIC GESTATION.[1]

BY

JAMES F. W. ROSS, M.D., C.M.,

Associate Professor of Gynecology, Toronto University,
Toronto, Canada.

(With seven illustrations.)

THE discussion of the subject of ectopic or extrauterine pregnancy is of interest to the medical profession and of value to the laity. The physician is anxious to make a diagnosis and the lay woman is anxious to benefit by it. A great deal has been written of late on the subject and there are many questions that require further consideration.

I made a careful search through many of the original monographs on the subject some years ago, and presented a paper before the American Association of Obstetricians and Gynecologists in 1892 together with a report of a few cases. I am now able to give a further report of my experience, and append to this paper a tabulated statement of the cases upon which it is based.

[1] Read before the Alumni Association of Detroit Medical College, June 4, 1902.

All writers on the subject are familiar with the work of Dr. William Campbell, who was a teacher of midwifery in Edinburgh and who published his monograph about 1842. He gave a large amount of material with but little attempt at good arrangement, says Tait. His work, however, is a landmark in the literature of the subject.

On this side of the Atlantic, Parry, of Philadelphia. published a very remarkable work on the subject in 1876. Again, later, the subject chosen for the Jeuks Prize Essay of the College of Physicians and Surgeons, Philadelphia, about the year 1889, was the diagnosis and treatment of extrauterine pregnancy, and the prize was awarded to John Strahan, of Belfast.

Tait, in 1888, wrote on ectopic pregnancy and pelvic hematocele. The work is based on an experience of forty cases.

Since the time when these writings were given to the public several points have been noticed: First, the less frequent rupture of ectopic pregnancy into the broad ligament than was supposed by Tait to occur; second, the ease with which the condition may be diagnosed before rupture; third, the frequency with which the disease occurs a second time in the same patient. It will be my aim to lay stress upon these three points in the present lecture.

I have a record of 45 cases (including one case of ruptured cornual pregnancy) operated upon. They include 3 cases operated on before rupture, 41. cases operated on after rupture, 1 case operated on after full time (ruptured cornual pregnancy), 5 cases after suppuration, 1 case of double ectopic gestation, 3 cases in which ectopic gestation occurred twice in the same patient, 1 case of interstitial pregnancy in its very earliest stage. I will endeavor to give you the outcome of this experience, not embellished in flowery language, but as a simple statement of facts. It will be well, however, to take the subject up systematically.

CLASSIFICATION.—The classification that I adopted in 1892 requires no change. Ectopic gestation may be met with in any part of the tube, from its intrauterine opening to its abdominal end. When the pregnancy is developed in the tube as it passes through the wall of the uterus, we call it interstitial or tubo-uterine; if developed in the middle portion of the tube, tubal; if developed at the ovarian end of the tube, tubo-ovarian or tubo-abdominal.

A pregnancy originating as an abdominal pregnancy has not

been proved to exist. Tait says that he cannot believe that a fertilized ovum may drop into the cavity of the peritoneum and become developed there, because the powers of digestion of the peritoneum are so extraordinary that an ovum, even if fertilized, could have no chance of development. If it is possible for the peritoneum to digest live structures so rapidly, why do we find intraperitoneal worms, and how can spermatozoa exist in this region? I have seen intraperitoneal worms free in the cavity of the peritoneum in fish, and I presume that it is the existence of life in the worm that prevents this digestion. The stomach wall is only digested post mortem. I feel, myself, that although abdominal pregnancy *per se* has not been demonstrated, there is no reason why it cannot occur.

A pregnancy originating as an ovarian pregnancy has not yet been proved to exist. Parry says "that if an ovarian pregnancy does occur it must be rare and will be curious; if it never occurs, so much the better." Bischoff and Barry are said to have discovered spermatozoa on the surface of the ovaries of bitches shortly after coitus. If it is possible for the spermatozoa to penetrate the wall of the ovary and produce an ovarian pregnancy, then, as a consequence of Bischoff's and Barry's observations, ovarian pregnancy should be frequently met with.

There are two conditions that must not be confounded in the classification of ectopic gestation. The first of these is pregnancy in a bifid or bicornuate uterus, and the second is a pregnancy occurring in a rudimentary uterine horn. These conditions must, however, be considered in the differential diagnosis of an ectopic gestation.

PATHOLOGICAL ANATOMY.—After the impregnated ovum has become arrested in the tube, a decidua serotina, if not a decidua vera, is formed; the chorionic villi develop. This development is beautifully shown in an early impregnated uterus of the rabbit. I have a slide prepared from such a uterus while a student in Zurich. The tubal wall, into which the chorionic villi push themselves, becomes thinned, and this is well shown in one of my specimens of unruptured tubal pregnancy. The specimen had not ruptured, but was on the point of rupturing.

Still further changes now take place. Blood vessels become increased in size and in numbers, the parts become very much congested, and the swelling of the tube, as seen in several of these specimens, closely resembles a small myoma in its interior. A decidua is formed in the interior of the uterine cavity; this de-

cidua forms early, but is not likely to be shed until after the
death of the ovum takes place or the tube has ruptured. I show
here a specimen taken from a woman who died at our Union
Station a few months ago. She died from intraperitoneal hemorrhage that was produced by rupture of a tube containing an
ectopic gestation.   Even though the pregnancy was of short
duration, the decidual lining can be distinctly seen.

A tubal pregnancy is frequently injured by the rupture of its
own vessels; blood is thus poured out around the ovum into the
interior of the tube. The progress of the condition now depends
largely upon the site occupied by the impregnated ovum. The
spot in which earliest rupture takes place is near to, or in, the

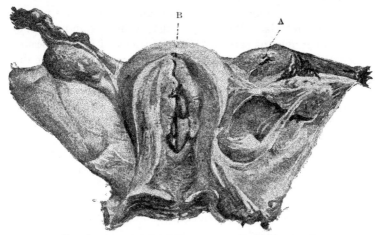

FIG. 1.—A, ruptured tubal pregnancy; B, decidua *in situ*.

uterine wall where the tube pierces the muscular structure of
this organ. The middle portion of the tube allows of much
greater distension, and, as a consequence, the pregnancy in this
situation will proceed further without rupture. When the ovum
is situated toward the abdominal ostium of the tube, tubal abortion is liable to occur through the fimbriated end. This leak may
only be small, or, in other words, a tubal "drip."

Rupture of the sac may occur at any of the sites liable to be
occupied by the impregnated ovum, and the result may or may
not be fatal to the mother and may or may not be fatal to the
fetus.

The ovum survives the rupture in only a very few cases. The
site of rupture in the interstitial variety may be so small as al-

most to escape detection, as is shown in the specimen here exhibited (Fig. 2) and reported in the table as No. 34.

Tait says that rupture may occur as early as the fourth week. I think I have seen it occur earlier. In THE AMERICAN JOURNAL OF OBSTETRICS, October, 1895, one of my cases is recorded that ruptured at a very early stage—I thought about two- or three-weeks gestation. A plate is there given, drawn from nature, but the plate does not exactly represent the size of the tube at the uterine end. It was smaller than it is there represented and corresponded more nearly with the condition of the tube on the distal side of the rupture.

The bleeding from an ectopic gestation may be either intraperitoneal or extraperitoneal. Intraperitoneal hemorrhage may

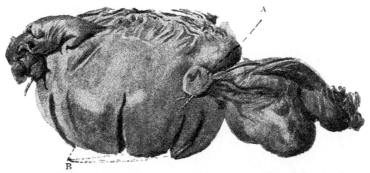

FIG. 2.—Interstitial pregnancy, very early rupture (Case 34). A, site at which uterine wall was ligated to control hemorrhage; B, cervical portion of uterus cut at various points.

occur in two ways: first, by direct rupture of the tube into the peritoneal cavity; second, by the tubal drip or a leakage, drop by drop, of blood through the fimbriated end of the tube. When extraperitoneal it becomes so as a consequence of rupture through the mesosalpinx into the layers of the broad ligament. A great deal of stress has been laid upon this latter form of rupture, but in my experience I have not met with it.

In the table it may be noted that I found distension of the broad ligament on a certain side after opening the abdomen, but that the sac was peeled out as the operation proceeded. Had the rupture been into the layers of the broad ligament it would have been impossible to have peeled out the sac in this way.

On superficial examination many of these cases will simulate a mass in the broad ligament, just as those cysts do that were formerly recorded, and that are perhaps still recorded, by the in-experienced as intraligamentous cysts. The cysts referred to are now known to be under the broad ligament— subligamentous and not intraligamentous. They can be readily distinguished owing to the fact that the tube will be found stretched along their upper surface. On closer inspection they will be found doubled under the ligament, but intimately associated with it. I do not for one moment deny that hemorrhage into the broad ligament does not occur, but I must insist that very few of these cases are brought to the operating table.

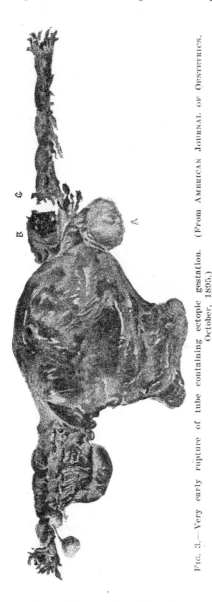

FIG. 3.—Very early rupture of tube containing ectopic gestation. (From AMERICAN JOURNAL OF OBSTETRICS. October, 1895.)

I take it that the bleeding from an extrauterine pregnancy may be either slow or rapid. When slow the blood coagulates; when rapid it does not coagulate to such an extent. When the blood coagulates it produces a mass; when it does not coagulate no such mass is produced. When the hemorrhage is slow and the blood coagulates adhesions are rapidly formed around the site of the hemorrhage, and in a short time just as much tension will be produced in this way as can be exerted by the loose layers of the broad ligament. After a time the amount of blood will be increased by fresh hemorrhage and the adhesions will no longer be able to retain the mass, and, as a consequence, free blood will be poured into the peritoneal cavity, and, if in any large quantity, will be found as high up as the liver and spleen. When the blood flows slowly the patients have attacks of syncope and of pain, and if the hemorrhage ceases for a time they resume apparent good health. The mass continues to increase in the pelvis so long as the hemorrhage continues intermittently.

In support of his argument in favor of broad-ligament rupture, Tait says that peritonitis rarely occurs in cases of broad-ligament rupture and that the talk about collections of blood becoming encysted is the veriest nonsense. I beg to assert that the blood does become encysted and that I have removed such encysted blood many times. It is not difficult to understand how we may have the organization of this blood clot without an appreciable amount of inflammation. Such organization of the blood is not a result of inflammation. Campbell recognized this feature years ago, and said in his book that the connection with the original mass—meaning the poured-out blood—through time, with the adjacent parts becomes so intimate that, when superficially considered, the ovum may seem to be involved by the layers of the broad ligament.

Tait considers that, in many cases after other operations upon the tubes, the mass that occasionally forms is an intraligamentous hematocele. There has been no proof adduced that these masses are intraligamentous hematoceles. Secondary hemorrhage is a well-recognized occurrence after the ligature of the blood vessels in other parts of the body, and among these friable, dense, and edematous structures in the pelvis there is no reason why secondary hemorrhage should not also occur. When these hemorrhages do occur it is difficult to understand why they should select the layers of the broad ligament instead of the pelvic cavity itself. I am satisfied that oozing may take place from the stump of an amputated ovary and tube into the general peritoneal cavity among the intestines, and that this oozing may cease and the blood clot may be absorbed or require vaginal section for its removal (as in a case of Dr. E. O'Reilly, of Hamilton).

Tait says in his "Lectures," on page 37: "Thus I tied the pedicle of one ovarian tumor with catgut and the patient died on the fourth day after operation. I found a large intraperitoneal hematocele, due to the gestation and loosening of the ligature." He states that these hematoceles produced by rupture into the broad ligament produce stricture of the rectum; and in recording such a case, the only evidence that he brings to bear to prove that the effusion of blood was in the left broad ligament is the fact that the floor and the posterior wall of the abscess were found to consist of old laminated blood clot. In his zeal to establish the new theory he goes so far as to state that effusion of blood into the broad ligament may be produced by a sudden arrest of menstruation, and, further, that numbers of cases in which this effusion occurs do not think it worth while to ask for medical assistance and get quite well without it. "And, still further," Tait says, in discussing a case, that was supposed to be one of ovarian pregnancy, reported by Hildebrand, "the very fact that it was discharged by the rectum is conclusive evidence that it rested in the broad ligament."

Such is the argument he uses to prove his case. Do not abscess of the ovary and abscess of the tube burst into the rectum without going through the diverse channel of the broad ligament? I have reported one case, in the Transactions of the Michigan State Medical Society, 1892, of secondary suppuration of an ectopic gestation that ruptured directly into the abdominal cavity itself, and I feel satisfied that these intraperitoneal hemorrhages, producing organized masses, may rupture either into the rectum, bladder, or abdominal cavity at will, and that they are not influenced in any way by the presence or absence of the broad ligament.

If the fetus dies and the placental structures become inactive, recovery may occur whether the hemorrhage has been into the layers of the broad ligament or into the peritoneal cavity, as a consequence of absorption of the masses. If the placenta remains active, a further hemorrhage either into the broad ligament or into the pelvic cavity may occur and serious and dangerous symptoms may supervené. Or, further, suppuration may take place with the formation of a pelvic abscess.

If the fetus lives it may develop in the abdominal cavity, in the layers of the broad ligament, and—but very rarely—in the tube itself. When it develops in the abdominal cavity the fetus is really surrounded by amnion, though it may be difficult to make it out. In one case on which I operated the fetus had escaped from a bicornuate uterus that had ruptured. The pregnancy reached full time and a secondary rupture of the sac occurred at the end of the ninth month. Primary rupture did not take place into the broad ligament. The sac surrounding the fetus might easily have been mistaken for broad ligament at the time of operation. The placenta after rupture may remain within the main gestation sac, or it may be partially extruded and, with the continuance of its growth, may spread out over the neighboring viscera.

When tubal abortion occurs the placenta is of course extruded into the abdominal cavity, and under such circumstances it seems hardly probable that it can have any power of taking on new adhesions to continue its life. If the placenta remains entire within the gestation sac after the extrusion of the fetus, there will then be two sacs, one containing the fetus and the other the placenta, and the cord will pass through an opening communicating from the one to the other.

SOME OF THE RARER CONDITIONS.—*Interstitial pregnancy* is but rarely met with. I have met with it in one case, of which the following is a report: Mrs. S. (No. 34 in table). Patient of Dr. Bryans, of Toronto. She had missed one period; had slight hemorrhage from the uterus. Before the doctor saw her she had fainted three or four times. Had been taken ill at noon on the previous day with sudden, severe pain in the abdomen. She was sent into the hospital under my care, and the case was, unfortunately, not correctly diagnosed by the house surgeon, as he thought the patient was threatened with a miscarriage. In the morning, when I saw her, she was almost moribund. Operated, however, and found the abdominal cavity full of blood. It was very difficult to make out the point from which the hemorrhage was coming. Drew up one tube, found it healthy; drew up the other tube, found it healthy, and was for a moment at a loss to know what to do. On raising the uterus I found a small spot on its anterior wall behind the junction of the round ligament with the uterine fundus. On sponging this off I could make out distinctly a small cavity about the size of a small pea, with dark edges, and from which blood oozed. It was evidently a rupture of an interstitial pregnancy of but very short duration. The patient died the same afternoon and I have here the specimen to show you (see Fig. 2).

Interstitial or tubo-uterine pregnancy may, however, continue to grow for several weeks, up to the end of the fourth month, or even longer. Rupture may take place either downward into the cavity of the uterus or upward into the abdomen. We have no positive evidence that a downward rupture has ever taken place without coincident rupture into the abdomen, but rupture into the abdomen alone has been met with. Very severe hemorrhage is one of the main features of this form of extrauterine pregnancy. Taylor met with but one case in his series of 42, Lawson Tait met with but one case in his series of 40, and I met with but one case in a series of 45.

Intra- and Extrauterine Pregnancy.—My friend Dr. Strathy, of our city, has met with such a case. He has kindly furnished me with the following notes: The patient's first child was born after an ordinary labor of a few hours. Another child was then felt to be in the abdominal cavity. It could be easily made out and the fetal heart sounds could be heard. The abdomen was not opened until the following day, when the child was removed without trouble. The placenta was found situated posteriorly over the psoas muscle and was not removed. Hemorrhage began at the time of the operation and could not be controlled, and the patient died four or five hours after.

Such an occurrence emphasizes the fact that it is extremely dangerous to operate during the life of the fetus.

Double Extrauterine Pregnancy.—I have met with one case of double extrauterine pregnancy, of which the following is a report: Mrs. E. (No. 42 in table). Patient of Dr. Andrew Eadie. Was taken ill one night with sudden, severe fainting spells while lying in bed. Was not seen by Dr. Eadie until the morning, when, on examination, he found a large mass in the pelvis behind and to the left of the uterus. I saw her at once and from her appearance judged that the case was one of ruptured ectopic gestation. She had the peculiar coloring of the skin so frequently noticed and a collapsed appearance. On further inquiry it was found that in August she had menstruated. In September she had seen very, very little; in October again but little was seen. Some pieces of decidua had come away from the uterus, but they were not preserved. The breasts indicated pregnancy. On examination, found blood clot, breaking down under the finger. Was satisfied that the case was one of ruptured extrauterine pregnancy.

On November 1, 1901, in the Toronto General Hospital Pavilion, assisted by Dr. Eadie, I opened the abdomen in the median line and found the abdominal cavity full of blood. On passing the fingers down to the right side, found a small mass; on drawing this up, found it to be omentum with an ectopic-gestation sac under its folds, running up to the surrounded Fallopian tube. On removing this sac the Fallopian tube was torn off; ovary and

tube on this side were ligated with silk. As soon as this gestation sac was disturbed a great deal of fresh blood was poured
out. The fingers were then passed down to the other side as a
matter of routine, and to my surprise I found another gestation
sac connected with the left tube. This was rapidly removed
from its adhesions, and on its removal it burst and the liquor
amnii escaped, together with a three-and-one-half-months fetus.
The two gestation sacs were, therefore, of different ages, and
the right one, though smaller, was certainly active as well as the
left. The pedicle was then tied off on the left side, a portion of

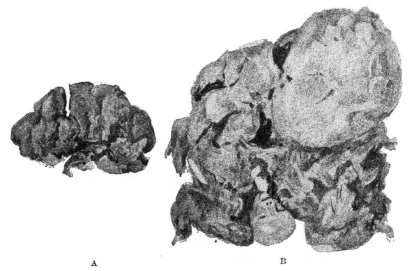

A   B

FIG. 4.—Case 42. Double tubal pregnancy. A, right side, eight weeks; B,
left side, twelve or fourteen weeks.

the ovary. being left to continue menstruation.   Abdominal
cavity was washed out rapidly and the patient almost sank on
the table. Subcutaneous injections of salines were given under
the breasts, the arms and legs bandaged, a drainage tube was
placed, and the wound closed with silkworm gut.   The patient developed pleurisy with effusion into the left chest, from
which I removed twenty-eight ounces; but, notwithstanding this
fact, she made an excellent recovery.
    The fact that both sides were active proved to me that it is
quite possible to have pregnancy occur in one tube and then, at a
subsequent date, occur in the opposite tube while the first is still

developing. The pregnancy in one tube, in this case, was evidently of three and one-half months' duration, while the pregnancy on the other side, we judged, was of about two months' duration.

Ectopic Gestation Occurring Twice in the Same Patient.—My experience with cases occurring twice in the same patient is as follows (three cases):

CASE I.—Mrs. H., æt. 24 (No. 3 in table). Operated on July 6, 1891. Had no children, but thought she had miscarried. Had passed three weeks over her monthly period, and had become unwell and remained so for seven weeks. The flowing then ceased and commenced again two or three weeks after. Severe pains, like labor pains, appeared; she became collapsed. The collapse disappeared and on June 30 she walked to the hospital. On examination a mass was found in front and to the right side of the uterus. Returning, two days later, to the hospital, I operated and found the abdomen filled with old dark liquid, and not clotted, blood. The woman had evidently been going around with this blood in her abdominal cavity. Removed ectopic gestation from the right side.

(Table, No. 9.) On October 10, 1895, I saw her again with Dr. Noble. Found her collapsed, pale, with all the appearance of internal hemorrhage; precordial uneasiness. Patient looked anxious and very ill. She had gone two weeks past her period. A sudden pain came on shortly after she wakened in the morning. No elevation of temperature. A mass was felt in the cul-de-sac of Douglas and broke down under the examining finger. Removed an extrauterine pregnancy from the left side. Patient recovered. This case was reported in THE AMERICAN JOURNAL OF OBSTETRICS, February, 1896.

CASE II.—Mrs. L., æt. 26 (table, No. 14). Referred by Dr. McMahon. Was nursing child 17 months old. Did not miss a monthly period. Was quite regular until she began, after one period, to flow continuously. This continued for four weeks. Patient was sent to my office, and I found the left tube and ovary normal, right ovary normal, right tube enlarged at its outer end and lying in front of the uterus. Two days after (August 14, 1896) I removed an extrauterine pregnancy, unruptured, from the right tube. Though the tube was unruptured, the abdomen contained old blood, and blood could be seen to ooze from the fimbriated end of the tube when it was drawn up, drop by drop, coming very slowly (tubal drip).

On September 28, 1898 (table, No. 27) saw the patient again with Dr. Eadie. Had missed a monthly period and gone a few days over. Irregular hemorrhage from the uterus and cramp-like pains in the lower part of the abdomen and chiefly on the left side. The two physicians who had seen her formerly saw her again and found a mass to the left side and behind the uterus. I examined her and found the ovary to be close to the uterus and normal in size. Next day removed an extrauterine pregnancy from the left tube. The ovary formed a cyst that had evidently been taken for the gestation sac, and the gestation sac had been taken for the ovary, being hard and firm and unruptured. The chorionic villi were penetrating the tube wall, and the wall might have ruptured any moment. There was no blood present in the abdominal cavity. There was no evidence of ligature or stump of tube on the opposite side, removed two years before. The wall of the uterus was smooth from the fundus downward. Patient recovered. This was reported in THE AMERICAN JOURNAL OF OBSTETRICS, volume xxxviii., No. 6, with the names of the attending physicians.

CASE III.—Mrs. R. (table, No. 20). This case has not been previously reported. Her physician was Dr. Fletcher, of Euclid avenue, Toronto. She had not missed a period, but uterine hemorrhage came on and continued for three weeks. She then had a sudden attack of faintness and became bathed in perspiration. Had pains of irregular character in the lower abdomen. On examination a mass was found behind the uterus.

On January 14, 1898, shelled out an ectopic-gestation sac with the clots found subsequent to rupture. Left tube and ovary were incorporated in the mass and were removed. Patient recovered.

(Table, No. 38.) In June, 1901, saw the patient again with Dr. Fletcher. She had indefinite pelvic pains and had come back on account of these, as we had advised her. On careful examination the doctor found a little nodule, he thought, on the right tube. I examined and found the same. The patient had a slight flow of blood from the uterus. We sent her to her home in the country and advised her to return in two weeks. She did so, and we examined her again and found the mass had increased to double its size, and concluded the case was one of extrauterine pregnancy on the other side.

On June 21, 1901, I opened the abdomen and found a hematoma of the right ovary; drew up the right tube and found an ectopic gestation the size of the end of the little finger. It was the earliest unruptured ectopic gestation I have ever seen. Removed tube and ovary on that side.

When making my first report of Case 1, in which ectopic gestation occurred twice in the same patient, I looked up the literature of the subject and found but five similar reports that entirely satisfied me as to the correctness of the diagnosis in each case. It cannot be possible, however, that I have had an exceptional experience in this respect. Taylor says that upward of fifty such cases have been recorded. In his own case I find, however, that the first ectopic gestation was not demonstrated by surgical operation or postmortem examination, and, in view of what I have to relate later regarding conditions that simulate ruptured extrauterine pregnancy, I am not prepared to accept reports without such surgical or postmortem verification. In my cases the pregnancy occurred first on the one side and then on the other.

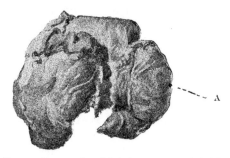

FIG. 5.—Very early unruptured tubal pregnancy at A (Case 38).

Coe has reported a case in which a lithopedion was found on the same side as that on which the ectopic gestation was situated at the time of operation. This demonstrated the fact that ectopic gestation can occur twice on the same side.

Ectopic Gestation Followed by Conditions Simulating Ectopic Gestation and Requiring Operation. CASE I.—In the table this case is reported as No. 1. Was operated on for extrauterine pregnancy December 24, 1886. She had good health and bore one child. Returned again and was operated on December 10, 1889, and a hematosalpinx, the blood of which was uncoagulated, was removed from the other side. There was no evidence to indicate that this was the result of impregnation. The symptoms on the second occasion were a continued flow from the uterus together with a mass on the left side.

CASE II.—This case is recorded in the table as No. 32. Operated on January 5, 1900, for extrauterine pregnancy. She returned on April 24, 1902, and was operated on April 26, when a tubo-ovarian cyst on the left side was removed. She complained, on the second occasion, of pains in the abdomen, chiefly on the left side. Had missed one week, but had no uterine hemorrhage. The mass could be felt on physical examination.

CASE III.—Case No. 13 in the table was operated on for extra-uterine pregnancy December 24, 1895. She returned again and was operated on October 19, 1896, for a hydrosalpinx on the left side.

CASE IV.—This case is reported in the table as No. 17. Operated on for extrauterine pregnancy on July 13, 1897, when the right tube and ovary were removed, together with gestation sac on that side. Left tube and ovary looked healthy. She returned again on March 25, 1898, and at the operation I removed a hematosalpinx on the left side.

Cases of Previous Operation for Other Conditions, Followed by Ectopic Gestation. CASE I.—Mrs. McC. (No. 22 in table). In July, 1897, I removed a small cyst of the right ovary. Patient made an uninterrupted recovery. In February, 1898, removed ectopic gestation after rupture of the sac on the left side.

CASE II.—Mrs. R. (No. 44 in table). Was operated on May 4, 1890, for large ovarian tumor. Secondary hemorrhage occurred, and the patient was reopened the same day. Recovered with some inflammatory symptoms. On January 28, 1902, operated again and removed an extrauterine pregnancy after rupture of the sac, from the opposite side.

The experience with these cases goes to prove that ectopic gestation follows the woman who has once had a pelvic inflammation. The report shows how difficult it is to be certain that a condition giving certain symptoms is undoubtedly ectopic gestation.

I operated on the wife of one of our leading practitioners for a ruptured ectopic gestation. She subsequently became pregnant and bore a living child, but in the interval, before pregnancy occurred, she was suddenly seized with all the symptoms of a ruptured ectopic gestation. No surgical operation was performed and she made a good recovery. Can I state, in such a case, that the patient undoubtedly suffered from extrauterine pregnancy on two different occasions? I have refrained from including this case in my table of ectopic gestation occurring twice in the same patient, owing to the uncertainty that existed, but I find that there have been many similar cases recorded without any greater amount of proof.

ETIOLOGY.—Ectopic gestation seems to be intimately associated with inflammation of the tubes. It has been stated that the inflammation has been followed by desquamation of the epithelium lining the mucous membrane, and that, owing to this fact, the ovum has been allowed to settle in an abnormal position.

Another cause of the disease is undoubtedly mechanical obstruction to the progress of the ovum through the oviduct. This mechanical obstruction may be caused by pressure from without or within the tube, by growth, or as a consequence of distortion of the tube produced by adhesions. It has been stated that atrophy of the tube is a cause of extrauterine pregnancy, but I have not noticed such atrophy in any of my cases. The tubes have always appeared to be healthy and normal on the opposite side. It is evident that they were not healthy or they would not have required subsequent operative interference.

My experience does not coincide with that of Taylor, who states that he does not believe that ectopic gestation is produced by a result of previous inflammation of the tubes. I have almost always been able to elicit the history of a previous attack of inflammation from these patients, and this inflammation has frequently been followed by a period of sterility.

I have met with ectopic gestation in a young unmarried woman, and once in a bride of seven weeks who was, I believe, a virgin when married.

SYMPTOMS.—The symptoms of ectopic gestation must be considered: first, before rupture; second, at the time of rupture; third, after rupture.

Symptoms before Rupture.—History of a previous attack of inflammation and sterility; a missed period, more or less subsequent, more or less continuous discharge of blood from the uterus; pelvic discomfort; bearing-down pains, paroxysmal in character, but not severe; soreness or enlargement of the breasts.

Physical Signs.—On examination, with or without an anesthetic, a small mass to be made out in the tube on one side of the uterus, firm in consistence, rounded, regular, and not pitted like the ovary, and at the same time the ovary can be made out as separate and distinct from it.

Symptoms at the Time of Rupture.—The symptoms present before rupture will have added to them the following: sudden, severe pain; collapse with cold perspiration; precordial uneasiness; pale and anxious face; rapid, thin pulse and dilated pupils; shifting dulness as the intraperitoneal blood shifts with the change of position of the patient; visibly increased vermicular action of the intestines; great restlessness; suppression of urine or great diminution in the quantity of urine; a desire to defecate without the ability to do so.

Physical Signs.—On examination there may be but little to be felt. It will be difficult to make out any small mass in the tube. Examination under these circumstances may give no clue as to the nature of the trouble.

Symptoms after Rupture.—In addition to the symptoms given before and at the time of rupture, we have the following: sallowish, faded-leaf color of the skin from absorption of blood pigment and loss of blood; slight puffing of the abdomen, without much tenderness and without rigidity of the abdominal muscles; recurrence of severe symptoms from time to time; slight elevation of temperature, irregular variations of pulse; irritability of the bladder may be present.

Physical Signs.—Pelvic examination discloses a mass on one side of, or behind or in front of the uterus. The blood clot may be felt to break down under the finger. There is a boggy feeling 'of the parts. The uterus is found slightly enlarged. A decidua may be discharged entire or in pieces.

I have not found the presence of the decidua of value in diagnosis. It is generally extruded too late and only after serious symptoms have set in. When it is extruded the case very closely simulates one of miscarriage and may be mistaken for it.

Tait says that he saw only one case of unruptured extrauterine pregnancy, and Parry says that it is very rarely that an opportunity is obtained to examine an unruptured cyst. I have brought three or four such specimens to exhibit here to-day. When the symptoms before rupture are more carefully studied and more carefully taught, unruptured extrauterine pregnancy will be more frequently met with. The unruptured cases with which I have met have occurred in the practice of those who have discussed the subject very carefully and who have been thoroughly familiar with the very earliest symptoms and physical signs. The diagnosis has, therefore, been made by them and only subsequently confirmed by me.

These are no "society utterances or library paper expressions," as Tait dubs them, but a statement of facts.

2

For many years a great deal of difficulty arose owing to the fact that writers endeavored to separate into two what was really one disease. They gave long tables of the symptoms of hemato-

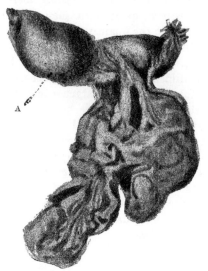

Fig. 6.—Unruptured tubal pregnancy at A.

cele on the one hand and ectopic gestation on the other. We now know that hematocele is, in most cases, due to ectopic gestation and that, therefore, the symptoms of hematocele are practically the symptoms of ectopic gestation subsequent to rupture or leakage.

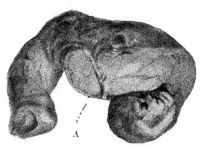

Fig. 7.—Unruptured tubal gestation (Case 26). A, site at which rupture was imminent.

DIFFERENTIAL DIAGNOSIS.   *Before Rupture.*—A diagnosis must be made from the following conditions: first, abortion; second, myoma, sarcoma, carcinoma of the tube; third, hematosalpinx;

fourth, hydrosalpinx; fifth, pyosalpinx; sixth, cyst, fibroid, or hematoma of the ovary.

In abortion there will be no mass felt in the tube. The uterus will, in all probability, be larger than in ectopic gestation. In growths of the tube there will be no symptoms of pregnancy; no period will have been missed. In hematosalpinx and hydrosalpinx, as well as in hematoma of the ovary, the symptoms will closely simulate those of ectopic gestation. From the cases recorded it will be seen that it is impossible to make a differential diagnosis until after the abdomen has been opened. In cases of pyosalpinx there will generally be a history of inflammation with an elevation of temperature and an absence of the symptoms of pregnancy. A small cyst of the ovary will frequently produce uterine hemorrhage, coming on after a missed period, but without any of the other symptoms of pregnancy. The cyst can generally be readily made out; it is too dense and rounded and fluctuating to be a tubal pregnancy. The ovarian ligament assists us in coming to a conclusion as to whether the enlargement is tubal or ovarian, and, furthermore, the ovary on that side will be found wanting.

In two of my cases I was enabled to diagnose unruptured ectopic gestation owing to this very fact. The enlargement of the ovary led to the diagnosis of extrauterine pregnancy; the mass in the tube was mistaken for the normal ovary. Fortunately, in each case the abdomen was opened, and, though the enlarged ovary had been mistaken for the gestation sac and the gestation sac had been mistaken for the normal ovary, the patients were readily relieved from what could have been serious danger.

A fibroid of the ovary may be made out by feeling the ovarian ligament, and the irregular and hard outline of the growth itself is its chief characteristic. It is not likely to be accompanied by uterine hemorrhage.

At the Time of Rupture.—Differential diagnosis at this time must be made, first, from acute poisoning; second, from rupture of the bladder; third, from rupture of the stomach or intestines; fourth, from intraperitoneal hemorrhage from some other source, such as ruptured uterus in a case of normal pregnancy, rupture of a pregnant bicornuate uterus, or rupture of a pregnant illdeveloped uterine horn; fifth, acute gonorrheal endometritis; and, sixth, attempted abortion.

In acute poisoning there may not be the symptoms of pregnancy or hemorrhage from the uterus. Rupture of the bladder is a very rare occurrence and generally associated with traumatism; symptoms of pregnancy will not be present and there will not have been uterine hemorrhage. Perforation of stomach or intestines, not due to traumatism, may closely simulate ectopic gestation at the time of rupture. Symptoms of pregnancy and uterine hemorrhage will be absent and there will, in all probability, have been symptoms of pre-existing inflammatory or other disease. Except in cases of perforation of a gastric ulcer, the patient is not, in my experience, greatly collapsed. Intraperitoneal hemorrhage from some other source cannot be definitely diagnosed from a ruptured ectopic gestation. Acute gonorrheal endometritis will very closely simulate ruptured extrauterine pregnancy. It is accompanied by fever and frequently by a discharge of blood from the vagina in which pus is found, and a discharge of either pus or blood from the urethra on stripping the same with the finger. There is often inflammation of the external genitals. Collapse is not marked; great abdominal tenderness is present. There will be no symptoms of pregnancy and the patient will not have missed a monthly period. Vomiting is often present, as well as rigidity of the abdominal walls.

In cases of attempted abortion there will be found some good reason why the patient does not wish to have a child. Symptoms of pregnancy will be present; temperature very high; pulse of inflammatory type; collapse not marked; rigidity of the abdominal walls. Patient gives evasive answers, though she may acknowledge having passed an instrument.

In the address on "Midwifery" read at the twenty-ninth annual meeting of the Canadian Medical Association, held at Montreal, I presented the table on page 21, that may be of interest.

Intraperitoneal hemorrhage may occur in a small amount and still give rise to severe symptoms. One of the patients on whom I operated for extrauterine pregnancy became pregnant subsequently. After she had missed two periods she was taken suddenly with severe pain in the side, in the lower abdomen, and felt as if something had given way. She had a large hernia from the packing that had been used at the time of the previous operation to check the terrible hemorrhage. I opened the abdomen, fearing that a loop of intestine might have become caught or that some bands had been torn, and feeling that I could, at the same time, repair the large hernia and place her in a better condition.

	Acute Gonorrheal Endometritis.	Ectopic Gestation.	...ed Abortion.
Previous health.	Good.	Perhaps history of ... this attack of inflammation and sterility.	Good. Very likely had children fast, if married.
History of discharge.	Mattery discharge, perhaps swelling of ...	No ...ary discharge.	Leuc... No swelling of labia.
Menses.	Menstruation ... commencing perhaps at an irregular time, and lasting for ten ... to three ... No period missed. ... not offensive.	A period missed, then irregular discharges of ..., more or less profuse. Discharge not offensive.	A period missed, perhaps only one or two days. Then discharge of blood lasting indefinite ..., as instrument is often introduced at frequent ... desire to bring ... away. Patient toward last becomes ... desperate and uses more ... foe. Discharge often offensive.
Pain.	Gradually ...	Spasmodic. At times very acute. Spreads over a considerable portion of ... Sometimes only one ... severe ... Often collapsed at ... of rupture and at ... successive hemorrhage.	Sudden pain, p...ps followed by spasmodic pains over a considerable period of time.
Collapse.	Not collapsed.		A partial condition of collapse. If from ... of irritating fluid injected into uterus through Fall... pla... ..., definite collap... ..., but it does not ...
Temperature.	Elevated. Often simulates typhoid.	Not very high	Very high.
Pulse.	Not rapid, unless general peritonitis present.	Varies. Rises with each hemorrhage into peritoneum. Goes up suddenly and comes down quickly.	... hard, inflammatory. ... up.
Rigor.	No rigors as a rule. Not ...	No rigors at this period. ... Pupils generally dilated.	Rigors present.
Appearance—Face.		Sallowish. Intermittent perspiration. At ... bathed in perspiration.	Anxious. Often slight delirium. Flushed, as if in high fever.
" —Skin.	No ... at first. Dry skin.		Intermittent perspirations, coming chiefly after chill.
" —Abdomen.	Distended, if peritonitis general. Muscles ... tender.	Slight puffing. Perhaps resistance from ... clot. Shifting dulness as clot shifts with patient's change of position. Not very tender. Increased vermicular action of ... may be s...	Slight puffing at this stage. ... localized tenderness simulating, if on the right side, appendicitis.
" —Breasts.	No enlargement. No change	Perhaps enlarged and changed. Often had a period of sterility.	Perhaps enlarged and changed. Often still nursing last child.
Position.	On ab... Feet ... up. Does not care to ... much. At first not persistent unless general peritonitis.	Restless. Turns from side to side.	Assumes any position. Perhaps dragging pain if lies on one side.
Vomiting.		Not a marked sign.	Irregular vomiting after taking food. Not persistent. Vomiting may ... be present ... as a consequence of pregnancy.
Onset of symptoms.	Definite ... as patient ... has no idea of ... of trouble.	Definite history given. No ... Not usually definite. No particular anxiety at non-appearance of menses.	No definite history given. Evasive answers. Contradictory statements. Though ... tallies cl...s ... with that of ... gestation, it lacks definiteness. Occasionally, if carefully questioned, ... shows that she was anxious at non-appearance of menses.
Digital examination.	Matting of parts on ea... beside of uterus. ... fixed. Uterus ...	Mass on one side of ... and behind. Clot may occasionally be felt breaking down under finger. Boggy feeling. ... perhaps slightly enlarged.	Mass usually on left side of ..., I think from use of right hand in passing ..., thus perforating ... at left side. No b... feeling.
Bladder.	Frequent history of irritability of bl...		No clot felt.

It was only after she was anesthetized that I was able to make out intrauterine pregnancy.

After the abdomen was opened I found a small quantity of blood and a large adhesion binding uterus to the pelvic struc-tures, that had been torn through. She was delivered later on, in the fifth month, in the early morning, and I saw her at 3 in the afternoon. I never had such difficulty in removing a pla-centa; it was universally adherent. She recovered.

I met with one other case of severe vomiting of pregnancy and collapse that simulated a case of ectopic gestation with rup-ture. The patient was threatened with a miscarriage and there-fore had uterine hemorrhage after having missed a period. The pregnancy had been allowed to go on until the condition from ex-cessive vomiting was extreme. Sudden pain and faintness set in. Upon careful examination, however, a correct conclusion was come to and a miscarriage induced, and even then we feared that the patient would succumb. A few days ago I saw the patient again in a similar condition and was struck with the close re-semblance to a case of ruptured ectopic gestation.

After Rupture.—Differential diagnosis must be made from, first, inflammatory disease; second, from tumor of the ovary; third, from pelvic abscess; fourth, from myoma uteri; fifth, from cornual pregnancy; sixth, from pregnancy in an ill-developed horn; seventh, from malignant disease.

The mass discovered in the inflammatory disease is usually situated on both sides of the uterus. It is harder and more sen-sitive to touch. Great elevation of temperature is noted. Tumor of the ovary is not accompanied by symptoms of previous rup-tured ectopic gestation unless it has been twisted on its pedicle. An ovarian tumor, pelvic in situation, that has been accompanied by uterine hemorrhage, and which has become fixed and inflamed as a consequence of a twist of its pedicle, will be difficult to diag-nose from a mass left in the pelvis from ruptured ectopic gesta-tion.

Pelvic abscess often results from ruptured ectopic gestation and breaking-down of the clot. Perhaps ectopic gestation is one of the most frequent causes of pelvic abscess. If of inflammatory origin, the history will assist in making a differential diagnosis.

Myoma uteri is usually more solid in consistence and rounder in outline, and the nodules on its surface are a great assistance in making a diagnosis. There will have been no sudden onset of severe symptoms.

It is difficult to diagnose cornual pregnancy, but the severe symptoms of rupture will, in all probability, have been absent. The same may be said of pregnancy in an ill-developed horn. If either of these have ruptured it will be impossible to distinguish from ectopic gestation after rupture. In malignant disease there will not have been any sudden onset of severe symptoms. The disease is accompanied by more pain and is of longer duration.

I had a curious experience with a case having an ill-developed uterine horn. The patient was 41 years of age, mother of four children. Had pain in the abdomen off and on for some time. It began in the left iliac region and passed in various directions. In September, 1891, had what she called typhoid fever and peritonitis; pain continued after this and came on chiefly at the menstrual period. When the patient was only 21 years of age she had had a lump, that appeared the size of a goose egg, to the left of the linea alba, in the lower pelvic region. A poultice was applied to it and it finally opened externally two or three inches below the umbilicus. The abscess remained as a chronic abscess for two years and then healed up. Owing to her indefinite symptoms when I saw her some years later, I decided to open the abdomen, and on April 9, 1892, this was carried out at the Toronto General Hospital. I found a bicornuate uterus; the mass to be felt to the left was one horn apparently only slightly attached to the cervix. This was determined by the situation of the round ligament joining its outer angle and the absence of broad ligament between the two uterine masses.

A year or two later I was called to see the patient with Dr. Rowan, of Toronto, and found her suffering from severe paroxysmal pains and obstinate constipation. She had been suffering from these pains for some weeks. The rectum was obstructed and a large mass was to be felt in the pelvis and could be felt above the pubes. I knew that the patient had a rudimentary uterine horn and decided that this mass must be retained menstrual fluid. She was not living with her husband. Upon puncture through the vagina a large quantity of black, tarry blood, resembling retained menses in cases of imperforate hymen, escaped. Had I not known the exact nature of the case I would have taken it to be one of pelvic hematocele caused by a rupture of an ectopic gestation into the broad ligament, but would have been puzzled by the tarry appearance of the blood.

Cornual Pregnancy.—In cornual pregnancy the round ligament will be found to run to the outer side of the mass, whereas

in tubal pregnancy the round ligament runs to the inner side of
the mass toward the median line.

Differential Diagnosis at Full Time before Death of Child.—
The diagnosis must be made at this time between ectopic gestation and *(a)* a normal intrauterine pregnancy with a very thin
wall; *(b)* displacement of the pregnant uterus by a fibrocystic
or myomatous tumor; *(c)* bifid uterus with pregnancy in one
chamber. I have met with several cases of thin uterine wall with
intrauterine pregnancy that felt as if the pregnancy must be outside of the uterus, but on more careful examination I was able
to satisfy myself that the condition was a normal one. In cases
of displacement of the pregnant uterus by a myomatous tumor
I have never had any difficulty in making a diagnosis.

I have met with one case of bifid uterus with pregnancy in one
chamber, and the report is as follows: Miss E., æt. 23. Had
menstruated and had a discharge of blood from the uterus.
Menstruation then ceased and she had seen nothing for two
months. There had been no abdominal pain and there was no
history of collapse. Patient looked in good health. I was so
uncertain as to the diagnosis of the case that I decided to use the
uterine sound. This passed in toward the right a distance of
about three inches. A tumor could be distinctly made out, to the
left side of the uterus, as large as a pregnancy at about three and
one-half months. I felt satisfied that the patient was pregnant
and decided that, as the uterus was empty, the pregnancy must
be an extrauterine one. There was milk in the breasts. Operation was advised and the abdomen opened on November 22, 1900.
I found a tumor that looked red and exactly like a pregnant
uterus. The sound was passed again and it went in, as before,
toward the right the same distance. On careful inspection the
case was found to be one of a pregnancy in one horn of a uterus
bicornis unicollis. Abdomen was closed and the patient went on
to full time and was attended by my friend Dr. McIlwraith, of
our city, who found the septum present at the time of delivery.

Differential Diagnosis at Full Time after Death of Child.—
The diminution in size of the abdomen, the false labor, and the
show that occurs are characteristic of this condition. The cervix is oftentimes found to be open, and in my own case (No. 45 in
table) the finger could be readily passed up into the uterine
cavity and the bicornuate condition of the uterus could be readily
made out. The diagnosis must be made at this time between
(a) slow-growing cancer, *(b)* fibrocystic tumor of the uterus,

and *(c)* tubercular peritonitis. In slow-growing cancer the increase is steady, and if there is any great increase in the growth the temperature chart will show evidence of suppuration, and this suppuration will be most likely to accompany an extrauterine pregnancy. A diagnosis between extrauterine pregnancy at this time and a fibrocyst of the uterus must be a difficult one.

I know of a case of tubercular peritonitis with the nodules floating about in the encysted fluid, simulating fetal parts, mistaken by an able surgeon for a case of extrauterine pregnancy after the death of the fetus. It was only after an exploratory operation had been performed that the diagnosis was settled.

TREATMENT. *Operation.*—Tait's first operation was performed in 1883. Operation is now the accepted method of procedure. It is called for to control the hemorrhage, to remove débris that may be dangerous to life, and to overcome the septic conditions that may present themselves.

Some have stated that the great impediment to the adoption of this treatment is the uncertainty of diagnosis. Tait laid down the dictum, however, that when the patient is found in danger of death from conditions within the abdomen which do not seem to be clearly of a malignant nature, but a correct diagnosis of which is impossible, the abdomen should be opened and the diagnosis made certain and thus successful treatment made possible.

He concluded "that in the great majority of cases of *extra*peritoneal hematocele, even when due to ectopic gestation, the disease may generally be let alone, being rarely fatal, and that it is to be interfered with only when suppuration or extreme hemorrhage has occurred. That, on the contrary, *intra*peritoneal hematocele is fatal, with almost uniform certainty, that so soon as it is suspected the abdomen must be opened and the hemorrhage arrested."

I must take exception to this opinion. I am satisfied that the cases of intraperitoneal hematocele are not uniformly fatal, and I have operated on cases that I feel satisfied might have recovered without operative interference, and have left unoperated on other cases, that have recovered, that had been collapsed and almost moribund at a considerable distance of time before I saw them. The fact that the patients had presented all the symptoms of intraperitoneal hemorrhage showed that such cases can recover without operation and that they need not necessarily be cases of hemorrhage into the broad ligament.

But it seems to me that such fine distinctions cannot serve any good purpose. If a diagnosis can be made before rupture—and that it can frequently be made is now beyond dispute—the abdomen should be opened, either through the abdominal wall in front or through the vagina below, and the unruptured tube should be removed. It is not necessary to remove the ovary if it is healthy. This will be a very simple procedure and the mortality, in skilled hands, should be almost *nil*. When rupture has occurred operation should be undertaken without delay. I have in one instance taken the patient in my carriage at once to the hospital at 1 A.M. in order to save delay. I have never regretted rapid action in these cases, but in two cases I have regretted delay. We should not attempt to quiet our fears by endeavoring to decide between tubal drip or weeping, and tubal rupture into the peritoneal cavity or the broad ligament. If your experience tallies with mine you will not often find the rupture into the broad ligament.

If you will do me the honor of carefully reviewing my table, you will see that the lowest mortality accompanies the early operation. When puzzled over these cases one should send immediately for further advice. We should not wait until the next day. If one consultant cannot be obtained owing to the lateness of the hour, another should be procured. Waiting means increased risk to the patient and increased difficulties for the operator. An operation is the only form of treatment in such cases.

The terrible contingencies that sometimes arise when the condition is allowed to proceed are particularly exemplified in Case 28 of the table (Mrs. J.). In that case, after opening the abdomen I found the uterus pushed forward; it looked like a uterus containing a six-weeks pregnancy. Adhesions of the omentum were broken down and these bled very freely. An enucleation of the mass was then started. After a time the finger burst into it and fluid escaped. Then portion of old clot came out. With the finger through the opening a fetus could be distinctly felt and this was extracted. The placental adhesion was now reached and blood gushed out immediately. It came so fast that, in a moment of desperation, I clamped the right uterine artery and then clamped the left one. And decided that it would be necessary to perform hysterectomy in order to get at the hemorrhage. Hemorrhage from these adhesions was terrible. The patient almost died on the table during the operation. Gauze was packed into the pelvis after the surface, from which the placenta had been removed, had been touched with persulphate of iron. The blood seemed to come from hundreds of spots and to well up from them. Pressure was applied externally, rectum packed with gauze, vagina packed with gauze, and a firm bandage placed *in situ*. Notwithstanding the fact that the uterus, tubes, and ovaries had been removed with the mass, the bleeding continued from the surface of the cul-de-sac of Douglas and the surrounding parts, so that gauze had to be used in the aforementioned manner. The patient lived for three days.

Such an experience should be sufficient to warn us to wait, in such cases, until after the death of the child or until full time. It is very easy to lay down this rule, but it is not so easy for us to observe it. The life or death of the fetus is difficult to determine, and many operators find themselves face to face with a live fetus and an active placenta, owing to this very difficulty. They would like to draw back, but are forced to go on.

When the pregnancy is advanced vaginal section should give way to abdominal section. Tait believed that vaginal section is an unsatisfactory method for the purpose of saving the child. There are many cases recorded in which great difficulties were met with in getting the child out, and only two cases were known to him in which the child had been extracted alive. His experience is similar to mine and was sufficient to deter him from making another attempt to deliver the fetus in this way. He wrote that he would never, under any circumstances, attack a subperitoneal pregnancy from the vagina. He considered that the child could not be dragged out without tearing tissues in which large sinuses have been abnormally developed, and through structures unyielding as they are this can only be done with much force and with the likelihood of losing its life. If large vessels be torn it is simply impossible to find them and secure the bleeding points.

In one case, that of Mrs. J. (No. 19 in the table), I operated in this way. The following is the history of the case: The patient had been ill five weeks. Had missed a month and then had gone five weeks after that and then went six weeks. Sudden, severe pain in the abdomen came on, and when I saw her, after she had been ill for five weeks, she was profoundly septic. Uterus was pushed forward by a mass as large as an adult's head, and I was satisfied the case was either one of suppurating hematocele from ectopic gestation or retained menstrual fluid in an undeveloped uterine horn.

No.	Name.	Age.	Doctor.	Labors.		Menses.		Irregular hemorrhages.	Other symptoms.
				No	Last.	Not missed.	Missed.		
1	Mrs. A.	38	J. F. W. Ross.	7	4 yrs.	....	Frequently went 2 weeks over.	Menses occasionally stop six weeks Dark Chocolate Color, fetid, profuse. Commenced Dec. 22, lasted till 24th. Came on December 28, lasted till January 4.	....
2	Mrs. W.	31	A. Lynd..	5	3 yrs	....	10 days over.	Regular to December, since then profuse. June 12 went ten days over. Severe pain some weeks after. Had to lie down. Discharge copious. Unable to get up since. Very weak	No signs of pregnancy. Case sent as one of probable hematocele or pelvic abscess. My diagnosis was either rupture of ectopic into broad ligament or uterine pregnancy and fibroid.
3	Mrs. H.	24	Hospital service.	0	......	....	3 weeks over.	March 20, 1891, unwell; went seven weeks, and again unwell June 9. Taken with pains like labor pains and flowing. Thought had a miscarriage. Collapse. Hot cloths and went to bed. Bleeding continued.	None ....
4	Mrs. L.	30	G. G. Rowe.	1	7 yrs.	.... ..	Went 7 weeks.	Doctor thought she had a miscarriage and curetted. July 18, menstruated; then went seven weeks, saw slight show.	Thought she was pregnant. After the curetting temperature went to 103°, pulse 120. Temperature rose suddenly. Violent diarrhea. Peritonitis.
5	Mrs. M.	28	C. R. Cuthbertson.	Only married 7 months.		....	5 days......	None	No other symptoms of pregnancy. No similar attack before marriage. Removed to hospital to be more closely watched. While there sudden severe attacks of peritonitis and determined to operate at once.
6	Mrs. G.	31	R. A. Stevenson and W. P. Caven.	None.....		....	3 weeks.	After missing three weeks had discharge of blood for three weeks.	Had a miscarriage three years before. Temperature and pulse normal until five days after first attack, when pulse was 130, temperature 102°.

Pain.	Physical examination.	Operation.	Result.	Remarks.
Pains on lifting, coughing, sneezing. Dyspareunia.	After examination per Vaginam, I left the house. Hastily called back. Patient collapsed.	Done on second or third day after rupture. Found ruptured tubal pregnancy. Thought probable hematosalpinx, know was pregnancy. Abdomen full of clotted blood.	Recovered.	
Severe. Could not sit or stand. Came on suddenly and simulated labor pains.	Tumor felt in right inguinal region. Very tender. Vaginal examination: Cervix up under pubes. Passed sound four inches, went to left. Uterus moved independently of mass.	Done about thirteenth or fourteenth week. Mass found apparently in broad ligament and not removable. Ectopic gestation. Opened and washed out sac and drained. Hemorrhage at intervals for nearly six months from drainage tube opening.	Recovered.	
Pain like labor pains. Collapse.	June 30 walked to hospital. Examination found mass. To return in two days. Under Chloroform a movable mass felt dropping into cul-de-sac. and hard, not boggy.	Operated about ninth or tenth week. Abdomen filled with liquid, not Clotted, blood. Blood grumous. Evidently there several days.	Recovered.	Operated at Toronto Hospital July 6, 1891.
After seeing slight show, taken ill with pain in right groin and across abdomen, not very severe. Pain in head and limbs. Put to bed Pain increased. Went out week after; went to doctor's house. Pain recurred in three days, severe; in bed; appeared weak. Pulse 90 to 120, then up and down. Poulticed. Simulated labor pains. Doctor told her she was pregnant.	Large mass extending nearly to the level of umbilicus, dull on percussion and fluctuating. Uterus three and a half inches in length, empty and in centre of pelvis, pressed by the mass back against sacrum. Diagnosed suppurating hematocele, but not sure whether due to ectopic gestation or not.	Done after five weeks of suppuration. Patient profoundly septic. Washed out clots from abdomen and removed fetal sac of about twelfth week from among intestines and unconnected with tube. Clots in abdomen had become encysted by inflammatory adhesions of intestines and had then suppurated.	Died.	
Five months after marriage seized with sudden pain, right side, low down in abdomen. Went to bed, sent for doctor. Cold sweat. In bed one and a half days. Up and around again. Recurrence of pain. Went to bed again.	Small mass felt on right side of abdomen, low down, in front of uterus and apparently between uterus and bladder. not movable or fluctuating. Diagnosis obscure; thought might be pus tube.	Found secondary rupture of a suppurating semi-organized old ectopic gestation clot. Purulent peritonitis.	Recovered.	
Abdominal pain, uncomfortable but not severe, lasted two weeks. Was straining at stool when sudden severe pain seized, low down in right side lower abdomen. Crawled to bed, got up a few hours after, pain recurred. Three attempts to walk. Pain came each time.	Pelvis filled with a mass. Diagnosed ruptured ectopic gestation, commencing suppuration in the blood clot.	Eighth to tenth week. Abdomen filled with blood, grumous, Coffee-ground-colored, and stinking.	Recovered.	

No.	Name.	Age.	Doctor.	Labors.		Menses.		Irregular hemorrhages.	Other symptoms.
				No.	Last.	Not missed.	Missed.		
7	Mrs. M.	34	Rowan and Burgess	3	5 yrs.	Regular.	....	....	Feeling poorly for a week.
8	Mrs. P.	34	T. S. Wiley.	......	......	....	1 mouth, and unwell 6 weeks after.	First hemorrhage that morning. On day before operation husband brought me complete deCidual Cast of uterine CaVity.	Two weeks preVious-ly suddenly taken with faintness. DoCtor found her in semi-Collapsed Condition; cold perspiration and rapid pulse. Afterward Complained of irritability of reCtum; distension. ImproVed and was up Taken ill, and doCtor thought hysterical. Again improVed, and then another attaCk when I saw her.
9	Mrs. H. Second operation.	28	T. Noble.	......	......	....	2 weeks oVer time.	....	Tender on pressure. Lips pale. Hands and feet felt Chilly. Looked ill.
10	Mrs. R	29	Hospital serViCe.	.....	.....	....	....	....	... .
11	Miss G.	...	J. T. Fotheringham	.....	......	....	2 weeks and began to lose blood.	....	No symptoms of pregnancy. Out walking when suddenly seized with pain in abdomen. Felt faint and could not walk. Immediately taken to hospital.

Pain.	Physical examination.	Operation.	Result.	Remarks.
Suddenly taken with severe pain. Doctor found her cold to elbows, pulse thready, Very pale, evidently collapsed. No pain of any account previously.	Found rapid, thready pulse, knees drawn up, and evidently extravasation in peritoneal cavity.	Could not finish operation at first attempt, owing to great collapse. Could only use ether and ethyl chloride. Ectopic gestation, about two weeks' duration, in left tube. Tube completely severed from uterus. Difficult to reach bleeding spot. Tied in a portion of cornu of uterus in ligature. Only removed left tube. Abdomen full of blood clot, scooped out by handfuls. Almost collapsed on table.	Died.	
....	At once concluded it was ruptured extrauterine pregnancy. Felt a mass of blood clot in pelvis. Looked very ill. Decided to wait couple of days to prepare her, but suddenly took worse, and decided to operate immediately. Commencing tympanites. Pulse 120.	Peritoneum opened and enormous quantity of blood in cul-de-sac of Douglas. Peeled out ectopic-gestation sac of about third month. Rupture through fimbriated end of tube. Tube end clamped with forceps to stop hemorrhage Fetus not found. Placental tissue. Enlarged tube, size of small orange. Clots washed out and drainage tube inserted. Tube tied with silk.	Recovered.	
In morning suddenly taken with pain in abdomen and nauseated. Pain increased.	Under anesthetic felt blood clot break down under my finger in vagina. Outer end of tube felt somewhat enlarged.	Operated inside of an hour after first seeing her. On opening abdomen blood gushed out. Enormous quantity unclotted blood free in peritoneal cavity. Left tube and ovary tied off. Right had been previously removed, washed out, and drained.	Recovered.	
....	....	Found tubal gestation ruptured into broad ligament on left side, and removed. Also cyst of ovary and dilated tube on right side; peeled out dense adhesions and ligated. Hemorrhage, morning after operation, through drainage tube Dr. Temple (in my absence) after consultation opened and found right pedicle ligature had cut through and abdomen full of blood.	Died.	Operation Toronto General Hospital November 13, 1895.
....	Cold hands, depressed pulse, pale lips, all appearance of intraabdominal hemorrhage. Found blood clot in abdomen on examination.	Ectopic gestation in right side Placenta extruding through rupture in tube. Tied off pedicle. Fetus about one inch long. As soon as peritoneum cut through, blood spurted out. Enormous clots and fluid blood removed. Washed out and drained. Left tube and ovary not removed.	Recovered.	On examination of specimen large rent found in tube on right side. Through rent placenta seen half extruded. Fetus escaped into abdomen. Bleeding free until pedicle ligated.

No.	Name.	Age.	Doctor.	Labors.		Menses.		Irregular hemorrhages.	Other symptoms.
				No.	Last.	Not missed.	Missed.		
12	Mrs W.		J. A. Amyot.	......	......	....	....	In November went two weeks over time. December 25 began to flow; flow then ceased a little while in January, but has been flowing ever since (March 19).	....
13	Mrs. F.	36	Hospital service.	......	..	....	......	....	....
14	Mrs. L.		T. F. McMahon.	......	17 mos.	Regular.	....	After one month's sickness began to flow and continued to flow four weeks.	....
15	Mrs. S.		J. W. Rowan.	......	15 mos.	....	Menstruated once since confinement and then went 5 weeks.	....	Pulse somewhat improved by stimulants.
16	Mrs. Y.		M Wallace.	......	......	.... ..	....	....	....
17	Mrs. R.		W. J. Fletcher.	.. .	......	....	2 months, and then began to flow. Never regular since first baby.	Menstruated in January and February. Missed March and April. In May regular, but small quantity and very painful, and faint spells when walking or sitting quiet.	Heart beat heavily with least exertion or excitement. Swelling of limbs and pains from knees downward. Appetite poor. Frequent desire to urinate, and pain on micturition.
18	Mrs. W.		T. Webster.	......	...	....	3 days	On May 21 unwell and continued until June 27. Well for a few days and then came on profusely. Operated July 30	Tenderness. When sitting felt discomfort of something, especially when riding bicycle. Painful urination. Some pieces like clot came away. No breast symptoms.

Pain.	Physical examination.	Operation.	Result.	Remarks.
Two or three days previous to when I saw her, had severe pain in abdomen.	... .	Found mass down behind uterus near fimbriated end of right tube. Drew up ectopic gestation. Ligated and removed tube and ovary. Washed out and drained on account of oozing.	Died.	
....	....	Ectopic gestation, size of large apple, Curled on left broad ligament. Ruptured some time from tube Ovary and tube and sac removed. Sac inactive, but looked ready to break down. Drained	Recovered.	Operation Toronto General Hospital July 13, 1896.
....	On examination found right tube small at uterine end but enlarged at outer end and lying in front of uterus.	Ectopic gestation of right tube tied off No adhesions. Abdomen full of tarry and unClotted blood. Tube not ruptured, but blood Could be made to ooze out by pressure on fimbriated end. Washed out and drained	Retied off Recovered.	
Sudden, Violent pain in abdomen, and fainted. Quite well previously. This occurred at 3 P.M.	I saw patient at 12:45 P M. Hands cold. Pallid, anxious appearance of faCe. Pulseless at wrist. PreCordial uneasiness lying on side. On turning on baCk dulness in front disappeared, showing eVidenCe of fluid in peritoneal CaVity Feeling of fulness in cul-de-sac of Douglas, and blood Clot.	Peritoneal caVity full of blood. Washed out enormous Clots from behind uterus. Tube Containing ten or twelVe days' pregnanCy removed. Tube had slit open near uterine cornu. Saline enemata ordered and legs and arms bandaged.	Recovered.	
....	....	Found large mass lying in left broad ligament. Tied off left tube and oVary, and removed old ectopic gestation. Extremely diffiCult enucleation. Right tube and oVary somewhat fixed and during examination began to bleed, therefore removed them also.	Recovered.	
Pain came on suddenly and lasted two hours. Very seVere. Pain aCross baCk and aching aCross bowels. Could not bear Clothes to touch her after pain Ceased. Pain CommenCed with flow and increased eaCh day. Fainted. RetChing during time of pain. Continued for two weeks before operation.	Found mass in front of uterus on right side.	Removed tube and oVary on right side. PregnanCy well out toward infundibulum. Tube Very small oVer surfaCe of placenta. Large quantity of blood esCaped from fimbriated end of tube and old clot in pelVis.	Recovered.	
Intense pain about four weeks preVious to operation. Three weeks preVious, seVere pain, and continued for these three weeks Pain like discomfort from gas.	Under anesthetiC found mass to left side, and ConCluded extrauterine pregnanCy.	Drew up ectopic gestation, ruptured to a slight extent on under surface. Several clots but no blood in general peritoneal CaVity. Tied off mass. Washed out and drained.	Recovered.	

No.	Name.	Age.	Doctor.	Labors.		Menses.		Irregular hemorrhages.	Other symptoms.
				No.	Last	Not missed.	Missed.		
19	Mrs. J.	..	Vrooman.	....	......	....	1 month. Then went 5 weeks. Again went 6 weeks.	. ...	....
20	Mrs. R.		W. J. Fletcher.	....	.....	Regular.	....	Came on and lasted three weeks.	Sudden attack of faintness and bathed in perspiration. Very weak.
21	Mrs. P.	...	R. J. Dwyer.	......	....	... ..	1 month before went 2 weeks over time.	None	Some milk in breasts.
22	Mrs. McC.	33	J. F. W. Ross.	......	.	.	....	Missed 1 montbly sickness by 2 weeks. Then came on and continued 2 weeks..	....	Tenderness in neighborhood left ovary and tube. Increased peristaltic action of bowels noticed through skin. Endeavored to get up, but fainted three times. Vomited. Puffing of abdomen. Pulse not increased. Temperature elevated to 99°
23	Mrs. S.	29	T. McKeown.	......	......	.	....	.. ..	....	....
24	Mrs. McT.	29	C. McKenna.	.....	...	....	Missed 1 period.	Some....	When doctor ;saw her, almost pulseless.
25	Mrs. C.	38	Hospital Case.	....	... ..	....	....	....
26	Mrs. B.	..	J. F. W. Ross.	.....	..	...	.. ,.... .	....	....
27	Mrs. L.	30	A. Eadie.	......	... ..	....	....	Second operation for ectopic gestation.

Pain.	Physical examination.	Operation.	Result.	Remarks.
Sudden, seVere pain in abdomen.	Very ill. Profoundly septic Uterus pushed forward by mass size of adult's head. Opened cul-de-sac Small pailful of clots in three stages of decomposition.	Broad ligament filled with mass, and felt fetus five and a half months. Packed CaVity of hematocele with gauze. Pulse 140. Almost died on table. GaVe unfaVorable prognosis. Had to open abdomen to assist in extraCtion of fetus.	Died.	
Pains of an irregular character in lower abdomen.	Mass found behind uterus, filling cul-de-sac of Douglas, and extending from right to left side.	After difficult manipulation of fingers in cul-de-sac of Douglas. intestinal adhesions broken down and blood Clot and ectopic gestation sac shelled out. Tube and oVary also removed. Washed out and drained.	Recovered.	
Sudden attacks of pain and fainting.	....	RemoVed eCtopic gestation at fimbriated end of tube on left side. RemoVed tube and oVary and as much of sac, or organized Clot, as possible. Drained.	Recovered.	
Pain in spasms, so intense that it could scarcely be controlled by morphine. Slight pain in left breast. Pain on micturition.	Urethra on examination showed no pus or redness CerVix uteri had a peCuliar graYish appearanCe.	Ectopic gestation at outer end of tube on left side, eighth or tenth week; removed. Tube removed by Chain Catgut suture, but this slipped, then tied with silk. Peritoneum darkened. Intestines CoVered with blood; pelVis full of blood OVary not removed, although small fibroid nodule on surfaCe. Clots washed out. No drainage.	Recovered.	
....	....	Shelled out eCtopic gestation rapidly. SCooped out handfuls of blood Clot. Intestines dark-Colored. Washed out. Drained.	Died third day after.	
While in store suddenly taken with pain in abdomen and fainted.	Two or three daYs after abdomen swollen, dulness on percussion on side been lying on. Per vaginam Could feel blood Clot break down	EctopiC gestation on right side Tube and oVary removed. Left ovary cystic and removed together with tube. Almost half pailful of blood Clot scooped out of peritoneal cavity. Washed out and drained.	Recovered.	
Pain in pelVis..........	Lump found. History indefinite.	Old ectopiC gestation sac easily removed. No drainage.	Recovered.	Operation Toronto General Hospital June 27, 1898.
....	....	RemoVed ectopic gestation of right tube, also tube. Left oVary behind. Left tube and oVary adherent and diseased and remoVed.	Recovered.	Operation St. Nicholas Hospital JulY 1. 1898. Unruptured
....	....	Ectopic gestation of about eighth week in left tube. Tube and oVary removed. Also CYst of oVary.	Recovered	Unruptured.

Name.	Age.	Doctor.	Labors.		Menses.		Irregular hemorrhages.	Other symptoms.
			No.	Last.	Not missed.	Missed.		
Mrs. J.	29	Dr. Gray.	......	..	.... ..	4 months..	None	Breasts enlarged and milk in them. Faintness, sickness at stomach. I thought she was almost four months pregnant.
Mrs. L.	38	Hospital service.	4	6 yrs.	....	1 period ...	Some after missing period.	Three fainting attacks.
Mrs. C.	42	S. G. Parker.	......	......	....	1 week over period.	Hemorrhage about two weeks previously. Doctor thought a miscarriage and Cureted.	Nipples looked dark. Faintness. Almost died from this. Went from one faint to another. Elevation of temperature to 102° after currettement.
Mrs. W.	39	G. Elliott.	......	......	Not missed.	....	Menstruated continuously five weeks.	In few days taken with sudden collapse and faintness. Doctor decided rupture had taken place, but she refused operation until my return.
Mrs S..	34	G. Gordon.	......	......	Not missed.	....	Some...	Enlarged breasts. Milk in them. Symptoms of pregnancy.
Mrs. K.	28	A. Eadie.	......	......	.. ...	A few days past period.,	....	Doctor found her almost pulseless. Collapsed. In two or three days, after rallying, taken home.
Mrs. S.	..	W. F. Bryans	......	......	....	1 period ...	Slight hemorrhage..	Fainted three or four times. Beads of perspiration on forehead. Pulse thin.

Pain.	Physical examination.	Operation.	Result.	Remarks.
... .	Uterus packed high up, somewhat enlarged. Passed sound two and a half inches. Uterus pressed forward and distinctly felt on outside of abdomen.	Uterus pushed forward, looked like Contained six weeks fetus Broke down adhesions of omentum, bled freely. When mass burst into, fluid and portions of old Clot escaped. Fetus felt with finger and with placenta removed. Blood gushed out immediately placenta touched. Uterine arteries clamped preparatory to hysterectomy. Portion of left ovary left behind. Hemorrhage from adhesion terribly profuse. Almost died on table. Necessary to pack with gauze after touching surface with iron. Pressure externally. Rectum packed and Vagina partially packed.	Died.	
Irregular pains........	Mass felt in pelvis.....	Ectopic gestation and large mass outside of tube. Hole in side of tube quite large. Removed mass. Bowel folded in over site of old clot.	Recovered.	Operation St. Michael's Hospital Aug. 5, 1899.
No pain for some time, when it suddenly came on.	Colostrum on right side on pressure.	Sac firmly adherent to omentum and abdominal wall. On peeling, frightful hemorrhage. Rapidly passed Clamps to each broad ligament and removed sac. Hemorrhage continued from anterior abdominal wall. Forceps applied. Pus came up with blood at first. Left tube removed. Almost died on table. Saline beneath breasts. Drainage.	Recovered.	
In side....	Found small mass. As I was leaving town advised them not to wait should severe symptoms arise.	Extrauterine pregnancy about sixth week. Ruptured tuboabdominal. No free blood in abdominal cavity, but Clots around tube end. Removed No drainage.	Recovered.	
Cramp-like pains, paroxysmal.	Mass on side of uterus.	Removed ectopic gestation from right broad ligament size of Cocoanut. Hemorrhage Considerable. Necessary to pack in gauze to control. Subcutaneous injections under each breast.	Recovered.	
Taken suddenly with pain while in Church. Carried to a house and fainted. Could not go home for Couple of days.	Two weeks after when I saw her, found mass filling pelvis, semi-fluctuant. Temperature elevated to 102°.	Omentum adherent in front. Pulled up and out gushed quart or more of blood. Removed left tube and ovary. Gestation near uterine end of tube. Gauze packed to control oozing.	Recovered.	
Taken ill at noon previous day with sudden, severe pain in abdomen.	....	Abdominal Cavity full of blood. fluid and Clots. Point of hemorrhage difficult to find. Removed tubo-ovarian Cyst on one side. Blood oozing drop by drop from small spot where tube enters uterine wall. Congested appearance of Vessels indicated very early ectopic gestation, interstitial and of a few days' duration. Salines injected, arms and legs bandaged, foot of table elevated everything to sustain life; almost Collapsed on table.	Died same afternoon	

Name.	Age.	Doctor.	Labors		Menses.		Irregular hemorrhages.	Other symptoms.
			No.	Last.	Not missed.	Missed.		
Mrs. L	..	N. H Merritt.	......	......	....	1 period ...	Then slight flow.....	Elevation of temperature after second attack. 102°. Pale lips, quite pallid when I saw her at night
Mrs. A.	...	R. C. Griffith.	......	......	....	A year ago missed 4 months.	....	Poor health for some time. Some years previous had attack of inflammation. Jolting in going to hospital brought on inflammation. Sore and distended. Elevation of temperature
Mrs. P.	35	A. Eadie.	......	......	....	....	Not as much as usual in November. Then came on, and then again when I saw her in December.	Hernia on left side..
Mrs. R.	..	W. J. Fletcher.	......	......	Not missed.	....	Some....	Operated previously for same condition.
Mrs. J. L.	30	A. Eadie.	......	......	.... ..	....	Menses came on and lasted four days longer than usual. Again one week after, only part of day.	No symptoms of pregnancy. Bathed in cold perspiration during attack.
Mrs. B		W. R. Walters	......	......	Not missed.	....	Began to flow........	Thought she was pregnant. Considerably distended.
Mrs. L.	..	T. Noble	......	......	Regular.	....	... .	No symptoms of pregnancy or ectopic gestation.
Mrs. E.	..	A. Eadie.	......	....	....	....	In August menstruated; in September but very, very little; October very slightly. Some pieces of decidua had come away.	Taken ill night previous with sudden, severe fainting spell while lying in bed. Breasts looked like pregnancy.
Mrs. T.	..	G. H. Carveth	Only married 7 weeks.		....	1 period ..	Some	No breast symptoms. Very weak and prostrated. Managed to drag herself upstairs and lie down.
Mrs. R	40	F. Dawson.	......	.. ..	.	3 months ago missed 10 days.	Began to bleed and Continued four weeks Doctor says he saw placenta and that she had a miscarriage.	Three months ago had sickness at stomach, pain. Previously operated on twelve years before for ovarian tumor.

Pain.	Physical examination.	Operation.	Result.	Remarks.
SeVere pain. While away was giVen hypodermatic morphia. Went home and had another attack.	....	RemoVed gestation sac, four to six weeks' duration, tubo-abdominal. Large amount of Clot remoVed.	Re-cov-ered.	
...................--------	Mass, eVidently CYstic, in pelvis.	Found adherent mass behind uterus. large amount of old suppurating Clot. Ruptured eCtopiC gestation about a Year ago and suppurated. VerY seVere hemorrhage, but finallY CheCked. Drained through Vaginal opening.	Re-cov-ered.	
Three attaCks of seVere abdominal pain at interVals.	Mass behind uterus and satisfied blood Clot poured out by ruptured eCtopiC gestation.	Large blood Clot behind uterus Gestation sac in tube setting up to left on top of Clot, about twelfth week. Hemorrhage in tube beYond produCing hematosalpinx. This leaked into peritoneal CavitY in small quantities, owing to adhesions. RemoVed tube and Contents. Drained.	Re-cov-ered.	
Indefinite pains........	Found small nodule first examination. AdVised waiting two weeks. Then found enlarged to double size.	RemoVed hematoma of right oVarY, also eCtopiC gestation of right tube size of end of little finger, unruptured.	Re-cov-ered.	Unruptured.
One slight attaCk of pain when evacuating bowels. Three weeks after, seVere attaCk of pain while lYing in bed.	BoggY-feeling mass in pelVis.	ECtopiC gestation end of right tube, abdominal. RemoVed Cleaned out Clots.	Re-cov-ered.	
SeVere pain in abdomen.	Mass behind and to left side of uterus.	RemoVed eCtopiC gestation of left tube, tubo-abdominal. Also large mass of blood Clot. Washed out with salt solution. Drainage tube.	Re-cov-ered.	
Sudden, seVere pain in abdomen while walking on street. Managed to crawl into store.	Thought there was an internal hemorrhage.	Small ectopiC gestation, from ten daVs' to two weeks' duration, in left tube. RemoVed with oVarY Abdomen full of blood. Washed out.	Re-cov-ered.	
....	PeCuliar Coloring of skin and Collapsed look. Felt blood Clots breaking down Mass chieflY to left side.	Abdominal caVitY full of blood. ECtopiC gestation sac under folds of omentum and running up to surrounded Fallopian tube. RemoVed this and while doing so tore off tube. RemoVed tube and oVarY. Fresh blood poured out. also gestation sac in left side about three and a half months Portion of left ovary left. Washed out and drained. Saline injected each breast. Arms and legs bandaged.	Re-cov-ered.	
A week before had sudden, seVere pain. Cold! perspiration. Had'another attack.	....	On opening abdomen a stream of blood. thickness of finger, spurted in air. Full of blood ECtopiC gestation of four or five weeks in right tube, remoVed with tube.	Re-cov-ered.	
....	Mass down behind uterus, pushing it forward.	Tubal eCtopic gestation with rupture into peritoneal cavity. Flakes of organized clot covered intestinal wall. RemoVed sac.	Re-cov-ered.	

No.	Name.	Age.	Doctor.	Labors.		Menses.		Irregular hemorrhages.	Other symptoms.
				No.	Last.	Not missed.	Missed.		
45	Mrs. H.	30	Dr. Mc-Dermott.	2	5 yrs.	....	....	One misCarriage. Menstruated July 1, 1886, beCame ill. Pain September 26, 1886. Lost quantity of blood one week. Then Ceased end of September.	End of September a swelling, size of large orange, to be felt in right iliac region. DoCtor in Constant attendance for bearing-down pains. In bed two months. Large with child when she got up. Legs swelled. Felt life in left side. Breasts large and hot. Felt life before Christmas and again in April.

Opened the posterior cul-de-sac through the vagina and removed a small pailful of clots. These clots were in different stages of decomposition. It was found to be impossible to deliver the fetus, and, as a consequence, I was forced to open the abdomen. After the abdomen was opened I was able to remove the fetus, about five and one-half months, and hastily close the opening and pack the cavity of the hematocele with gauze. The pulse had now reached 140. The patient did not stand operation well. Gave a very unfavorable prognosis and left for home. She died within a week. There was not much hope of recovery in this case, owing to the profoundly septic condition of the patient, and she died from this prolonged sepsis and not as the result of operation.

I mention this case to show that even after operation has been done through the vagina it may be impossible to deliver the fetus safely in this way.

At Full Time.—Tait thought it advisable not to operate before the child is likely to be viable, provided the delay necessary does not jeopardize the mother; and, further, that after the death of the fetus operation should be done without delay. I think that this is very sound advice.

Any attempt to destroy the fetus by medicines or the electric current is to be condemned. Many instances in which this has been attempted have resulted fatally. After the death of the child growth of the placenta may continue. I had one such case in which the woman bled through the drainage tube for a period of two months after operation. The fetus was removed, but it

WITH RUPTURE.

Pain.	Physical examination	Operation.	Result.	Remarks.
April 15, 1887, severe pains came on. Sent for doctor. Pains ceased and did not return. but instead a soreness of stomach. Previously been ill off and on for two or three weeks. Doctor expected delivery of child.	Discharge of blood from vagina under examination, with clots and débris like placenta or decidua. Constant pain. External palpation gave fetal parts. Found uterus bicornis unicollis.	Preperitoneal fat very abundant. Opened peritoneum and stopped all bleeding points. Firm adhesions toward pubes in front, bled freely. On pressing above, fluid gushed out Sac wall ruptured. Liquor amnii in abdominal cavity. Fetus full time removed. Fastened sac to abdominal wall Cord drawn out. Drained cavity. Placenta untouched.	Recovered.	

was not considered advisable to remove the placenta. Whether this bleeding occurs as a consequence of growth of the placenta, or of a single detachment of portions of the placenta, it is difficult to say. A piece of placenta retained *in utero* produces frequently grave hemorrhage for two or three months after miscarriage, and yet the placenta does not increase in size or grow, and when removed it looks organized, but not putrid, and does not give rise to the idea that it is active. I presume the same condition may exist within the abdomen after what corresponds to a partial miscarriage is effected by means of operative interference and the fetus has been removed. One thing is certain, that surgical interference in the fourth and succeeding months, when the fetus is alive, is extremely dangerous, and surgical interference in the fourth, fifth, sixth, and seventh months is more dangerous than it is toward the end of gestation; and that surgical interference at any time before the death of the child is much more dangerous than it is after the death of the child.

Full Time after Death of Child.—There is danger to any woman who carries an encysted fetus. Abscess may form at any time and the fetal parts may be extruded through the vagina, through the rectum, or through the bladder. But such a condition need not be incompatible with a long and useful life, provided that no abscess forms.

I saw a lithopedion removed by Prof. Billroth, when I was a student in Vienna, that had been carried in the abdominal cavity for a number of years. The patient died as a result of the operation. She had not been greatly inconvenienced by her condition and I have always felt that it would have been better to have let her alone.

Treatment of Placenta.—In the case on which I operated the placenta was left *in situ*. The opening into the wall of the sac was fastened to the abdominal opening and a Ferguson's speculum was passed in to act as a drainage tube. Symptoms of sepsis developed and irrigation of the sac was carried out at frequent intervals. The placenta came away piecemeal. The sac finally closed and the patient made a good recovery, though the convalescence was tedious.

Tait considered that the umbilical cord should be divided close to its placental origin, that the placenta should be emptied, as far as possible, of blood, and that after washing and cleaning the sac it should be hermetically sealed by closing the opening into it with stitches; and, further, that if symptoms of septicemia arise the sac should be reopened and drained. He had, however, treated three cases in a manner similar to that adopted by myself. They all survived, but only after going through a process of offensive suppuration that lasted for months and that nearly killed them all. Theoretically, the method of closing the sac ought to give good results, but in practice I am afraid subsequent suppuration will be found to occur.

And now, gentlemen, allow me to thank you for your patient hearing. This evening's address has given you the result of part of my lifework. Records have been carefully kept for this purpose and I cannot, in my lifetime, reduplicate them. Lawson Tait, my brilliant and much-admired master, has already passed into the great beyond, but not before he had instilled into me, and into others who had the benefit of his teaching, the habit of keeping accurate records of cases requiring abdominal operations. To this habit you owe the presentation of these cases and the lessons to be drawn from them.

I feel that I have been greatly honored by your Association and will always carry with me a pleasant recollection of its session in 1902.

481 SHERBOURNE STREET.

ON THE ETIOLOGY, HISTOLOGY, AND USUAL COURSE OF ECTOPIC GESTATION.[1]

BY

SAMUEL WYLLIS BANDLER, M.D.,

Adjunct Gynecologist to the Beth Israel Hospital, New York.

(With illustrations.)

OF the cases examined in series sections, these three are taken as types representing the important forms and stages.

I. THE COLUMNAR TYPE OF TUBAL GESTATION.

The following specimen (Fig. 27) presents an oval body, measuring one-third of a centimetre in its greatest diameter, situated on the mucous folds of a tube removed because of the

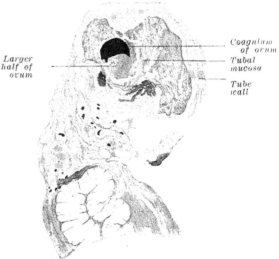

FIG. 27.—Very young ovum situated on the tip of the folds of the tubal mucosa in a case of ectopic gestation accompanied by an old intraperitoneal hemorrhage.

diagnosis of ectopic gestation (on operation the abdomen contained clotted blood). The tube was stained *in toto,* embedded in celloidin, and cut in series sections. Fifty slides from the

[1]Continued from p. 818, June JOURNAL.

middle area of the tube contain sections of this oval-shaped structure (Fig. 27a).   A section through its greatest diameter shows
it to be composed of two unequal halves: a smaller half consisting
of a blood coagulum, and a larger half composed of closely
grouped cells, of protoplasmatic cells and masses containing one
or more nuclei, and of villi.   Villi are also found, but sparsely,
about the coagulum (Fig. 28).

Sections through the smaller diameters show the coagulum
diminishing in size and extent, with an actual and relative increase in the extent and area composed of closely grouped cells

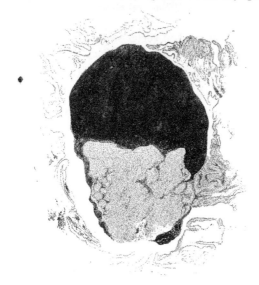

FIG. 27a.—Ovum of Fig. 27, showing division into two halves and an intimate
connection with the tubal mucosa on the right.   (Section through the greatest
diameter.)

and villi, furnishing, then, a centre composed of cells and a
periphery in which are villi (Fig. 29).

The more external sections are continually smaller (Fig. 30),
and the central cell area diminishes in size, so that the small and
most external sections present only villi (Fig. 31).   In all the
sections the villi are in the periphery of the centrally situated
closely grouped cells. .

By reconstruction, then, we obtain a solid, oval-shaped body
possessing a covering composed of protoplasmatic cells and villi.
Within this covering are closely grouped cells, and in the interior, although eccentrically situated, is the coagulum.   We are

dealing with an ovum in which the amnion, umbilical vesicle, and the central cavity are obliterated by blood, while the tro. phoblast and villi are preserved. This ovum, as we may view it,

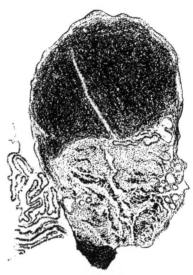

FIG. 28.—Another seCtion through ovum of Fig. 27, showing in one half tro. phoblast cells, Villi, and VeiY dark sYncYtial masses.

is adherent on one side to folds of mucosa which evidence a proliferation of their epithelial covering. On the epithelial covering, and between the folds, are rows of round, structure.

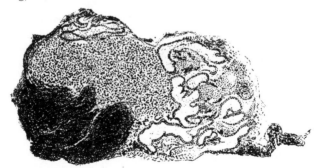

FIG. 29.—A more peripheral seCtion, showing trophoblast cells and Villi and VeiY little of the blood coagulum.

less bodies densely grouped, and the same are found at numerous points covering the ovum, except at the end opposite to the coagulum. In other words, on and between the mucosa folds in

contact with the ovum is seen a plasmatic substance distinctly
excreted by the epithelium, and in it are also red blood cells and
leucocyte nuclei.

The tube wall facing the other end of the ovum presents
mucosa folds, whose epithelium is interrupted at various points,
while at other points are proliferations of epithelium and round
cells. The stroma of many of the folds is absent, while others
possess dilated capillaries and vessels, and still others are filled
with blood extravasations. The tube wall itself is covered with
epithelium, and in the wall are extravasations of blood, and
dilated arteries and veins. *At no point in the tube wall or in
the mucosa is there any decidual change or any condition representing an entrance of trophoblast cells or of villi.* The ovum
is surrounded by a plasmatic substance which I have observed
on uterine and cervical polyps covered with epithelium and in

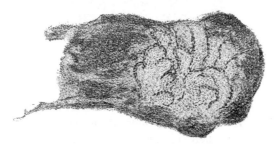

FIG. 30.—A still more peripheral section, showing only villi.

active growth. It is not a deposit from the blood, as such, but
one actively secreted or produced. This same element is found
on the mucosa folds in immediate contact with the ovum. The
adhesion of the ovum at these points is a firm one. It is well
preserved and therefore in active contact with some nutrition-
producing tissue. The shape and character of the oval body,
together with its other characteristics, prove it beyond doubt to
be an ovum. If not entirely surrounded by the tips of the
mucosa folds, it was probably situated among them near the
tube wall, but not on or in the wall.

The other end, with the numerous trophoblast cells, plasmodial
elements, and villi, was probably surrounded, too, by mucosa folds,
and here, too, an intervillous space, containing blood coming from
the capillaries of the mucosa, was probably present. Although we
shall see that this end was infiltrated by maternal blood, I cannot

forbear, in this connection, to mention the possibility that the ovum obtained nutrition from the epithelium of the mucosa at the point of adhesion, which represents to me the reflexa or capsularis composed of tubal folds.

(In the placentæ of many animals it is found that the blood extravasated from the uterine vessels is made use of by the fetus, in that the degenerating products of the extravasated blood cells are taken up and absorbed by the ectoderm cells. According to Strahl, in Galago, a Madagascar lemuride, numerous extravasations are found in the uterine mucous membrane, and their products lie in the connective tissue in the form of larger and smaller yellow granules. The epithelia of the glands near this extravasated blood are more or less filled with granules resembling these. He considers them to be rests of the blood cells which are taken up by the gland epithelium and made use of by

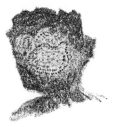

FIG. 31.—Most peripheral section, showing a villus only.

the latter in furnishing an iron-containing secretion. The gland epithelia here perform a function which in other placentæ is performed by the fetal ectoderm. In Galago fetal villi are always in contact with the uterine epithelium and obtain nourishment from it. Between the uterine epithelium and the epithelium of the villi are seen strands which represent the uterine milk taken up by the villi. Thus the fetus gains the greatest portion of its nourishment through the chorionic epithelium.)

The main cell body is composed of cells, without distinct cell boundaries, containing nuclei of varying form and staining darkly. At various points are found paler cells with a distinct nuclear membrane which unite in groups of three or more. More external, in the region of the villi, the cells are more distinct and the nuclear membrane is more clear and nucleoli can be distinctly seen (Fig. 32). The more external these cells are found the larger and the more swollen and the paler do they become, and a

homogeneous intercellular substance is present.   In the centre
of those sections where the cells are so densely grouped (Fig. 29)
are minute, darkly-staining granules whose identity at first was
not distinct.   In the more peripheral areas, however, their character is evident; for they are only found where red blood cells are
present and they are therefore leucocyte nuclei.   The nearer we
approach the circumference the more do we find blood in the in-
terstices between the cells, at first as isolated cells or groups, and
later in larger spaces containing red blood cells.   Wherever blood
in small amount is present, the cell nuclei become dark and
change their form, becoming long spindle-shaped, arranged in

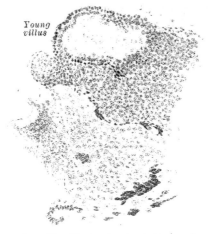

Young
villus

FIG. 32.—An area from Fig 28. showing trophoblast cells, their transition to
the chorionic epithelium in the upper part, and to syncytial groups in the lower
part.

single strands or in longer parallel groups.   Where, however,
blood in larger amounts is present, protoplasmatic masses containing numerous round or spindle nuclei may be observed.   Near the
circumference the number and extent of the round protoplasmatic groups and the number of the darker or longer spindle-
shaped nuclei increase, and the latter seem to invade the sections
described from the exterior toward the interior.   In the exterior of the sections are villi covered with a double layer of
thin syncytium with flat nuclei.   The centre is composed of embryonal connective tissue staining blue and containing branching.
cells (Fig. 32).   Other villi, some of which are quite long, have a
centre composed of round nuclei with nucleoli which are very

closely grouped, and transitions from these cells to syncytium may be distinctly observed, as in Fig. 32. These villi, as well as the others, are found only in the external area or near the coagulum. Knobs of syncytium and so-called syncytial giant cells are present about these villi, connected by a pedicle or lying apart. In the central areas no connective tissue can be observed. In the external layers, however, as said before, it is evident in the form of a structureless substance between the cells, giving these areas a

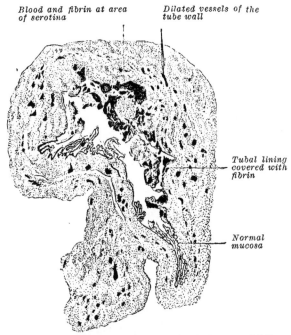

Blood and fibrin at area of serotina

Dilated vessels of the tube wall

Tubal lining covered with fibrin

Normal mucosa

FIG. 33.—Section of tube, showing normal mucosa in the lower and left area, while above and to the right is the area of attachment of the ovum, giving a typical picture of the tube after tubal abortion.

pale appearance (Fig. 32). It is not present in the younger villi and is only evident in the fully formed ones.

II. THE INTERCOLUMNAR TYPE OF TUBAL GESTATION.

A further stage of development of a tubal ovum is well represented in Fig. 33. The examination, in series sections, of this specimen, known clinically as tubal abortion, divulges numerous interesting features. One half of the circumference of the tube lumen is of a normal character; the other half is in a torn, infiltrated condition which involves not only the mucosa folds but also the submucosa up to the muscularis. Close examination evidences the fact that the ovum was situated on the tube wall, compressing and destroying the mucosa folds at the situation

Muscular fibres of tube wall

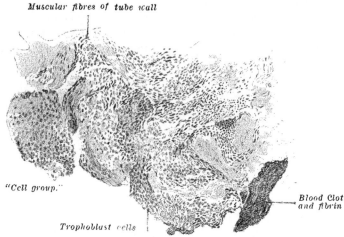

"Cell group."

Blood Clot and fibrin

Trophoblast cells

FIG. 34.—Portion of serotinal area of Fig. 33, showing pale trophoblast Cells and cell groups and the darker syncytial cells.

known as the serotina. On either side of this point the mucosa folds were evidently united about the ovum, forming a pseudo-reflexa. The capillaries and large vessels at the serotinal point

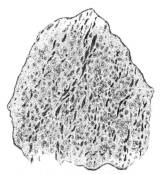

FIG. 34a.—Typical area in Fig. 34, Commonly mistaken for decidua. showing pale trophoblast Cells and dark syncytial Cells.

are filled with blood (Fig. 33), and many evidence larger or smaller injuries and invasions of the wall. At the serotinal portion and for some distance on either side is observed in the submucosa a tissue resembling at first sight decidua.

On close examination we find oval, very closely grouped cells, consisting mainly of nuclei and possessing each a nucleolus (Fig. 34). They are extremely closely grouped and between them are found no capillaries or spaces. This tissue rests not only on the free surface of the tube wall, but invades it at many points to a

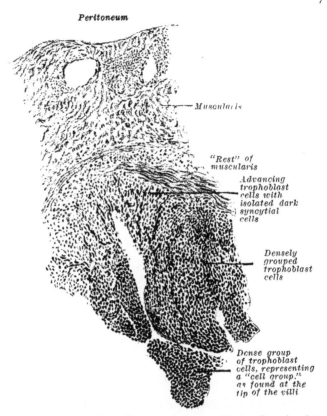

FIG. 35.—Section through tube wall at serotinal area, showing the paler character of the adVanced trophoblast cells and tbe darker character of the densely grouped trophoblast cells near the oVum. TYpical field formerlY mistaken for decidua, but differentiated by the dark spindle-shaped sYncYtial cells. This drawing shows that in tubal abortion the "rests" are of the same nature as in uterine abortion.

considerable depth (Fig. 35). The invasion of the tube wall is not an even one, for at some points it forms a continuous deep layer like the decidua, at other points it enters the submucous tissue in irregular branches and projections, and at other points, through lateral infiltration, is separated from the free surface of the tube wall by a considerable space of normal submucous tissue.

These cells are found about the smaller and the larger vessels, invading and infiltrating their muscular walls up to and into the lumen of the vessel.

The character, arrangement, and structure of these cell masses leave no doubt that they are trophoblast cells. In addition they may be identified by the fact that at almost all points, especially those points near the inner surface of the tube, they are accompanied by isolated, long, spindle-shaped protoplasmatic cells, by groups of polynuclear protoplasmatic masses, and by long, often parallel bands of the same character (Figs. 34a and 35a). These are the syncytial cells, absolutely identical with the same

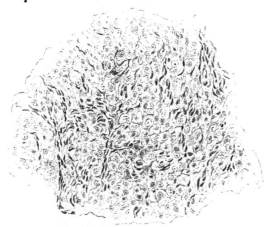

FIG. 35a.—Another area from Fig. 35, showing the "adVance guard" of infiltrating trophoblast and sYnCytial cells.

elements observed in all the previous specimens, especially those seen in the first tubal ovum.

These cells may be further identified as trophoblast cells by the fact that they are found, at the tip of some adherent villi, extending directly into the tube wall. These trophoblast cells enter into the submucosa and muscularis, forming the tissue which so many investigators have called decidua. These complexes of trophoblast and syncytial cells, especially the groups found at the tips of the villi, are not yet filled out with mesoderm, but are to form future villi.

At no point do the connective-tissue cells of the tubal folds or of the submucosa evidence any change resembling, in the slightest

*degree, those changes occurring in the uterine mucosa which re-
sult in the formation of decidua cells.*

*At no point do the epithelial cells of the mucosa evidence any
change of a so-called syncytial character.*

III. THE CENTRIFUGAL TYPE OF TUBAL GESTATION.

Figure 36 represents a tubal gestation, containing a fetus, in
the sixth or seventh week. The tube wall is preserved in its entire
circumference, with the exception of two minute areas where the
chorionic villi *have actively perforated it.* Projecting into the

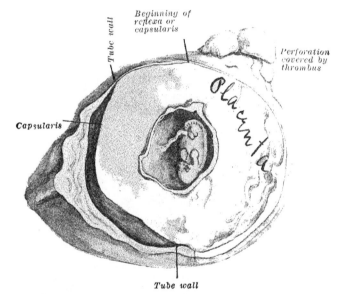

FIG. 36.—Tubal gestation with fetus attached by umbilical cord, showing a
perforation by the growing villi closed by a thrombus.

dilated lumen of the tube, and almost touching the mucous lining,
is the outer covering of the fetal sac, the capsularis. One half of
the circumference of the tube is invaded, infiltrated, and
stretched by the other half of the fetal sac wall, that is, the placenta. On both sides, at the junction between the infiltrated tube
wall and the preserved but decidedly stretched tube wall which
surrounds that half of the fetal sac which projects into the tube
lumen, the mucosa of the latter passes over upon the fetal sac
and can be followed upon it as a covering of the latter for a
certain distance. The summit of the sac is covered by a tissue

composed of fibrin, trophoblast cells, leucocytes, etc.   The ovum possesses, then, a capsularis composed in part of fetal folds and submucosa.   This capsularis is, strictly speaking, no reflexa.   It must be called a pseudo-reflexa or capsularis.

The area of the tube circumference entirely filled by villi is the true placental site, and here is found a real intervillous·space bounded on all sides by the point of union of the tube wall with the base of the capsularis.   The remainder of the circumference of the fetal sac evidences villi, but the space between the cap-

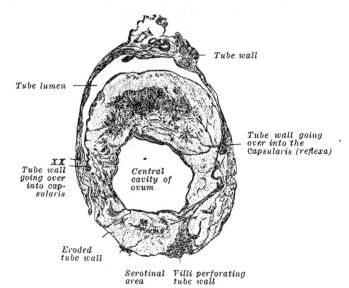

FIG. 36a.--Tubal ovum with perfectly developed capsularis.   Tube wall passes on both sides over into the capsularis.   Major portion of placenta is at the lower border, where tubal tissue is eroded and perforated by the villi.   This area is the intervillous space.   Between the tube lumen and the central cavity of the ovum is the capsularis filled with blood and blood crystals.

sularis and the inner lining of the sac is mainly filled with blood and blood crystals.   At the real placental site almost no remnants of the tube wall can be found.   At this half of the tube wall there are nothing but villi, trophoblast cells, syncytial cells, and a sea of maternal blood (Fig. 36a).

The process involved in this invasion of the tube wall and the process involved in the formation of the villi can, in each section, be extremely well judged on either side at the point of junction of the capsularis with the tube wall (Fig. 37.).   Here, on either side, there extend into the gradually thinning tissue of the tube villi, cell groups, and syncytial cells which invade the muscularis in what may be called a concentric path. We observe, at the tips of fully formed villi, the typical trophoblast cell groups. We see them extending into and between the muscular fibres, changing into and accompanied by syncytial cells and masses of every kind and form yet described (Fig. 38). *At no point is there the slightest evidence of any decidua or of any decidual reaction.* The trophoblast cells invade the vessels

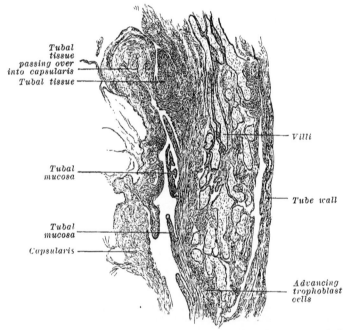

Tubal tissue passing over into capsularis

Tubal tissue

Tubal mucosa

Tubal mucosa

Capsularis

Villi

Tube wall

Advancing trophoblast cells

FIG. 37.—Area *XX* of Fig. 36 magnified, showing the reflexa or Capsularis and the infiltration and invasion of the tube wall by the trophoblast and villi.

of the tube wall, and the villi themselves enter the tube wall and, with the trophoblast groups at their tips, enter the vessel lumina.

At the main placental site are found trophoblast cells with the clearest and most distinct change into various forms of independent syncytial groups and into the syncytial covering of the villi (Fig. 39). They are likewise seen to pass over gradually into the layer of Langhans, which at all points resembles the syncytial layer to such an extent that it might be said that the

covering of the villi consists of a double layer of syncytial cells
(Fig. 39). The villi have actively perforated the tube wall individually and in groups, so that the intervillous space communicated with the abdominal cavity at these points.

*This stage is the exact macroscopic and microscopic counter-
part of the stage seen in Fig. 19.*

*If no interruption take place, the capsularis unites with the
mucosa of the enveloping tube wall in the same way that this
process is exemplified in the uterus.*

The various steps in the succeeding months of development of

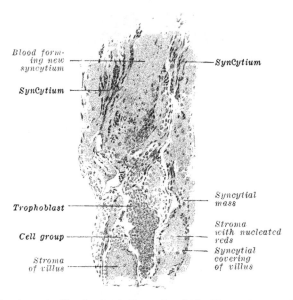

Blood form-
ing new
syncytium

SynCytium

SynCytium

Trophoblast

Cell group

Stroma
of villus

Syncytial
mass

Stroma
with nucleated
reds

Syncytial
covering
of villus

FIG. 38.—Area of adVancing trophoblast cells of Fig. 37, showing transition of
trophoblast cells to sYnCYtial groups and to the sYnCYtial CoVering of the Villi.

a tubal gestation may, so far as the development of the placenta,
the fetal sac, and the fetus is concerned, be considered as
identical with the same processes in the uterus; for over ninety
cases of full-term ectopic gestation with viable fetus are recorded.

The various steps in the development of the tubal placenta,
depending as they do mainly on the cells of the ovum itself, the
trophoblast cells, are the same as in the uterus. The difference is mainly in the different character of the base or trophospongia. We may draw the following conclusions:

(1) In tubal gestation no decidua or trophospongia develops. The mucous lining of the uterus is really a lymph tissue; the sub-mucosa of the tube is not.

(2) Fetal cells, in tubal gestation, may at any time enter the maternal circulation.

(3) As·regards the trophoblast, the syncytium, the villi, the formation of blood by the trophoblast cells, and all other par-ticulars, the processes depending on and originating in the ovum are the same in both uterus and tube.

Certain investigators have described ova embedded in the tube wall, where a capsularis, was present containing muscle fibres passing out from the tube wall into the base of the capsularis.

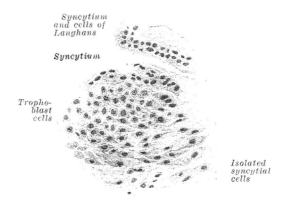

Fig. 39.—Drawing from serotinal area of Fig. 36*a*, showing trophoblast cells. going over into isolated syncytial cells and into syncytial masses.

The ovum was found entirely under the entire thickness of the tube wall, lying on the vessels of the ligamentum latum—the so-called pseudo-intraligamentous form.

CONCLUSIONS.

In the tube, the embedding of the ovum and the development of the placenta, then, is found to follow three fairly distinct forms: (1) the columnar, (2) the intercolumnar, (3) the centri-fugal.

1. In the columnar type of development (Fig. 27) the ovum is. surrounded by mucosa folds only. Here an invasion of the capil-laries of the tubal mucosa occurs. Such a columnar situation makes abortion easy and of little danger. Very soon after the entrance of the ovum tubal bleeding may result; the ovum dies.

and further hemorrhage expels it. The tube may return to a normal state without any evidence of the previous condition, or else a hematosalpinx may be formed if the abdominal end of the tube is closed. The ovum may, theoretically, develop to a much further degreé and press the folds against the tubal wall. If development continues the villi may extend into it, and the connection of the ovum and the villi with the surrounding tissue is a loose one, as in the case of Abel and of Wyder and in the specimen Fig. 27.

2. In the intercolumnar form (Fig. 33) the ovum may rest on the wall of the tube. Any tubal fold beneath it will be compressed, but epithelium may be present in a depression. Other folds may form a capsularis, which consists then of mucosa alone; if such a capsularis be firm an intervillous space may develop. The villi at the placental site enter into the wall; here a hemorrhage may result through this invasion of the wall and of the vessels and through an invasion of the capsularis by fetal cells; or, since the capsularis does not undergo decidual change and is therefore less yielding, the capsularis may rupture. If it be torn, or if it be not closely adherent, the intervillous space is opened. Abortion, complete or incomplete—usually incomplete —is the general rule, but rupture might occur. If the abdominal end be closed a hematosalpinx or a tubal mole may represent the final outcome.

3. In the centrifugal form (Fig. 36a) the ovum sinks into the wall of the tube and an invasion of the wall and vessels by the villi may take place even up to the serosa. The capsularis is formed by muscularis and mucosa. It may rupture at its summit. The invasion of the vessels entering the intervillous space may cause hemorrhage. The villi which extend up to the serosa may cause bleeding, though their penetration is so gradual that these points are usually covered with thrombi. Finally a rupture may take place at the placental site through multiple perforations producing an arrosion. The ovum practically eats up the wall. Even though the tubal diameter be large enough to give sufficient room, this occurs. It is not the result of pressure, as may be seen in gestation at the fimbrian end, where rupture also can result. Villi which perforate the serosa may cause a very decided hemorrhage into the peritoneal cavity. When no rupture has occurred and the abdominal end of the tube is closed, only the microscope may divulge the source of such an intraperitoneal bleeding. Such minute perforations may cause

collapse through hemorrhage, even though the opening be no larger than the head of a pin. Even after the death of the ovum the villi can grow, and an active tubal mole is found with continned bleeding. If they do not grow, hemorrhage continues, since no contraction can take place, as is the case in the uterus. The centrifugal form furnishes the majority of tubal ruptures. But the vast majority of these so-called tubal ruptures are either erosions or due to erosion by the perforating villi.

THE USUAL COURSE OF ECTOPIC GESTATION.

The theory that the tube ruptures because the ovum is too big is, as a rule, wrong for cases in the first three months. The various interruptions of ectopic gestation are all the result of hemorrhages primarily minute. The usual ending, clinically, of the gestation begins with bleeding in the tube. The invasion of the vessels of the mucosa and the tube wall and the invasion of the serosa furnish the causes for hemorrhage. The death of the fetus, as in the case of the uterus, brings about changes which result in bleeding. The primary cause is a lack of decidua. In a mucosa previously affected, when many large vessels are changed by the fetal cells and invaded by villi, an increase in tension through contraction of the tube walls furnishes an easy explanation of this hemorrhage. In the uterus the vessels are firmly embedded in the thick decidua and take a twisted course; in the tube the vessels are straight and embedded in loose connective or fetal tissue. Bleeding on the part of the capsule is possible and of frequent occurrence, since it does not undergo decidual change and may be invaded by fetal cells. The contraction of the muscle fibres on either side of the capsularis renders the rupture of this pseudo-reflexa easy because of the absence of decidual changes, and the point of rupture is usually at the summit of the capsularis. If the capsularis be composed of tubal folds the intervillous space is easily involved. If the capsularis be composed of muscularis and mucosa a decided bleeding may result if only the summit of the capsularis be torn.

Rupture of the tube almost always takes place at the placental site, which is the seat of old and new hemorrhages. The hemorrhage and loosening of the ovum which represent the clinical ending of these cases is not the first bleeding, for older ones are usually present. The various processes depend upon the ovum, the condition of the tube before pregnancy. the character of the union of the ovum with the tube, the place of union, and trauma. The reaction of the tube is limited to the area of the ovum; and in this we find the main difference between tubal and uterine gestation. The uterus undergoes early independent growth, the tube does not. With the development of the ovum the uterus grows hand in hand, while in the tube the ovum makes room for itself and obtains its nourishment by the invasion of the tube walls. It may stretch the circumference of the tube so that its wall, as in the case of Abel, may be reduced to a layer of connective tissue so thin that rupture may result at any point.

Ampullar cases usually end in abortion, generally with hematocele. There is no obstruction, unless decided adhesions are present, and the blood is generally poured out quickly into the pelvic peritoneum or into the sac of Douglas. Such an abortion may be complete or incomplete. Rupture in this situation occurs, but very rarely. The majority of tubal gestations are situated in the isthmus tubæ nearer the uterine end. In those cases we have (1) abortion without rupture, complete or incomplete, with bleeding from the abdominal end of the tube. Generally a hematocele is found at the abdominal end. The tubes are often so curved that it is difficult for the blood to make its way to the fimbriæ, and the oozing is of a slow character. The blood extends rarely more than a very short distance toward the uterine end, because of the numerous short curves present here. (2) We may have single or multiple microscopic perforations of the tube wall by villi, causing even decided hemorrhage without apparent cause. (3) We may have macroscopic perforations or "erosions" of the tube wall, covered or not by thrombi, and causing great hemorrhage. (4) We may have abortion with rupture either into the free abdominal cavity with no hematocele at the abdominal end of the tube, or with partial encapsulation, in which event there may be hematocele at the abdominal end if the tube is open. (5) We may have an intraligamentous tear with hematocele at the abdominal end. In these latter cases the placental site is always on the inferior surface of the tube and the ovum has descended centrifugally to the vessels of the ligamentum latum. These are by far the most difficult cases surgically, and may require hysterectomy to remove the mass *in toto*.

CASE I. (Fig. 27).—Twenty-eight years of age, married thirteen years. One labor eleven years ago. Divorced ten years ago, and operated vaginally at Mt. Sinai for pelvic abscess, since which time periodical attacks of pain on the right side every three months. Married again twenty months ago. *One year ago, pain, fainting spells.* Three months before admission, pain. Two months before, only stains instead of menstruation. ONE WEEK BEFORE, SEVERE CRAMPS, FAINTING SPELLS, following a metrorrhagia of several weeks. Operation showed plenty of old blood in the pelvic cavity. Tube distended, clot at fimbrian end. Other tube normal. Microscope, columnar type, with evidences of a previous old ectopic gestation.

CASE II. (Fig. 33).—Twenty-seven years old; four children. last nine months ago. Nursing. Four weeks of abdominal cramps and uterine hemorrhage. Well for one week and then symptoms returned up to admission, on which day she fainted three times on account of pain.

Operation.—Much blood; right tube distended and clot at fimbrian end. Ovarian cyst. Incomplete tubal abortion. Intercolumnar type, villi and cells of Langhans and syncytium in the wall. Reflexa consisted probably of folds involving one half the circumference of the tube. The other half of the lumen normal.

CASE III. (Fig. 36).—Old blood clots in the abdominal cavity showed the cause of the increasing attacks of pain with intervals of relief to be due to bleedings from perforations of the tube wall which were closed at times by the formation of thrombi.

CASE IV.—Patient 32 years old; two children, last three years ago. Skipped two menstrual periods. Two weeks later examined because of abdominal pain. Examination showed left-sided tumor, elastic, with pulsating vessels on the left side of the vagina. Uterus enlarged. Next day signs of hemorrhage, pale, pulse 120.

Operation showed much blood, dark clots and bleeding from the tubal end. Incomplete tubal abortion, placental mole, slight involvement of the wall. No Graafian follicle in the ovary.

CASE V.—Twenty-five years old; three children, last fifteen months ago. Three months ago first menstruation (probably nursing). Two months ago skipped menstrual period. For four weeks metrorrhagia and cramps lasting fifteen to twenty minutes and recurring as often as three to four times a day.

Operation.—Vaginal celiotomy. Little free blood. Microscope. Ovum, disintegrated by blood and surrounded by villi and tubal folds, found in the tube. Folds also present in the wall at many points. Organized clot adherent at one point. Intercolumnar and partly centrifugal, for muscularis and mucosa

extend on either side partly over the mole. Organized tubal
mole. No fresh bleeding.

CASE VI.—Thirty-seven years old; married eighteen years; six
children, last three years ago. Last menstruation four months
ago. Operated because of abdominal pains. No blood in the
peritoneum. Tube and ovary free. Continued bleeding into
the tube, which was full of fresh blood. Probably would have
broken through the closed abdominal end. Incomplete tubal abortion of the type of hematosalpinx. Placental mole. Decided involvement of tubal wall. Large vessel in the periphery going
over gradually into the intervillous space.

These cases point to the decided danger from continued bleedings involved in tubal abortion. The general view is that tubal
rupture gives much more pronounced symptoms and a much
more decided hemorrhage than tubal abortion. When we consider that incomplete abortion means that villi are left in the
tubal wall and that so-called complete tubal abortion means the
retention of trophoblast cells, we may readily understand that
bleeding may continue for an indefinitely long period. It is a
fact, however, that even complete abortion may cause decided
symptoms. Mandl reports two cases from the clinic of Schauta,
accompanied by pronounced collapse and decided hemorrhage.
In the first case no villi were found in the tube wall (see
Fig. 33). In the second case, although villi were found in the
blood clot in the tube, none were found in the tube wall. Like
cases of tubal abortion, with symptoms as severe as are frequently
the rule with tubal rupture, have been reported by Klein, Zedel,
Piering, and others. It seems to me these histological and clinical evidences are of sufficient weight to destroy the view, prevail-
ing in many minds, that tubal rupture should be treated by extirpation of the tube and that tubal abortion demands only conservative treatment. The proportion of tubal abortion to tubal
rupture is probably 8 or 10 to 1. In this connection it is quite
sufficient to mention the dangers arising from hematocele. The
injury to the peritoneum, the adhesions which take place, and
above all the by no means infrequent occurrence of subsequent
purulent degeneration of such an accumulation of blood, are only
some of the injurious results avoided by prompt removal.

The possibilities are represented by the processes of abortion,
microscopic perforation, macroscopic perforation, rupture, hematosalpinx, and tubal mole. In 99 cases of interrupted tubal
gestation in the clinic of Schauta, a hematocele was found 60

times—55 after abortion, 5 times after rupture.   If the bleeding be very slow, the blood forms a capsule (due to peritoneal adhesions) into which the subsequent hemorrhages enter, the so-called secondary hematocele.   If adhesions are present at the abdominal end of the tube they may form a portion of the capsule.   The resulting hematocele *after* rapid bleeding furnishes the primary or diffuse form.   The secondary hematocele occurs much more frequently than the primary.   In the 60 hematoceles found among 99 cases in the clinic of Schauta, only 4 were diffuse.   Of the abortions found in the same clinic, 75 were incomplete and 6 were complete.

THYROID EXTRACT IN PAINFUL MENSTRUATION, ETC.

BY

J. COPLIN STINSON, M.D.,
San Francisco. Cal.

THYROID extract is a comparatively new remedy.   It has been used in myxedema, cretinism, psoriasis, goitre, exophthalmic goitre, obesity, chronic melancholia, fractures, fibroid tumors of the uterus, menorrhagia, amenorrhea as a part of obesity, hemorrhages dependent upon flexions and versions, keloid, chlorosis, gout, rickets, diabetes, acromegaly, deafness of the myxedematous, sclerosis of the middle ear, as a galactagogue, and in recurrent cancer of the breast.   The writer has been studying clinically the action and uses of thyroid since it was introduced to the profession, and in this paper takes up the action of this animal extract in dysmenorrhea and ovarian neuralgia, etc.   The difficulty in curing these cases depends upon the fact that their impressions of pain become more and more marked as time goes on, and nothing so much increases their susceptibility as the use of opiates.   The abuse of opium, other narcotics, anodynes, and stimulants is widespread; and furthermore these drugs, after routine use, induce conditions of the nervous and other systems that are more difficult to cure than the original disease.   Having determined the conditions of the uterus, ovaries, etc., in all cases wherein an examination is justifiable, the treatment is commenced. For the pain many remedies have been used—*e.g.*, pulsatilla, cimicifuga, salicylates, guaiacum, mercuric bichloride, potassium iodide, viburnum prunifolium, caulophyllum, viburnum opulis, bromides, gelsemium, cannabis indica, nitroglycerin, antipyrin, apiol, opium, etc.   Opium in some form is most frequently used. No remedy is more abused nor should be prescribed less frequently, as more harm than good has been done by its administration.   It is very easy to get into the habit of using it, and only in very extreme cases should it be used, and then it should preferably be given in the form of a suppository.   Of course all cases of dysmenorrhea are somewhat relieved by rest, recumbent posture, hot applications to the lower abdomen, and hot douches, but there are many patients who cannot afford to lay up for several days each month.   In thyroid we have a remedy of much value in these cases.   It supplies material to the system which influences metabolism, is carried in the plasma to the tissues and organs, and has a specific action upon the vasculo-motor nervous mechanism of the uterus and ovaries.   Reaching these organs, it takes part in the process of metabolism, becomes loosely incorporated with the anatomical elements of the parts, and in passing through them takes part in their activity, modifies their action, and lessens the blood supply to the pelvic viscera.   As the sensibility to uterine and ovarian pains is readily diminished by thyroid extract, it is thus a uterine and ovarian anodyne and sedative, as it arrests the afferent impressions at their formation. It belongs to that class of nervous depressants that paralyze the medulla before consciousness is destroyed—i.e., the same class group as aconite.   It is an indirect anodyne, as it does not act immediately through the brain, but attacks the pathological cause of the pain in the uterus, upon which it then acts as a specific anodyne.   Thyroid, possessing a powerful and peculiar action like this, can fully deserve the name of a uterine and ovarian alterative anodyne and sedative.

Marked systemic effects are produced by medium doses of thyroid.   The nervous and vascular systems are considerably affected, the pulse rate is increased, arterial tension lessened, the cerebrum is somewhat stimulated, loss of weight shows increased tissue waste, and the normal functions of the skin, uterus, and presumably other organs of the body are re-established.

In April, 1901, the writer was treating a patient for painful menstruation.   For years she had suffered severely with pain at each period, during which time she had to cease her work, go to bed, apply hot applications, and use internally hot drinks, household remedies, whiskey, paregoric, opium in several other forms, and many other remedies without much relief. Examination of her pelvis and abdomen showed the uterus and ovaries in normal position and good condition. I prescribed for her suppositories of belladonna and opium, and gave in addition internally belladonna, chloral hydrate, viburnum, and paregoric. These afforded her some relief. I also several times at my office dilated the cervix uteri, using metal dilators. These produced considerable pain, but relieved the severe menstrual pains somewhat. A few months later, on account of considerable obesity, I put her on a diet, exercise, and extract of thyroid internally. She had been using the thyroid for several weeks when her menstruation came on. She continued the thyroid during this time, and she afterward reported to me that she had gone through her period without any pain at all, whereas at all other times she had suffered severely. She reduced her weight twelve pounds by using the thyroid, and she has since then been relieved at each period of dysmenorrhea by the administration of thyroidin, one grain in capsule three times a day, given for two days before menstruation, and increased to two grains three times a day during menstruation. (*Formula of thyroidin:* dried extract sheep's thyroid, one part represents six parts fresh gland; whitish powder.) She was and is thus completely relieved of pain without producing any disagreeable symptoms; furthermore, the thyroid appears to act also as a general tonic, increasing muscular and nervous energy. Since this case the writer has repeatedly used thyroidin in painful menstruation with most pleasant results, affording nearly perfect relief in over eighty per cent of cases. Thus it is evident that thyroid extract is efficacious; administered as above described, does not produce thyroidism, as the drug is not taken long enough at a time to produce untoward symptoms. During the intervals constitutional and local treatment may be required. This implies correction of all defective hygienic conditions, greatest care in diet, bathing, dress, exercise, and mental exertion, and regulation of the bowels. Moderate sexual intercourse has a favorable influence. Pregnancy and childbirth often cure the disease. Reduced iron one-half grain, arsenic one-sixtieth grain, strychnia one-sixtieth grain, gentian one-quarter grain, and cascara one-half grain, in pill or capsule, taken three times daily or more frequently, is of value in the anemic. The general nutrition should be improved by malt extract and a full diet. All excitement, both local and general, as well as excessive sexual intercourse, dancing, and the prolonged use of the sewing ma-

5

chine, should be avoided.   All pathological lesions of the uterus, adnexa, and vicinity should be remedied by proper medical and surgical treatment.   Any disturbances of digestion and excretions should receive appropriate diet and treatment.   If during the interval there is pain (neuralgic) in the uterus or adnexa, I find that thyroidin, one to two grains, administered twice or thrice a day, acts splendidly in relieving pain without producing any untoward symptoms.   Cases not relieved by thyroid or other medical treatment should be subjected to surgical operation, *i.e.*, thorough dilatation of the cervix uteri and whatever other additional operations are required.

533 SUTTER STREET.

BIBLIOGRAPHY.

KINNICUTT: Internal Secretions. Triennial Congress of Physicians, Washington, D. C., 1897.
BRUCE: Journal Mental Sciences, 1895, p. 41.
GAUTHIER: Semile méd., July 14, 1897.
POLK: Med. News, July 3, 1897, and January 14, 1899.
STAWELL: Intercolonial Med. Journal.
JOUIN: Gynécologie, October, 1897.
WHITE: Armour & Co.'s Booklet on Thyroid Gland.
STEHMAN: Armour & Co.'s Booklet on Thyroid Gland.
PAGE AND BISHOP: Lancet, May 28, 1898.
KEATING AND COE: Clinical Gynecology.

FURTHER NOTES ON THE USES OF THE WAX-TIPPED CATHETER IN THE DIAGNOSIS OF STONE IN THE KIDNEY OR URETER,

AS WELL AS THE IMPORTANCE OF RETROGRADE CATHETERIZATION WITH THE WAX-TIPPED BOUGIE IN SOME CASES.

BY

HOWARD A. KELLY, M.D.,

Baltimore, Md.

(With two illustrations.)

I HAD almost come to the conclusion about a year ago[1] that the introduction of the X-ray was destined to render unnecessary any further use of my wax-tipped catheters in the diagnosis of renal and ureteral calculi.   I now find, however, that this is not

[1] AMERICAN JOURNAL OF OBSTETRICS, October, 1901, p. 441.

the case, and under various important conditions the scratch-marks on wax-tipped catheters or bougies may still afford precious information which on the one hand either is not given by means of the X-ray plates, or, on the other hand, is confirmatory in cases in which the X-ray diagnosis is doubtful. Moreover, when stones are lodged in the posterior pelvic half of the ureter the bougie may correct an erroneous inference from the photographic plate.

In the case of an X-ray photograph taken about one year and a half ago at the Johns Hopkins Hospital, the stone appeared close to the brim of the pelvis, while the examination with the renal catheter showed that it was quite low down on the floor of the pelvis. At the operation I opened the peritoneal cavity and discovered the stone just back of the right broad ligament, embedded in a mass of adhesions; unable to extract it without great hazard by the abdominal route, I displaced it by thrusting it forward until it could be felt through the vault of the vagina, where an incision was made into the ureter and the stone extracted. The wound closed of itself in the course of several weeks and the patient went home well. She died some months later of an acute intestinal obstruction due to adhesions of the ileum around the site of the inflammatory focus. The wax-tipped catheter, upon being introduced into the left side, showed no scratch-marks, but on the right side, almost immediately upon entering the ureter, the wax-tipped catheter was engaged in a partial obstruction and was pushed on to the kidney with some difficulty throughout. On withdrawal of the stylet fifteen cubic centimetres of urine collected in thirty-five seconds, sixty cubic centimetres in from seven to ten minutes. Pressure over kidney, and particularly straining by patient, caused the urine to shoot out of the catheter in a continuous stream. On withdrawal of the catheter it engaged until within twelve and one-half centimetres of the external orifice and one side of the wax tip showed several deep gouges.

Another class of cases in which the X-ray diagnosis is often made with difficulty, but which are easily accessible to the wax-tipped bougie, is that of stout people where the entire thickness of the abdomen over the regions to be photographed is over nine inches. In such cases the shadow-throwing power of the ray is impaired by the distance of the tube as well as by the distance of the plate from the stone, and the danger from its use is enhanced by the closer proximity to the body, the patient being more liable

to be burned.   I had an interesting case of this kind in association with Dr. Halsted (loc. cit., Case 8).   The patient, a very
stout woman, had a calculus in the left kidney, as revealed by
scratch-marks on my wax-tipped bougie.   Dr. Halsted made an
incision in the side, exposing the kidney, and opened its pelvis
through the dorsum; being unable to discover the calculus, he
freely incised it from end to end, and was still unable to find the
stone.   As I was at the hospital at the time he was operating, he
requested my services in consultation.   Feeling sure of the diagnosis based on the scratch-marks, and at the same time satisfied
that the calculus could not still be lodged in the kidney after so
thorough an investigation, I heated the wax mass, dipped the tip
of the catheter into it, and then carried the catheter with its

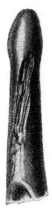
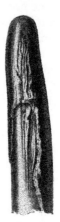

FIG. 1.   FIG. 2.

coated, polished, easy-to-be-scratched surface down the ureter in
a retrograde direction from the pelvis of the kidney to the bladder.   Upon withdrawal of the catheter scratch-marks were plainly found again, and upon a careful vaginal examination the calculus was felt through the left vaginal vault, lodged in the ureter
in front of the broad ligament.   At Dr. Halsted's request I then
made a longitudinal incision through the vagina and through the
ureter and removed the calculus.   The linear wound was drained,
but soon closed spontaneously, and she left the hospital completely recovered.

A further case, showing still better the value of the wax-tipped
bougie, was a patient, 59 years of age, with severe renal crises.
When she first came to me I passed in the wax-tipped catheter

and secured at once the distinct wax-marks or gouges as shown in Fig. 1. An X-ray examination was then made for confirmatory diagnosis, but, owing to the stoutness of the patient and the character of the stone (uric acid and urates), no satisfactory shadow was obtained; the utmost that could be said was that, in view of having secured the scratch-marks, there was a spot in the region of the pelvis of the kidney which might be viewed with suspicion.   In order, then, to render assurance doubly sure, I passed up another wax-tipped bougie with the result as shown in Fig. 2.

At the operation the kidney was opened and its pelvis thoroughly explored, but no stone could be found.   Four weeks later, during the convalescence, however, after a series of attacks of pain following the direction of the ureter, a stone was found between the lips of the labia majora just outside of the urethra. Since that time, now two months ago, the patient has been entirely free from pain and has recovered from her right side pyelonephrosis.

I would further record a case of right renal crises which I examined by the wax-tipped catheter, passing the instrument up both ureters and finding no scratch-marks. I injected the right kidney through the catheter, over-distending it, and this brought on a typical attack of the characteristic pain, demonstrating beyond doubt that the pains felt in the side were due to renal crisis. An X-ray picture showed, to our astonishment, the right side free, but a small calculus in the left ureter down in the bony pelvis.   I at once made a vaginal examination and found a phlebolith, about five millimetres in diameter, in the left vaginal vault.

To recapitulate briefly, the wax-tipped bougie as a means of diagnosing stone in the urinary tract still has a field for itself, under the following conditions:

(a) The scratch-marks afford a valuable confirmation of the findings of the X-ray plates.

(b) The wax-tipped catheter serves to distinguish phleboliths about the vault of the vagina and in the pelvic veins from ureteral calculi.

(c) In the cases of stout women, where the X-ray findings are unsatisfactory and the repeated use of the X-ray is dangerous.

(d) In cases of uric acid and uratic calculi, where the X-ray shadow is faint, leaving doubt as to the diagnosis.

(e) In extemporized hurried investigations when the X-ray

apparatus is not conveniently accessible, and more especially in retrograde catheterization from the pelvis of the kidney downward in the course of a renal operation, to determine whether there are any calculi lodged in the ureter.

(f) In fibrous or old inflammatory thickenings about the renal pelvis, which give a shadow on the photographic plate exactly like a stone. An instance of this kind has occurred in the practice of Dr. Douglas, of Nashville, Tenn.

THE MEDICAL SIDE OF GYNECOLOGY.[1]

BY

EDWARD W. JENKS, M.D.,
Detroit, Mich.

I HAVE been prompted to write a brief paper on the subject announced, and dealing only with generalities. by the remark made to me by one of our distinguished Fellows. that "there is no such a thing as medical gynecology."

We all know that since the organization of this Society the methods of the gynecologist have changed, great advances in surgery have been made, new surgical operations have been devised, and the mortality succeeding surgical procedures greatly diminished. The general surgeon has invaded the field of the gynecologist, while the gynecologic surgeon, in turn, not infrequently operates upon anything operable, be the patient male or female.

The many prolonged lives consequent upon the evolution of gynecologic surgery is a matter for congratulation and deserving of the highest commendation, not alone by the entire medical profession, but by altruists also. The brilliant achievements of accomplished abdominal and gynecologic surgeons have had an additional effect in bringing into existence many surgical and gynecological neophytes who attempt the kind of professional work that only masters are equipped for. Often these men acquire an excellent surgical technique, but wholly ignore valuable and ancient landmarks; they are men to whom prognosis is a lost art and diagnosis is only determined after a use of the knife. A

[1] Read at the meeting of the American Gynecological Society in Atlantic City, 1902

few years ago mutilation of women by surgeons of this class in every hamlet and country crossroads was of common occurrence. The *éclat* of surgical operations put conservatism in the background; recoveries from operation were counted as cures, but the many neurasthenic, insane, and utterly miserable women, needlessly or too much operated upon, even yet continue to afford abundance of evidence that recovery and cure are not synonymous terms. The results of such gynecologic surgery in full swing a decade ago are still apparent, as there seems to have grown up, in consequence, what may be termed a new school of gynecologists, who look upon the literature of the past as rubbish, all of its pathology faulty, and its teachings pernicious. To them libraries are no longer of value, and only recent publications of surgical exploits, damp from the printer's ink, are worthy of consideration. Materia medica comes in for more than its share of ridicule by this newest school, they seeming to forget that a thorough knowledge of the treatment of diseases of women, which implies a certain degree of familiarity with materia medica, is an essential prerequisite for the thoroughly equipped gynecologist.

The distinction of making many surgical operations often brings reputation, and pecuniary compensation out of all proportion to the rewards of patient labor in the field of pathology and therapeutics. For these reasons it is not wholly surprising that medical gynecology has failed to be an attraction to many, for genius has exhibited its triumphs more frequently in surgical gynecology.

It is true that in the past, in private practice and in the medical wards of our hospitals, many gynecologic cases have been treated by medicines only, and have died, that if met with at the present time would be treated and cured by surgical means. It is also true that many gynecologic operations are successfully made by general surgeons, but that does not make them accomplished gynecologists.

It may be of some interest, as bearing upon this point, to note that one of our Fellows has had made for him quite recently an investigation of the results of a year's work of surgical gynecology in nine large hospitals, and that the mortality of the cases in the hands of general surgeons was 6 per cent, while in the hands of gynecologists it was 3.8 per cent.

There is a medical side to gynecology which cannot be ignored, for a special training, together with a thorough knowledge of general medicine, are essential prerequisites for the making of the ideal gynecologist. At least one-half of the women seeking for advice and relief for disorders peculiar to their sex are suffering from some deranged condition of the eliminative organs, as shown by constipation or defective elimination of solids in the urine. Even where there are lesions in the pelvic organs, no relief from distressing symptoms can be secured until underlying constitutional causes of pain and general poor health are first ascertained and removed. The rheumatic and gouty diatheses are responsible for many of the uncomfortable and distressing symptoms, with or without pathological changes within the pelvis, for which the aid of the gynecologist is sought. There are many derangements of the system which closely resemble diseases of the pelvic organs. For instance, pain in the back, the commonest complaint of women, may be due to coccygodynia, or myalgia, or chronic malarial toxemia, or other constitutional causes; pain in the abdomen, sometimes attributed to the ovaries, may be due to habitual constipation or to an atonic condition of the large intestine.

We recognize the fact that chronic constipation, with the consequent pressure upon the left ovary, is one of the most frequent conditions giving rise to ovarian pain with many reflex symptoms, such as sympathetic sciatica, so closely resembling ovarian disease as sometimes to be thus designated.

Upon another point it has recently been aptly said: "No gynecologist of experience is likely to undervalue the retroactive effect of the nervous and mental symptoms upon the one hand with the pelvic organs upon the other; but such a man will always realize the rarity with which neurasthenia, or similar affections of pelvic organs, are disassociated from distinct pelvic symptoms."[1]

Hepatic disorders may frequently be mistaken for uterine, while the reverse holds true. Other constitutional diseases coming under the care of the gynecologist because the subjects are women, with symptoms indicating some pathological changes in the pelvic organs, require no surgical interference, but medicinal treatment only. Other conditions frequently arise where a clear and definite acquaintance with the diseases of the chest and a practical knowledge of auscultation and percussion are essential to a complete diagnosis. · Many of the disorders of menstruation can be best treated medicinally—and that they are common no one can gainsay..

[1]Dr. Edward Reynolds.

It is not my purpose in this paper to attempt to specify diseases or conditions for which medical treatment rather than surgical promises the best results.

I am convinced that some of the medical schools are somewhat responsible for the neglect of medical gynecology. Surgical technique is taught in all its refinements, but symptomatology, differential diagnosis, and the treatment of diseases of women amenable to medicinal remedies cannot receive adequate attention in the brief time devoted to them, if one can judge by results. I have myself known of several ordinary practitioners of medicine, tiring of the routine of general practice, to spend a few weeks taking a post-graduate course of instruction and then announce themselves as gynecologists. They had the best of teachers, from whom they acquired a knowledge of technique and surgical operations they did not before possess, but otherwise seemed to have acquired no new knowledge. The treatment of disease by other means than surgical seemed to possess no attraction for them and was of minor importance. The glamor of gynecologic surgery had obscured the commonplace, but equally important, study of gynecologic medicine.

The experience of all gynecologists who are not interested solely in operating will bear out the assertion that the first essential qualification to successful practice in this specialty is a wide and extensive knowledge of disease, but more especially chronic constitutional disorders.

It is true that gynecology is, in part, surgical, and without surgery it would be relegated to the position it occupied three-fourths of a century ago. Surgical procedures are in many ways more satisfactory than other methods of treating disease, by reason of the brilliancy of execution and the more speedy certainty of results—to say nothing of higher remuneration. But in all candor may it not be asked, "Are not surgical matters being cultivated to the exclusion of medical?" Pathology, symptomatology, diagnosis, prognosis, together with clear and definite ideas of the physiological action, range of application, and the expected results of medicinal remedies prescribed, are as essential to the gynecologist as is dexterity in surgical operations.

Mill, in an address to the University of St. Andrew some years ago, said: "It is the utmost limit of human acquirement to combine a minute knowledge of one or a few things with a general knowledge of many." This general knowledge of medicine and surgery, and the application of it in his special work, makes the accomplished and skilful gynecologist.

"The future of gynecology," very aptly says Dr. Reynolds in his recent address to the Maine Medical Association, "lies in the careful, thorough, and scientific study of every agency which bears upon the pelvic organs of women, and of all the agencies which may be employed for the relief of pelvic disease, medicinal, hygienic, and psychological, as well as the merely surgical."

There are, for obvious reasons, those whose entire time is absorbed by operative work, and who, by reason of their surgical skill, add to the glory of gynecologic surgery; of such men it is unbecoming to say a word in derogation, but everything that is possible in commendation. The aim of this brief and imperfect paper is not to criticise, but it is a plea for the medical side of gynecology and that it be not relegated to obscurity in our zeal to advance gynecologic surgery. I wish also to enter my protest against so many calling themselves gynecologists who plough only in one furrow of the field of gynecology, while the field itself is only a part of the great domain of medicine and surgery.

It seems to me proper in this connection to say a few words concerning the function of this Society in equalizing, if it may be so termed, the practice of gynecology. The transactions of this Society are not for its Fellows only; its utterances are authoritative, for within its fellowship, from its organization to the present time, American gynecology has had its best representatives. Their influence is educational and far-reaching in moulding the thoughts and influencing the actions of very many in the profession who aspire to perfect themselves in practical gynecology.

As pertinent to my theme, I conclude by quoting from the address of one of our honored Presidents, who during his lifetime was distinguished alike for his skill as an operator and the profundity of his knowledge in every department of medicine:

"This Society, as the name in its broadest sense implies, comprehends all that pertains to obstetrics and the diseases peculiar to women, and hence have to deal with the most complex structures and functions manifested in the universe. It follows, therefore, that, while a thorough knowledge of the special subject is an absolute necessity, a certain familiarity with all collateral branches of medicine and surgery is highly essential to the accomplishment of the ends and aims of all who claim fellowship here. If a man devotes his whole time to the practice of one branch of medicine or surgery, he should not expect to be excused if he lacks a general knowledge of all the great principles of the science of medicine. On the contrary, the one is required as a basis for the other.''[1]

84 LAFAYETTE AVENUE.

AN ANENCEPHALIC, HEMISOID MONSTER.[2]

BY

A. ERNEST GALLANT, M.D.,

Professor of Gynecology, New York School of Clinical Medicine, etc.

(With three illustrations.)

THE specimen herewith exhibited was recently presented to the writer by Dr. James A. Campbell, accompanied by the following history: ''The mother of this monster, Mrs. R., about 40 years old, a healthy, robust Russian weighing about 250 pounds; her anatomy was normal; XIIIpara (five miscarriages, six full-term children, two monstrosities). Her husband is a strong, healthy, hard-working Russian, a metal-roofer by trade.

''The mother reports that the previous (twelfth) birth was also a monster, like a snake, in no respect resembling the genus *homo;* was premature, occurring at the fifth month.

''This, her thirteenth pregnancy, was at full term. Labor occurred on March 10, 1901, and was normal in so far that it went through the regular stages, but the midwife in attendance was unable to deliver. On my arrival the os was found dilated and a hard body with a cavity in the centre presenting, the nature of which I was unable to determine, but supposed I was dealing with the cranial cavity. The sac was filled with cerebrospinal fluid. By judicious traction on the sac delivery was soon accomplished. At no time was any brain tissue found in the liquor amnii.

''I have examined all the monstrosities in the various museums in Paris, Dublin, London, etc., but have never seen anything like this, which I think is unique.''

This specimen is remarkable chiefly from the absence of the

[1]Alexander J. C. Skene, Presidential Address, 1887.

[2]Presented to the New York Academy of Medicine, Section on Obstetrics and Gynecology, March 27, 1902.

whole of the right half of the trunk and upper and lower extremities, and in the peculiar curvature of the trunk, by which the left lower extremity occupies the place of the right shoulder (Figs. 1 and 2). This process of non-development on the right and attachment of the left side must have taken place very early in fetal life and prior to the fourth week of gestation.

The head presents the usual features common to anencephalics: absence of calvarium, cerebrum, cerebellum, and medulla,

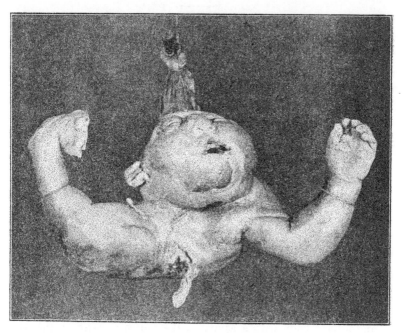

FIG. 1.—Anterior view.

and represented only by a fibrous sac, the contents of which have not been determined.

The face, the nose, eyes, mouth, and base of the skull are those of a well-developed child, and teeth can be felt and seen through the gums of the upper jaw (Fig. 1).

A depressed nipple occupies the site of the left breast, and a similar depression is seen on the lower part of the neck of the opposite side.

The anal opening is represented by a shallow dimple at the posterior part of the rima. On the inner side of the thigh a cutaneous "tab" marks a rudimentary, unformed scrotum and determines the sex.

The extremities are those of a well-formed, fully-developed fetus, as shown by the following measurements: Trunk, axilla to groin, 7.5 centimetres. Upper extremity—arm (length) 8, forearm 6.5 centimetres; (circumference) biceps 10, forearm 10 centimetres. Lower extremity (groin to external condyle) 15.5 centimetres; (circumference) thigh 15, calf 9 centimetres.

The X-ray plate taken by Dr. W. J. Morton is the result of

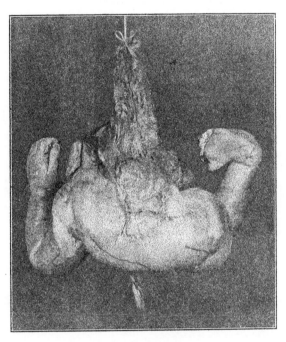

FIG. 2.—Posterior View.

exposing the specimen to a moderately soft tube, for sixty seconds by the stop-watch, at a distance of twenty-two inches. They reveal most distinctly the humerus articulating with the scapula; the clavicle in its normal position; the ulna and radius and all the bones of the hand and fingers complete. The femur articulates with the cotyloid cavity; the ilium, ischium, and pubis still ununited. The tibia and fibula and the carpal, metacarpal, and phalangeal bones for each of the seven toes are quite distinct (Fig. 3).

On the left (lower) side the ribs present, though distorted by the abnormal bending of that side of the trunk.

The base of the skull is well formed. the vertebræ bent into a sickle shape with its convexity toward the left.

The trunk presents but one opening, the umbilicus. one-half inch in diameter (Fig. 1). On introducing my little finger the heart can be made out in its normal position and of usual size— apparently the only occupant of the single cavity, there being no septum to distinguish thoracic from peritoneal cavity, nor are there any evidences of liver, intestinal tract, or lungs. Under

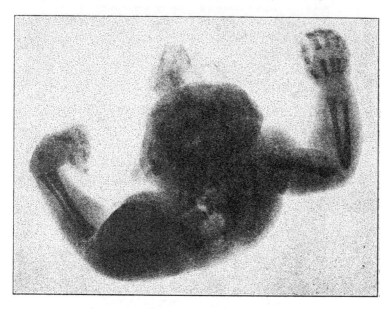

Fig. 3.—Radiograph.

these circumstances it was impossible for this fetus to live after the cord was severed.

From an etiologic standpoint the recent statistics of Georghiu bearing on the question of infection of the parents and mal- formation of the progeny are of profound interest.[1] "He found that there was scarcely an infant showing arrest of development or a malformation which did not possess a mother or father, or both, suffering from some infectious condition, such as typhoid fever, tuberculosis. scarlet fever, syphilis, measles, etc. The

[1] L'Obstétrique, 1900, v., p. 63; American Year Book of Medicine, 1901, p. 310.

more intense the infection the more probable was it that the infant would show malformations. Multiple malformations generally pointed to a very marked maternal infection. The infants were generally born slightly prematurely and below weight. There was rarely a history of traumatism or of maternal impression, and in only one instance was there consanguinity. Georghiu thinks that there is undoubtedly a relation of cause and effect between the infection and the malformations, but there are other circumstances which intervene.''

Summarizing, we have a *single monster,* characterized:

1. By defect: *(a)* absence of calvarium and brain (anencephalus); *(b)* absence of right half of the body and extremities (hemisus); *(c)* absence of lungs, liver, intestinal tract, and genital organs (heart in normal position); *(d)* absence of diaphragm; thoracic and peritoneal cavities one sac.

2. By abnormal position: left hip occupies the site of right shoulder.

3. By numerical excess: seven toes (polydactyl).

4. By deformity: talipes equino-varus.

60 WEST FIFTY-SIXTH STREET.

PSEUDO-PREGNANCY.

REPORT OF CASES.[1]

BY

W. S. SMITH, M.D.,

Professor of Gynecology at the Maryland Medical College ; Gynecologist
to the Franklin Square Hospital,
Baltimore, Md.

WHEN we bear in mind the fact that in many instances the diagnosis between true and false pregnancy is by no means easy, and think of the frequency with which the symptoms of gestation are either simulated or obscured by disease, not to mention the possibility of the condition being deliberately and wilfully feigned, it should not be necessary to insist upon the necessity of greater caution than is sometimes shown by medical men in answering the simple query, ''Am I pregnant or not?'' Upon our reply to that apparently innocent question may obviously

[1]Read at the annual meeting of the Medical and Chirurgical Faculty of Maryland, held in Baltimore, April 22-24, 1902.

depend the good name of a young woman, the happiness of a
wife, or the reputation of a physician.   Indeed, there is perhaps
no complaint which, when misunderstood and mismanaged, may
give rise to greater trouble to practitioner as well as patient than
pseudo-pregnancy, and none in the diagnosis of which mistakes
are more commonly made.   I think I am justified, therefore, in
saying that the subject is deserving of more than passing attention or merely theoretical interest.   In the pre-aseptic days, before the present perfected technique in abdominal surgery had
been evolved, and when operations within the peritoneal cavity
were attended with such danger, the differential diagnosis of pregnancy was a matter of supreme practical moment.   The surgeon
who opened the peritoneum in search of a supposed tumor, only
to find a physiological tumor—the pregnant uterus—had ofttimes made a serious and costly error.   At the present day, when
exploratory celiotomy has become a comparatively safe procedure
and is so often employed as a diagnostic resource, this phase of the
subject has far less practical significance.   Conversely, however,
the differentiation of the various intra-abdominal and intrapelvic conditions which may present a more or less complete
mimicry of pregnancy is still of very considerable importance,
involving, as it does, either an entire omission or an indefinite
postponement of treatment when the indications for remedial
measures may be imperative.

   In view of these facts, and of the scant attention accorded the
subject in the obstetrical and gynecological text books, I have
thought that it would not be unprofitable to bring this topic before the Faculty.   If, in doing so, I should succeed in eliciting
some discussion of pseudo-pregnancy, and above all in giving
never so little additional emphasis to the importance of being less
hasty in diagnosticating pregnancy where in most cases its non-
existence can be easily established, my purpose will have been accomplished.

   The frequent occurrence of pseudocyesis as a climacteric condition has been pointed out. especially by those engaged in dispensary and hospital practice.   This fact may have led some who
have given little or no attention to the subject to associate it
almost exclusively with that period of a woman's life.   Such an
impression is altogether erroneous.   Pseudo-pregnancy may occur at any period from puberty up to and beyond the menopause.
I need only refer to the varied forms of disease by which

pregnancy may be counterfeited, some of them occurring in youth as well as in old age. Any morbid condition which causes an enlargement of the intraperitoneal cavity, such as ascites and visceral tumors, and especially solid and cystic growths of the uterus and the ovaries, may give rise to difficulties in diagnosis. Less frequently, physometra, or gaseous distension of the uterus, hematometra, the so-called "phantom tumor," and molar pregnancy may be encountered. In some of these conditions—such, for instance, as hematometra, myxomatous mole, and intramural fibroid tumors of the uterus—not alone the symptoms but many of the signs of normal gestation may be present in such array that the most careful observations and the most thorough diagnostic skill are required to arrive at a correct conclusion.

Of the differential diagnosis of these conditions it is not my purpose now to speak, particularly since it must be said that they are relatively infrequent, and that the largest number of cases of false pregnancy are found in women, approaching or beyond the menopause, in whom there is no gross lesion of the intrapelvic organs, and since also it must be acknowledged that it is in just such cases that the proper diagnosis can most easily be made. The two cases about which I shall speak belonged to this class. One of them was Mrs. C., residing in the southern section of the city, who called me from the house of a neighbor and made a statement substantially as follows: She was 35 years old; had been married about ten years, but had no children. Her previous personal history was good and she had enjoyed excellent health. She was pregnant; of that she was sure. She not only felt that she was pregnant herself, but a physician had told her about three months previously that she was in the seventh month of gestation. She desired to consult me because she had been suffering greatly with gastric disturbance, had little or no appetite, could not sleep at night, was extremely nervous, and, besides, the movements of the child caused her a great deal of discomfort. Moreover, the time of her expected confinement had already passed and that had begun to create no little anxiety. She simply wanted to know what was wrong, if anything, and in what way relief could be obtained. In reply to questions from me she said that she had menstruated regularly up to ten months before, at which time the menses became very scanty, and that they had finally disappeared entirely. At about the same time she began to suffer from nausea, her breasts became larger and were painful, her appetite was capricious, and her nervous sys-

6

tem markedly deranged.   Several months after the beginning of
the symptoms enumerated (she could not say definitely just
when) she began to notice the movements of the child, which had
gradually become stronger, until at that time they were extremely vigorous and persistent.   About this time, also, her abdomen commenced to enlarge and had continued to increase in
size somewhat rapidly.   Her friends had noticed the marked
change which she had undergone, and of course agreed with her
physician and herself that she was pregnant and joined in the de-
lightful anticipation of her approaching maternity.   I was told
by a mutual friend and neighbor that unusual preparations had
been made for the anxiously-awaited event and that baby clothes
in great abundance had already been completed.

Such were the circumstances and such the condition of the woman at the time of my call.   I told her it would not be possible
for me to advise her intelligently without first making an examination, to which she readily consented.   Her abdomen was
bared from symphysis to sternum and hastily explored.   It was
quite as large as that of a woman at the end of pregnancy, but
was not tense.   The enlargement lacked the definiteness of outline, the prominent ovoid shape which we are accustomed to observe in advanced gestation, but was more generally distributed
and more uniform.   The umbilicus was not prominent, but retracted; there was little or no pigmentation of the linea alba, and
no evidence of the so-called lineæ albicantes or striæ gravidarum.
Percussion gave a note that was flat in the lower portion of the
abdomen and semi-resonant above.   On grasping and lifting the
abdominal wall between my hands, very great thickening was
made out and much of the swelling disappeared.   Auscultation
did not disclose fetal heart sounds, but did reveal marked gur-
gling due to imprisoned intestinal gas.   On making a vaginal examination my reserved diagnosis was abundantly confirmed.
The vaginal walls were not discolored, were not unusually moist,
thickened, or redundant, and, above all, the cervix was long,
conical, and hard.   On pushing the cervix backward in the direction of the posterior vaginal fornix and lifting it up on my
forefinger, while the outstretched fingers of the other hand were
as far as possible pushed beneath the roll of fat and held firmly
against the lower abdominal wall, I was able to palpate the body
of the uterus, which was apparently undersized.   I promptly
told Mrs. C. that she was not pregnant, but she evidently did not
believe me; so I suggested that, in order to make "assurance

doubly sure," I would call again the next day, bring my instruments, and give her an even more thorough examination. To this also she agreed. However, I received a terse note from her the next morning in which she said that it would not be necessary for me to call again. Strange to say, this lady was visited shortly afterward by a prominent physician, who also eliminated pregnancy, but advised her to go at once to a hospital to be operated upon for an ovarian cyst. She followed his advice, was very properly and wisely examined under anesthesia at the hospital, when it was discovered that the so-called cyst had "silently stolen away." The diagnosis was eventually made of a premature menopause, a great excess of abdominal and omental fat, and dystrypsia associated with a great deal of gaseous distension of the bowels.

The case of Mrs. E., living on Eutaw street, was somewhat similar. She was also sterile, about 32 years of age, and had menstruated regularly up to nine months before. At that time she stopped menstruating, began to suffer from nausea, noted enlargement and tenderness of the breasts, followed some months later by great increase in size and what she assumed to be fetal movements. She had convinced herself and her husband that she was pregnant, and, after waiting for the expiration of her time, actually believed labor to be coming on and sent for a monthly nurse. Labor, however, did not progress to her satisfaction, and, after several days of anxious waiting, she sent for me. I did not examine her abdomen, but found the vaginal indications of a non-gravid uterus sufficiently definite to warrant a positive conelusion. The vagina was pale; the cervix was small, conical, and firm; and while the uterus was not clearly palpable, it was evidently not enlarged. I communicated the very unpleasant information to her, but her young husband had been so anxiously and so cheerfully awaiting the advent of an heir that, after my departure, she concluded she would not undeceive him; so, with the assistance of the nurse, and in his absence, she procured a young baby, which he found on his return snugly ensconced by her side, and which has since, so far as I know, successfully filled the rôle of the genuine article—the real prince.

It is remarkable with what exactness the symptoms of pregnancy may be counterfeited in many of these cases. Occurring, as they so often do, in women who are approaching either a premature or a normal menopause, who are very desirous of having offspring, and who perhaps have familiarized their minds with

everything relating to the subject, it is not surprising that the
unwary physician is made to share in the opinion so confidently
expressed by the deluded woman.   In this way it is that we may
have not only the various nervous and sympathetic disturbances
supposed to indicate pregnancy, but also such symptoms and
signs as morning sickness, enlargement of the breasts and areolar
papillæ, and even the secretion of a lactescent fluid.   If at the
same time the abdomen becomes gradually increased in bulk,
whether from an excessive deposit of fat in its walls and in the
omentum, from intestinal distension caused by fetal accumulations and by flatus, or from any of the various diseased conditions to which I have referred, the position of the practitioner
may become an eminently delicate and undesirable one.   For the
same reasons, also, it can truthfully be said that spurious pregnancy is often psychical as well as physical in its origin.

I have already adverted to the great difficulties which may be
experienced in differentiating various disorders from true pregnancy, especially early pregnancy, even when the most thorough
physical exploration is made by the most skilful hands.   The
class of cases of which the two given may be taken as examples
is not so difficult of recognition, and embarrassments only occur
either when no examination is made at all or when perhaps an
incomplete survey of the breasts and abdomen is all that is attempted.   The breast signs and the auscultatory abdominal signs
should not, in my humble judgment, be depended upon by the
average practitioner, since the sources of error are so numerous.
The most generally valuable and reliable diagnostic test, it seems
to me, is that afforded by a properly conducted vaginal and
vagino-abdominal examination, telling us, as it does, the position,
shape, size, and consistence of the cervix, giving us valuable information in regard to the color and character of the vaginal
walls, and enabling us in most instances to map out with greater
or less definiteness the body of the uterus.

I have therefore selected my two cases designedly, belonging,
as they do, to that variety of pseudo-pregnancy most frequently
met with, in which the psychical element plays a conspicuous
part, in which the physician would do well always to be on his
guard, and in which, above all, the results of simple diagnostic
methods are so convincing and satisfactory.   To epitomize my
remarks, then, or rather to reduce them to their ultimate analysis, would be to say that my experience leads me to believe that a
closer study should be made of the vaginal indications of true and

false pregnancy, that a greater reliance should be placed upon such indications, and that a more frequent resort should be had to the vaginal and vagino-abdominal method of examination in cases where there is the slightest reason for the entertainment of a doubt.

412 CATHEDRAL STREET.

CORRESPONDENCE.

A NOTE ON THE OPERATION FOR CYSTOCELE

DESCRIBED IN AMERICAN JOURNAL OF OBSTETRICS, JUNE, 1902.

To THE EDITOR OF THE AMERICAN JOURNAL OF OBSTETRICS, ETC.

SIR:—A further experience with my operation for cystocele, described in your last number, demonstrates two great advantages not referred to in the original description. A restoration of the muscle of the urogenital trigonum (Waldeyer), the homologue of the compressor urethræ in the male, cures the distressing incontinence of urine with which so many middle-aged women are tormented. Further, the repair of the injury to all four of the vaginal sulci makes a much more perfect restoration of the vaginal introitus than can be secured in any other way. In the average case the oval denudation of Martin between the triangular denudations in the anterior vaginal wall may be omitted.   Very respectfully,

B. C. HIRST.

TRANSACTIONS OF THE
AMERICAN GYNECOLOGICAL SOCIETY.

First Day—Morning Session.

The Society convened in the ballroom of Hotel Rudolph under the presidency of DR. SETH C. GORDON, of Portland, Maine.

An address of welcome was delivered by DR. PHILANDER A. HARRIS, of Paterson, N. J., which was responded to by the President.

DR. THOMAS A. ASHBY, of Baltimore, Md., reported a

CASE OF WANDERING SPLEEN PACKED IN THE PELVIS, COMPLICATED BY TYPHOID FEVER; SPLENECTOMY, WITH RECOVERY.

The author directed attention to the anatomy and function of the spleen, and said its size was influenced by bodily nutrition, the organ being large in the well-nourished and small in the poorly-fed individuals. In 1887 McCann reported 19 cases of splenectomy with 13 recoveries. These cases were reported by 18 different surgeons. Sixteen were observed in women and 3 in men. In properly selected cases he thought there was no doubt that the spleen could be removed with as good results as those which followed the removal of the uterus, the ovaries, or the kidney.

The chief interest in the case detailed by the essayist was from the standpoint of diagnosis. The patient, a young woman, had lived all her life in a malarial section of country and had had repeated attacks of malarial fever. She had contracted a malarial spleen which, from its increased size and weight, had exerted such traction upon the splenic ligaments as to permit the spleen to wander down into the pelvis, where it became impacted behind the uterus and filled the pelvic basin. How long it had remained in this position there was no way of determining. In the meantime she became infected with the typhoid organism and developed typhoid fever. In the initial stage of the disease her temperature took a high range and pelvic pains were soon felt. Her family physician, being called in at once, palpated the abdomen and, finding a large mass in the pelvis well above the brim, with marked tenderness and high temperature, concluded that he had a large inflammatory tumor to deal with. At this time there were no typical symptoms, and there were no typhoid cases in her family or neighborhood. He at once brought her to the hospital for treatment. At the time of Dr. Ashby's first examination the physical signs were markedly those of an inflammatory mass in the pelvis. There was pain on pressure, a doughy sensation to the touch, and the skin over the region of the tumor was so red and shiny that the surface indications were those of a suppurating mass ready to break through the skin. When anesthetized the following morning, the physical signs had markedly changed, and his diagnosis, before opening the abdomen, was that of an ovarian cyst or myomatous tumor. He determined to make an incision to find out the true character of the growth, and to remove the same. As soon as the incision was made the spleen was discovered and its removal at once decided upon. The enlarged size of the organ, length and weakness of its ligaments, made an attempt at its restoration and attachment to its normal position a matter of physical impossibility. The only safe course was to remove the organ, and this was done without the least difficulty, as its pedicle was not larger than one's little finger at the point of its attachment under the diaphragm. It was ligated in sections and the stump well covered with peritoneum.

The subsequent behavior of the patient's temperature could not be accounted for until a typical typhoid reaction was obtained some six or seven days after the operation. From that time on the typhoid condition was regarded as the primary disease and was treated accordingly. The abdominal section presented no features to occasion the least alarm. She ran the regular course of the fever and her convalescence was uneventful. Her health since her recovery has been much better than prior to the attack of typhoid fever.

DR. I. S. STONE, of Washington, D. C., stated that he had reported a case in the *Annals of Surgery* some two years ago similar to the one narrated by the essayist, the only difference being, so far as he could judge, that there was no history of typhoid fever following the operation. The patient, a woman, was admitted to the hospital about eight years ago. At that time he discovered that she had a mass in the pelvis which felt like a soft myoma, with symptoms of menorrhagia. She had a cystic ovary. An operation was done, without the least thought of the spleen being displaced. It was found and left, as he thought it best at that time not to remove the spleen, because there were no symptoms in the history of the case directing his attention to that organ, and he thought a splenectomy would complicate the recovery. A large cyst of the ovary was removed; the patient recovered from the operation and from the menorrhagia. About five years later she was readmitted with symptoms of peritonitis, and a large tumor filling the left half of the abdomen, but not extending quite as high as the ribs, there being more of the mass in the pelvis than under the ribs. He realized then that the woman had a large growth of the spleen. Splenectomy was done.

With reference to splenectomy, he thought there was no longer any danger from hemorrhage in properly selected cases. This had deterred many men from performing the operation. In his own case the recovery was uneventful. Patient had none of the so-called symptoms of voracious appetite, and she had remained in a normal condition ever since.

DR. WILLIAM T. HOWARD, of Baltimore, Md., said that the paper of Dr. Ashby proved beyond cavil or question that splenectomy was a dangerous operation. Of 9,361 gynecological cases at the Johns Hopkins Hospital, splenectomy had been done three times successfully by Dr. Kelly. In each of the cases, according to the report, which may be found in a recent number of THE AMERICAN JOURNAL OF OBSTETRICS AND DISEASES OF WOMEN, an incorrect diagnosis was made. In one case the spleen was mistaken for a cyst of the kidney; in the other two cases it was mistaken for an ovarian cystoma. He thought the diagnosis could have been made with care in all of these cases. As to dislocation of the spleen, it did not follow that because this organ was displaced splenectomy was indicated. He held that it was not called for in many cases. He said that Dr. William Osler speaks, in the fourth edition of his ''Practice of Medicine,'' of two cases in which the spleen was dislocated, and that his colleague, Dr. Halsted, had pushed the organ back into its normal position and had kept it there by bandages and gauze packing until adhesions had formed, and the organ had remained in its normal position for eighteen months afterward, in these two cases, so that it did not by any means follow that because a spleen was dislocated it should be removed. He was inclined to think that there was too great a tendency in modern times to resort to unnecessary operations.

DR. A. LAPTHORN SMITH, of Montreal, reported a case of splenectomy, the operation having been done last summer. He said there was no possibility of an error in diagnosis in this case, because the spleen was so large that it could be lifted up and stood on itself much like an enormous mushroom. He could feel the sharp edge of it. The woman was watched carefully for over a year. The condition of her blood had improved, but her life was rendered miserable by the size of the tumor, and he thought he would risk performing an operation. Splenectomy was done, which proved to be exceedingly easy. He was almost certain the woman would recover. He took every precaution with the stump; he tied it in two halves; sewed up the edge with running catgut; he clamped it with pressure clamps, so that he was almost sure there would be no hemorrhage—yet during the following night hemorrhage occurred and the woman died at 5 o'clock the next morning. He opened the abdomen and found about twelve ounces of blood in the abdominal cavity. He did not feel discouraged by the fatal results in this case, and in a similar one he would again resort to splenectomy.

DR. R. STANSBURY SUTTON, of Pittsburg, thought in suitable cases, where the spleen was not very much enlarged and wandering, it would be a good idea to open the abdomen, seize the spleen and rub it well with a piece of plain sterilized gauze, push it back into place, stitch it, and trust to the inflammation excited by the rubbing to conduce to the formation of adhesions there; and probably it might have a good effect by establishing a sort of collateral circulation or an additional circulation similar to that which we were able to get by uniting the omentum to the abdominal wall in cases of abdominal dropsy due to disease of the liver. This was merely a suggestion that had occurred to him. Certainly, he would try this in preference to removing a small or slightly enlarged spleen.

DR. A. PALMER DUDLEY, of New York, had seen three cases of enlarged spleen, two of the spleens having been removed by himself and the other by a fellow-practitioner. One was the case of a boy from whom he removed the spleen, which was really the result of leukemia, as he afterward learned, and lost the case. His second case recovered, it being one of prolapsed spleen, the organ lying behind the uterus. The third case was supposed to be one of enlarged cystic tumor, either of the pelvis or of the pancreas. In this case a blood test was taken and leukemia was not found to be present. He made a diagnosis of sarcoma of the spleen. The right edge of it rested on the right iliac fossa; it filled the pelvic cavity and extended quite up to the diaphragm. In order that he might not make a mistake, he invited a colleague to examine the case, and he had a blood test made for his consultants. An exploratory incision was advised and made, going down nearly to the median line, which confirmed the diagnosis of an enlarged spleen, supposed to be sarcomatous. The growth was so large and the adhesions so extensive about it that he thought he would sacrifice the patient's life in removing it. While the abdomen was open he thought he would introduce his hand and forearm around the spleen and remove some of the splenic contents, providing it were cystic, and have it examined. So he took a hypodermatic needle which is used in cases of spinal anesthesia, and withdrew about half an ounce of the contents of the spleen, sent it to the Post-Graduate Laboratory for examination, and a diagnosis was made of sarcoma of the spleen. He sewed up the abdomen, expecting that the patient would die. She removed to Pennsylvania shortly afterward; had recovered from the exploratory incision, and, much to his surprise, he asked her brother about two months ago how long the woman lived, and he replied, "She is perfectly well, and is visiting over at my house in New York City."

DR. J. WESLEY BOVÉE, of Washington, D. C., had learned a valuable lesson in operating upon a leukemic patient with a twelve-pound spleen. The spleen was in its normal position. The woman died on the table. Since that time he had done two splenectomies, one for malarial hypertrophy and the other for marked idiopathic hypertrophy. As regards the necessity for an examination of the blood previous to operation, he learned the importance of this in his first case, in which he did not have a blood examination made, but operated, and the case terminated fatally. As to what had been said by Dr. Sutton with reference to the possibility of fixation of the spleen, he thought it was a questionable procedure. The Germans had done what is called splenopexy, which consisted in incising the peritoneum and making a sort of sac, putting the spleen into it and inserting a few sutures on the edges of the incision to hold the organ in place. This held the spleen out of position; it modified the circulation of the blood to such an extent as to cause trouble in the spleen in the future.

DR. JOSEPH E. JANVRIN, of New York, recalled a case that came under his observation some three years ago which he thought was attributable entirely to malaria. The spleen weighed between seven and eight pounds. He had no difficulty in removing the organ. The patient suffered from malarial symptoms and nothing else, except from the extreme size of the spleen, which caused more or less discomfort. He thought there was not over one ounce of blood lost during the operation. There was apparently no shock. The patient seemed comfortable after being placed in bed; but at about 1 o'clock the following morning he was hastily summoned and found the patient in a very weak, prostrated condition, and within one hour she died. What she died from he did not know, and never did know. In opening the abdomen after death he found that everything was perfect in the abdominal cavity as he had left it. He attributed death to what is sometimes called secondary or surgical shock.

Dr. ASHBY, in closing the discussion, said that the physical signs in his case were those of a marked cystic or soft tumor, and, with the high temperature which the woman had for some days, he was satisfied that there was some inflammatory condition within the pelvis and therefore made an exploratory operation. After opening the abdomen he found the condition of the spleen he had described, with the long pedicle, and the question of restoring the organ to its former condition was a matter of physical impossibility, and the only thing to do was to remove the organ, which was done.

Dr. EDWARD W. JENKS, of Detroit. Mich., read a paper on

THE MEDICAL SIDE OF GYNECOLOGY.[1]

Dr. EDWARD REYNOLDS, of Boston, said that he who considered the whole woman as well as the case, the constitutional condition as well as the lesion, was likely in the end to be the most successful man.

Dr. JOSEPH TABER JOHNSON, of Washington, D. C., said that the Society had had several papers on the medical side of gynecology since its organization, and it took a brave man, in the presence of so many surgeons possessing so much surgical skill and ambition, to say a word on the side of medical gynecology. Dr. Barker, in his inaugural address to the Society, spoke of medical gynecology, while Dr. Thomas, in his presidential address before the Society, took the opposite view. Dr. Skene had even written a book on the subject of medical gynecology. He thought it was true that, as operators, very frequently the medical points in connection with cases were neglected to the injury of the patients. The gynecologist was startled once in a while by hearing that a patient died on the table, and hearing the operator say afterward that proper care was not taken in determining whether the patient had a weak heart or not, or in making himself acquainted with the fact as to whether or not a weak heart existed. Similar complaints were made relative to the kidneys, their condition not having been ascertained previous to operation. He urged that greater attention be paid to the medical side of surgical cases.

Dr. GEORGE J. ENGELMANN, of Boston, regretted that there were not more papers read bearing on the medical side of gynecology. Some twenty years ago he was severely criticised at a meeting of the St. Louis Medical Society for saying that the future of gynecology was in the knife. Unfortunately, the knife had been used so much that other phases had been neglected. He thought the results of surgical work were by no means always to be considered successful for the patient, and no matter how unattractive other phases of gynecology were, gynecologists

[1]See original article, p. 70.

would have to devote more attention to them in the future than they had in the past.

LACERATIONS OF THE CERVIX UTERI AND PELVIC FLOOR.

Dr. W. L. BURRAGE, of Boston, Mass., read a paper on this subject in which he made an eloquent plea for their more careful study, their diagnosis and treatment. He said the glamor of successful abdominal surgery had left the less dangerous and less showy plastic surgery in the background.

He urged the members of the Society to stand by the principles enunciated by Emmet and to devote their energies to perfecting details of operative technique, rather than to invent or advocate operations which involved principles diametrically opposite to those of Emmet.

Dr. WALTER P. MANTON, of Detroit, Mich., thought the majority of cases of laceration of the cervix that came to the gynecologist were in such a condition that an amputation of the cervix was almost necessary. If the cicatricial tissue was the cause of the reflex or local trouble, the gynecologist should not only cut out a wedge-shaped piece from the angles of the wound, but he should trace the ramifications of the cicatrix with the scissors. In order to do this successfully, one, in a proportion of cases, almost found it necessary to amputate the cervix.

Of the reflex phenomena resulting from cervical lacerations, he had had abundant opportunities for observation. He had operated on many women who had been brought to the verge of insanity as the result of chronic lacerated cervices; he had operated on a large number of insane women who had been materially helped toward mental recovery, if not entirely restored. and he did not think he exaggerated the importance of this condition. He had found, in a number of cases of laceration of the pelvic floor, very little laceration of the perineum, and it had always seemed to him that the most important function of an operation was to bring together the separated or lacerated fibres of the levator ani muscle. This had more to do with a successful result than the mere union of a tear of the perineum.

Dr. HERMAN J. BOLDT, of New York, said the essayist had called attention to the repair of lacerated cervices by means of trachelorrhaphy in preference to amputation of the cervix. He thought there were a great many instances where trachelorrhaphy was not applicable; that the gynecologist in such cases had better resort to cervical amputation, particularly in those instances where there were stellate lacerations, where there were large cervices with highly inflamed uteri in connection with them.

Dr. HUNTER ROBB, of Cleveland, Ohio, agreed in the main with the essayist. He could not agree, however, with the intermediate repair operations recommended by Dr. Dickinson for either complete or incomplete tear of the pelvic floor, of the perineum, or of the cervix. He had under observation a number of cases and it was his experience that when operation was done immediately after labor, particularly in cases of laceration of the perineum or of the pelvic floor, the chances of infection were much less than when the gynecologist waited for the intermediate stage. If one waited for the intermediate stage, bacterial decomposition had abundant opportunity to take place and cause the tissues to break down. If stitches were passed in the intermediate stage, the tissues would be found to be extremely friable, and the chance of infection would be much greater than when the repair was done immediately. The danger of infection was much greater in the intermediate stage than in the early or late repair of the cervix or perineum.

DR. PHILANDER A. HARRIS, of Paterson, N. J., indorsed the position taken by the essayist, and he was glad to know that he objected to doing amputation of the cervix. He had a case under observation at the present time which he had tried to get better by other means, in which the item of painful menstruation seemed to have followed amputation of the cervix. The removal of badly diseased tubes afforded no relief, and a serious dysmenorrhea had followed cervical amputation. Another case which he had in mind presented also a serious train of symptoms which had not been relieved by good men who had had the case under their care, so that he thought amputation of the cervix, as it was practised a few years ago, was a good thing to avoid to a considerable extent in the future, unless there were special reasons or indications for its performance. A mere laceration of the cervix, no matter if the rents were multiple, was no indication for lopping off a considerable part of the cervix and producing so much mutilation.

DR. I. S. STONE, of Washington, D. C., spoke of cancer in cases of laceration of the cervix, saying that the essayist had only mentioned it as a possibility, but it had seemed to him a very important matter. The other day it was brought to his mind by a well-educated woman, who had referred to the neglect of a very excellent practitioner in not immediately repairing a laceration of the cervix for the purpose of preventing cancer. The woman referred to was a physician, who had said that a practitioner had been derelict in not having repaired a lacerated cervix immediately after its occurrence, in order to prevent cancer from taking place, and from which the patient was now dying. He was not aware that the pathology of cancer had been so well established that one could say any man was derelict in the performance of his duty for not making an immediate repair of a lacerated cervix. However, in looking over his experience he was able to say, that many cases of carcinoma began in the sulcus or little tear in the cervix. He would be very glad to have an expression from those present on this subject.

DR. WILLIAM T. HOWARD, of Baltimore, did not think it was necessary to operate for the repair of all lacerations of the cervix. He mentioned the case of a negress who was sent to him a number of years ago, she having been delivered of a hydro-cephalic child. The cervix was lacerated; the entire vaginal insertion was torn off completely, a space not larger than his forefinger left, so that it was easy to see the viscera behind the uterus. The whole vaginal roof was covered over by granulations. The woman was in no condition to be operated upon. He kept her in the hospital under antiseptic treatment, built up her general health, until the vaginal insertion had become united again in a normal way. A large vesico-vaginal fistula, which extended an inch and a quarter from the urethra up toward the vaginal junction, had healed entirely with the exception of a small space. He thought many cases of laceration of the cervix occurred in which healing would take place if the parts were kept clean and antiseptics used, such as carbolic acid in two and a half or five per cent solution.

Dr. CHARLES JEWETT, of Brooklyn, emphasized the importance of the postponed operation. He thought every obstetrician must have had many imperfect results from attempts to repair the pelvic floor immediately after labor. It had been his practice in hospital cases to defer operation. He had not, however, found it necessary to leave it four or seven days. He thought the following day was the best time to operate for the repair of these lacerations. He had operated at all stages, with satisfactory results. By repairing a laceration the following day there was very little danger from infection, and he had seen no objections to the method of postponed operation from that standpoint.

Regarding suture material, he had used ten-day chromicized catgut almost exclusively of late, the great advantage being that it did not have to be taken out. It was a decided advantage over the permanent or non-absorbable suture.

Dr. A. PALMER DUDLEY, of New York, thought it was an easy matter to sew up a lacerated cervix of any extent immediately after delivery or as soon as the placenta was expelled. Among the reasons given by him were that a six- or eight-pound child had dilated the pelvic structures, the uterus had emptied itself, and the broad ligaments, which previous to delivery were extensive, were amenable to traction. He always delivered a woman on the left side in Sims' posture, and the patient did not change this position until the cervical injury was repaired. (Here Dr. Dudley demonstrated on the blackboard his method of repairing a laceration of the cervix.)

Dr. J. WHITRIDGE WILLIAMS, of Baltimore, Md., said that his experience had taught him that it was inadvisable to operate for the repair of a cervical tear immediately after labor, unless there was considerable hemorrhage. When there was considerable hemorrhage an operation should be performed in every instance. The genital tract of a woman after childbirth should not be repaired, unless it is absolutely necessary, as every exploration added materially to the danger of infection. Laceration of the perineum, on the other hand, should be repaired immediately after childbirth, unless the condition of the woman is too serious to allow it. He did not believe in the intermediate operation. If a primary operation could not be done, it was much better to let the woman wait until the end of three or four weeks and do a secondary operation. Then we had a condition of affairs which was favorable, and the operation would undoubtedly effect the desired result. If a secondary operation was done the parts were often relaxed, and quite frequently after the operation was completed one might have an unsatisfactory result and be compelled to do the operation a second time. He saw a woman recently whose perineum he had repaired immediately after labor. Healing had taken place by first intention; yet, in spite of that fact, the levator ani muscle had stretched, and the probabilities were that in the near future the woman would need another operation.

Dr. J. Riddle Goffe, of New York, asked Dr. Williams how many of his primary operations on the perineum he regarded as failures because some of them had to be done a second time and some of them were cured. He thought much depended upon the proportion of cures and failures as to whether the cases should be let go for a secondary operation. Every woman who could be prevented from undergoing a secondary operation was saved from an unfortunate experience. Personally, he was a strong believer in the primary operation.

Dr. Williams said, in reply, that he believed every perineum that was lacerated should be repaired immediately at the close of labor. The point he desired to make was this: that instead of getting perfect union, so far as healing was concerned, the woman a month afterward very frequently would have a relaxed outlet, due to the fact that the operator had not succeeded in bringing together the torn fibres of the levator ani muscle. The parts above it had not been restored to their normal condition. No one insisted more on the necessity for immediate operation than he did, but the results were not always satisfactory.

Dr. Goffe said he would regard an operation as a failure if the levator ani fascia was not restored.

Dr. E. E. Montgomery, of Philadelphia, stated that too much importance could not be attached to the leaving of a sufficient portion of undenuded surface to prevent subsequent contraction which took place in the progress of involution. This was the great difficulty in the earlier primary operations, that the orifice was so contracted that there was subsequently deficient drainage; the patient suffered from secondary conditions which involved the tubes and ovaries and pelvic peritoneum.

He could not agree with the writer as to the infrequent performance of amputation of the cervix in preference to trachelorrhaphy. Where a laceration was extensive and Nature had made an effort to repair it, where there had been a large amount of cicatricial tissue deposited, the lips widely everted, it was just as important to remove the cicatricial tissue in the central as in the lateral surfaces. Where the surfaces could be brought together by sutures a marked impression was made upon the central portion, giving rise to subsequent reflex disturbance similar to that induced by the presence of cicatricial tissue in the lateral lines, and in such cases he thought it was far preferable to resort to amputation of the cervix. In such an amputation, however, it was not necessary to do extensive removal of issue, but to remove merely the cicatricial tissue at the expense of the inner flap and leave a long external flap, doing practically a Schröder operation in combination with that of Emmet.

DR. ROBERT L. DICKINSON, of Brooklyn, said that one of the most important reasons for deferring the primary operation in cases of laceration of the cervix and of the perineum immediately after labor had not been mentioned. All were agreed as to the minor injuries of the cervix. These did not need touching. It was the severe injuries that required operative measures. A minor injury of the perineum could be repaired without an anesthetic. A severe injury of the cervix extending into the broad ligament or down the vagina, or a severe injury of the perineum tearing through the sphincter ani, needed good surgery, time, anesthesia, and a good operator. A patient who had received a severe tear was one who had passed through a severe labor, who was exhausted and suffering from inertia uteri, and an operation performed upon such a patient immediately after labor was usually done in a hurried and careless manner. It seemed to him more preferable to operate the next day or three or four days later, when thorough and careful work could be done.

DR. A. LAPTHORN SMITH, of Montreal, said he was frequently asked by women in his office whether, if they had their cervices repaired, he could give them a guarantee that the cervix would not be torn at a subsequent confinement. In a considerable number of cases in which this accident had happened at a subsequent confinement, the women had refused to undergo another operation because they thought there was no use of having it done. These women had also heard of a number of cases of severe labor during which women had suffered during the first stage from having the cervix previously sewed up. These considerations had induced him to give up Emmet's operation for lacerated cervix if the woman was likely to have children again. He expressed himself as being in accord with the essayist that there ought to be decided opinions advanced as to whether a lacerated cervix predisposed to cancer. He was perfectly convinced himself that it did, and he thought the Fellows could not make the impression too widespread, because so many cases of cancer had evidently resulted from lacerated cervices. He drew attention to the advantage of cervical amputation over the Emmet or Schröder operation in those cases where there was great thickening of the end of the cervix.

DR. WILLIAM E. ASHTON, of Philadelphia, spoke of the preliminary treatment of cases of laceration of the cervix. He believed that if treatment were directed toward the hypertrophy of the cervix, induration, cystic degeneration, and the eroded condition of the cervix—in other words, pathological conditions dependent upon cervical laceration—for several weeks prior to deciding upon operative measures, in a number of cases it would not be necessary to do trachelorrhaphy or resort to cervical amputation, whereas at the time the patients were first seen either one of these measures might have been indicated. There could be no doubt whatever that where there were pathological conditions of the cervix, the result of laceration, the Emmet operation did not effect the best results; in other words, he thought there was no use of repairing a cervix if it was the seat of cystic degeneration. Under such circumstances operations of the Emmet type were failures. In the same way the Emmet operation was not indicated in a case of indurated or hypertrophied cervix. He felt reasonably certain that if many of these cases were properly treated for weeks by the means familiar to the Fellows, in the course of that time a number of the cases which would have been selected for cervical amputation originally would now come within the line of trachelorrhaphy.

He expressed his disbelief in the immediate operation for lacerated cervix, also in the intermediate operation, and agreed with Dr. Williams that the less manipulation done high up in the vaginal canal after labor the better for the patient, on account of the danger of infection.

DR. FRANCIS H. DAVENPORT, of Boston, said there was one point with reference to immediate repair of the perineum that had not been brought out, and that was the question whether it was possible to completely repair the perineum at that time. His experience had been that many women came to him who had been handled by good men and their lacerations sewed up, yet there was still a giving way or loss of substance of the perineal body, due to the separation of the fibres of the levator ani muscle. The external perineum, so to speak, had been repaired, but other tears had been overlooked. When this fact was told women, they would say, "Doctor, I was sewed up at labor," and the question arose whether the accoucheur was not at fault. He did not think the accoucheur was at fault, because there were many cases where it was impossible to demonstrate a lesion or tear at the time which occurred subcutaneously. There was a separation underneath the mucous membrane, and this could not be repaired accurately at the time of labor. To get the ends of the muscles and fasciæ together would require considerable denudation or opening of the mucous membrane, which, of course, could not be done, so that many of the cases could not be adequately repaired at the time of labor, but must be repaired at a later stage. He did not think an intermediate time —that is, a time within a few days or even a few weeks after labor—was the best time, as the tissues were not in a condition favorable for the best healing.

DR. JOSEPH E. JANVRIN, of New York, spoke of the occurrence of cancer as a result of laceration of the cervix. He said the question of cancer at the present time was one concerning which there was great diversity of opinion. However, he thought the profession was fairly well agreed that any injury to any part of the uterus, to any part of the breast, to any part of the glandular structures was very apt to be a provocative cause of disease, and that disease was generally of a malignant type. Therefore he believed, from his own experience and observation, that in a good percentage of cases of lacerations of the cervix we ultimately had the occurrence of carcinomatous degeneration. This degeneration, however, did not occur, as Dr. Stone had said, in the sulcus where the cicatrix formed any more than it did in the lacerated lips themselves. He thought it was just as likely, perhaps more so, to occur away from the sulcus. He never performed immediate repair of the cervix except in cases of considerable hemorrhage. He agreed with Dr. Williams that in perineal tears it was wise to operate immediately, and when this was done the results were usually successful.

DR. R. STANSBURY SUTTON, of Pittsburg, said the late Mr. Lawson Tait used to say that there was no surgical operation so worthless as Emmet's cervix operation, and twenty years ago there was not an operation done so frequently in Germany as biconical section of the lacerated cervix. Martin, who did six or eight operations a day sometimes, in answer to the speaker's interrogatory stated that he had seen a number of cases where no laceration of the cervix existed and where the patients had not previously been pregnant. His own experience had revealed but one case of epithelioma of the cervix in a virgin. With that one exception, all the cases of epithelioma of the cervix which he had seen had been associated with cervical laceration. He recalled the cases of several women whom he had urged to have their lacerated cervices repaired, and as an argument he said to them they were in danger of having cancer later on. Three of the women, who had refused to have their cervices repaired, died subsequently of cancer of the cervix. So that, in his opinion, cancer of the cervix was associated with traumatism of the cervix; and, so far as he knew, the disease did not begin in the cicatricial tissue in the cleft, but it began at the junction of the pavement or flat epithelium with the ciliated epithelium just at the margin of the external os prior to the laceration.

DR. BURRAGE, in closing the discussion, said the debate had brought out one fact—the importance of teaching every physician who confines a woman, and before he gives up the case, to make a diagnosis as to the condition of the cervix and pelvic floor. He should explain the condition he finds to the patient and advise what he thinks ought to be done, if an operation be necessary, and should not leave the case and let it run for luck and later on have the case pass into the hands of some other practitioner or specialist.

First Day—Afternoon Session.

SYMPOSIUM ON RETRODISPLACEMENTS OF THE UTERUS.

Dr. Matthew D. Mann, of Buffalo, N. Y., discussed the

ETIOLOGY, PATHOLOGY, AND SYMPTOMS.

He believed the round ligaments were important factors in holding the uterus in place, and that they acted in the manner pointed out by Kellogg. If the ligaments be stretched the uterus fell behind the centre of gravity, and the round ligaments were not able to pull it far enough forward, so that intra-abdominal pressure fell on the posterior wall with every effort to increase backward displacement; and as time went on the case became worse. Weakening of the pelvic floor, or relaxation of the pelvic outlet as the result of childbearing, with or without rupture of the perineum, would allow the uterus to sag downward and the fundus to fall backward. Relaxation of any of the supports of the uterus tended to backward and downward displacement of the organ, and if the ligaments and pelvic floor were relaxed then eventually there would be prolapse to a greater or less extent, dependent upon the amount of relaxation. He spoke of the utero-vesical ligament as having a considerable influence in producing uterine displacement. He mentioned other factors which caused the uterus to become displaced backward, one of which was rupture of the perineum, which enabled the vaginal walls to sag. If these came down, with cystocele or rectocele, then the vaginal wall, dragging upon the cervix, would pull the organ downward and tip it over backward.

In displacement of the uterus the circulation and nutrition of the organ were interfered with, so that in a short time the woman would get a chronic congestion, with thickening and enlargement of the connective tissue of the uterus. This might be called, for want of a better term, a chronic metritis.

Another cause of displacement of the uterus was laceration of the cervix, which allowed the organ to sink down into the pelvis, to turn slightly backward, the displacement going on from bad to worse. The speaker had seen two cases of displacement of the uterus, one following whooping cough in an adult, the other from straining at stool. In the latter case the uterus was forced outside of the body from constant straining at stool. although the hymen was intact.

As regards the symptoms of retrodisplacement of the uterus, among them he mentioned backache, bearing-down pains in the pelvis, etc. He did not believe that every case of posterior displacement of the uterus caused symptoms, but he did believe that the majority of cases of backward displacement of the uterus did produce symptoms. A woman with a backward displacement of the uterus would not continue to remain well; she might be well for the time being, but eventually he thought she would suffer. He did not believe a backward displacement of the uterus could exist for any great length of time without the woman suffering more or less. Besides the symptoms familiar to the gynecologist, he thought there were a great many reflex symptoms. A woman with a retrodisplaced uterus might suffer considerably from reflex symptoms without the presence of pelvic symptoms. He cited cases in point.

DR. F. H. DAVENPORT, of Boston, followed with a paper entitled

NON-OPERATIVE TREATMENT OF RETRODISPLACEMENTS OF THE UTERUS.

The author discussed three points: first, the methods of non-operative treatment; second, the indications for their employment; and, third, the results.

The only important method of non-operative treatment was that by pessary. Twenty-five years ago it was practically the only method, and for that reason it was developed to a remarkable degree, not only as regards the variety of displacements, but also the numerous forms of pessaries devised for their relief. Massage, electricity, and general tonic treatment could not properly be called methods, but were merely adjuncts. The choice, then, lay between treatment by operation and that by pessary. With the development of surgical procedures, that by supports was thrown into the background and neglected. There were cases, however, which were well adapted to the pessary treatment. Such were, first, cases of simple retroverted uterus without complication, which had presumably lasted only a short time; second, retroversion following childbirth; third, cases complicating neurasthenia as a result, where operation was inadvisable until the patient's health was built up.

The pessary treatment was not applicable to cases in young girls where local treatment of any kind was inadvisable, to cases complicated with lacerations, or to cases of long standing where secondary changes in the circulation of the uterus had followed. Many of those which should be operated on refused operation and chose the pessary. What, then, were the chances of cure? The writer's own statistics had shown that of all cases treated by pessary about one-third were cured, either anatomically or symptomatically, by the use of a pessary for from one to two years. In selected cases the showing would be far better. Such success, however, presupposed close study of the case, care in the selection of the pessary, and constant supervision while it was worn.

The only displacements which needed correction were prolapse and retrodisplacements, and the latter might be usually corrected by one of two varieties of pessaries, the Langford and the Albert Smith. The treatment by pessary, therefore, while it should be scientific, was simple.

Dr. CLEMENT CLEVELAND, of New York, read a paper on

THE ALEXANDER OPERATION.

The author described this operation in detail. Although usually performed for retrodeviations of the uterus, he had found it useful in the cure of forward displacements. The selection of cases, however, was very important. In cases where adhesions existed it was better to follow some of the other methods or resort to the vaginal route. In cases where the Alexander operation was not indicated he preferred the operation devised by J. Dougal Bissell, and styled by him "internal shortening of the round and broad ligaments," with which the writer had had many good results.

To obtain the best results in the Alexander operation a pessary should be worn before, and for two months after, the operation. It was also advisable that the patient should wear one for a few months after confinement. She should be kept in bed for three weeks after the operation, and the dressings should be changed daily. The main point in the performance of this operation was to reach the external ring with a clean cut from the surface. To a beginner a great stumbling block was the mistaking the superficial fascia for the aponeurosis of the external oblique. The writer believed that by including in the first suture the pouch of the peritoneum or infundibuliform process, it not only strengthened the attachments of the ligaments, but added to the support of the uterus. Sterilized iron-dyed silk was recommended to hold the ligaments. Hernia as a result of this operation was rare, and, when met with, was due either to faulty technique or suppuration. The chief causes of failure were (1) suppuration in the wounds, and (2) the too tightly tying of the ligament sutures.

In comparison with other methods, the writer preferred the Alexander operation for an uncomplicated case of displacement. In his opinion the vaginal method of operation should be confined to women who had borne children.

ABDOMINAL SUSPENSION.

In speaking of the advantages, disadvantages, and results of suspension of the uterus, Dr. HUNTER ROBB, of Cleveland, Ohio, insisted that suspension and fixation were not interchangeable terms, the latter procedure being always undesirable.

Before we were able to speak with certainty as to the results, we must have more accurate data, which could only be obtained by a more rigid classification and a subsequent analysis of sufficiently larger series of (1) uncomplicated cases of malposition; (2) those cases of malposition in which other pathological conditions were present, but in which the malposition was the indication for operation; (3) those cases in which the suspension was only a supplementary operation.

Robb believed that in suspension we had a method of permanently relieving a large percentage of patients suffering from obstinate retroflexion. Difficulties in future pregnancies were mainly the result of fixation operations and not of suspension. Hernia of the abdominal wall, adhesions, and localized or general sepsis were due to faulty technique and should not occur.

INTRA-ABDOMINAL SHORTENING OF THE ROUND LIGAMENTS PER VAGINAM FOR THE CURE OF RETRODISPLACEMENTS OF THE UTERUS.

Dr. J. Riddle Goffe, of New York, read a paper on this subject. He said that gynecologists were uniformly agreed that the ligament which served the most important function in supporting the uterus was the sling of tissue reaching from the promontory of the sacrum, known as the utero-sacral ligaments, to the posterior wall of the cervix, plus the utero-sacral ligament reaching from the anterior wall of the uterus to the symphysis pubis. This was reinforced by the cellular tissue and ligamentous structure in the base of the broad ligament. So long as the utero-sacral ligaments retained their proper tone and length, swinging the cervix high in the hollow of the sacrum, retroversion of the uterus was impossible. It was for some malign influence affecting the utero-sacral ligaments, therefore, that we must look for the cause of retrodisplacements of the uterus, and it was consequently to the repair or the recovery of function in the utero-sacral ligaments that gynecologists must look for restoration to a normal condition. Unless the indirect result of any operation for maintaining the uterus in its normal position was to enable the utero-sacral ligaments to involute and recover their tone and sustaining power, that operation became a failure. That this could be secured by direct operative procedure upon the utero-sacral ligaments themselves he was convinced from his experience.

The next most favorable tissue to utilize for this purpose was the round ligament. This was attested by the results secured by many operators upon the round ligaments in various ways. Alexander and others had demonstrated that the round ligaments, when shortened at the external abdominal ring, were efficient in maintaining the uterus in its normal position when applied to cases of retrodisplacement uncomplicated by inflammatory process. Olshausen had shown that the round ligaments, when caught up near to the uterus and attached at the edges of the abdominal incision, were efficient and satisfactory in restoring the uterus to its normal position. Wylie, Mann, and many of their followers had experienced complete satisfaction in simply doubling the round ligaments upon themselves and stitching them in that position through an abdominal incision. Dührssen, Wertheim, and Vineburg had presented most conclusive statistics bearing upon the efficiency of shortening the round ligaments through a vaginal incision by catching them up near the horns of the uterus and stitching them into the vaginal wall. The same German operators. Dührssen, Wertheim, etc., and, in this country, Byford and the essayist, attest to the equal efficiency of operating through the anterior vaginal fornix and doubling the ligaments on themselves in accordance with the Wylie-Mann suggestion. He had not found a method which had given him such universal satisfaction as this.

He reported 130 cases that he had subjected to this procedure during the past sixteen years. and he knew of only three failures; and these were due to some departure from the regular procedure in which a modification was attempted. Among these cases, 10 were known to have become pregnant and 8 had gone to full term, the pregnancies resulting most comfortably and satisfactorily, the uteri retaining their normal position thereafter. Of the miscarriages, one was in a syphilitic negress, and in the other the cause could not be learned.

The value of this method over others depended, therefore, upon the general question of the superiority of the vaginal route of attack over the abdominal route, and the incomparably wider field of application as compared with the Alexander operation.

Among the author's cases he found six of congenital retroversion in young, unmarried women whose ages ranged from 19 to 27 years. In these cases, although the vagina was small and the hymen intact in all of them, he was able to perform this operation and effect a complete cure in all.

The last paper of the symposium was read by Dr. J. Wesley Bovée, of Washington, D. C., entitled

OPERATIONS ON THE UTERO-SACRAL LIGAMENTS IN THE TREATMENT OF RETROVERSION OF THE UTERUS.

He recounted briefly the surgical treatment of the uterosacral ligaments. His first operation for shortening the uterosacral ligaments through the vagina was done June 28, 1897, and since that time he had had seven other cases, all successful. By the abdominal route he began shortening these ligaments February 21, 1900, and since then on three other occasions had the operation been done.

The method of shortening these ligaments through the vagina, as he had planned and practised it, was to place the patient in the extreme lithotomy or Simon's position, and, with a self-retaining perineal retractor in place, the posterior lip of the cervix is grasped with a volsella forceps and drawn forward. The antero-posterior incision is made through all the structures of the posterior vaginal fornix, except the peritoneum, and extending approximately from the cervix to the rectum. By careful dissection the ligaments are brought plainly into view. Then, grasping one of them with a forceps midway between the extreme points to be united and loosening the traction on the cervix at the same time, the fold of the ligament is brought down into the vagina; then a curved needle, armed with kangaroo tendon, is passed through the ligament at the extreme points noted, and another through the loop thus formed and through the posterior portion of the cervix below the insertion of the ligaments. When the other ligament has been treated in a similar manner, the two deep sutures are tied and then the others. The wound is now spread well open and the two ends of it approximated by a continuous kangaroo-tendon suture. When the wound is closed it appears to have been originally a transverse one. Sometimes the writer had modified it by separation of the anterior vaginal wall from the uterus and converting the wound into a longitudinal wound or by transplanting the wall higher on to the uterus. When adhesions have been thought to exist in the retrouterine space, the cul-de-sac has been entered and the adhesions separated. In all instances he had shortened the round ligaments through the anterior fornix.

By the abdominal route the plan he had followed was to use the Trendelenburg position, remove the intestine and omentum from the pelvis, and by the use of a specially long retractor hold the uterus and appendages well forward and upward. Then, tracing the utero-sacral ligaments with the fingers to properly locate them, a longitudinal incision is made through the peritoneum near the inner margin of one of them. The ligament is then partially dissected loose and is treated much as by the vaginal route. The peritoneum is closed by a purse-string suture or by the plan of closing the vaginal wound. The other side is similarly treated and the abdomen closed. He had in a few instances shortened the round ligaments at the same sitting. The results of the various operations for shortening the utero-sacral ligaments were good. The author's own work in shortening the utero-sacral ligaments consisted of eight vaginal and four abdominal operations. As to the advantages of the operation, the extraperitoneal shortening of these ligaments with the adjoining portion of the vaginal wall was practically devoid of danger and was frequently indicated.

The abdominal route was less frequently required; yet, with the abdomen open, perhaps for some other purpose, shortening of these ligaments would be very little extra risk for the patient or extra tax upon the part of the surgeon. It did not have the same conditions incident to ventrosuspension and ventrofixation which were considered by some as real dangers, and it was supporting Nature's supports to this important reproductive organ.

(To be continued.)

TRANSACTIONS OF THE
OBSTETRICAL SOCIETY OF LONDON.

Meeting of April 2, 1902.

The President, PETER HORROCKS, M.D., *in the Chair.*

PRIMARY TUBERCULOSIS OF THE CERVIX SIMULATING CANCER.

DR. A. H. N. LEWERS read a paper on a case of primary tuberculosis of the cervix simulating cancer, and which he had treated by vaginal hysterectomy.

The patient was a married woman, 36 years of age, who had never been pregnant. For nine months before she came under observation there had been a vaginal discharge which was blood-stained and slightly offensive. Bleeding had been noticed after coitus and also after using a vaginal syringe. She had had slight pain in the left iliac region for about five months. This did not appear to have been at all severe. The catamenia had been regular, lasting three or four days only, and not attended by any special pain. The patient's general health had been good up to twelve months before she came under observation. Then she found herself beginning to get weak and disinclined for exertion, and to suffer from the local symptoms above mentioned. She did not think she had lost flesh. One of her aunts died of consumption, but otherwise the family history was unimportant.

On vaginal examination the condition of the vaginal portion of the cervix seemed identical with what is found in many cases of cancer. The vaginal portion appeared to be the seat of ''a growth'' which was friable and bled readily on examination. The uterus was freely movable. Believing that the case was one of cancer of the cervix suitable for radical operation, he performed vaginal hysterectomy on January 30, 1896. The patient made a good recovery. He had seen her several times since, and had a letter from her on November 20, 1901. in which she said that she ''enjoys fairly good health and has had no return of the bleeding.''

While she was in the hospital there was no evidence of any disease in other organs.

When portions of the supposed malignant growth were sent to the Clinical Research Association for examination, the report came back that there was no evidence of cancer, but that the structure was tubercular.

Brief reference was made to the writings of Pozzi, Cullen, and Whitridge Williams, from which it appears that primary tuberculosis of the cervix is an exceedingly rare condition.

Specimens of tubercular disease of the body of the uterus, the cervix and vagina were shown by Dr. Russell Andrews, Dr. Williamson, Mr. Targett, and Dr. Croft, and discussed in connection with Dr. Lewers' paper.

Dr. Handfield-Jones narrated a case which had come under his observation in which the patient, a multipara aged 30, had suffered for several years with strumous disease of both hands. Several fingers and parts of the metacarpal bones had been removed at different times, owing to the presence of tubercular disease of the bones and joints. For months the patient had been suffering with excessive menstrual losses and in the intervals from a foul vaginal discharge. Examination showed that the cervix was deeply excavated by tuberculous ulceration and that the mischief had extended to the upper part of the vaginal wall on the left side. As the patient would not submit to any radical operation, the ulcerated cervix was thoroughly scraped and then Paquelin's cautery freely applied to the base of the ulcer. Cicatrization followed, and two years later the patient was found to be free from any further spread of tubercular disease in the genital tract, but she had commenced to develop tubercular lesions in her lungs. The good effect of the curettage and use of the actual cautery was very manifest, and might certainly be used with advantage for cases in which extirpation of the uterus was deemed undesirable.

Dr. E. O. Croft remarked on the importance and difficulty of diagnosing cases of tuberculous cervicitis. There was a closer resemblance of the symptoms in Dr. Lewers' case to those of cancer than in the case described by himself. Dr. Lewers' patient had had bleeding, pain, and some offensive discharge. Dr. Croft's case had absolute amenorrhea for many months, bleeding only taking place when examined. The growth was softer than in cancer and did not break away in the same crumbling manner. The papillary masses were easily detached and were more of the consistence of mucous polypi than of the vegetations of cancer. Dr. Croft, on his first examination of the case, concluded that the growth was not of the nature of any of the ordinary forms of cancer of the cervix, but kept in mind the possibility of an early condition of botryoidal sarcoma, or myxoma of the cervix. The tuberculous nature of the lesion was, however, established by microscopic examination before operation was decided on. In reply to a remark of Dr. Lewers, Dr. Croft said that tubercle bacilli had not been definitely demonstrated.

The President said he was surprised to hear that tubercle in the uterus in the majority of cases was confined either to the cervix or to the body; for, in the only two cases that had come under his observation, the whole mucous membrane from the os externum to the top of the uterus was affected, and he had thus been led to think that tubercle differed essentially in this respect from cancer.

Also, in his own case and in Dr. Lewers' case, the patients had

never been pregnant.   He was surprised to hear Mr. Targett say
that it was easy to diagnose tubercle.   Certainly it might be in
the lungs, either clinically or post mortem with the naked eye;
but in tubercle of the uterus he thought it was difficult, and
even where a piece had been cut out and investigated microscopically it had been pronounced to be sarcoma.   He was under the
impression that the specimen shown by Mr. Targett from the
Guy's Hospital Museum was the same one to which he had referred.

She was in a medical ward, and he (Dr. Horrocks) had seen
her and had diagnosed from the condition of the swollen cervix,
which seemed filled with ovula Nabothi, a follicular inflammation
of the cervix.   She was transferred to the care of Dr. Galabin,
who cut a piece out, and, after careful microscopical investigation, came to the conclusion that it was sarcoma and removed
the uterus by vaginal hysterectomy.   The whole of the uterine
mucous membrane was greatly thickened and diseased throughout.   It was examined at the Royal College of Surgeons by Dr.
Goodhart and some one else, and tubercle bacilli were found.

PSEUDO-INTRALIGAMENTARY CYST.

DR. FAIRBAIRN showed a unilocular ovarian cyst containing in
its wall large solid masses undergoing necrotic change.   The
cyst itself showed no evidence of any twisting of the pedicle, and
was in fact a sessile cyst enucleated from underneath the broad
ligament.   The solid masses were of a deep purple color and
projected into the interior as a number of rounded bosses; on
section they were very firm and hard, and cut more like a fibroma
than the solid adenomatous structures of an ovarian cyst.   When
fresh they were full of blood and had an appearance very like
that of liver.   Microscopically they proved to be adenomatous,
with a papilliferous arrangement.   There was a very extensive
extravasation of blood and thrombosis of vessels into the necrosed
parts.   The partial necrosis affecting only the solid masses is
somewhat difficult to explain.   As there was some calcification at
the base of the cyst, this may have interfered with the blood
supply.

TUBAL GESTATION.

DR. AMAND ROUTH showed a specimen of a Fallopian tube
ruptured toward its fimbriated end in two places.   The patient
was a multipara, aged 25, who when about six weeks pregnant
was seized with collapse and all the signs of intra-abdominal
hemorrhage.   When the abdomen was opened the peritoneal
cavity was found to be full of blood, and the ovum in its intact
membranes was found to be adherent to the edge of a rupture
on the posterior aspect of the right Fallopian tube near the
fimbriated end.   The tube was ligatured off and removed, and
was then found to be ruptured both anteriorly and posteriorly.
The patient rallied well from the operation and made an easy
convalescence.

When examined the ruptured tube showed the following features: The tube measures 7 centimetres in its long axis. At the cut uterine extremity it is normal in size for one centimetre of its length, but its lumen is impervious. One centimetre from the cut end the tube widens out into a thin-walled sac, the distension reaching as far as the fimbriæ, which appear as so many finger-like processes proceeding from the sac; the abdominal ostium having been closed, it is no longer traceable. The tubal gestation sac measures 6 centimetres in length by 2.5 centimetres in width through its greatest diameter. The sac tapers at either extremity, being more or less fusiform in shape. The walls of the sac have ruptured both anteriorly and posteriorly, the one tear in the distended condition measuring 1 by 2 centimetres, the other being 2 by 2 centimetres in extent. Both tears proceed to within 2 centimetres of the fimbriated extremity of the tube.

DR. RUSSELL ANDREWS having shown a photograph, two drawings, and the pelvic organs from a case of congenital, or rather infantile, prolapse of the uterus associated with spina bifida, DR. BLACKER commented upon the case.

DR. WILLIAMSON showed a specimen of umbilical cord containing four umbilical arteries and only one umbilical vein, and DR. McCANN showed a specimen of a tubal mole.

Meeting of May 7, 1902.

The President, PETER HORROCKS, M.D., *in the Chair.*

DR. JOHN S. FAIRBAIRN read a paper on

FIVE SPECIMENS OF FIBROID TUMOR OF THE OVARY, WITH OBSERVATIONS ON THEIR PATHOLOGICAL ANATOMY.

Attention was first directed to the descriptions of these growths as given in the text books and monographs on the subject. The general statement was that these tumors are formed by hyperplasia of the whole stroma, so that the organ is converted into a hard tumor retaining more or less the original shape of the ovary. Five specimens, varying in size from a small growth the size of a hen's egg up to a large tumor of over four pounds in weight, were described in detail. In all of them the new growth had arisen within the ovary, and affected only a portion of the stroma, leaving a considerable part of the organ as a separate and easily recognizable structure. The microscopic appearances were also noted, and a short clinical history of the cases from which they were obtained was added.

After looking through a large number of recorded cases of fibroma and fibromyoma of the ovary, some fifteen or sixteen were selected as similar to those described in the paper and a short abstract of them was given. When such specimens have been shown at societies they have given rise to some discussion from the unusual persistence of a portion of the ovary. The number of instances quoted, together with the five specimens under review, was sufficient to show that the descriptions usually given were misleading.

While the difficulty of detecting unstriped muscle cells among fibrous tissue cells was acknowledged, the evidence of a comparative examination of sections from these tumors appeared to be in favor of their being considered fibromata. The sections provided a very good opportunity of contrasting the minute structure of the growth with the ovarian stroma from which they had originated; the results of such a study were adduced in favor of considering these firm, hard growths of the ovary as simple fibromata, and not as fibrosarcomata. The question of these tumors arising from a chronic oöphoritis was discussed very briefly, and the importance of the tunica albuginea in forming a strong covering to ovarian growths was pointed out.

In conclusion, the fibromata of the ovary were divided into three classes for purposes of description.

1. The ovary is entirely replaced by the new formation. This occurs in small as well as large growths, and therefore does not depend on the size to which the growth has attained.

2. A local growth of the stroma leaving part of the ovary unaffected, except by compression. The growth tends to remain within the capsule of the ovary.

3. Pedunculated fibromata like subperitoneal fibroids of the uterus. These may either have originated in the stroma and later been extruded, or they may be growths of the tunica albuginea.

MR. ALBAN DORAN maintained that the three specimens which he exhibited that evening in relation to Dr. Fairbairn's important paper implied that fibroma and myoma of the ovary were distinct diseases.

The section of the large fibroma showed perfect wavy white fibre, as did the section of the little solitary fibroma not half an inch in diameter. The myoma, unlike the two fibromata, was closely related to the ovarian ligament, which included muscular tissue derived from the uterus. On section it showed plain muscle cells, precisely as seen in a section of a myoma of the uterus.

Edematous fibroids were once taken for sarcomata of the ovary; subtracting these suspected malignant growths from the malignant solid tumors of the ovary, we should probably find that carcinoma of the ovary was much more common than sarcoma, as Martin had demonstrated, whilst fibroma, innocent even when looking malignant, was by no means rare. There were plenty exhibited that night. Mr. Doran noted how the tube and mesosalpinx often underwent little or no hypertrophy in fibroma, so that when the tumor was large it was rather difficult to get at the pedicle.

MR. BLAND-SUTTON congratulated Dr. Fairbairn on establishing the fact that the encapsulation of the tumor could be relied upon as a generic and distinguishing feature.

When the fibroid was of moderate size, as in the smallest specimen of his series, the disproportion between the ovary and the tumor was not so marked; but when the mass had a circumference of 20 or even 30 centimetres, or more, then the small bud-like remnant of the ovary at the uterine end of the tumor appeared very incongruous.

The leading features of these tumors could be summarized thus: encapsulation, ovoid shape, intense hardness, and the whorled disposition of the tissue as displayed on the cut surface. These were a group of signs presented by no other tumor of the ovary, and their clinical value was equal to their simplicity.

There was an important feature by which ovarian fibroids were distinguished from similar tumors in the uterus. It was well established that uterine fibroids did not arise after the menopause, whereas ovarian fibroids occurred in the aged, and on two occasions Mr. Bland-Sutton had successfully removed them at the ages of 64 and 66, and the clinical histories indicated that the tumors had only been noticed two years before removal.

The extreme hardness of these tumors was a valuable clinical sign, and in one of the cases in Dr. Fairbairn's series Mr. Bland-Sutton was able to accurately diagnose the character of the tumor from this sign alone.

The paper was a valuable one, even if only regarded from the point of view that its author had rescued a genus of tumors from a group notorious for containing members with extremely bad characters.

DR. GRIFFITH fully agreed with the conclusion arrived at by Dr. Fairbairn in his interesting paper. He had endeavored to show, in the paper referred to by Dr. Fairbairn, that all tumors of the ovary, whether cystic or solid, were, in the main structure of their solid parts, connective tissue, derived from and having the essential character of the spindle-celled stroma of the normal organ.

Corpora fibrosa were physiologically the ultimate stages of the corpora lutea, and where they were enlarged their structure appeared to remain of the special character of the normal bodies, and not spindle-celled.

DR. BRIGGS said that amongst his original cases and amongst recent ones he had figured and noted circumscribed growths to which Dr. Fairbairn had paid conspicuous attention. The early writers were correct in alluding to both diffuse and circumscribed growths.

Dr. Briggs suggested that Dr. Fairbairn had shown a want of courage in selecting fibroids, and not fibromata, as the title of the paper founded on the five cases he had described. Mr. Alban Doran's specimen exhibited that night, if not actually a myoma, was the nearest approach in its microscopical characters to a myoma of any he had ever seen. Dr. Briggs thought that would be a general opinion which meanwhile, in the face of so much evidence to the contrary, might be held in reserve.

The main danger had been, as Mr. Bland-Sutton said, in ascribing malignant properties to cellular structures without adequate clinical proof. In Dr. Briggs' experience this impeachment was not limited to gynecologists.

The proof of the innocence of cellular growths described as fibromata of the ovary had been substantiated by Mr. Alban Doran and himself in the published paper referred to by Dr. Fairbairn. Dr. Briggs cited the case in which he operated almost immediately after he had published his paper. In a girl aged 17 there was a large, brain-like solid growth of the ovary. The girl now lived and was an active hospital nurse. The tumor was proved to be a highly cellular growth, a myxoma.

The rarity, as alleged, of fibromata of the ovary was not justified by facts which had now accumulated. Dr. Briggs added that all his patients from whom he had removed these tumors still lived.

Dr. Herbert Spencer was surprised at the number of writers cited by the author who regarded ovarian fibroids as diffuse growths involving the whole of the ovarian tissue. His own experience was opposed to such a view, for, out of five cases under his own care, in four the growth was very definitely limited to a portion of the ovary, and in the fifth (a large tumor) he thought possibly the tumor was so limited, but without spoiling the museum specimen by a series of thin sections it was impossible to settle this point. Ovarian fibroids were certainly benign growths and had much in common with uterine fibroids. The latter did not involve the whole tissue of the uterus, but sometimes displaced and compassed it to a remarkable extent. It seemed to him most unlikely that such a benign fibroid growth would invade and destroy the whole of the tissue of the ovary, and, as a matter of fact, in the five cases alluded to, and in several others he had seen, it did not do so. A most interesting point in connection with these growths, not alluded to by any speaker, was their origin. Two of his cases suggested, and a third he thought clearly demonstrated, the origin of an ovarian fibroid in the tunica fibrosa of a Graafian follicle. This mode of origin had been mentioned by Rokitansky, though he did not know upon what evidence. Patenka's corpora fibrosa were, as Mr. Doran had pointed out, merely degenerated corpora lutea and were entirely different in structure from the fibroids.

The President pointed out that these tumors and also sarcomatous and malignant tumors generally differed from fibroids in that the cut surfaces remained flat like a cut raw potato, whereas fibroids always became slightly convex on the cut surfaces immediately on being incised, and this convexity gradually increased in quantity owing to the shrinking of the elastic and muscular fibres.

He considered that it was of great importance to be able to say that a given tumor was a fibroma and innocent, or a sarcoma and malignant, and he hoped the work of Dr. Fairbairn would assist in this direction. He mentioned a case he had shown himself, where equally competent observers had expressed diametrically opposite opinions regarding the microscopic sections.

So far as he had gathered, the chief distinction seemed to be that in fibromata the blood vessels were much more clearly defined, but he wished to know if this could be relied upon in deciding.

DR. RALPH VINCENT made a communication on

LYMPHANGITIS MAMMÆ,

an affection of the breast arising about the tenth day of the puerperium, with well-marked clinical features. He brought forward the notes and temperature charts of six cases illustrating this condition. These cases showed the following clinical signs: There is a wedge-shaped area of inflammation, the apex being at the nipple, the base being at some part of the junction of the breast with the chest wall. This wedge-shaped area is red, slightly edematous, hot to the touch, tender and indurated, the induration being distinctly outlined and definitely corresponding with the redness. The inflamed area is raised above the general breast surface, but the inflammation is confined to the superficial structures and does not involve the mammary gland. During the development of this condition the temperature rapidly rises, the patient complains of pain in the breast and of headache, whilst constipation is frequently present. The treatment required was simple: the infant was taken from the breast, hot fomentations were applied to the inflamed part, and the patient was freely purged. Within about forty-eight hours the affection disappears. He attributed the condition to an infection conveyed to the nipple from the lochia serosa.

DR. AMAND ROUTH asked if the author was sure that some of his cases were not small mammary abscesses which had opened suddenly into one of the larger milk ducts, thus accounting for the sudden cessation of all the symptoms.

Specimens of fibroma and myoma of the ovary were shown by MR. ALBAN DORAN, MR. STANLEY BOYD, and MRS. STANLEY BOYD. DR. VICTOR BONNEY showed a specimen of very early twin pregnancy, with fetuses of different dates, also a specimen of early pregnancy. DR. TATE showed a sarcoma of the uterus complicated by glycosuria and removed by vagino-abdominal hysterectomy.

Meeting of June 4, 1902.

The President, PETER HORROCKS, M.D., *in the Chair.*

MR. ALBAN DORAN read a paper on

PREGNANCY AFTER REMOVAL OF BOTH OVARIES FOR CYSTIC TUMOR.

A woman aged 25, after bearing one child, underwent ovariotomy for a multilocular adenomatous cystic tumor of the left ovary. She then bore four more children, and afterward, when 39 years of age, came under the author's care, and he removed a similar tumor of the right ovary. The base required enuclea- tion. part of the capsule was ligated like a pedicle with silk and the greater portion cut away, but in that part no trace of the Fallopian tube could be detected. A small tubercle on the left of the uterus was the sole remnant of the left appendages. After convalescence the period recurred, and continued till the patient became pregnant and bore a child at term two years after the operation. The period then returned, and ceased ab- ruptly when the patient was 45. The consequent menopause symptoms were distinct. though mild.

The author briefly reviewed a few cases, already reported. where pregnancy ensued after the removal of both ovaries for tumor or chronic inflammatory disease.

1. Schatz. Both ovaries removed for cystic tumor; one tube and a piece of ovarian tissue were purposely left behind. Five years later the patient gave birth to a child at term.

2. Stansbury Sutton (Pittsburg, Pa., U. S.). Both ovaries removed for cystic disease: right pedicle severed by cautery. left by scissors. Patient twice pregnant afterward.

3. Gordon (Portland, Me., U. S.). Removed both tubes and ovaries for inflammatory disease; patient delivered of a child two years later. Other reported cases were doubtful.

The presence of ovarian tissue was essential in these cases. In the author's case it was probably a detached area lying in the right ovarian ligament; the cyst itself was certainly enucleated entire. The author suspected that the Fallopian tube escaped ligature and removal altogether, the base of the tumor being enucleated from the posterior layer of the broad ligament. The condition after operation would then be as in Schatz's case, the tube remaining entire. It was not absolutely certain, however, that the tube was not included in the ligature and in part re- moved. This occurred in Stansbury Sutton's and Gordon's cases, and reference was made to a case where pregnancy oc- curred after Cesarean section and ligature of both tubes with silkworm gut for "sterilization" (Galabin-Horrocks). The ligature might either loosen or perhaps ulcerate through the tube. which manages to heal behind it without stricture of its canal. The tube might then resume its functions, even if re- duced to a stump.

MR. BLAND-SUTTON observed that Mr. Doran's interesting communication really raised two important questions for con- sideration, namely, the occurrence of pregnancy after double ovariotomy and the effect of a ligature on the continuity of the lumen of a Fallopian tube. Probably no one in England had studied so closely the "fate of the ligature" after successful ovariotomy as Mr. Doran. and he certainly was the first to study the changes which took place in the stump of the pedicle after intraperitoneal ligature.

It was now quite certain that when a Fallopian tube was ligatured in continuity it did not necessarily permanently obliterate the tubal lumen. In his Cesarean section for pelvic contraction, Mr. Bland-Sutton in 1891 tied the Fallopian tubes with thin silk within an inch of the uterus; this patient had remained sterile. On a subsequent occasion, where it was deemed prudent to induce labor for uncontrollable vomiting and epileptic seizures, an attempt was made to sterilize the patient by drawing out each tube and transfixing the mesosalpinx with a needle armed with thin silk and then tightly tying the tube near its middle. This failed, for the patient quickly conceived again and had reconceived many times, though her constitutional condition had never allowed a pregnancy to go to term. Since this experience Mr. Bland-Sutton had always tied the tubes in two places and exsected a piece of the tube when it was desirable to sterilize a patient.

Doran's suggestion that "the ligature may perhaps ulcerate through the tube, which then healed behind it without stricture of its canal" was probably true, and the following case in a measure supported it:

In 1898 Mr. Bland-Sutton removed an ovarian cyst; its very slender pedicle was tied with thin silk. Although recovery was uneventful, the patient complained during many weeks of cramp-like pain on the side from which the cyst had been removed. The pains gradually passed away, and ten months later, during menstruation, the patient accidentally noticed on her napkin a tiny loop of silk, which she saved. This was the loop of silk used to secure the Fallopian tube; it had ulcerated into the tube and had been very slowly conducted into the uterus and so escaped. A silk ligature applied to the cut end of a ureter in the course of a nephrectomy is sometimes conveyed to the bladder in the same manner. Mr. Bland-Sutton was glad to have the opportunity of stating that the opinion he expressed to the Society in 1892 had not been borne out by subsequent experience, and it is now abundantly clear to all that the mere application of a silk ligature to the Fallopian tubes could not be depended upon to permanently obliterate their lumina and thus prove an obstacle to pregnancy.

Dr. Galabin said that he had met with two cases in which the attempt to sterilize by tying the Fallopian tubes had failed, and which were those referred to by the author. In that in which Dr. John Shaw had tied the Fallopian tubes with silkworm gut in performing Cesarean section, it was certain that the ovum had passed by the tube on which the ligature appeared to remain *in situ;* for on the side on which the ligature had cut through and the tube was divided the divided ends were absolutely closed. In the second case he had himself, in performing Cesarean section, tied the tubes with kangaroo tendon, and the patient

8

became pregnant again within a year or so. Taught by the experience of these cases, he had since then adopted the plan of cutting a piece out of the tubes between two ligatures, then pulling out the stump on each side as far as possible and cutting it off, so that the open lumen was left at the bottom of an inverted cone of cellular tissue. None of the patients so treated had become pregnant again, and he was inclined so far to regard this as a reliable method.

Mr. BUTLER SMYTHE asked Dr. Herbert Spencer if he could give any information relative to the pregnancies of Mr. Bland-Sutton's patient. She had attended the Samaritan Hospital and stated that subsequent to the operation she had twice miscarried with twins, which rather surprised her, inasmuch as all her previous pregnancies had been single. He also wished to know if the fits had been benefited by the operation.

THE PRESIDENT had expected to hear a hot discussion on how pregnancy could have taken place when both ovaries had been removed. But Mr. Doran had frankly admitted that a piece of ovarian tissue had been left behind at the second operation, so that there was nothing strange about the case. He was surprised to hear Mr. Doran advocate the removal of both ovaries entire when it was possible to leave a healthy piece. He thought it better to leave some ovary whenever possible.

DR. AMAND ROUTH thought that sufficient cases could now be collected to explain the occasional occurrence of menstruation and ovulation after double ovariotomy, and he observed that in most of the reported cases a latent period of a few months, or even years, elapsed before menstruation again appeared. He thought it likely that a small piece of the hilum of one ovary might be left, containing no Graafian follicles sufficiently developed to immediately come to maturity. He believed that such a piece of ovarian stroma, together with the follicles, became in a few months further developed, and ovulation and menstruation then recurred.

DR. BOXALL remarked on the impossibility of making absolutely sure that sterility will necessarily result from ligature of the Fallopian tubes. The importance of the question often arises when operation is undertaken and the tubes are at the same time ligatured with the object of rendering the woman sterile; but may also arise when, from disease of the appendages, operation is indicated. For instance, he has recently met with a case in which, owing to long-continued and recurrent attacks of inflammation, it became necessary to urge surgical interference with the appendages. To this procedure objection was raised both by the patient and by her husband solely on the ground that complete removal of the appendages would entail sterility. In that event cohabitation would be forbidden by their church. Eventually the symptoms became so urgent that operation was rendered imperative. Fortunately it was found possible to retain a healthy part of one ovary, in consequence of which the menses have not been discontinued.   And, notwithstanding that the greater part of both tubes, as well as one ovary and part of the other, was of necessity removed, no occasion arose for the separation which they both so much dreaded, for it was possible to assure them that impregnation was not, by the operation at any rate, put beyond the bounds of possibility.

Mr. ALBAN DORAN, in replying, said that he was much interested in the discussion on attempts to sterilize a patient by tying or cutting the Fallopian tubes.   He believed that in his own case a trace of healthy (not cystic) ovarian tissue was left in the right ovarian ligament.   It was easy to extirpate all ovarian tissue when the ovaries were taken away with the uterus, and not difficult when a pedunculated ovarian cyst was removed, as the ovarian ligament was elongated and very prominent.   But when the base of the cyst burrowed and lay close against the uterus, the ovarian ligament could rarely be distinguished.

In one case where Mr. Doran was obliged to remove the uterus with the burrowing adherent tumor, he found on examining the specimen that it would have been practically impossible to leave the round ligament or part of a pedicle without leaving also ovarian tissue, morbid or healthy.   As it was with a cystic tumor, so it was with inflamed adherent appendages, and so it very often was with an ovary removed to check the growth of a uterine fibroid.

In all these cases the operator dared not cut the pedicle sufficiently short to remove all ovarian tissue, for he knew that if he did so the ligature would probably slip.   Hence it was not very hard to understand that in some cases menstruation, or even pregnancy, occurred after removal of both ovaries.   In his own case the ovarian ligament with some healthy tissue had probably been flattened against the uterus and had thus escaped the ligature.   After-histories of all abdominal operations were valuable, especially as to the fate of ligatures which were shed sometimes eight or ten years after they had been applied.

Mr. MAYO ROBSON contributed a short communication on a case of

PRIMARY OVARIAN GESTATION.

He pointed out that though he had operated on about fifty cases of extrauterine gestation, the present specimen was the only one of the series in which he had been able to prove primary ovarian gestation.

Doubtless many of the cases described previously as ovarian pregnancy had been of that nature, but this was apparently only the fourth case in which absolute proof had been furnished by showing an early embryo in its membranes and contained in a sac in the ovary.

Martha C., aged 24, was admitted to the Leeds General Infirmary on April 11, 1902, in a state of profound collapse.

History.—She stated that on the previous night, six weeks after her last menstrual period and a fortnight after missing her menses. she was seized with a sudden pain in the right side while engaged in blackleading a grate. She became very faint and pallid and soon vomited. She was put to bed, but the pain continued during the night and was much worse next morning. The pallor also increased. She was seen by her doctor (Dr. H. Towers), who diagnosed extrauterine gestation and advised her removal to the Infirmary. She said she was a married woman. but had never had any children. and her husband had been abroad for some months. On admission the patient was very pale indeed. Temperature 98°, pulse 130, respirations 48.

She complained of pain on the right of the abdomen, which was distended and did not move on respiration. It was very tense and tender. rendering palpation difficult, but a fluid thrill could be obtained on flicking with the finger. No tumor could be felt. Examined per vaginam, the uterus was found to be fixed and Douglas' pouch was prominent. There was no history of bloody discharge from the vagina. A diagnosis of ruptured extrauterine gestation was confirmed and immediate operation advised.

The patient was wrapped in warm blankets and taken to the theatre. where she was put on a heated operating table and anesthetized with ether. The skin of the abdomen was then quickly washed and purified and a vertical incision made above the pubes. When the peritoneum was opened there was a sudden gush of blood and clot. The right appendage was at once seized and clamped as bleeding was going on. but before it could be brought to the surface it was necessary to detach the Fallopian tube, which was firmly adherent to the bottom of Douglas' pouch, the ovary projecting above the tube. to which it was not adherent in any way. On the top of the ovary there was a firm mass surrounded by clot, and on lifting this from the ovary a cavity was found in the ovary itself into which the small ovum would easily fit. The left ovary and tube were examined and found to be healthy. The mesometrium was then transfixed and the tube and ovary removed after ligature.

For the following description of the specimen, which is in the Royal College of Surgeons' Museum, thanks were due to Mr. S. G. Shattock: "The parts removed are those of an ovarian pregnancy. They comprise the fimbriated end of the right Fallopian tube. the ovary and the ovum partly surrounded by and embedded in recent blood clot. Connected with the fimbriated extremity of the tube are two small pedunculated cysts, the larger about half an inch in diameter. The ostium is crossed by a thin membranous band of adhesion, beneath which a black bristle has been passed. The tube was firmly adherent to the bottom of Douglas' pouch and quite free of the ovary, the highest part of which projected above its level. At the inner pole of the ovary is a partly collapsed cavity about three-quarters of an inch in diameter. This cavity is widely open through a sharply defined semicircular rent of recent origin; in the thin summit of the lid-like portion there is a second narrow, less regular slit half an inch in length. Over the cavity in the ovary lay the lens-like recent clot, which is mounted separately in the preparation. The clot is about an inch and a quarter in diameter and of concavo-convex form; in its concavity, partly embedded in it and partly free, there lies a villous chorional sac. The sac has been opened in the right half of the clot and the membranes everted; connected with the everted membranes there is displayed a minute embryo about four millimetres in length.''

From the position of the right tube, the fimbriated extremity of which was firmly fixed to the bottom of the pouch of Douglas, leaving the ovary free above it, it seemed probable that the spermatozoa must have reached the right ovary through the healthy left tube.

DR. ARNOLD W. W. LEA showed a rare type of malignant ovarian tumor, and DR. LOCKYER brought forward a uterus which showed rapidly growing epithelioma of the cervix. Specimens of extrauterine gestation were shown by the PRESIDENT and DR. WILLIAMSON.

DR. LEWERS demonstrated some sections of cancer of the cervix in which from four to fifteen years had elapsed without recurrence.

REVIEWS.

MANUAL OF ANTENATAL PATHOLOGY AND HYGIENE: THE FETUS. By J. W. BALLANTYNE, M.D., F.R.C.P.E., F.R.S. Edin., Lecturer on Midwifery and Gynecology, Medical College for Women, Edinburgh; Lecturer on Antenatal Pathology and Teratology in the University of Edinburgh; Examiner in Midwifery in the University of Edinburgh; Assistant Physician, Royal Maternity Hospital, Edinburgh; Honorary Fellow of the Glasgow Obstetrical and Gynecological Society and of the American Association of Obstetricians and Gynecologists. Pp. 526. With 14 colored plates and 55 figures in the text. Edinburgh: William Green & Sons, 1902.

Dr. Ballantyne's numerous contributions to antenatal pathology have made him so well known that no introduction is necessary to those in the medical profession who have kept at all in touch with the recent developments of a subject destined to be of tremendous importance for the future of the individual and the race. Antenatal pathology is preventive medicine in its most hopeful aspect, yet it is practically unexplored. A chart showing our present knowledge might be compared with a map of our own country of a century and a half ago. The coast lines and the adjacent lands are shown with an approach to correctness, a few prominent features of the interior are marked out along the easier lines of exploration, but most of its vast expanse is marked arid desert. As, in the history of our own country, the march of events has continually narrowed this desert area, so will the research of the future reveal to the antenatal pathologist fertile valleys and teeming mines of knowledge where now we can imagine only barrenness.

Dr. Ballantyne is one of the most persistent and successful explorers in the antenatal field, and the present volume gives the results of his labors along the lines of Fetal Physiology and Pathology. A succeeding volume will treat of Teratology and Morbid Heredity.

After defining his subject and indicating its various subdivisions, the author discusses in the first three chapters the relation of antenatal pathology to other branches of study, devoting considerable space to the antenatal factor in gynecology. The fourth chapter takes up the physiology of antenatal and neonatal life, including the physiological and anatomical readjustments at birth and their influence upon the character of the maladies of the new-born infant. Types of these maladies are described illustrating the intrusion of the antenatal factor. All of this may be considered in the nature of an introduction to the subject of antenatal pathology itself, which, with a wonderful variety of phenomena, fills the balance of the volume. The chapters include the Anatomy, the physiology, the pathology of the fetus; Transmitted fetal diseases; Ill-defined morbid states of the fetus; Idiopathic diseases of the fetus; Traumatic morbid states of the fetus; Intrauterine death of the fetus; Diagnosis of fetal morbid states; Therapeutics of fetal diseases; Hygiene and Therapeutics of fetal life.

The work evidently represents years of research. In many particulars it is a most original book. There is much of practical value, much to stimulate thought, and much toward the solution of the riddle of antenatal death, disease, and deformity. It presents a subject upon which we all need instruction, and presents it in a way to merit the appreciation of our profession.

B. H. W.

PROGRESSIVE MEDICINE. A Quarterly Digest of Advances, Discoveries, and Improvements in the Medical and Surgical Sciences. Edited by HOBART AMORY HARE, M.D., assisted by H. R. M. LANDIS, M.D. Vol. I., March, 1902, pp. 462. Vol. II., June, 1902, pp. 442. Philadelphia and New York: Lea Brothers & Co., 1902.

In Volume I. the surgery of the head, neck, and chest is under the charge of Charles H. Frazier, whose abstracts include one of a paper by Koplik on aspiration by lumbar puncture in five cases of cerebro-spinal meningitis with symptomatic relief; an interesting discussion of the surgery of the trigeminal nerve; the relation of the parathyroids to goitre; advances in cardiac surgery; a discussion of decortication of the pleura and other operations upon the lung. Under infectious diseases, by Frederick A. Packard, are a number of articles worthy of perusal, chiefly prophylactic measures in typhoid, papers on bubonic plague, diphtheria, malaria, yellow fever, and dysentery. Floyd M. Crandall has devoted some space to the subject of the new-born infant, but infant-feeding naturally occupies the leading place among single subjects. These, with the consideration of individual diseases of children, fill 56 pages. L. Hektoen has undertaken in pathology a very extensive task. The most recent work, that on the formation of antibodies, is of course the most striking feature, while a number of papers on tumors are abstracted. Laryngology and rhinology complete the subjects in this volume.

Volume II. is of especial interest as containing the sections on abdominal surgery and gynecology, which together occupy 238 pages. Detailed discussion of such extensive contributions is impossible. William B. Coley again furnishes the chapter on abdominal surgery, and John G. Clark that on gynecology. Alfred Stengel has a broad field in diseases of the blood, chiefly in connection with serum pathology, blood plaques, and granular degeneration of erythrocytes. Ophthalmology is included in this volume.

THE PRACTITIONER'S MANUAL. A Condensed System of General Medical Diagnosis and Treatment. By CHARLES WARRENNE ALLEN, M.D., Consulting Genito-Urinary Surgeon to the City Hospital; Consulting Dermatologist to the Randall's Island Hospital; Professor of Dermatology at the New York Post-Graduate School, etc. Second Edition, revised and enlarged. Pp. 888. New York: William Wood & Co., 1902.

This, as its name indicates, is a book constructed on a plan of selective condensation from many authors, and affords a quick method of securing the views of the leaders in medical thought. Diseases are arranged alphabetically, and under each heading are discussed briefly diagnosis, differentiation, prognosis, and treatment. Many prescriptions and methods are given, each credited to its own author. The necessity for the early appearance of a second edition is evidence of the favor with which the work has been accepted.

DISEASES OF WOMEN. A Manual of Gynecology Designed Especially for the Use of Students and General Practitioners. By F. H. DAVENPORT, A.B., M.D., Assistant Professor in Gynecology, Harvard Medical School. Fourth Edition, revised and enlarged. Pp. 400. With 154 illustrations. Philadelphia and New York: Lea Brothers & Co., 1902.

This little work holds almost the same place in gynecology that King's "Manual" does in obstetrics. It is brief, clear, and practical, and intended as a help to the general practitioner in treating his every-day gynecological cases.

SYPHILIS. A Symposium. Pp. 122. New York: E. B. Treat & Co., 1902.

This little book is a reprint of a series of articles upon the

subject of syphilis written for the *International Medical Magazine*. In general the articles are brief, though the power of concentration of the various writers is well shown in a series of
answers to a set of questions, the answers of some requiring only
half a page while others consume as much as seven.

MANUAL OF CHILDBED NURSING, with Notes on Infant Feeding.
By CHARLES JEWETT, A.M., M.D.. Sc.D., Professor of Ob-
stetrics and Diseases of Women in the Long Island College
Hospital. Pp. 84. Fifth Edition, revised and enlarged. New
York: E. B. Treat & Co., 1902.

Primarily written for the nurses of the Training School at the
Long Island College Hospital, the object is to furnish an aid in
remembering the important practical teachings of the hospital
training. The present edition has been rewritten and adapted
for general use by nurses and mothers.

THE INTERNATIONAL MEDICAL ANNUAL. A Year Book of Treatment and Practitioner's Index. Pp. 688, 1902. New York:
E. B. Treat & Co.

This medical annual appears for the twentieth time in its customary dress and arrangement. The subject matter is divided
into two parts, the first on therapeutics, the second on medicine
and surgery. In the latter abstracts of articles upon subjects in
all branches are placed together in alphabetical order. Among
the American contributors are Drs. Abbe, Chapin, Hammond,
Loomis. and Schley, of this city.

TRANSACTIONS OF THE SOUTHERN SURGICAL AND GYNECOLOGICAL
ASSOCIATION. Vol. XIV. Pp. 430. Published by the Association, 1902.

This handsome volume contains the forty papers and the discussions that were brought to the attention of the Association at
its fourteenth annual meeting, held at Richmond, Va., on November 12, 13, and 14, 1901. They cover a wide field, ranging from
the treatment of painful menstruation, the prevention of perineal laceration, and puerperal sepsis. to operations for penetrating wounds of the abdomen, prostatic hypertrophy, Pott's disease. and hepatic drainage. Some of the gynecological papers
have appeared in the pages of this JOURNAL and show the standard reached by the Association. '

BRIEF OF CURRENT LITERATURE.

OBSTETRICS.

Cicatricial Atresia of the Vagina Necessitating Cesarean
Section.—The patient of E. Lévêque *(Ann. de Gyn. et d'Obst..*
Jan.) was first seen at the fifth month of pregnancy, suffering
from severe burns of the vagina. vulva, perineum, anus. and ad-

jacent regions, the result of a douche of sulphuric acid. After separation of large sloughs, cicatricial contraction occurred to such an extent as nearly to occlude the vagina. The pregnancy was allowed to continue, with the intention of operating just before term. Labor commenced unexpectedly and Lévêque performed Cesarean section, followed by complete removal of the uterus and appendages, as the vaginal atresia was so complete as to have prevented the discharge of the lochia had the uterus been preserved. Both mother and child were saved.

Laparatomy during Pregnancy.—Doléris *(Comptes-rendus de la Soc. d'Obst., de Gyn. et de Ped. de Paris,* Dec.) adds another case to the list of operations during pregnancy. His laparatomy was performed for adherent retroversion at two and one-half months. After breaking up adhesions the uterus was drawn forward and the round ligaments shortened intra-abdominally. Delivery occurred at term. Twelve days later the uterus was found in good position, but rather low in the pelvic cavity.

Pustular Dermatitis Transmitted to Fetus.—Immediately after birth Lop *(Bull. de la Soc. d'Obst. de Paris,* Feb. 20) observed a pustular dermatitis upon the child. The mother had had a similar eruption fifteen days before labor. Staphylococci were found in the pus and blood of both mother and child. Lop concludes from this that the infection occurred in utero through the maternal blood, not from examinations by septic hands. The child died as a result of the infection on the seventh day.

Prophylaxis of Ophthalmia Neonatorum.—It having been suggested that potassium permanganate was a specific for ophthalmia neonatorum and that its use by all midwives should be made compulsory in France, a report was requested from the Committee on Hygiene of the Academy of Medicine of Paris. This was furnished by A. Pinard *(Ann. de Gyn. et d'Obst.,* Jan.), who quotes the statistics of several writers as showing that, although the gonococcus is the usual exciting cause, purulent ophthalmia of the new-born may be due to the pneumococcus, Weeks' bacillus, bacillus coli, streptococcus, staphylococcus, and other organisms. He shows that the infection usually takes place while the eyes are in or emerging from the genital canal—a primary ophthalmia; or subsequently from contact with infected persons and objects—a secondary ophthalmia. The report contains the statistics of the Baudelocque clinic in regard to the use of 1 :1000 solution of potassium permanganate as a prophylactic. From November 10, 1900, to June 25, 1901, the eyes of all children were washed immediately after birth with soap and water, then with this solution. Among 1,316 children there were 23 cases of ophthalmia, 1.4 per cent; 7 of these occurred within four days after birth, 16 at a later period. These figures, with others, are offered as demonstrating that potassium permanganate is not an infallible prophylactic; and that all statistics show that, in spite of any agents employed and any technique, some cases of ophthalmia will occur. The importance of preliminary disin--

fection of the maternal canal, and of early application to the child's eyes of whatever prophylactic measures are used, is strongly emphasized.

Hysterical Contraction of the Uterus during Pregnancy.— In the case reported by Guillermin *(Bull. de la Soc. d'Obst. de Paris,* No. 8, 1901) severe uterine contractions began at the fourth month, after a fright. They continued at intervals during the next month, in spite of treatment, yet without affecting mother, child, or cervix. Stigmata of hysteria were then found, hypnotism tried, and the contractions ceased after suggestion.

Large Placenta.—Perret *(Bull. de la Soc. d'Obst. de Paris,* No. 8) describes a placenta 64 centimetres in circumference, 6 in thickness, and weighing 1,850 grammes. Examination showed that it was hypertrophied and macerated, but no vascular lesions suggestive of syphilis were found.

Diabetes Mellitus and Dystocia.—The occurrence of dystocia due to unusual size of the fetus in two cases, coincident with diabetes mellitus of the mother, suggests to Chambrelent *(Bull. de la Soc. d'Obst. de Paris,* No. 9) that there is some causal relation between this disease and the increased fetal development. In each of his cases the fetus weighed nearly $5\frac{1}{3}$ kilogrammes.

Cesarean Section.—The method of Fritsch of performing Cesarean section with a transverse incision of the fundus is approved by D. Jurowski *(Cent. f. Gyn.,* No. 5), who reports three cases operated upon in this way with favorable results.

Acetonuria in Pregnancy, Labor, and the Puerperium.— Stolz *(Arch. f. Gyn.,* Bd. lxv., H. 3) has studied 97 cases—32 of these during pregnancy, 71 at the time of labor, and 64 during the puerperium—in regard to the excretion of acetone in the urine. He finds that during pregnancy the physiological acetonuria is changeable and increased. It is usually increased during labor, being more constant and more marked the longer the duration of this event, and particularly in I- and IIparæ. During the first three days of the puerperium there is increased acetonuria. This is not a reliable sign of fetal death, but rather a physiological occurrence.

Permanent Results of Conservative Treatment of Interrupted Extrauterine Pregnancy.—Von Scanzoni *(Arch. f. Gyn.,* Bd. lxv., H. 3) finds, by reviewing the cases at the Leipzig clinic. that very favorable results follow the conservative treatment of interrupted extrauterine pregnancies of not more than a few months' duration. Those so treated were discharged fourteen days sooner than the cases submitted to laparatomy. The expectant treatment showed an ability to return at once to housekeeping in 25 per cent, while only 16 per cent of those treated by the vaginal and 3 per cent of those by the abdominal route could do so. Ability to do heavy work within six weeks after leaving the clinic were seen in these three classes in 40, 22.5, and 14.5 per cent, respectively. Subsequent capacity for conception was greatest in the cases treated conservatively. Laparatomy is indicated only for signs of persistent internal hemorrhage and increase in size of the hematocele.

Partial Edemas in Puerperal Infections.—This is the term applied by P. Budin *(Bull. de la Soc. d'Obst. de Paris,* Jan. 16) to a localized edema occurring some time after the onset of a severe puerperal infection and ascribed by him to the presence of toxins. In a case described in his paper delivery had taken place on November 16. On the 20th there were constitutional and local signs of uterine and vaginal infection. The uterus was digitally curetted and swabbed out. False membranes appeared on the cervix and vaginal walls. All local lesions disappeared under treatment by the 30th, but slight fever was still present. On December 7 there was slight edema of the right foot, and on the 8th pain in the upper part of the right thigh, more marked upon pressure than motion. The neighboring portion of the abdomen was edematous, and there was a tender point over the femoral vein in Scarpa's triangle. On the 9th the edema had extended downward to the malleoli and dorsum of the foot. The leg was put at rest, as phlegmasia alba dolens was suspected, but on the next day the edema had entirely disappeared at the lower third of the thigh and upper third of the leg, and had increased in its lower portion and foot. Four days later the foot alone remained swollen and the left foot was similarly involved, and for four days more both were swollen, white, and painless. On the 18th the left foot showed improvement and in a few days both were normal. Several similar cases are mentioned by Budin as showing that the presence of a purulent collection must not be inferred from the occurrence of such localized edema in cases of puerperal infection. In the discussion, Boissard thinks it more likely that such an edema is more probably the result of thrombosis of limited extent in small vessels, due to toxins or bacteria in the circulation. The involvement of the second foot, as in the case reported, is seen in cases of phlegmasia and suggests a feeble, limited, and temporary affection of this kind. Maygrier recalls a case of such edema after puerperal infection, and Bar agrees with Budin that the lesion is probably caused by toxins. These cases are of interest from the points of diagnosis from septic processes resulting in pus formation and the consequently different prognosis.

Treatment of Rupture of the Uterus.—On the basis of the literature and personal statistics of 77 cases, C. Cristeanu and Draghiesco *(Ann. de Gyn. et d'Obst.,* Feb.) advocate for complete rupture total abdominal hysterectomy, with vaginal drainage after irrigation, and sponging the peritoneum as in other cases of peritoneal infection. Such infection is so common in these cases that they assume it to be the rule. For incomplete ruptures they favor extraction of the child by the natural route, without any other manipulations than the application of forceps, followed immediately by laparatomy and total hysterectomy. If the child has penetrated the tear in the uterine wall and lies in a

peritoneal pouch, they make no attempt to deliver by the natural·
route, but extract through the abdomen.   If there are manifest
signs of peritonitis, hysterectomy is followed by the same procedures as in cases of complete rupture.   Usually, however, they
do not irrigate, and close the peritoneal cavity with catgut without drainage.

A. Brindeau *(Bull. de la Soc. d'Obst. de Paris,* Jan. 16) advocates in case of uterine rupture with severe hemorrhage, laparatomy, whether the rupture is complete or incomplete.   If incomplete, he would incise the peritoneum over the tear, so as to
permit removal of clots, and then treat the case as one of complete rupture.   In the latter case the wound may be sutured if
the tear is complete but the woman not infected.   If the mother
is infected or the fetus in the abdominal cavity, supravaginal
hysterectomy is indicated, with abdomino-vaginal drainage if
labor has been prolonged or liquor amnii or meconium has entered
the peritoneal cavity.

Retained Placenta.—L. Tissier *(Bull. de la Soc. d'Obst. de
Paris,* Feb. 20) records the expression of a placenta, showing no
signs of putrefaction, sixty-nine days after labor.   There had
been only very slight losses of blood until the sixty-eighth day,
when a severe hemorrhage occurred.   This was attributed by
Tissier to separation of the placenta.

A. Brindeau *(Bull. de la Soc. d'Obst. de Paris,* Jan. 16) reports
two cases which illustrate the difficulty which is occasionally experienced in recognizing this condition.   In each case the fetus
had been expelled and the uterus, which was supposed still to
contain the placenta, seemed upon examination to be entirely
empty.   Careful exploration showed that in the first instance the
placenta was completely adherent and, after contraction of the
uterus, seemed to line it entirely, except near the internal os,
where the free border of the membranes could be felt and separated.   In the second case careful search showed a pouch on the
anterior wall which contained the whole adherent placenta.   The
pouch was due to local inertia, for as soon as the placenta was
extracted this depression disappeared, leaving the interior uterine
surface perfectly smooth.

Symphyseotomy for Persistent Brow Presentations.—Wal-
lich *(Comptes-rendus de la Soc. d'Obst., de Gyn. et de Péd. de
Paris,* Jan.) discusses the value of symphyseotomy in the treatment of brow presentations, upon the basis of 7 cases so managed
and 12 in which the operation was not performed.   All were persistent brow presentations and all in Pinard's service.   All
temporary brow presentations are omitted as tending to destroy
the value of the statistics.   Of the 12 cases not treated by
symphyseotomy the maternal mortality was 16 per cent, the fetal
58 per cent.   The 7 cases with symphyseotomy gave no maternal
mortality and a fetal of 28.5 per cent.

Ovariotomy during Pregnancy.—The statistics, including 148
cases compiled by Orgler *(Arch. f. Gyn.,* Bd. lxv., H. 1), show a

mortality of 2.7 per cent for ovariotomy during pregnancy. The latter was interrupted by the operation in 22.5 per cent of the cases. The earlier in pregnancy the ovariotomy is performed the less is the probability of abortion.

GYNECOLOGY AND ABDOMINAL SURGERY.

Complete Inversion of the Uterus.—J. A. Amann, Jr. *(Monats. f. Geb. u. Gyn.,* Bd. xv., H. 1) describes an interesting case of complete inversion in a woman 41 years of age, who had had two labors, the last fourteen years before. Eleven years ago menstruation, previously regular, became irregular. There had been dragging-down sensations for years, and one year ago the uterus prolapsed but could be replaced by the patient. After a sudden strain, fourteen days before, the tumor reappeared and increased in size, with symptoms of infection and loss of weight. A long, narrow tumor, continuous above with the everted vaginal wall, presented near its lower end the uterine opening of the left tube, and was here continuous with a large, rounded tumor which was connected above with the everted posterior vaginal wall. The fingers could be passed between the round tumor and its anterior pedicle, the inverted uterus. After removal of the entire protruding mass, the rounded mass proved to be a submucous uterine myoma. This had evidently been protruded through the cervix and had become adherent to the posterior vaginal wall. In falling downward it had inverted the uterus and also dragged the portion of the posterior vaginal wall to which it was adherent downward, forming a posterior pedicle. Death from pyemia.

Prolapse of the Urethra.—A case of prolapse of the urethra in a healthy and well-developed girl of 5½ years is reported by Bente *(Münch. med. Woch.,* No. 53, 1901). The common predisposing factor—general debility and relaxation—certainly could not be invoked to account for the causation of the trouble. It seemed dependent upon constipation causing straining at stool and upon coughing. Medical treatment was unsuccessful and operation was required and gave good results.

Uterine Fibroids.—R. Olshausen *(Cent. f. Gyn.,* No. 1) again advocates enucleation of even multiple myomata when it is possible. During the last two years he has been able to apply this operation in 27 per cent of his 136 cases. In some of these he has removed six, nine, or more tumors with success.

Ventrofixation.—J. C. Cameron and F. A. L. Lockhart *(Jour. of Obst. and Gyn. of the Br. Emp.,* Mar) report six cases of labor following ventrofixation—five of their own cases and one of W. C. Mills. Of these six cases three were instrumental and three were not. In five cases the uterus was found in good position some months after labor, but in one case, that of a single woman, the retroversion returned. In one case the fixation was so strong that it prevented the head being driven into the pelvic cavity. The head was against the symphysis pubis and forceps were applied. The uterus was inclined to the left side and fixed by the adhesions. The good results of these cases he attributes to, first, the care with which the sutures were passed across the anterior surface of the fundus in the middle line; second, to inclusion of the peritoneum only of the anterior wall, and at times the urachus; third, to the stretching of the false ligament. Cases of this variety should be carefully observed for untoward symptoms, so that labor may be produced at the end of eight months in the interest of the child.

Hypertrophy of the Breasts at Puberty.—The literature of this subject is enriched by a case report of E. Pflanz *(Cent. f. Gyn.,* No. 2). The woman's breasts had shown abnormal development even when she was a child. At 14 she began to menstruate and the breasts increased in size with great rapidity, reaching at 16 the size which they retained at the age of 30, when the case was seen. At this time they hung down to the level of the umbilicus and their greatest circumference was respectively forty-eight and forty-seven centimetres. Although married twelve years, she had never been pregnant. Her brother also had greatly-developed breasts.

Results of Operation in Sixty Cases of Malignant Disease of the Breast.—A. Marmaduke Shield *(Lancet,* Mar. 8) comes to the following conclusions from a careful survey of sixty cases of malignant disease of the breast: That the risk of removing cancer of the mammæ by extensive operation is small and should not amount to more than one or two per cent; sepsis is preventable and when it occurs is due to the surgeon. That early and free removal gives prospect of years of freedom, and, in a good percentage of cases, of good health and enjoyment of life. That the cases which do badly are: (1) soft, rapidly-growing cancer in young and vascular women, and (2) cases of long continuance before operation, where skin and cervical glands are widely infected. That in certain cases visceral cancers and cancers in the liver coexist with, or rapidly follow, operation, and the explanation of these is uncertain. That the practice of early exploration by incision of small nodules and indurations in the breast is of the first importance and should be strongly urged upon the profession generally, especially upon those in general practice who so often see these cases in their early beginnings and upon whom the great responsibility of prompt diagnosis falls. No one should undertake an operation for mammary cancer unless he is capable, and has had sufficient operative experience to remove all lymphoid tissue from the axilla; the leaving of infected glands toward the apices of the axillary spaces being a common source of failure in the results of this operation. The prognosis is still dubious, as we sometimes get just the opposite result from that expected. Operate early and extensively.

Ovarian Opotherapy.—Paul Dalché and E. Lépinois *(Bull. gén. de Thérap.,* Jan. 8) have studied six cases treated by ovarian opotherapy, and find that administration of ovarian extract causes polyuria and an increase of phosphoric acid and certain other solids. Under this treatment the ratio of uric acid and of phosphoric acid to urea became approximately normal. In the treatment of chronic rheumatism with deformity, which they attributed to ovarian dystrophy, they obtained diminution of pain, while the joint lesions, though not decreasing in extent, did not become greater. In women who had long passed the menopause ovarian extract was inefficacious. The improvement which occurred in a young man under this treatment suggests that the same alkaloid occurs in both ovary and testicle.

Intestinal Obstruction by Uterine Fibroids.—Operation for intestinal obstruction caused by uterine fibroids is rarely required. G. Chavannaz *(Rev. mens. de Gyn., Obst. et Ped. de Bordeaux,* t. iii., No. 12) has met with two cases in which it was necessary. In one there were symptoms of an acute intestinal obstruction caused by compression of the small intestine by a pedunculated uterine fibroma. Death occurred during the operation from asphyxia due to inhalation of fecal vomitus. In the second case there were symptoms of chronic obstruction, which became so marked as to require operation. The intestinal compression was caused by a fibroid, no larger than an egg, situated upon the posterior surface of the uterus. On account of extreme intestinal distension the formation of an artificial anus was the only procedure adopted. Recovery followed.

Treatment of Sepsis.—J. Wernitz *(Cent. f. Gyn.,* No. 6) warmly recommends the following procedure for the treatment of sepsis: Through a rectal tube a warm one-half to one per cent saline solution is allowed to run gently into the intestine by raising an irrigator in which it is contained. The irrigator is then lowered, allowing the return flow of the fluid. It is then alternately raised and lowered, changing the fluid as it becomes impregnated with fecal material. When the intestine has been cleansed in this way so as to leave its walls free to absorb, the alternate raising and lowering of the irrigator are so timed as to permit more to enter than to flow out. In an hour about one-half to one litre of saline solution will be absorbed, causing marked increase of the quantity of urine, loss of thirst and dryness of mucous membranes, and profuse perspiration. The writer reports a successful illustrative case.

Vesicular Mole with Bilateral Ovarian Cysts.—Few cases of simultaneous occurrence of vesicular mole and bilateral ovarian cysts have been recorded. Baumgart *(Cent. f. Gyn.,* No. 4) describes such a case on account of its possible bearing upon the etiology of moles. He mentions, however, that it is uncertain to what extent the growth is directly attributable to the ovarian disease, and whether it is not the result of endometritis which had arisen from the circulatory disturbances associated with the ovarian lesions.

Pseudo-hermaphroditism.—H. Roger *(Presse Méd.,* Mar. 22) describes the findings at the autopsy of a supposed boy of 19. The external genitals were those of a normal male, except the arrangement of the pubic hair, which was like that of a woman. The penis was well developed, the scrotum normal but containing no testicles. The internal organs were a normal uterus and small vagina, the latter opening at the veru montanum of a urethra of the male type. There was no prostate. The uterine appendages of the right side were present, the ovary being cystic, as was shown by microscopic examination. There were no tube and ovary on the left side and no testicles. The case is remarkable on account of the almost perfect male type of the external organs. while a single ovary was the only genital gland present.

Treatment of Ureteral Lesions during Laparatomies.—Weinreb *(Arch. f. Gyn.,* Bd. lxv., H. 1) records a case in Landau's clinic in which a portion of the right ureter was removed during a radical abdominal operation for carcinoma of the cervix. In this case Landau ligated the proximal end of the divided ureter without unfavorable results. Weinreb considers this and other instances mentioned as showing the advisability of this procedure when so large a portion of the ureter has been removed as to make implantation into the bladder impossible. If a secondary nephrectomy should be required the results would be better than from a primary operation of this character.

Parametritis Posterior.—A. Müller *(Cent. f. Gyn.,* No. 9) considers the affection described by others as parametritis posterior. etc., usually a disease of the rectum with subsequent extension through the utero-sacral ligaments to the uterus. The uterus is seldom involved primarily, except in gonorrheal cases. The trouble usually begins in childhood with abdominal pains, painful defecation, and constipation. Later are added weakness of the back, backache, dysmenorrhea with scanty or profuse flow. The rectal wall becomes the seat of chronic inflammation and thickening, with subsequent contraction, and then accumulation of hard fecal masses above the stenosis. There is often alternating constipation and diarrhea. The chronic inflammatory process may extend from the rectal wall, which becomes bound down by bands, to the adjacent tissues and uterus. The treatment must be primarily that of the rectal condition. laxatives and enemata. The bands binding the rectum to the uterus should be stretched by vaginal massage.

Tuberculosis of Vermiform Appendix and Right Appendages.—Many cases of inflammation of the uterine appendages of the right side and of secondary involvement of the vermiform appendix, or *vice versa*, have been reported. Tuberculosis of the tube may later involve the neighboring peritoneum and appendix. In a case described by Emil Kraus *(Monats. f. Geb. u. Gyn.,* Bd. xv., H. 2) the primary seat of the disease was in the vermiform appendix, with subsequent extension to the uterine appendages.

Uterine Castration.—Under this name L. Pincus *(Cent. f. Gyn.,* No. 8) treats of another use to which he has been able to apply atmocausis. He recommends it for artificial sterilization of incurable invalids in whom the prevention of pregnancy is of great importance. In a case of phthisis in which he employed this method the uterine cavity was completely obliterated above the internal os. In a case of nephritis the upper half of the cavity was entirely destroyed. No accidents attended either case.

Dysmenorrhea.—The cause of dysmenorrhea is the subject of a paper by A. Theilhaber *(Cent. f. Gyn.,* No. 3). Only a small proportion of the cases of menstrual pain owe their trouble to anatomical defects. Submucous fibromyomata may act as foreign bodies and cause severe expulsive pains. With perimetritis the physiological uterine contractions cause pain by traction upon the inflamed peritoneum. About three-fourths of all cases of menstrual pain are of the class of so-called "essential dysmenorrhea," or those not due to anatomical causes. Theilhaber attributes the pain in these cases to tetanic contraction of the circularly placed muscle fibres in the region of the internal os. Menge thinks the pain arises from contraction of the longitudinal layer of the uterus, which is not perceived in healthy women, but is translated into menstrual pain in hysterical or neurasthenic women even when their genitals are normal. In opposition to this view Theilhaber states that contractions of voluntary muscles are not painful in neurotic persons, that contraction of longitudinally placed non-striated muscle is constantly occurring in the viscera without pain.

Effect of Menstruation upon Psychical or Convulsive Disorders.—Viallon *(Ann. de Gyn. et d'Obst.,* Feb.) has studied the effect of menstruation upon a number of inmates of the Bron asylum. His conclusions are that the toxic condition induced by menstruation is caused in some cases by various functional troubles, most commonly gastro-intestinal or urinary disturbances. Under these conditions menstruation may be accompanied by distinct rise of temperature, mental troubles characterized usually by mental confusion, or convulsive seizures in epileptics and general paralytics.

Traumatic Granuloma of the Urinary Bladder.—Without any reference to having made any pathological examination of his cases, G. Kolischer *(Cent. f. Gyn.,* No. 10) describes as a distinct type a group of cases in which, after traumatism, there are desire to urinate, feeling of congestion in the region of the bladder, frequent profuse hemorrhages from the bladder, and the presence of phosphates in granular form in the urine. Cystoscopic examination shows a bright-red mass resembling granulation tissue over a scar, bleeding easily upon contact, not sensitive itself but surrounded by a sensitive area. The treatment is removal of the growth.

Pain is felt in these only when tetanic contraction of circular fibres occurs. If it were the result of simple hyperesthesia of the uterus it would be difficult to explain its disappearance after birth of the first child, as this seldom cures hysteria. The flow

9

of blood from the uterus is so free, except in the small proportion of cases in which it is clotted, that the presence of an obstacle to discharge of the menstrual fluid can hardly be invoked
as the cause of pain. During labor the circular fibres of the
internal os are stretched and torn, and the effect is probably
similar to that in other cases of spasmodic contraction of circularly placed muscle, e.g., vaginismus. The pains associated
with submucous fibroids are like those of labor; those connected
with perimetritis are also intermittent, as they continue only
during the uterine contractions.

Inversion of the Uterus.—Paul Bar (Bull. de la Soc. d'Obst.
de Paris, Jan. 16) calls attention to the sudden collapse which
may occur not only at the time of inversion of the uterus, but
during attempted reduction. He describes two cases of sudden
death at this time. His paper also discusses the subject of what
ligaments limit the prolapse of the inverted uterus. These
seemed to be chiefly the infundibulo-pelvic and to a slight degree
the utero-sacral ligaments and bladder. The paper also discusses the treatment of the condition, from simple reinversion
of the uterus to hysterectomy.

DISEASES OF CHILDREN.

Abnormal Psychical Conditions in Children.—George F.
Still (Lancet, Apr. 12, 1902) thus sums up his study of the
subject: A morbid failure of moral control is not uncommon
in children with general impairment of intellect—there is, in
fact, a congenital limitation of the capacity for the development
of moral control associated with a similar limitation of the general intellectual capacity; that, except in the lower grades of
idiocy and imbecility, where the cognitive relation to environment is absent or extremely defective, there is not necessarily
any direct proportion between the moral limitation and the general intellectual limitation; that no particular type of idiocy
or imbecility can be specially associated with moral defect; nor
is there any evidence, so far as can be judged from a clinical
study of these cases, that any particular gross lesion of the brain
is requisite to the limitation of moral control.

Adenoid Vegetations and their Influence on the Palatal
Arch.—Frederick H. Millener (Phil. Med. Jour., Apr. 12, 1902)
does not wish to make the assertion that the irregular or V-
shaped maxilla is caused entirely by the pressure of these
growths upon the formed or forming superior maxilla. Nor
does he wish to state that the pressure of the muscles of the jaws
causes this deformity. These are plausible hypotheses, but he
does think that all cases of adenoid vegetation can and do cause
a tremendous alteration in the facial expression, such as the
atrophy of the antra of Highmore owing to the closure and disuse of the nasal passages. This, in connection with deficient
oxygenation of the blood and the general sickly condition of the
subject, has a tendency to cause an irregular arch as well as poor

teeth. He thinks that the V-shaped palate and irregular teeth are caused by breathing insufficiently, and under-development caused by non-oxygenation of the blood. Before the teeth of a person from 10 to 18 years of age are regulated, or before we attempt to treat their ears or any ear trouble, we should first ascertain that they are not mouth-breathers and that there are no adenoid vegetations present. If these are found they should be promptly removed. The diagnosis is simple, merely placing the finger in the nasopharynx. Almost anybody with but little experience can diagnose their presence or absence, and even without this the enlarged faucial tonsils and facial expression are sufficient. Of course there are still surgeons living who object to removing adenoids, as there are still some who deprecate the removal of the faucial tonsils, on the ground that children will grow out of them. But it ought to be remembered that even if tonsillar hypertrophies do become reduced with advanced age, the subjects have in the meantime *grown into their symptoms,* and these are found every day in cases of deafness. The wide-awake dentists have an unusual opportunity to detect these symptoms and conditions, and with this opportunity comes a duty to add to their already useful vocation that of aiding parents to see the importance of subjecting their afflicted children to operative interference and freeing them from these conditions with their long train of attendant symptoms and serious results.

Bacterium Coli Commune in Cow's, Goat's, Ass', and Human Milk, On the Vegetation of.—Cozzolino *(Archiv. f. Kinderhk.,* vol. xxxiii., Nos. 3 to 6), finds a marked difference in the growth and increase of the bacterium coli in human milk and in that of the cow, goat, and ass. During the twenty-four hours following its inoculation into human milk the bacterium undergoes an inhibition of growth, and even a decrease in numbers. In the other milks, on the contrary, it increases rapidly. After about forty-eight hours the difference has grown less or has ceased to exist. It would seem that breast milk is not so good a culture medium for this organism from four to forty-eight hours as are the other varieties of milk. This circumstance, together with the much smaller acidifying power of human milk, may explain the diminished frequency and severity of gastro-enteric disturbances in the breast-fed infant as compared with the bottle-fed child. Finally, it must be remembered that in the gastro-intestinal canal the milk comes in contact with the colon bacillus only after the digestive juices have acted upon it.

Cigarette Inebriety.—J. M. French *(Quarterly Jour. of Inebriety,* Jan., 1902) says that it is impossible to study the cigarette habit intelligently without at the same time considering the whole subject of the effects of tobacco upon the human system. Its chief peculiarities, as distinguished from the other forms of the use of tobacco, are three in number: 1. It is indulged in to a very great extent by young and growing boys. 2. The cigarette,

being only "a little cigar" and mild and pleasant in its immediate effects, is in some instances smoked almost constantly.
3. Also because of its mildness, it is the common practice to in-
hale the smoke, thus largely increasing the poisonous effects of
the nicotine, which is the chief deleterious agent in tobacco.
Investigation has shown that there is no truth in the sensa-
tional stories of poisonous ingredients contained in tobacco, nor
in the charges that insanity and crime are caused by their use.
Whatever harm is done by the cigarette is done by the tobacco
which it contains, and not by the rice paper in which it is
wrapped, nor any foreign poison.   As to the effects of the use of
tobacco on immature or growing boys, there is plenty of evidence
of an unimpeachable nature.   It has been found in Yale College,
Amherst, etc., that the non-users of tobacco gain during the college course in weight, height, chest girth, and lung capacity
more than the users of tobacco.   In France, at the Polytechnic
School, the non-smokers took the highest rank in every grade,
and the smokers constantly lost grade.   In an experimental observation of 38 boys, of all classes of society, who had been using
tobacco for periods of from two months to two years, 27 showed
severe injury to the constitution and insufficient growth, and 32
showed irregularity of the heart's action, disordered stomachs,
cough, and a craving for alcohol.   Within six months after they
had abandoned the use of tobacco one-half were free from their
former symptoms, and the remainder recovered by the end of
the year.   Impaired vision, especially color blindness, is a common result of the habitual use of tobacco.   A New York oculist
describes a peculiar disease, the symptoms of which are dimness
and film-like gatherings over the eye, which appear and disappear at intervals.   This is known as the cigarette eye.   The
injurious effects of tobacco on the heart are well known.   Dr.
Cathett declares that inflammatory affections of the nose and
throat are more persistent and recover more slowly in excessive
users of tobacco than in other persons.   He adds that a scratch,
pimple, blister, or wart, or a sore lip, mouth, tongue, or throat,
may be made cancerous by keeping it constantly bathed in
tobacco juice or smoke.   In order to determine, with any claim
to scientific accuracy, the nature and effect of tobacco upon the
human system, it is necessary to observe its action, not only upon
the individual user, but also upon his descendants.   Tested in
this manner, the statement may safely be made that among
those strong and vigorous men who have used tobacco habitually
and constantly for many years without apparent injury, in not
a single instance will their children, especially those born after
the habit had been long indulged in, possess an equal degree of
vigor and endurance; and particularly in not a single instance
can they indulge in the habitual use of tobacco without ex-
periencing those injurious effects which their fathers escaped.
But whatever may be the verdict with reference to the use of
tobacco by healthy adults, there exists no difference of opinion

among physicians or scientific men as to its effects upon young and growing boys. All agree that none of these ought, for the sake of their own development, physical, mental, and moral, to use tobacco in any form. It is its effect upon this class which constitutes the essential reason why the cigarette habit is properly regarded as a menace to civilization.

Congenital Syphilis, Parrot's Pseudo-Paralysis in.—Scherer *(Jahrb. f. Kinderhk.,* vol. lv., No. 5) studied two cases of pseudo-paralysis of the upper extremities in syphilitic infants. At autopsy the bones were found to be intact. He observed the pseudo-paralysis in eleven of fifty cases, or twenty-two per cent. Microscopic examination of the spinal cord showed the blood vessels to be dilated and containing many streptococci: some of the capillaries had real streptococcus emboli. There was no reaction outside the vessels. The cocci were present in all the viscera. It is probable that in those cases of congenital syphilis where the bones and nervous system are intact the pseudo-paralysis is due to toxins, either of the luetic poison or of other bacteria present in the blood. Congenital syphilis predisposes to secondary infections which cause death.

Contribution to the Symptomatology of Cretinism and Other Forms of Idiocy.—Henry Koplik and Jacob Lichtenstein *(Arch. of Ped.,* Feb., 1902) describe an anatomical sign or stigma which they have for some time carefully studied, and which they have observed on certain patients. While demonstrating the peculiarities of the skin and conformation of the hand of cretins, they were struck with a prominence in the region of the antithenar eminence and over the situation of the os pisiformis. It is immediately adjacent to the groove which separates the palm of the hand from the forearm, and, viewed from the side, rises abruptly from the above groove, giving a bayonet-like appearance. It is apparently an over-development or hypertrophy of the small muscles of the inner border of the hand, attached to the os pisiformis, as well as perhaps an enlarged condition of the bone itself. It has been observed in a cretin only three months old, and can therefore not be a hypertrophy due to crawling on the floor and supporting the weight on the inner border of the hands. The infants in which this prominence has been seen are idiots, cretins, microcephalic idiots, and children who are congenitally deficient. It has not as yet been met by the authors in Mongolian idiots. It has been found in all cases of cretinism.

Diphtheria of the Conjunctiva Treated by Antitoxin.—L. Emmett Holt *(Arch. of Ped.,* May, 1902) reports the case of an infant 6 months old suffering from diphtheria of the right eye: 2,400 units of antitoxin were administered. Ice compresses were applied and a solution of atropine dropped into the eye. The progress of the case was rapid and uneventful. In twenty-four hours the temperature had fallen from 102° to 100⅘° and in forty-eight hours to normal. Improvement in the eye began almost immediately, and in twenty-four hours a very decided change was seen. On the third day the swelling had so far diminished that the child could open the eye, and the membrane was almost gone. It did not disappear entirely until the sixth day. Diphtheria bacilli were found by cultures as late as the seventh day, but on the tenth day the eye was entirely well. No more convincing demonstration of the value of antitoxin can be found than in cases like this, which formerly, under any treatment known, almost invariably went on from bad to worse, ending in the destruction of the eye.

Epilepsy, The Use of Dormiol in.—Hoppe *(Münch. med. Wochens.,* vol. xlix., No. 17) employed a mixture composed of equal parts of chloral and amyl hydrate, in eleven cases of status epilepticus in children. The remedy was given per rectum, a solution of 1:15 being administered in doses of two to three tablespoonfuls in one-quarter to one-third of a litre of lukewarm water. It was readily absorbed and caused no local irritation. While the drug is of questionable value in the regular treatment of epilepsy, it is decidedly of service in these cases of status epilepticus and of very frequently repeated convulsions in which rest is needed for a time.

Etiology of Noma.—A. Trambusti *(Il Policlinico,* January, 1902) has isolated a micro-organism in noma which, under suitable conditions of association, is capable of reproducing the disease. He considers it probable that other micro-organisms which have been isolated by other investigators might also be capable of producing the disease, but no one seems to have attempted to do it. It remains to be proved which of the associated microbes (staphylococci, streptococci, protei, etc.) found in the gangrenous mass is of chief importance in association with the micro-organisms found at the margins of the gangrenous area. The author thinks it allowable to conclude that noma is not to be considered as a specific disease, but as a form of gangrene which may be determined by various pathogenic organisms in association with certain microbes found in the cavity of the human organism communicating with the external world.

Frequency and Cause of Death in Sick Infants Treated in Institutions.—Schlossman and Peters *(Archiv. f. Kinderhk.,* vol. xxxiii., Nos. 3-6) give the results obtained during the year from July 1, 1900, to June 30, 1901, in the Children's Polyclinic at Dresden. Of 300 infants under one year of age, 53 died. All the deaths occurred in bottle-fed children, while 93 breast-fed infauts developed no case of serious illness. Twenty-five deaths occurred during the first three days following admission and before the treatment in the institution could prove of service. Eight fatal results were due to diseases which were hopeless from the outset; 20 followed diseases not prognostically hopeless, and were, therefore, not prevented by the treatment. Among the latter were pneumonia, nephritis, general atrophy, and gastro-enteritis. The material treated was of the worst, and the hygienic conditions in the institution not very good. The good results achieved in spite of these drawbacks were largely due to the fact that breast-feeding was extensively used. It must prove to be an indispensable factor in every hospital for infants.

Gangrene of the Lung.—Francis Huber *(Arch. of Ped.,* Mar., 1902) reports three fatal cases seen in the Vanderbilt Clinic. In one, a boy of 7, the physical signs led to the conclusion that both sides were implicated. No autopsy was permitted. In the second, a child of some 3 years of age, seen at irregular intervals, there was a large cavity on the right side, and, though the breath was extremely fetid, the amount of trouble on the other side was considered to be of such a grave nature that operation was not thought advisable. In the third case, a child of 4 years of age, considerable improvement took place under the use of guaiacol and tonics. The family was opposed to operation, and it was learned subsequently that the child had died rather suddenly and unexpectedly. No autopsy. A fourth case terminated more favorably under tonic treatment. Another, a child of 3 years, was operated on with good results.

Walter Lester Carr (ibid.) reports a case in an infant a year old. There was never any fetid odor of the breath nor of the expectoration. The sputa were white or yellowish white, had no green nor brown tinge, and were not streaked with blood. The baby raised more than was usual for one of its age. The character of the temperature curve, and also the general condition, pointed to a septic process, but this could not be definitely determined to be a gangrene in addition to a septic broncho-pneumonia. The case was fatal, and at the autopsy there was found to be pulmonary gangrene.

An editorial (ibid.) says: Gangrene of the lung is met with infrequently, and from the description of Rilliet and Barthez in 1843 to the present there has been no absolute symptom, nor set of symptoms, that discloses the destructive character of the disease or separates its features from many that are common to septic pneumonia, empyema, and bronchiectasis, with any one of which the gangrenous process may be associated. When gangrene of the lung is observed in the course of an epidemic, such as measles, the symptomatology is so complex that the gangrenous invasion of the lung is masked and its course is unlike that which follows the presence of a foreign body in a bronchus. The physical signs are not always distinctive of consolidation, and when a pneumonic area is present a focus of gangrene which has undergone softening will produce sounds similar to those of a tubercular process. Infarcts near the site of destructive necrosis may cause sufficient consolidation to disguise the character of the gangrenous softening. Pneumonia and gangrene are usually associated and the separation of the physical signs due to the latter process is not always easy. As the gangrene is a destruction of lung tissue, some help may be gained by an inspection of the sputa. Thus these are seen as blood-streaked, rusty, greenish, and frothy in children whose ages would indicate that they could not expectorate except by violent effort or after a great accumulation of material in the upper air passages. Unfortunately, however, the expectoration is frequently wanting, as are the gangrenous odor and sweetish breath, which are described as distinctive when detected in older patients. The septic picture is a dark one, and perhaps it is best stated that the constitutional symptoms are out of all proportion to the physical signs. Blood examinations have not been satisfactorily recorded, so that we have nothing to help us differentiate the disease except a high leucocytosis. It is to be supposed that the results of examinations will show blood counts similar to those of gangrene in other parts of the body. The bacteriology is not fully established, but Seitz found that any one of the pyogenic group of bacteria may be present in the gangrenous areas. Where a diagnosis can be made the success of treatment is not in medication, but from surgical interference. Over sixty per cent of a series of cases recorded by Herczel were saved by radical measures.

"Habit Tic" in a Child Two Years and Three Months of Age.—John H. W. Rhein (*Ann. of Gyn. and Ped.*, April, 1902) reports a case in which there was a spasmodic affection of the muscles around the eyes and of the right side of the face. The twitchings recurred frequently, and indeed at first were continuous. The only abnormality that could be found was a redundant foreskin which had a pin-point meatus. There was in the eyes a total refraction error of $+3$ dioptres on each side. Circumcision was performed, and the fluid extract of cimicifuga was ordered in increasing doses until five drops three times a day were given. Five days after the operation the twitching lessened greatly, and in two weeks' time there was scarcely any movement visible. A slight photophobia remains. The writer is not at all sure that the inflamed prepuce was the whole cause of the tic. Many of the cases of this sort arise from some refractive error, and his present opinion is that the primary cause in this case was the ocular defect, which alone was insufficient to cause any symptoms until the further nervous irritation due to the inflamed prepuce and glans penis was added. He has little doubt that the symptoms will return sooner or later, when it will be necessary to resort to some measure to relieve the ocular irritation.

Hysteria in Childhood, A Case of.—Leick (*Deut. med. Wochens.*, vol. xxviii., No. 20) describes the case of a boy 9 years of age, brought for treatment because he had been unable to write for several days. A sudden attack of vomiting had followed the compulsory eating of some soup which he had refused at first. After that he could neither stand nor walk for a day; and on the disappearance of the "paralysis" his handwriting underwent a marked change, in that it was illegible and covered with blots, as though the fingers were unable to hold the pen. As chorea could be excluded, a diagnosis of hysteria was made. Two minutes' application of the faradic current to the hand effected a marked improvement in his writing, and after a second application of the electricity it was as good as ever. Subsequent observation proved the cure to be a permanent one. The boy was over-joyed at his rapid recovery.

Muscle Juice and Raw Meat in the Treatment of the Pulmonary Tuberculosis of Children.—Albert Josias (*Revue d'Hygiène et de Médecine Infantiles*, No. 1, 1902) says that the best way to obtain muscle juice at home is to macerate the meat in about a quarter of its weight of water for three-quarters of an hour, then to place meat and water in a home press and use all the force possible; this will give for 100 grammes of meat about 15 to 20 cubic centimetres of juice slightly diluted by the water which has been added. The fluid obtained is reddish, with but slight taste, and putrefies in a few hours; it must therefore be prepared just before using, and in summer, if one is obliged to wait an hour before serving it, it must be kept on ice. The children treated by the author with this juice have taken it readily, without anything having been added to disguise the taste. The daily dose given to children weighing from 20 to 25 kilos (44 to 55 pounds) was the extract from 500 grammes of raw meat, together with from 100 to 200 grammes of chopped raw meat and the usual food given in hospitals. The results justify the following conclusions: When the lesions present are due to the tubercle bacillus alone, this treatment causes a decided improvement; the weight increases, the general condition improves, and auscultation shows that there is an arrest in the extension of the tuberculous process. Time only will show whether this amelioration is lasting. But when the tuberculous lesion is invaded by all the microbes which vegetate in the softening lungs and in the cavities, when the organism is profoundly affected by the poisons circulating in the blood, the treatment cures exceptionally, ameliorates sometimes, but most often has no appreciable action on the disease. Raw meat and muscle juice do not appear to have any direct action on the microbes or on their poisons, but act by increasing the resistant powers of the organism.

Operative Treatment of Chronic Bright's Disease.—A. Primrose (*Can. Jour. of Med. and Surg.*, March, 1902) reports the case of a boy of 10 years apparently cured of Bright's disease by stripping the capsule of the kidney. This truly is a remarkable and satisfactory result, but the explanation thereof is still quite obscure. The treatment has thus far been purely empirical. The fact that stripping the capsule of the kidney relieves the condition of albuminuria was stumbled upon accidentally, and it has gradually dawned upon us that we may possibly possess an effective method of treating chronic and acute nephritis. Nothing we know of the physiology and pathology of renal secretion will adequately explain the results obtained in this operation. There is here provided a field for valuable research work, and, no doubt, investigation will proceed forthwith in the experimental laboratory. The questions which have to be solved are: how can this operation produce such an effect upon the secretory activity of the kidney as to increase the amount of urine secreted and to diminish the amount of albumin, and how are these effects so far-reaching as to remove edema and ascites? Mr. Reginald Harrison has suggested an explanation which appeals to the writer as reasonable if applied to certain classes of cases. He believes that renal tension is relieved by splitting the capsule, and thus the kidney is permitted to perform its normal function. That renal tension exists in acute nephritis no one will deny; such rapid swelling of the organ has occurred that post mortem the capsule has been found to have actually burst. Well-recognized principles of surgery may therefore be employed here, and an incision of an acutely inflamed kidney may, by relieving tension, afford relief and effect a cure, just as a glaucoma is relieved by iridectomy, or an acute orchitis is relieved by incision. These are comparisons suggested by Mr. Harrison, and cannot but agree that the arguments he advances along these lines for incision of the capsule of the kidney in acute nephritis are logical. The explanation is, however, not adequate for those cases of albuminuria of long standing which are relieved by simple nephrotomy. Mr. Harrison's successful cases are those of post-scarlatinal nephritis; nephritis contracted by exposure to cold; nephritis after influenza and that of traumatic origin. He has also observed the disappearance of albumin after operation in calculous nephritis.

Ophthalmia Neonatorum.—Reynolds Wilson (Phil. Med. Jour., Apr. 12, 1902) says that the demands in the matter of treatment are met by the following method of procedure: 1. The antepartum care of the birth canal. 2. The scrupulous cleansing of the lids following expulsion of the head, and constantly thereafter in suspicious cases. 3. The non-invasion of the palpebral sac by separation of the lids before the appearance of typical discharge. 4. Prompt and absolute isolation upon the appearance of conclusive signs of specific inflammation. 5. Thorough and systematic irrigation. 6. Astringent application of silver nitrate in cases of prolonged suppuration. In conclusion, as an important adjunct to local treatment, attention should be given to the general condition of the child in cases of debility and malnutrition. The measures directed toward the care of the infant are comprised in cod-liver oil inunctions, small doses of whiskey internally, and breast-feeding. At the same time the mother should receive some form of tonic treatment.

Pertussis with Cerebral Engorgement.—J. F. Rinehart (Pediatrics, Jan. 15, 1902) reports the case of a child of 5½ years who suffered from such prolonged spasmodic attacks of cough that a set of symptoms referable to the brain itself developed— drowsiness, inability to fix the attention upon a subject when aroused, irregular muscular twitchings and sharp neuralgic pains affecting first one part of the body and then another. The

rational method of procedure in such cases is to remove the cause
—*i.e.*, the prolonged forcing of blood into the brain caused by
cough—and, second, to use derivatives to cause the absorption of
whatever serum may have been already forced through the vessel walls and into the brain substance. The first is best accomplished by the following prescription:

℞
Tincturæ stramonii seminis............................ ℥ ij.
Ammonii bromidi .... ℥ ij.
Elixir simplicis....................................q.s. ad ℥ ij.

A teaspoonful of this is given in a little water every two or
four hours, as may be needed to quiet the cough. This is the
strength ordinarily required for a child of 5 years. After-
treatment consists in the administration of the above mixture
often enough to keep the cough within bounds, and of 2½-grain
doses of carbonate of ammonia every three or four hours as an
expectorant, together with milk and whiskey at short intervals.
The recovery of the case reported was prompt.

Primary Intestinal Tuberculosis in Children.—David Bovaird
(*Arch. of Ped.*, Dec., 1901), from his investigations on the subject, reaches the following conclusions: 1. That English reports
alone show any considerable number of cases of primary intestinal tuberculosis. 2. That primary intestinal tuberculosis is
a very rare affection among children in or about New York, little
more than 1 per cent of the cases of tuberculosis having this
origin. 3. That the proportion of tuberculous cases found at
autopsy in New York is lower than that of European observers.
4. That the evidence connecting tuberculosis among children
with the consumption of the milk of tuberculous cows is very
scant.

Pyloric Stenosis in Infants.—E. W. Saunders (*Arch. of Ped.*,
April, 1902) concludes, from the increasing number of cases of
hypertrophic pyloric stenosis published annually, that this anomaly is by no means rare. The clinical phenomena are fairly
uniform and typical, and the diagnosis offers little difficulty in
the later stages. After a certain interval from birth, varying
from a day to three months, the infant, without apparent cause,
begins to vomit. This is usually attributed to simple indigestion
or to some fault in the mother's milk. Under careful regulation
of the diet and the administration of antemetics, improvement,
if it occurs at all, is only temporary. The vomiting becomes
worse and is projectile. Large quantities of milk are thus
ejected, more than can be accounted for by the previous feeding.
Obstinate constipation ensues. The infant more or less rapidly
loses in weight. The physical signs may be entirely negative in
the beginning. A palpable tumor at the pylorus is exceptionally
found. Progressive dilatation of the stomach occurs. On inspection of the abdomen the upper zone will be observed to be
bulging and contrasts strikingly with the depressed lower zone.
The bulging of the epigastrium subsides visibly after a paroxysm

of vomiting. Peristaltic waves are visible over the epigastrium after the abdominal walls become attenuated. Examination of the gastric contents reveals the fact that the stomach does not empty itself in one or two hours. In some cases hydrochloric acid is in excess, but more often it is diminished or almost absent. Coincidently with the gastric dilatation the signs of gastric catarrh may become manifest. The contents of the stomach show evidences of decomposition; the organic acids, lactic and butyric, being present. Large quantities of mucus are vomited, perhaps once in twenty-four hours or once in two days. The condition of the infant grows steadily worse, the distress is more severe, and the fatal issue is inevitable. Post mortem the pylorus is found to be very much thickened. The pyloric lumen is stenosed to a varying degree. The hypertrophy at the pylorus is composed principally of circular muscular fibres, but the longitudinal layer, the mucous and submucous coat also partake of this overgrowth.

As to treatment, medicinal and dietetic measures should in all cases be first employed. The indications are as follows: *First.*—The administration of some medicinal agent which shall overcome to a greater or less extent the violent contractions of the pylorus. Among the drugs to be recommended are belladonna, bromides, and chloral. Opiates should not be given, as the motor function of the stomach is thereby impaired. *Second.*—The treatment of the secondary gastric irritation. This results from the stagnation of food and should be treated by washing out the stomach and by giving the stomach rest; rectal feeding should, therefore, be resorted to from time to time, and for twenty-four or more hours nothing but water given by the stomach. When food by the mouth is again allowed, the stomach should be washed out occasionally to remove a possible residuum of undigested food. *Third.*—The diet of the child should consist of food which forms no coagulum in the stomach. This point has not been sufficiently insisted upon. Milk or any food containing undigested casein will not answer, consequently the mother's milk is usually unsuitable, while the milk of a wet-nurse in advanced lactation will succeed. Whey or peptonized milk, or a mixture of both, is generally the best food. The deficiency in fat should be supplied by cod-liver oil. A very small percentage of cream can be gradually added. If the coagulum formed by the cream causes distress or increases the vomiting, it must be completely predigested. A mixture of whey and predigested milk perfectly agreed with the patient last named. It is well to aid the motor power of the stomach by gravity; hence, after nursing, the infant should be placed on its right side. If the diet is perfectly fluid some nourishment will ·pass through the pyloric opening. The end to be accomplished is hypertrophy of the gastric wall without dilatation, hence the quantity of food should not be large. Gaseous distension of the stomach should by all means be prevented. Large quantities of milk in the first stage must inevitably lead to ectasia. A stomach is not stronger when over-distended. When it is seen that the infant is failing in spite of rational treatment, surgical intervention must be advised.

Rheumatic Nodosity in Infants.—Herbert Josias (*Med. Press,* Apr. 30, 1902) says that there are two varieties of rheumatic nodosity: the first is dependent on chronic rheumatism, and is, as a rule, independent of articular inflammation; the second is an epiphenomenon of acute articular rheumatism, and forms with chorea one of the most curious sequelæ of infantile rheumatism. The author describes two cases of the latter disease. The first, a boy of 11 years, had nodosities on the pinna of the ear, which is an unusual situation, and in all 60 to 70 on the upper extremity of the right side, 80 on the left side; 60 and 70 on the right and left lower extremities. In size they varied from that of a grain of hempseed to that of a lentil and were slightly painful on pressure. In the second case, a boy of 13, the nodosities were numerous, easily movable, and attached to the deeper tissues. In both cases the heart was affected. Both recovered under treatment by sodium salicylate. The correlation of the attack of nodosities with cardiac disease in childhood requires of the physician a careful examination of the heart in every case of the disease. Endocarditis is the most common form of cardiac lesion found in these cases, its usual site being the mitral valves. The most plausible hypothesis of the disease is that which likens the subcutaneous nodosity to the nodosity found on the mitral valves in endocarditis. In both cases the cellular proliferation is due to the same cause. It is, however, strange that the appearance of the endocardial nodosities and of the subcutaneous ones does not synchronize. Endocardial nodosities may exist without any subcutaneous ones appearing. But subcutaneous nodosities are never present without a similar condition coexisting in the endocardium.

Rheumatism of the Jaw, Two Cases of Isolated.—Manasse (*Münch. med. Wochens.*, vol. xlix., No. 20) reports the case of an adult and that of a 9-year-old boy whose family history was good and who complained of severe pain in both ears after an exposure to cold. There was general weakness, but nothing was found on examining the ears. The region in front of the inferior maxillary articulation was red and swollen; in the mouth also. Mastication was painful. The temperature reached 38.5° C. on the evenings of the first two days. After remaining stationary for two days the symptoms disappeared in five days more. Treatment consisted of painting with iodine externally and within the mouth, and the administration of 0.25 of lactophenin four times a day. Disease of the nose, ears, teeth, and parotid gland could be positively excluded, and the success of the therapy employed speaks for the correctness of the diagnosis. Attention is called to the fact that in certain cases of earache it may be well to consider the possibility of rheumatism of the inferior maxillary articulation.

Scarlatinal Nephritis.—Baginsky *(Jahrbuch für Kinderheil-kunde*, vol. liv., No. 5) observed 88 cases of scarlatinal nephritis in his hospital during the past five years. The earliest day of the scarlatina on which the nephritis developed was the sixth, and the latest was the thirtieth. The majority of the cases began with fever, and those with marked fever proved to be especially dangerous. The quantity of urine was increased at first in some cases. In 18 children a chronic albuminuria remained, and in 5 of these unmistakable signs of chronic nephritis developed. Cases treated in the hospital from the onset ran a decidedly more hope-ful course than those admitted late. The cause of this is the treatment, consisting of four weeks' rest in bed and two weeks' absolute milk diet. Venesection is recommended for uremia, and tannin for long-standing hematuria.

The Serum Exanthemata in the Last Four Years, Experience with.—Von Rittershain *(Jahrb. f. Kinderhk.*, vol. lv., No. 5) observed that the serum exanthemata are much less frequent and less severe than they were formerly; thus there were 6.45 per cent of such eruptions in his service during the past four years, compared with 22 per cent in the year 1897. The diag-nosis of "scarlatiniform serum exanthem" may be very difficult, and is only allowable when a mixed infection with scarlet fever can be positively excluded. Otherwise it is better, at least from a prophylactic point of view, to look upon such a suspicious ery-thema as an abnormal case of scarlet fever and treat it accord-ingly.

Spindle-Celled Sarcoma of the Thorax in a Child.—Louis Fischer *(Arch. of Ped.*, May, 1902) reports the case of a boy of 8 years who had a tumor which occupied that region of the thorax usually occupied by the heart. The child's general con-dition was bad, the dyspnea so great that he had to sleep in a sitting posture. Prognosis was bad, and operation was resorted to, but the child died soon after. The tumor was found to be a spindle-celled sarcoma. These growths are rare in children. The interesting points about this case were: 1. The displaced heart—the heart being immediately behind the right nipple. The pulsations and apex beat could be distinctly felt and seen about two finger breadths below the right nipple. 2. The in-tense dyspnea caused by pressure of the tumor. 3. Constant cyanosis and edema of the limbs, due to interference with the return circulation to the right side of the heart.

Suprarenal Extract in the Treatment of Gastro-Intestinal Hemorrhage in the Newly-Born.—L. Emmett Holt *(Arch. of Ped.*, April, 1902) reports the case of an infant which began to vomit blood sixteen hours from birth, repeating the vomiting at intervals of a few minutes for about eight hours, when the writer first saw the case. The amount of blood vomited each time was from a few drops to a teaspoonful. Most of it was of a dark-brown coffee color mixed with mucus. The general con-dition of the baby was excellent. There seemed every reason for believing that the hemorrhage came from the stomach, and it was decided to try the effect of suprarenal extract. One grain of the saccharated extract was ordered every hour, suspended in water. This was given regularly for six or eight hours, after which the dose was reduced to half the quantity and the intervals were made longer. Twelve hours after beginning the suprarenal the hemorrhage entirely ceased and did not recur. The child then began to take its food normally and when forty-eight hours old was nursing as well as any child. By the fifth day the minute hemorrhages which had been seen beneath the skin had disappeared, as also those on the mucous membrane of the mouth. In all the child took twelve grains of the suprarenal, and of this ten grains were retained. The entire period of the hemorrhages lasted about thirty hours. The subsequent history of the child was uneventful. The solution of the active principle, adrenalin, is possibly to be preferred for internal use to the powder, as one grain of the extract makes a rather large dose for a young infant. Whether any marked effect upon general hemorrhages is to be expected by internal administration of the extract is problematical, but its local effect seems to be proved in the case reported.

Traumatic Tetanus Treated with Beechwood Creosote Hypodermatically.—George Higginson (*Nashville Jour. of Med. and Surg.*, May, 1902) was called to see a boy of 12 suffering from traumatic tetanus in marked form. He was placed in bed in a darkened room which was cool and well ventilated, and kept as quiet as possible. One-grain doses of calomel were ordered each hour until six were taken. Chloral to control the spasm was given by rectum, and morphine was administered hypodermatically morning and evening. Although the antitetanic serum was used in large doses, the patient grew rapidly worse. The author then tried carbolic acid hypodermatically in five-minim doses, morning and evening, for three days, without in any way affecting the disease. The patient was now in an extreme condition and he determined to use creosote in large doses. Twenty minims of beechwood creosote (Merck) were administered in a drachm of olive oil hypodermatically, morning and evening. The chloral and morphine were still used and in a short time distinct benefit was noticed. The patient would entirely relax for short intervals, relieving the dysphagia, and he could take nourishment and he continued to improve. This treatment was continued for twenty days, after which time the dose of creosote was diminished daily. The convalescence was very slow. A nourishing diet was ordered and small doses of strychnine were exhibited. The patient was able to stand up after twenty days' treatment with the creosote, but some rigidity persisted, especially in the abdominal muscles. In three months he was entirely well and has regained his flesh and strength. The beechwood creosote in the above-mentioned doses did not cause any untoward symptom, and at no time during its administration was the urine rendered dark and smoky. The antitetanic serum seemed to have no effect whatever.

The Treatment of Congenital Cleft Palate by Mechanical Appliances.—George A. Raymond *(Boston Med. and Surg. Jour.,* Feb. 6, 1902) states that he has been unable to find a single case where perfect speech ever resulted from a surgical operation. With a mechanical appliance carefully fitted and adapted with the greatest accuracy, however, he finds no difficulty in having even a child become so accustomed to it that it is worn with as much ease and comfort as a set of teeth is worn by an adult. One of the advantages of the appliance is that you can at any time meet the requirements made necessary by development, whereas in the case of operation what you may gain in childhood is lost when adult age is reached. In the matter of speech one does not look for perfection at once, but as soon as the patients become accustomed to the use of the appliance the tone is changed in quality as much as the tone of a violin with the sounding-post put back in position after having been taken out, or the bridge changed from the wrong to the right position. Speech can be improved very greatly at any age, but of course the younger the child the more nimble will be the tongue to imitate sounds.

The Value of Widal's Serum Reaction in the Diagnosis of Typhoid Fever in Children.— J. H. Thursfield *(Pediatrics,* Oct. 15, 1901) concludes from his experiences that in children's diseases a positive Widal reaction is trustworthy evidence of the presence of typhoid fever; that a negative reaction later than the tenth day of an illness is strong but not absolutely convincing evidence of the absence of typhoid fever; and that repeated negative reactions are trustworthy evidence that the case is not typhoid at all. So far from agreeing with Wentworth, he believes that the test is at least as reliable in children as in adults, and, indeed, of even greater value. In the first place, one can generally exclude in children the occurrence of a previous case of typhoid. In adults this has been a frequent cause of mistakes, for the reaction sometimes lasts months, or even years, after an attack of the fever, and so a positive reaction is obtained where there is no typhoid fever present. This source of error is far less likely to be active in children. Secondly, the author is inclined to think that the reaction occurs earlier in children than in adults. Again, there is among children a fever which, while strongly resembling typhoid fever, does not run the course nor present quite the symptoms of typhoid. This disease, whatever it is called, is sufficiently common to be recognized as one of the sources of error in the diagnosis of typhoid. It was formerly supposed that in many instances the disease was an abortive typhoid. The use of the Widal serum reaction has, however, shown that few of these cases are true typhoid. In fact, it has introduced certainty where there was confusion, and promises to give even better results than have been already attained, when we have learned more of the conditions which regulate it.

THE AMERICAN

JOURNAL OF OBSTETRICS

AND

DISEASES OF WOMEN AND CHILDREN.

| Vol. XLVI. | AUGUST, 1902. | No. 2. |

ORIGINAL COMMUNICATIONS.

THE TROPHOBLAST AND CHORIONIC EPITHELIUM, AND THEIR RELATION TO CHORIO-EPITHELIOMA.

BY

SAMUEL WYLLIS BANDLER, M.D.,

Adjunct Gynecologist to the Beth Israel Hospital, New York.

THE DEVELOPMENT OF EXTRA-EMBRYONAL TISSUES IN ANIMALS.

In discussing the histology of gestation it is important to note that in this field, as well as in that of embryology, many of the most important and valuable points have been learned through the study of like processes in animals. The results obtained in investigations in the latter have been applied more or less closely to the various developmental changes in the human being. Though ofttimes erroneously applied, they have been the source through which many vexed questions have been settled. More recent investigations, however, prove that it is not so much the erroneous applications of the results gained in the study of animals as it is errors made in these observations which have so long delayed a satisfactory conclusion concerning the various processes involved in human placentation. It is necessary, for that reason, to consider first the more recent studies concerning animal placentation, as reviewed by Selenka.

10

Marchand examined the placentæ of rabbits gravid from eight to sixteen days. In the earliest specimens he finds on the ovum a growth of ectoderm elements consisting of two layers: (1) a deeper layer of separated cells and (2) a superficial plasmodial. Since the latter is still covered in part by the zona, it is necessarily of fetal origin. In addition he observes *transitions from the cell layer of the ectoderm into the plasmodial.* The deeper cells become larger and are arranged in groups. Their cell boundaries disappear, and, through a union of these cells, a plasmodial layer is formed, covering the deeper ectoderm, but, as a rule, distinctly outlined from it. This ectodermal plasmodium unites with the syncytially-changed uterine epithelium, forming the first connection between the ovum and the uterine wall. In the placenta of nine to ten days Marchand finds blood (1) in the maternal vessels possessing an endothelial lining and (2) *in ectodermal spaces in the cell layer.* Into these spaces, which possess no endothelium, the blood from the maternal vessels enters. In the placenta of eleven days few of these unlined ectodermal spaces containing blood remain. Most of them are now lined with a continuous layer of elements rich in protoplasm, which Marchand considers originate from the maternal vessel endothelium (?), which has undergone a "syncytial change."

Maximow, in his investigations on rabbit placentæ, denies, in contrast to Marchand, the existence of a fetal ectodermal plasmodium as early as the eighth day. He believes that, when the ovum attaches itself to the uterine wall, the ectoderm consists of only *separated cells, which come in contact with the epithelium of the uterus and cause it to degenerate.* When the ectoderm, after disappearance of the uterine epithelium, reaches the maternal vessels, the glycogen-containing cells of the uterine connective tissue change to large polynuclear structures. In these cells he finds elements resembling red blood cells in form and color. Only later, when the ectoderm enters into the decidua, does it divide into two layers: (1) one with cell boundaries, the cytoblast, and (2) one without cell boundaries, the plasmodiblast. The latter is found only where the villi come in contact with the glycogen-containing cells, *at the walls of the maternal vessels.* It is not found where the villi grow into the connective tissue between the vessels. From the tenth day on, spaces filled with maternal blood are found in the fetal plasmodium and there develops an ecto-placenta, *into whose ectodermal villous formations the mesodermal elements bringing the allantoic vessels enter.*

Opitz finds in the rabbit a double ectodermal layer during the process of attachment of the ovum in the uterine wall: (1) an internal layer formed of separated cells, and (2) an external plasmodial layer. *The latter causes the uterine syncytium to disappear* and aids the attachment of the ovum to the uterine wall freed of epithelium. In the plasmodium spaces occur into which maternal blood empties from the eroded maternal vessels. From the ovum, ectodermal cell groups enter into this ectodermal plasmodium, *are vascularized, and later become also plasmodial.*

Those syncytial cells which Marchand considers as resulting from maternal endothelium, Maximow, however, views as ectodermal plasmodium when found in the fetal portion of the vessels, but considers them in the maternal portion to be endothelial. Opitz considers these cells *to be entirely of ectodermal origin.* It is to be noted that Maximow and Opitz mention the destruction of the uterine epithelium. Later fetal mesoderm with the allantoic vessels enters into the placenta and on its external surface the remnants of the ectoderm are found as flat covering cells. The epithelium of the uterus plays no part in the development of the placenta, *but forms a syncytium which is absorbed by the ectoderm cells.*

In Tarsius, Hubrecht finds that the uterine wall, through a change of the connective tissue, forms a trophospongia, *between which the glands degenerate.* On the growth of the embryonal ectoderm or trophoblast, a mixture of trophoblast and trophospongia occurs, with a decided increase in the volume of this early placental formation. Then the development of the mesodermal villous elements takes place, and the mesoderm villi surround themselves with a trophoblast covering. Between the trophoblast cells lacunæ form, into which maternal blood passes. Finally, the trophospongia becomes a thin layer which represents the boundary toward the deeper maternal tissue.

In Tupaja, when the ovum rests upon the uterine wall *its ectoderm causes the uterine epithelium to disappear.* The trophoblast grows decidedly, with the formation of giant cells, and occasionally forms a combined layer with the uterine epithelium in which maternal and embryonal nuclei lie in a common plasmodium. *The maternal portions degenerate,* but the ectodermal tissue is divided into (1) a deeper layer, the cytotrophoblast, and

(2) a superficial syncytial layer, the plasmoditrophoblast, which constitutes only a temporary differentiation. In the uterine wall, in the meantime, the connective-tissue trophospongia is formed; the border between ectoderm and maternal connective tissue disappears, for these tissues infiltrate each other. In this resulting union the trophospongia is overcome by the trophoblast and the maternal blood passes from the maternal capillaries into the embryonal trophoblast spaces. The mesodermal fetal cells then enter with the allantoic vessels and receive on their external surface a covering of trophoblast.

Although various investigations have shown that the variations in the development of the placenta in different animals are quite unexpected, and that among the individual mammalia, even when closely related, decided differences are found, yet the trend is more toward the view that, as a rule, the syncytium originates from fetal ectoderm. According to Strahl and Selenka, in quite a group of placentæ the uterine epithelium plays no unimportant rôle. On the other hand, Fränkel, as a result of extensive investigations, comes to the conclusion that *the higher the organization of the placenta and the more firm the connection between maternal and fetal tissues, so much the less is the maternal epithelium preserved.*

He finds that in the rodents and in the insectivora, whose placentæ, of all the animals he examined, stand nearest to the human placenta, *the uterine epithelium ceases at the border of the placenta.* Only in the pig does it remain. In the cow and sheep the epithelium in the cotyledo shows a tendency to degeneration. In the cat, rabbit, squirrel, guinea-pig, rat, mouse, and mole the uterine epithelium takes no part in the formation of the placenta. A so-called syncytial formation, however, he finds to occur in the most varying tissues. *The higher in the animal plane the animal stands, the more does the chorionic epithelium grow into the maternal connective tissue robbed of its epithelium.*

Opitz finds that in the guinea-pig the foundation for the placenta is the fetal ectodermal plasmodium vascularized by maternal vessels. The placentæ of the rabbit, the guinea-pig, and the human being agree in that earlier or later the ectodermal surface of the ovum comes in contact with the connective tissue of the uterine mucosa. Finally, between maternal blood and the fetal vessels found in the mesoderm of the villi only one layer of the ectodermal syncytium is left. The apparently great differences are to be explained by the fact that in the rabbit and guinea-pig the projections of ectoderm and mesoderm (the villi) come into union with each other, while in the human being they are always separated.

THE TROPHOBLAST AND CHORIONIC EPITHELIUM.

The great growth of the ectodermal cover in the ova of animals has been made known to us by Van Beneden, Duval, Nolf, and especially by Hubrecht, who gave it the name trophoblast.

In 1889 Hubrecht, in examining the placenta of the hedgehog, found a decided resemblance in numerous points to the human placenta. He asked then that the following questions with regard to the human ova should be studied:

1. Can, in the earliest stages of human ova, evidences be found of a trophospherical tissue between the villous covered ovum and the inner surface of the decidua reflexa?

2. Are there in this tissue blood vessels which receive their supply from those blood vessels which run in the reflexa?

3. Can evidences of a trophospherical tissue be found in the serotinal region?

The discussion of the histology of gestation in both uterus and tube shows that the various processes in the development of the human placenta resemble these observed in animal placentation.

It must be noted that these processes follow the steps observed by Hubrecht, Maximow, Opitz, etc. Yet there are still many diverging views as to the origin of the syncytial covering of the villi, as has been also observed in this regard in the investigations in animals.

Selenka and Strahl, in their examination of young human ova, find their views, gained in the examination of animal placentæ, sustained—namely, that the syncytial layer originates from the uterine epithelium. With this view Kossmann and Merttens agree. Eckardt finds that the syncytium originates from the maternal endothelium. Spee states that the syncytium develops from the connective-tissue cells of the decidua. Langhans considers the syncytial layer ectodermal, and the inner layer of Langhans mesodermal. Leopold and Gaisser consider the layer of Langhans to be of mesodermal origin *because they find these cells in the mesoderm of the villi*. Fränkel is uncertain as to the origin of the syncytium in human ova, and *finds transitions between the cell of Langhans and cells situated in the mesoderm of the villi.* Kastschenko, Minot, Van Heukelom, and Ulesko-Stroga-nowa consider both layers to be of fetal origin.

Eckardt, who holds that the syncytium originates from the maternal endothelium (?), states that the capillaries of the decidua which form lacunæ under the surface have a varying character. Many possess a distinct growth of the wall elements, which is often so great that he would consider these areas to be sections of glands, were it not for the blood therein contained. We know that, in the decidua menstrualis and graviditatis, blood may enter the glands between the epithelial cells or may break into the glands. The epithelium, which, especially in the neighborhood of the ovum, grows distinctly and shows an enlarged elongated protoplasm, resembles to a certain degree the syncytium. These cells, however, degenerate through the action of the blood and the glands are destroyed or pushed aside. From his description it is quite evident that Eckardt was describing such areas, which he mistook for a growth of maternal endothelium. With these remarks the views of Eckardt may be dismissed.

Merttens found in the particles obtained by curetting sixteen days after the last menstruation a few sections of an ovum with the enveloping decidua. He describes (1) the chorion and the villi. On the latter are cell groups, and between them are found spaces constituting the intervillous space. (2) The spongiosa, containing numerous glands, and (3) the compacta, a pale zone lying between 1 and 2 and containing large pale cells, between which are numerous darkly stained nuclei.

In the compacta he finds large cells and large spaces. Between the large cells syncytial masses are irregularly distributed. The cell spaces are round, long, or irregular, and often empty into the intervillous space. They contain blood and are lined with syncytial masses, which at some points are very thin and at other points quite thick. Where these spaces empty into the intervillous space the syncytial masses continue into the syncytium of the villi. Merttens does not know whether these spaces are glands, vessels, or lymph spaces. They are undoubtedly, however, the lacunæ of Hubrecht, Peters, and Opitz.

The epithelia of the glands are like beaker cells, and on their free tips is a half-moon of glycogen. The glands show papillary projections (compare Fig. 1). Merttens believes that the syncytium results through a change of the surface and gland epithelium (?). In his Fig. 8 Merttens represents, in the upper portion, the epithelium of such a gland, and the lower half represents syncytial masses. He believes that the latter result from these epithelial cells, which lose their cylindrical form and unite. From his descriptions and his drawings it is neither clear nor probable that the epithelium changes into these syncytial masses. Besides, this area is taken from decidua particles not connected with the ovum, and at no point can he find the epithelium of the glands contributing in any way to the syncytium of the chorion.

On the contrary, this ovum is at the stage where the trophoblast is almost consumed by the growth of the intervillous space, and the cell groups at the end of the villi, which Merttens calls points of union between the villi and the decidua, are simply the remains of the trophoblast.

In a very early ovum described by Spee the villi are covered with two layers. The inner, the cell layer of Langhans, he attributes to the ectoderm. The outer layer, the syncytium or adventitia of the ovum, he describes as follows: "This layer is often lifted off from the chorion ectoderm. It appears as a continuous thin streak of protoplasm with more or less closely grouped nuclei arranged in a single row. In the layers of the enveloping zone lying near the ovum are found cells which, through a diffuse staining of the nucleus and through the vacuolar character of the protoplasm, resemble the cell elements of the syncytium very much. In the space between the serotina and the ovum (intervillous space) we find them often close together and not distinctly separated, so that here the early stages of the polynuclear protoplasmatic groups are present. Such groups are also found united to the membrana chorii. Concerning their origin opinions differ. I have never observed a mitosis or an amitosis in their nuclei. The idea that the chorion ectoderm furnishes these masses may be set aside because of the sharp division between these two layers by a cuticula. These conditions prove that the syncytial formation does not increase through a division of the nucleus or the cell in the intervillous space. Since, however, an increase in the amount of the syncytial substance occurs within the intervillous space, this can only be explained through a wandering of already finished masses from the connective tissue of the compacta into the ovum. Epithelial cells cannot be considered as the source, since the maternal cavity surrounding the ovum, even in the earliest stages, shows no epithelial lining, although in the later stages closely pressed glands are present all about the ovum and their epithelium is preserved at least up to the end of the first month.'' It may be seen that Spee left out of consideration any possible action of the blood upon the ectoderm cells as an aid to the formation of syncytium. His decidua cells, resembling syncytium, are possibly changed trophoblast cells. Cells from without probably form the syncytial covering of the villi and of the membrana chorii, in his opinion. We think they are trophoblast cells of fetal ectodermal origin, acted on by the blood—a possibility which he left out of consideration.

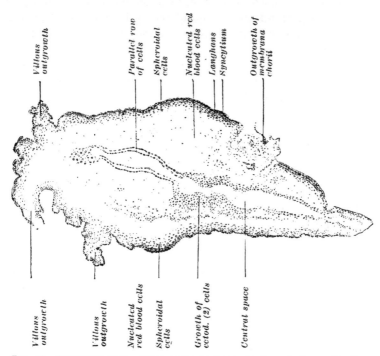

FIG. 40.—Transverse section through the fetal sac of a four- to five-weeks ovum.

Fig. 40 represents a transverse section through the greatest diameter of the ovum loosely connected with the decidua in the fourth or fifth week of uterine gestation. The centre is a space lined with a double parallel layer of cells arranged in single file. This also loses its parallel arrangement at certain points, where cells of the same character are found in groups several layers deep.

External to these cells, in the entire circumference of the sac, is a substance staining a deeper red and composed of extremely fine, granular, and thin-fibred, cotton-like material. In it, at numerous points, are isolated and grouped cells which look like nucleated red blood cells.

The next stratum is formed of round and oval cells, of the same character as the lining of the central space, but arranged in several somewhat parallel layers. Between these cells is a fine fibre-like substance, like the one just described, but taking a lighter red stain. The outer cells are rounder and more spherical than the inner, and the outermost cells, with a clear protoplasm and distinct nucleus, form a single layer of distinct cells with distinct cell boundaries.

The extreme external covering of the membrana chorii is of a plasmodial character, and contains nuclei of various forms and evidences many vacuoles (Fig. 41). Each vacuole represents

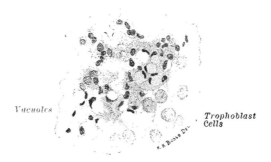

FIG. 41.—Vacuoles representing body of trophoblast cells, while the nucleus is a crescent in the circumference. From the membrana Chorii of Fig. 40.

the space filled by a trophoblast cell, the nucleus being compressed at one point into a small crescent. At certain points outgrowths are present which contain larger and smaller areas of granular and plasmodial character, the aforementioned distinct cells, blood, and protoplasmatic groups containing small pale cells, small dark nuclei, and nuclei undergoing degeneration. Attached to the membrana chorii and all about it are innumerable villi in all stages of growth, young and old. The older villi present the same structure and possess the same cells, including the nucleated red blood cells, as are found in the chorionic membrane.

The conclusion gained from a comparison of this specimen with the structure of the villi is the following: The single

layer of cells immediately under the plasmodium of the chorionic membrane, the spheroidal cells under it, the distinct cells
found in the outgrowths, the spheroidal cells in the young villi
and in the cell groups which form the new villi, and the cell
layer of Langhans, are identical and represent the ectodermal
trophoblast cells.   The villi are simply excrescences of the membrana chorii.

When the blood comes in contact with the trophoblast cells it
does not coagulate.   It does, however, exert a decided influence
on the nuclei.   Strahl found, in examining the placenta of
Galago, that the blood extravasated from the vessels of the
uterus is made use of by the fetus, in that the degenerating
products of the extravasated blood cells are taken up and absorbed.   These products are found in the form of larger and
smaller yellow granules in the gland epithelium, which the latter
uses in furnishing an iron-containing gland secretion.   In the
placenta of other animals the blood extravasated from the vessels of the uterus is taken up and absorbed by the ectoderm
cells, and in certain animals the fetus obtains its nutrition because the ectoderm, covering the villus, takes up the substance
given off by the uterine epithelium.   Merttens observes that
Lieberkühn in the placenta of the dog, and Strahl in the placenta of the mole, find ectoderm cells taking up and absorbing red
blood cells.   Peters states that Tafani, in the placenta of the
cat, found chorion ectoderm cells outside of the placenta taking
up red blood cells.   We find much blood—that is, red blood
cells—in the syncytium.   It is also found in the vacuoles.   Peters
believes that the blood takes part in the changes of the trophoblast nuclei and that its elements contribute to the formation
of the protoplasmatic masses known as the syncytium.   "Not
only the blood plasma, but also the nuclei of red and white
blood cells, pass into the composition of these masses."   It may
be seen in Fig. 11 that the red blood cells change into a detritus
and combine, so that finally small irregular areas containing small
nuclear remnants result.   A gradual destruction of red blood
cells takes place, and the presence of leucocyte nuclei may be
observed.   The plasma, when acting suddenly and in large
amounts, causes the trophoblast nuclei to shrink and take on a
dark stain.   When acting slowly it disintegrates them, flattens
them, so that in a resulting homogeneous protoplasm nuclei of all
forms may be found.   It is evident, then, that the protoplasm
of the syncytium is the product of the blood cells, the blood

plasma, and the protoplasm of the trophoblast cells. *The nuclei of the syncytium are the changed trophoblast nuclei.*

Wherever blood comes in contact with fetal cells syncytium results, whether in the decidua or in the intervillous space, so that *syncytium really plays the part of an endothelium* and at all periods, especially in the later stages, resembles endothelium so closely that it was naturally mistaken for it in nearly all the earlier investigations.

Many observers have noted a brush-like covering on the syncytium, though I have never found it. This striated surface on the syncytial covering of the chorion, and often observed on the isolated polynuclear protoplasmatic masses, appears to Spee to be a sort of fibrillation on the cell protoplasm. He believes that it originates through the influence of a sap current toward the ovum, because such a brush-like fibrillation is found in those places where a regulated transit of products through cells occurs, as in parts of the excretory ducts of the salivary glands and the kidneys on the side toward the connective tissue, and also perhaps in the osteoblasts in the Howship lacunæ of bone.

Tubal ova and the uterine ova furnish us with the following positive conclusions:

1. The human ovum possesses an ectodermal growth of cells, the trophoblast, consisting of closely-grouped cells.

2. When vascularized, a second external layer, consisting of plasmodial mononuclear and polynuclear elements, results.

3. Elements of the blood circulating in the spaces and lacunæ of the trophoblast contribute to the protoplasm of the syncytium. Among other elements, the secretion of the uterine or tubal epithelium may likewise contribute to the formation of the syncytial protoplasm. At any rate, much of the protoplasm (but none of the nuclei) is of maternal origin.

4. On the villi and the membrana chorii the plasmodial cells form the outer syncytial layer, while the closely-grouped cells beneath it furnish the single layer of Langhans.

5. The stroma of the chorionic villi is formed of mesodermal tissue in which are later found capillaries communicating with the umbilical vessels and containing fetal blood. Clear in almost every detail, then, a trophoblast formation, consisting of an inner layer of separated cells and an outer or plasmodial layer such as is found in the placental development of animals, is present in human placentation.

BLOOD-FORMING FUNCTION OF THE TROPHOBLAST.

In another particular. as I believe can be shown, this re-semblance is carried out still further—namely, the formation of blood by the fetal placenta.

In sections through the umbilical vesicle of Tarsius and Tu-paja, Hubrecht finds. polynuclear cells which he considers to be mother blood cells. Their nuclei result through fragmen-tation of a large nucleus. The individual nuclei within the mother cell then become surrounded with a special circle of plasma. When the original mantle of the protoplasm of the large cell is lost, the included cells are freed, forming embryonal nucleated red blood cells. During their circulation in the em-bryonal fetus the nuclear membrane disappears and the nucleus changes to a drop in which the chromatin diminishes, while the protoplasm begins to resemble the former nucleus. The cells become gradually smaller, and the final forms do not result from the protoplasm but from the nuclei of the cells. The blood cells originate, then, from the original nucleus of a mother blood cell. Hubrecht finds the same steps in the placenta of Tarsius as in the umbilical vesicle. He finds the same to occur in the trophoblast and in the maternal spongia, and even in the vessels which lie between the glands. In the placenta of Tupaja the same steps are noted, but, in addition. the epithelium, as well as the connective tissue of the decidua. is the seat of red blood cells derived from nuclei.

In his ovum v. H. Spee describes the mesoderm layer as follows: He finds two different cell forms occurring side by side and inter-mingled: (1) Branched cells, extending into fine threads which project in all directions and which may well be considered con-nective-tissue fibres. Where these cells occur singly—for in-stance. at certain points in the abdominal pedicle and in the villi—the mesoblast appears exceedingly poor in nuclei. Strong-ly-stained specimens are necessary to see the numerous fine, wavy, and sharply contoured fibres of the embryonal connective tissue. (2) Between these structures are found larger, strongly prominent spindle cells with oval nuclei, arranged sometimes closely together like bundles, and at other points separated from each other by wide spaces without evident contents. The course of these fibres follows, with noticeable constancy, the curves of the free mesoderm surface—that is, the surface covered with epithelium.

In our opinion many of the second form of cells are probably ectodermal. In an ovum described by Reichert, on the inner side of the chorion is a substance which he considers to be a mucoid-like deposit and which also extends into the villi. The cavity of the ovum is likewise filled with this substance. Spee considers this to be mesoderm tissue, although Reichert describes the contents of the ovum simply as a mucoid substance without cells. Spee says that the contents of the amnion and of the umbilical vesicle of ova hardened in alcohol never coagulate, but such a condition does take place in the wide mesoderm slit of dead young human ova.

Thus the early embryonal mesoderm tissue of the membrana chorii and of the villi is very poor in cells, and the description of Reichert, characterized by Spee as mesoderm substance, serves to characterize as mesoderm the non-celled material found between the central space and the external layers of cells seen in Fig. 40 and also found in many of the younger villi.

It has been mentioned that Langhans considers the cell layer to be of mesodermal origin, and that Leopold holds the same view because he finds *transitions between the stroma cells and the cell layer.* Fränkel, who believes that the cell layer and the syncytium are probably identical, finds the question difficult of solution *because of the numerous villi whose interior is composed of ectodermal trophoblast cells.* We have called attention to this occurrence as a frequent one, and have likewise observed the resemblance between the cell layer of the membrana chorii and the several layers of cells under it which are embedded, however, in mesoderm substance (Fig. 40). The origin of the villi, the fact that they are formed out of solid trophoblast groups, the fact that only later does mesodermal tissue reduce them to the generally single layer of Langhans, the fact that in this reduction to a single layer many trophoblast cells are left embedded in the stroma of the villi and the membrana chorii, and the numerous transitions between these cells and the cells of Langhans, prove that they are ectodermal cells situated in a basis of mesoderm substance in which only later mesoderm nuclei appear.

As the villi grow older, these ectoderm cells are crowded by the growing mesoderm tissue, so that some degenerate, while others take part in the following important changes—that is, THEY FORM RED BLOOD CELLS.

In the same manner that the external trophoblast cells, which come in contact with the blood, obtain from it a protoplasmatic envelope, while they themselves form the nuclei, in quite the same manner these cells situated in mesoderm are seen to gradually change their form, become darker, become surrounded by a red-staining granular protoplasm of the same character as the mesodermal tissue. They then represent nucleated red blood cells. They are often seen in stages where the nucleus becomes fragmented or divided into other cells. These larger and smaller nucleated reds are found isolated or in groups, often lying in spaces or slits of the mesoderm of the villi and membrana chorii. These spaces are often surrounded by very long, very dark, and spindle-like cells, evidently forming the endothelium of the future capillaries.

We have observed the statement that in animals the mesoderm, which enters the trophoblast groups and forms the stroma of the villi, carries with it the branches of the allantoic vessels. Vessels, however, are not present in the villi of the human ovum until the third week, and the villi are then filled with mesoderm or ectoderm cells, and it would be impossible for extensions of the allantoic vessels to enter into the innumerable extensions of the membrana chorii constituting the villi. The process followed, however, is probably the following:

Mesoderm does not enter as a distinct tissue into the trophoblast elements *after they have been reduced by the maternal blood to syncytium,* but is present between the trophoblast cells *from the very earliest period,* as may be seen in the description of the tubal ovum. When, therefore, a trophoblast cell group comes in contact with maternal blood, the outer cells are changed to syncytium, underneath which results the cell layer of Langhans, which in the still later periods disappears. The mesoderm substance, when increasing in amount, dilates the villus and forms the stroma. In the resulting stroma are left the remaining more or less scattered trophoblast cells. From these, nucleated red blood cells are formed, which lie in small slits or spaces, which spaces become lined with endothelium, thus forming capillaries. These capillaries gradually increase and finally become very numerous, having a tendency to lie close under the epithelial covering of the villi. Whether any of these trophoblast cells take part in the formation of the endothelium, it is impossible to say with certainty. These same processes are observed in the membrana chorii. These capillaries in the villi and in the membrana chorii later unite with the umbilical vessels which make their way through the abdominal pedicle.

The nucleated red blood cells, in their subsequent circulation through the fetus, become changed, and from the third month on ordinary red blood cells are found. In the membrana chorii of our uterine ovum the same stages of capillary development may be observed, but to a less extent than in some of the villi which already possess numerous and distinct capillaries. In the later stages this process is more marked in the membrana chorii

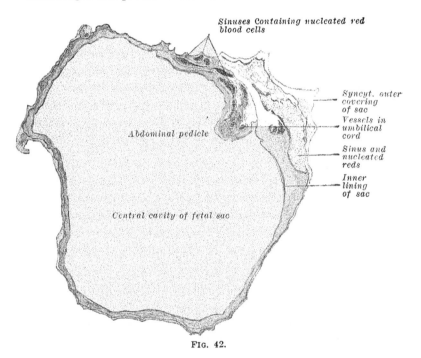

Fig. 42.

than in the villi, as may be seen from the following description of a tubal gestation with well-preserved fetus:

The fetus was lying in the central cavity of the ovum (Fig. 42), attached by an umbilical pedicle which entered the placenta at the site to be mentioned later. The fetus was one centimetre long; the abdominal wall was not yet closed, and the arm and leg formations were just evident as small pinhead knobs. The cavity of the ovum is lined by a membrane composed of flattened cells with distinct nuclei. At various points in the circumference of the membrana chorii, and especially at the point.

where the abdominal pedicle is attached, are numerous larger or smaller spaces, separated, sometimes, from the maternal blood by only a single or double layer of cells, which at many points are of a distinctly plasmodial character. The membrana chorii has at various points, and especially at the placental site, numerous villi attached to it and numerous small projections of the same structure as villi. These spaces, or sinuses, contain masses of round, red-staining protoplasmatic masses with dark central nuclei, many of which are undergoing division—nucleated red blood cells. It seems probable that many of these sinuses or spaces represent dilatations of the parallel row of cells observed in Fig. 40, wherein were noted, at various points, groups of cells of a trophoblast character. It is probable that those groups form the nucleated red blood cells observed in these sinuses.

The largest of these sinuses are present near the insertion of the abdominal pedicle, and all of them are separated from the maternal blood of the intervillous space, often by only a single layer. These sinuses represent, then, areas in the membrana chorii filled with nucleated red blood cells of placental trophoblast origin, which subsequently enter the fetal circulation.

In the pedicle itself a change to the subsequent non-nucleated red blood cells may be observed, for in its substance are fetal vessels and sinuses filled with cells of a different character. They are small, with a thin circumference of protoplasm and a dark nucleus filling out almost the entire cell body. These represent, then, the later stages of the red blood cells.

The resemblance of this process to the one noted by Hubrecht in Tupaja and Tarsius carries out still further the resemblance of the various processes in the human placenta to those in the placentæ of animals. That this theory and explanation, whereby red blood cells are formed of trophoblast ectodermal cells, is a rational one and proven by the examination of our specimens seems to me evident. In addition, it serves to explain the presence of trophoblast cells in the interior of the villi—a fact which has led many, who have considered them mesodermal because situated in the mesodermal stroma, to likewise call the cells of Langhans mesodermal. The formation of nucleated red blood cells from trophoblast cells, on the addition of a protoplasm of mesodermal origin, would serve to make their resemblance to syncytium very great; for the latter is composed of trophoblast nuclei with a protoplasm largely composed of maternal blood plasma. If, as many sections have suggested, the capillaries were lined by endothelium which is also formed of these trophoblast nuclei, the resemblance of this process to the formation of syncytium would be further increased; for the syncytium simply plays the part of endothelium, separating the other fetal cells at all times from the circulating blood.

THE RELATION OF THE CHORIONIC EPITHELIUM TO CHORIO-EPITHELIOMA.

There have been observed and reported over 150 cases of a uterine growth of exceedingly malignant character occurring after abortion and labor, or even after tubal abortion. The clinical symptoms are: (1) Pronounced uterine hemorrhage, recurring even after repeated curettage; (2) very early metastases, especially in the lungs and vagina; and (3) early death through hemorrhage, cachexia, or septic infection.

Macroscopically, these tumors are more or less localized, ulcerating, degenerating, hemorrhagic growths, frequently passing deeply into the uterine wall, or through it with involvement of the peritoneum.

Microscopically, these tumors are characterized by hemorrhagic areas, areas of degeneration, the presence of fibrin, and the involvement and invasion of capillaries and large vessels. They are especially characterized by the presence of (1) pale round and polygonal cells with pale protoplasm and pale nucleus, and (2) of large round and spindle-shaped cells with large dark nuclei, and also of large, irregular branches composed of polynuclear protoplasmatic masses.

These atypical growths have been variously described as sarcoma, carcinoma, carcinoma after abortion and labor, and as sarcoma and carcinoma causing abortion.

Sänger, in reviewing these cases, found a decided resemblance in their characteristic elements, and came to the conclusion that the decidua cells were the cause of the growth, giving it then the name of deciduo-sarcom or deciduoma malignum.

As a result of the investigations of Fränkel, and later of Marchand, attention was called to the fact that those cells which so closely resembled decidua cells were really of fetal origin and were, in fact, the cells of Langhans, while the spindle-shaped and grouped masses of polynuclear protoplasm were of syncytial origin.

From all sides, especially in England and Germany, this view was attacked. It was pointed out how baseless was the view

11

that fetal cells could produce a growth of this malignant character, differing from carcinoma only in the fact that metastases resulted through the blood channels instead of the lymph paths.

This controversy is to-day by no means settled, many holding the view that these tumors are sarcomatous, originating from the decidua cells. The giant cells and the protoplasmatic masses are referred, likewise, to changes in the decidua. Others hold that these growths result from the epithelial covering of the villi. That these cells, if they are of fetal origin, should be mistaken for decidua cells is a natural error, for we know that even in the normal processes a positive distinction is often very difficult. It is to be noted that many investigators have called the typical trophoblast cells in tubal placentation, too, decidua cells. Still others lean to the view that the stroma of the villi plays its part.

On the other hand, among those who hold that these growths originate from the chorionic covering a division of sentiment exists; for those who consider the syncytium and cells of Langhans to be of uterine origin class these growths as carcinoma and sarcoma of a somewhat atypical character. Those who believe, as we have shown, that the epithelial covering of the villi is of fetal ectodermal origin, and who therefore also class these tumors under the category of carcinoma, are introducing into pathology a new element.

A factor which has served to clear our views on these various disputed points is the knowledge that fifty per cent of these malignant uterine growths, commonly known as deciduoma, follow the presence of hydatid mole.

In hydatid mole we find the same elements as in normal placentation, only that these elements are excessive in number and size. Hydatid mole represents a hypertrophic growth of the chorionic covering, accompanied by dropsical swelling of the chorionic stroma. As is well known, the covering of the villi consists of two layers, an outer syncytium, an inner, the cell layer of Langhans. The growth concerns both the syncytium and the cell layer of Langhans. The abnormal element is the occurrence of very large cells with immense nuclei in large number, and a decided growth of the syncytium, accompanied by the formation in the latter of large vacuoles.

Leaving out of consideration those cases malignant because of the diffuse and deep infiltration of the uterine wall by the cystic villi, by no means are all hydatid moles of a malignant character. An attempt to distinguish between the benign and malignant cases was proposed by Neumann. He observed, in three cases subsequently resulting in the so-called deciduoma, large cell elements in the stroma of numerous villi which he considered to be infiltrating elements of the syncytium. He observed, further, an abnormal infiltration of cell groups through such syncytial elements. Investigation of subsequent cases shows that malignant forms are not always preceded by such changes in the hydatid mole, while others have found these changes and yet no malignant growth occurred.

Even the occurrence of metastases is no proof of malignancy, for Pick reported a case with a metastasis of villi in the vagina and yet the patient recovered. We know that fetal cells are given off from the normal placenta into the maternal circulation. Even the normal placenta, as Pick believes, may give metastases of villi, and these may (1) degenerate or (2) grow slightly or (3) produce the same syncytial growth as is observed in benign hydatid mole. (4) Primary malignant growths may originate, and have originated, from such metastases.

Malignancy, in the case of hydatid mole, is not then to be judged alone by the occurrence of metastases. Those cases which subsequently develop into the so-called deciduoma evidence their malignant character *by the ability of their cells to grow in an unlimited manner,* aided by the character of the tissue which permits or also aids this growth. Various theories have been propounded in explanation of this phenomenon. 1. Through the syncytium there is a constant exchange of products, and after hydatid mole, or on the occurrence of abortion or labor or any process causing the removal or death of the fetus, this exchange ceases. The fetal cells then, if in a favorable surrounding, are supposed to use this nutrition for themselves and increase until an unlimited growth results (theory of Marchand). 2. Ribbert considers the unlimited ability of certain malignant tissues to grow to be due to the separation of their mother cells from their normal connections. 3. As is well known, Cohnheim considered displaced embryonal cells to be the future source of many benign and malignant tumors.

An interesting power or potential retained by displaced cells is that of differentiation. We know that displaced cells, cells removed from their normal relations, are able, after an interval of many years, to grow and produce structures of varying form. This is best exemplified in the case of dermoid cysts, for their character distinguishes them from all other tumors. The later in the stage of embryonal development these cells are displaced the more simple is the structure of the resulting dermoid; the earlier in the period of embryonal development their displacement occurs the more differentiated are these cells. For that reason embryonal cells displaced in the early weeks produce tumors of complicated character, for their potential as regards differentiation is great. Cells displaced at a later period possess a lesser potential as regards differentiation, while those epithelial and connective-tissue cells displaced very late, as at points where the skin only remains to be united, and at the branchial clefts, produce only the simplest form of dermoid growth. They produce only cells of the same character and structure as the parent cell if the stage of complete differentiation had been already reached. If the displacement occurs before this period, such elements are found in the subsequent growth as the parent cells would have produced had they remained in their normal situation. Such early cells, however, reproduce far greater growths and far more extensive tissues than would have resulted had they not been displaced. This is evidenced by the fact that no loss of any normal tissue or structure results. In dermoid cysts of the ovary, for instance, very large and complicated tumors are found, resulting from the displacement of ectodermal and mesodermal cells by the Wolffian body, and yet the maternal body is otherwise normally developed.

In the genital tract, especially, we find numerous evidences of another cell potential, that is, the ability to first display accelerated growth after a lapse of many years. We find in the uterine wall, under the peritoneum, in the broad ligament, and in the ovary, generally after puberty, epithelial and glandular growths, sometimes of considerable size, resulting from the displacement of cells of the Wolffian body. In the fetus and in the newly-born, hundreds of uteri and appendages have been examined and yet relatively few such displacements of Wolffian-body cells can be found. This means that the displacement concerns simply embryonal cells of this organ, which even at a much later period possess the power to develop the same structures as the parent organ. This growth takes place, as a rule, at and after puberty, and the same is true in the case of dermoid cysts.

We find, then, that the general stimulation of tissue and cell growth occurring after puberty may influence such embryonally-displaced cells in the same manner.

We find, on close investigation, that almost all ovarian and parovarian cysts result from the continued growth of structures which in the embryo were functionating organs, but which in the fetus and in the adult are supposed to undergo regressive changes, namely, the epoöphoron and the paroöphoron, constituting the two divisions of the Wolffian body. Papilloma of the ovary, in all probability, also develop from cells of these supposedly regressive structures. Ovarian cysts also frequently show papillomatous changes. These are, strictly speaking, only huge increases of the characteristics of the primary embryonal organ.

Not infrequently these papillomatous growths are macroscopically of a malignant character, in that they break through the covering of the cyst or through the ovary, grow without restriction, invade the peritoneum, infiltrate the surrounding organs, and produce cachexia.

Such changes may also display the microscopic characteristics which we attribute to carcinoma—that is, a continued growth of the epithelium, a breaking through of the membrana propria, and an infiltration, microscopically, of the tissue surrounding the epithelial cells. In other words, we find a continued unlimited growth of cells, reproducing, even though in a changed relation, the character of the mother cell.

These smaller and larger reproductions of the Wolffian body, these cystic growths originating from the Wolffian-body cells, these papillary and malignant growths originating from the same source, as well as dermoid cysts, furnish us with evidence of the ability of regressive cells and organs, and cells removed from their normal relations, to undergo a more or less unlimited growth, even after lying dormant for many years. These cells, however, are cells of the patient and are open to the same influences as normally situated cells.

In the case of chorio-epithelioma, however, we find fetal cells, often only a few weeks old, possessing naturally no great potential as regards differentiation, but an exceedingly high potential as regards their ability to grow. The energy and potential of these cells may be appreciated from the fact that the earliest case occurred two weeks after the interruption of pregnancy, while the latest occurred nearly four years after hydatid mole.

The most prominent point of a ripening Graafian follicle is poor in blood supply and is called the stigma folliculi. It is here that the opening takes place which furnishes an outlet for

the ovum.   This opening is probably the result of the reaction or
chemical effect produced by the ripe ovum, for, in the newly-born
and in children, follicles of the same size and even larger ones
exist without bursting—the so-called atresic follicles.

After ovulation the ovum is thrown out into the abdominal
cavity, and then, influenced by the wave movement of the ciliated
epithelium of the tube, the fimbriæ of the ampulla, and the fimbriæ ovaricæ, finds its way into the uterus.   The wave movement
of the ciliated epithelium causes a current in the peritoneal
plasma which directs the ovum into one or other of the tubes.

A fecundated ovum embeds itself in the lining of the uterus
through centrifugal descent.   The ovum then causes a reaction in
the surrounding tissue and a dilatation of the surrounding lymph
spaces, so that a resulting localized edema takes place.   In addition a dilatation of the capillaries is produced.

The outer layer of the ovum develops into what is known as the
trophoblast, which is a product of the ectoderm, and from it
develop the cells of Langhans and the syncytium.

Shortly after the ovum is embedded in the mucosa a connection
between the trophoblast and the maternal blood takes place
through a rupture of the capillaries.   The maternal blood then
bathes the ectodermal trophoblast.   This opening of the maternal
vessels occurs, however, *before the formation of villi;* and the
cells of the trophoblast may therefore enter the maternal veins
at the very earliest period.

The compact layer of the decidua is the zone which envelops
the ovum.   The trophoblast at points may extend far into the
compacta, for *the cells have a decided power of wandering.*   The
trophoblast, therefore, invades the maternal tissues even at the
earliest period.

A gradual transition of trophoblast cells into syncytial cells,
and a gradual change of trophoblast nuclei to syncytial nuclei,
take place through the corrosive action of the maternal blood,
and elements of the maternal blood aid in forming the syncytial
protoplasm.   The syncytium does not originate from the maternal endothelium, nor from the uterine epithelium, nor from
the decidua cells.

Just as, in the early stages, the trophoblast invades the decidua, so, after the formation of villi, is the future course of the
ectodermal trophoblast and of the syncytial cells of a destructive
character so far as the decidua is concerned.   The trophoblast and
syncytium invade the maternal tissue and mingle with it.   They

infiltrate the decidua and bring it to destruction. The trophoblast and syncytial cells erode the capillaries and blood vessels,
the blood in turn changing fetal cells to syncytium.

The invading trophoblast and syncytial cells have at all times
a great power of wandering. They enter, between bundles of
muscular and connective tissue, into the lymph spaces and into
the blood vessels. At full term the uterine wall is infiltrated with
fetal cells of a syncytial character.

From the very earliest moment *fetal cells are continually entering the blood of the mother*, not only in the primary intervillous
space but in the fully formed intervillous space, as well as
through the vessels of the uterine decidua and wall.

CHORIO-EPITHELIOMA.

Under chorio-epithelioma we distinguish two forms, the typical
and atypical. In the typical form (Fig. 43) we find large, round,
polyhedral cells with strikingly large, very irregular, lobulated
nuclei which stain very deeply and often degenerate, forming
vacuoles. The protoplasm is relatively scanty. These cells are
capable of great wandering and are found more or less isolated
between the muscle and the connective-tissue bundles (Fig. 46),
in the lymph spaces and in the vessels. They form the advance
guard in the way of infiltration. There are, further, irregular
bridges of protoplasm containing scattered or grouped nuclei of
various sizes (Fig. 44). Many of these groups of nuclei are the
same large, irregular, lobulated nuclei as were observed in the
form just mentioned. In addition are found irregular masses of
protoplasm containing many small nuclei. The character of the
latter is identical with normal syncytium.

The irregular groups of protoplasm containing grouped nuclei
of various sizes are undoubtedly of syncytial character, for they
result through the blood surrounding and infiltrating the cells
of Langhans, and it is very evident that these cells form the aforementioned grape-like nuclei (Fig. 45). The isolated large cells
are likewise of syncytial character. They have generally been
mistaken for decidua cells. They may be distinguished from the
cells of Langhans, for the latter are pale, polyhedral groups of
distinctly epithelial character. They are rich in glycogen and
therefore often contain vacuoles. The nuclei are large but pale.

The cells of Langhans are better illustrated in the atypical
form (Fig. 47) where the syncytial elements are relatively in the
background. In fact, no more and no different syncytial cells are

present here than in normal gestation.   The trophoblast cells lie
closely grouped and are surrounded by syncytial elements in
quite the same manner as in normal gestation, or especially in
tubal gestation.   They are polygonal cells, concerning which
different views have been held.   They have been called decidua
cells.   No vessels of their own, however, are present in these
epithelial-like groups, and their character, their structure, and

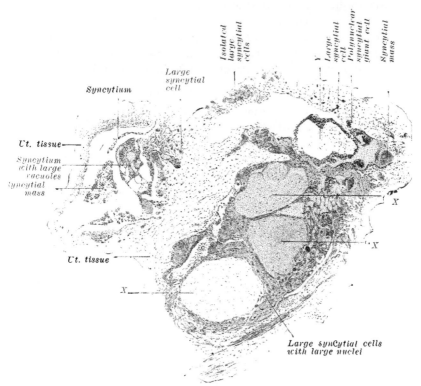

Fig. 43.—Low-power drawing of the typical form of chorio-epithelioma, showing the uterine wall invaded by chorionic elements.   *X X X*, three areas of dense
connective tissue surrounded by chorionic epithelial elements and resembling
chorionic villi.   *Y*, connective tissue centre surrounded by polynuclear syncytial
mass of considerable thickness, probably a villus.

their arrangement so closely resemble the trophoblast cells observed in normal gestation that any other view is not to be considered.   These epithelial-like cells and the syncytial masses of
various forms all originate from the trophoblast cells.

In these growths newly formed villi have not yet been found—
a proof of the limited power of differentiation possessed by the

trophoblast cells alone. It may be said, therefore, that two forms of this tumor exist, the first typical, the second atypical. The former cases are so characteristic that they cannot be mistaken. The latter have been so frequently called carcinoma by eminent au-

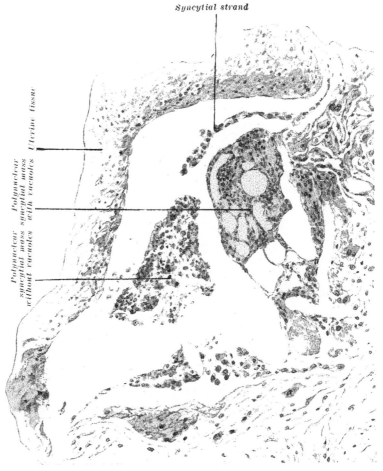

FIG. 44.—Upper left-hand corner of Fig. 43 highly magnified, showing the character of the polynuclear syncytial masses. Along the right and lower borders are larger isolated mononuclear syncytial cells.

thorities that our belief that many of these are overlooked and incorrectly diagnosed is certainly true.

A study of the histology of so-called deciduomata, and a comparison of their structure with the structure of normal placental elements, prove these tumors to be of fetal origin. The cells from which they develop are the cells which cover the chorionic villi. Since these are epithelial in character, these tumors, belonging as they do to the most malignant forms, should be called chorio-epithelioma.

We have, then, in the chorio-epitheliomata a reproduction of the same constituent elements as are found in normal placentation and as are observed in benign and malignant cases of hydatid mole. These cells exert the same influence and effect on the maternal tissues as do the fetal cells in a normal uninterrupted pregnancy.

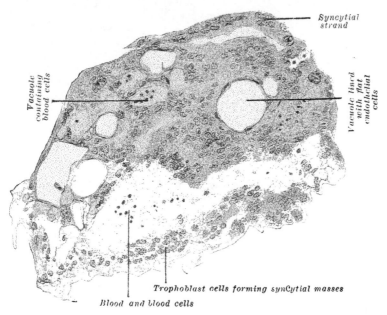

Fig. 45.—Highly magnified area of Fig. 44, showing finer characteristics of syncytial masses. Change of trophoblast cells *en masse* into polynuclear. vacuolar structures.

They invade, as do the normal trophoblast cells, the maternal decidua and destroy it. They infiltrate and erode the walls of the vessels. They invade and infiltrate deeply, too, the uterine wall. They advance either as distinct Langhans or trophoblast cells or as syncytial cells, or else they undergo in their advance a change from the former to the latter, especially when in contact with maternal blood, as in the case of placentation either uterine or tubal. Their invasion of the maternal vessels and capillaries gives them. from their earliest existence as malignant cells, the opportunity of invading the maternal circulation with a resulting early formation of metastases.   Their ability to erode the vessels causes profuse and constant bleeding.   Their ability to destroy the maternal tissue as they advance produces larger and smaller areas of degeneration and necrosis accompanied by the presence of much fibrin.   These cells preserve their ability to grow when they reach their new locations, with the result that they produce in the various organs, but most frequently in the vagina, malignant nodules of the same character as the parent growth.   In fact, these secondary nodules have in some cases been observed before the character of the uterine symptoms called attention to the presence of malignant conditions in the uterus.

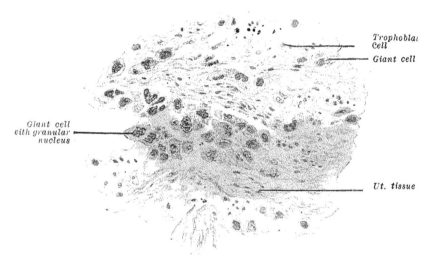

FIG. 46.—Highly magnified area of Fig. 43. showing character of isolated mononuclear giant syncytial cells and the infiltration by them of the uterine tissue and lymph spaces.

The fetal cells producing a chorioma are situated in the most favorable surrounding.   They have been performing practically malignant functions in that they have destroyed, even during normal placentation, maternal tissues, and have invaded maternal vessels, and have been carried off into the maternal circulation. When connected as part and parcel of an ovum, when feeding and nourishing the fetus with the products of the maternal blood which have passed through them, they are, so to speak, under control of the parent organism the ovum, yet when released from this connection they continue an independent growth of their

own.   It is quite probable that in hydatid mole the edematous
swelling of the chorionic stroma is due to interference with the
proper exchange between the fetus and the mother, due to a more
or less increased and independent growth on the part of those
cells whose function it is, normally, to aid and permit of this
exchange.   It is likewise probable that the growth of the chorionic
cells in chorio-epithelioma takes place during the pregnancy and
is rather the cause than the result of abortion.

We have observed in the development and change of trophoblast cells to syncytium that the closely grouped cells, when
vascularized, change to plasmodial or syncytial cells.   That the

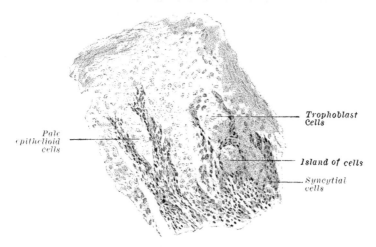

Pale epithelioid cells

Trophoblast Cells

Island of cells

Syncytial cells

Fig. 47.—High-power drawing of atypical chorio-epithelioma greatly resembling
carcinoma.

blood of the mother furnishes the greater portion of the protoplasm of these syncytial cells h'as been clearly shown.   Therefore
their production and growth, even in normal conditions, depends
upon their taking up from the mother essential elements, while
the trophoblast cells themselves furnish the nuclei.   Therefore
the growth of so pathological a tumor as a chorio-epithelioma is
not absolutely a reproduction of fetal cells, but is in a more or
less direct manner a maternal production also.

The invasion and destruction of maternal tissues in normal
gestation occurs within certain fixed limits, and the fetal cells
entering the maternal circulation undergo no future growth.
What preserves this balance?   What limits and controls the

potential of the parasitic fetal cells? In hydatid mole, and especially in chorio-epithelioma, the fetal cells are no longer held in check and they possess the power of unlimited growth. What has upset the normal balance?

When the fecundated ovum enters the uterus, it destroys the surface epithelium under it and descends actively into the decidua. It produces a decided reaction in its immediate circumference, so that even in its earliest stages it evidences a chemical power. When the maternal blood makes its exit from the capillaries it ought to coagulate, but does not. It circulates against the fetal cells which have the power to prevent coagulation. The trophoblast and syncytial cells are bathed by maternal blood and enter the circulation; therefore the ovum has a certain enzyme action and the fetal cells may be said to furnish or represent a placental secretion.

On the other hand, the blood contains elements which exert a corrosive action on the trophoblast cells, changing them to syncytium. The resulting syncytial cells then cover the villi; they play the part of endothelium (which they then greatly resemble) and protect the cells of Langhans and the stroma from the corrosive influence of the blood. That the individual cells in chorio-epithelioma have the power to grow without limit, and that the cells entering the circulation have the energy to produce malignant metastases, shows that *the decidua and the blood no longer have the power to limit and control their growth.*

In reviewing the anatomical and physiological characteristics of the female sex before and during pregnancy, and bearing in mind the normal changes of pregnancy (such as the cessation of menstruation, the act of labor, etc.), but especially the pathological states occurring almost entirely or exclusively in connection with pregnancy (such as osteomalacia, eclampsia, and chorio-epithelioma), we are forced to the conclusion which, while partly theoretical, is nevertheless logical.

Ovarian secretion has a great trophic influence upon the uterus. It stimulates the growth of the round cells of the stroma into decidua cells. The lining of the uterus is truly a lymphoid tissue, and it is the great development of the decidua and its secretion which prevents the involvement and macroscopical perforation of the uterine wall by the placental villi. Although it may be said that ovarian secretion stimulates the growth of the fetal cells and that certain elements in the blood hold their growth in check, it is probably the ovarian secretion in the maternal blood which aids the decidua in holding the placental development within normal limits, and which renders the trophoblast cells and the syncytial cells entering the circulation innocuous.

In normal placentation the human organism furnishes us with a process parallel to that occurring in certain bacterial infections, that is, the production of two opposing toxins or ferments: (1) a blood element, probably the ovarian secretion, and (2) the placental secretion.

In the normal woman the ovary is responsible for the periodical loss of blood known as menstruation. This process is due to a secretion furnished by the ovaries, for on their removal this process ceases and the reduction of oxygen exchange amounts to twenty per cent. This secretion stimulates various functions of the body, and at regular periods an outlet for this secretion occurs. Every menstruation represents, in addition, the birth of a non-fecundated ovum, that is, a labor *en miniature*.

When, however, fecundation and development of the ovum take place, the ovum and its enzymes nullify the menstrual stimulation of the ovarian secretion. The trophoblast cells invade the maternal decidua which is stimulated by the ovarian secretion, and likewise enter the blood of the mother. A normal gestation is accompanied by the stimulating effects of the retained ovarian secretion and these two enzymes are then opposed in their action. No menstruation occurs, for the placental secretion has nullified the action of the usual forces.

At the end of nine months, when the ovarian secretion is sufficient in amount or character to overcome the neutralizing action of the enzymes of the ovum, labor occurs, that is, the same process as is observed in a minuter degree in menstruation, for menstruation, as said before, is a labor *en miniature*.

Remembering the constitutional action of ovarian secretion, it may be said that if, shortly before, during, or after labor, there is an overwhelming superiority of the ovarian secretion over the placental or a mal-relation between ovarian and placental secretion, the constitutional involvement known as eclampsia results.

Following the analogy further, it may be said that chorio-epithelioma is due to the fact that the resistance to the fetal enzymes and fetal cells offered by the blood and the ovarian secretion is insufficient to hold the growth of the fetal cells in check. Chorio-epithelioma occurring generally after abortion or hydatid mole is certainly the cause rather than the result of the abortion. Chorio-epithelioma represents a more advanced stage than that of hydatid mole, but both of these conditions follow the normal processes in their course and growth. The only difference is the power of unlimited growth possessed by the chorionic cells in these pathological conditions. The difference in the resistance offered by the patient points to a constitutional element as an important factor in the etiology of chorio-epithelioma.

127 East Sixty-first street.

A CHANGE NEEDED IN OUR PRACTICE IN DEALING WITH CANCER OF THE UTERUS AND CANCER OF THE BREAST.

BY

A. LAPTHORN SMITH, B.A., M.D., M.R.C.S. Eng.,

Fellow of the American and British Gynecological Societies; Professor of Gynecology in the University of Vermont; Professor of Clinical Gynecology in Bishop's University, Montreal; Surgeon-in-Chief of the Samaritan Free Hospital for Women; Gynecologist to the Western General Hospital and to the Montreal Dispensary, Montreal, Can.

Ten years ago I had accumulated sufficient evidence to convince me that cancer was a contagious disease and that, contrary to the opinion generally held, it was not hereditary. I cannot give all the evidence here, but one or two instances must suffice. First, it has been the exception and not the rule for any of my cancer patients to have had a cancerous father or mother; second, it has been the rule that they have lived in the house with a cancerous husband or other person who was no blood relation to them, or, as in the case of two sick nurses, they attended a woman with cancer; third, many others were exposed to contagion in other ways, such as being examined by a doctor who had just examined a woman with cancer without disinfecting his finger. Although the tradition of the heredity of cancer is so deeply rooted in the popular mind, we should leave ourselves open to conviction, as there was just the same stubborn objection to the introduction of the belief in the contagiousness of tubercle twenty years ago, the belief in the heredity of which latter disease lasted many years after its contagiousness was absolutely proved. Believing, as I do, that cancer can be conveyed by contact, if the receiving soil is favorable, I think that every hopeless case of cancer should be isolated, or at least that precautions should be taken to limit the spread of the disease, such as the wearing of jute pads to collect the discharges, which pads should be burned; also, the frequent douching with formalin or permanganate of potash to destroy the cancer cells which are thrown off in the discharges; and the disinfection of the patient's own hands, as well as those of her attendants, whenever they are brought in contact with diseased surfaces. We shall never know how many cases of cancer owe their origin to contagion carried by the examining physician's fingers. When this possibility has been fully realized the same thing will happen, I believe, that has happened with puerperal fever—there will be a rapid decrease in the number of cases.

Cancer of the uterus, whether of the cervix or of the body, is in the beginning an absolutely local disease, and if operated on at this stage, and under absolutely antiseptic precautions against infecting the cut surfaces, the operation would give us one hundred per cent of ultimate recoveries. It seems difficult to get either patients or their physicians to realize that on one certain day in the history of the case there was no cancer and that on the next day the case was cancerous. More than once a medical friend in the country has brought me a case of cancer for operation, in an inoperable condition, six months after he had first seen the case and begun to treat it with nitrate of silver applied through a cylindrical speculum, telling me of his own accord that the lacerated cervix, which he took for an ulcer, looked worse every time he saw it. Such a course is little less than criminal. In one case the doctor's remorse for his delay in advising removal was truly painful to behold. Surely it must be time to make a change in our practice when the best operators all over the world now refuse to operate on from eighty to ninety per cent of the cases brought to them because they find that not one of these rejected cases would be alive in two years after removal of the uterus. I presume their reason for refusing is that an operation which does no good to the patient does harm to other patients with the same disease in a less advanced stage, who could be saved by operation, but refuse to undergo it because they have seen the bad results in others, who were not fit subjects for operation. Our only hope, therefore, is to get the cases as near the beginning as possible and then not to lose a day in having the diseased area removed. If the disease were not so awful or so fatal I would be satisfied to remove the cervix only, as I have had a few cases who not only remained well for many years, but also one who bore several children afterward; but, considering the terrible risk we run of thereby leaving a minute portion of diseased tissue above the internal os, I feel that the only safe course to pursue is to remove the whole uterus. Must we also remove the ovaries and tubes? A few years ago I would have answered, "Not unless the disease has reached the fundus." But having seen two cases of the disease recurring in the ovaries more than a year after extirpation of the uterus, at which time they were apparently healthy, I think we should, whenever we can do it without greatly increasing the primary mortality, remove the adnexa for the sake of insuring a good remote result.

Above I have expressed the opinion that if the uterus were removed at the very beginning, under strict precautions against infecting the remaining raw surfaces, there would be no recurrences. While I recognize the fact that many so-called recurrences are nothing more nor less than the same disease which has already extended to the broad ligament, continuing on its fatal course unhindered or even hastened by the operation, yet I think there are many others in which the disease was limited to the uterus and yet during the operation some of the cancerous juices got on to the raw edges and quickly inoculated them. We cannot, therefore, be too careful to cut away all ulcerating surfaces and then dry them up with the thermocautery before beginning the extirpation. The uterine cavity should then be carefully packed firmly with dry sublimated cotton to prevent any liquid from being squeezed out of the uterus during the manipulation. Merely sewing up the cervix is not enough, as I have proved by passing the water from the tap through the sewed-up cervix after the uterus has been removed. If my premises are correct, then the method, lately advocated, of splitting the uterus and removing it in two halves should be abandoned. If the diseased organ is too large to remove by the vagina, it would be better to free the cervix by a vaginal incision, clamping the uterine arteries, then opening the abdomen and tying off the broad ligaments, after which the uterus can be removed quite easily and without infecting the peritoneum, which latter is the cause of the high mortality after abdominal hysterectomy for cancer.

The primary mortality of the operation of vaginal hysterectomy for cancer in the most favorable cases is quite small; in fact, under certain conditions I believe it would be *nil*. These conditions are, first, that the operator be an expert who can complete the operation in from ten to fifteen minutes; second, that

12

there be no hemorrhage, either primary during the operation or later from slipping of the ligatures.   For this reason I prefer the magnificent clamps which Ségond brought to America four years ago, and which I procured soon after and have used ever since.   Although I have used catgut ligatures in a considerable number of vaginal hysterectomies, I have never felt sure that they would not allow the ovarian artery to slip out of the knot, especially in those cases where the uterus could not be well pulled down.   We are obliged to drag the uterus forcibly down in order to get the ligature on, and what then appears to be a very tight knot may become a very loose one when the tension is removed. When removing ovarian cysts by the abdomen I always take the precaution of relaxing the pedicle before putting the final strain on the first knot.   Jacobs claims that the woman is *brisée* (broken up) more when we use clamps than by ligatures, and I have noticed the same thing.   He thinks this is due to compression of the nerves by the clamps, while the ligatures only compress the arteries.   Even so, however, I consider the advantages of the clamps in greater speed and security from hemorrhage sufficient to give them the preference.   There is one point well worth remembering, namely, to put the clamp on the ovarian artery from above downward instead of from below upward, as there is then absolutely no danger of the top of the broad ligament slipping out of its bite.

Nothing short of a revolution in our present policy of waiting for more proof holds out any hope of improving our present wretched showing.   That the subject is worth while discussing is evident when we consider that over one hundred thousand people die every year from cancer in Europe and America alone, and that the uterus and the breast are the most frequent locations.   The prevention and cure of cancer offers the greatest field for our energies, excepting tuberculosis, of all the subjects in medicine and surgery.   Every one of these thirty-five or forty thousand women who die annually from cancer of the uterus might be saved if the following plan were faithfully carried out by every individual practitioner.   The first thing to do is to abolish laceration of the cervix, for the best time to save a woman from death from cancer is before she gets it; the preventive treatment of cancer begins at her first confinement.   Give Nature time to complete the first stage of labor absolutely without interference, unless it be to check its rapidity by the judicious use of opium so that the pains will be less frequent and less violent.

Were I to write the history of the several hundred lacerated cervices I have repaired it would make a sad record, for there are many among them in whom the forceps was applied without the shadow of an excuse an hour or two after the first pains of a first confinement; and Emmet, the greatest authority on lacerations of the cervix, has stated positively that he has never met with cancer of the cervix without a previous laceration, for even in a virgin who came to him with epithelioma of the cervix he found on investigation that she had had divulsion of the cervix performed for dysmenorrhea many years before. I believe that if one could make out a list of the various countries, according to the amount of belief their practitioners and specialists have in the importance of laceration of the cervix and the necessity for its repair, we would find that cancer was diminishing in those countries at the top of the list and increasing in those at the bottom. I have recently seen it stated that cancer of the uterus was increasing greatly in Germany and decreasing in the United States and Canada; and it seemed to me, during my visits to these two countries, that the German physicians thought that lacerations of the cervix were of very little importance, while the physicians of the United States were the most keenly alive to the necessity for their repair. For my own part, among the seven thousand cases on my records at the various hospitals and dispensaries which I attend, cancer of the uterus is becoming more and more rare. While, ten or fifteen years ago, a case presented itself almost every week, now I do not find a case once in two or three months, and this notwithstanding that I am looking out more carefully than ever for them and that I have a larger number of patients to examine. I attribute this to the fact that I have amputated or repaired every cervix sufficiently lacerated to have eversion of the lips and consequent ulceration and scar tissue. I also believe that all my medical friends who send cases to me fully realize the importance of following this plan. So that ninety-five per cent of the lacerations have been repaired, and even the few remaining ones are only waiting till their babies are weaned in order to have it done. There is one fallacy which I would like to controvert: that a woman with a lacerated cervix runs no risk of cancer until she is 45 years of age. I have seen several women under 30 die from cancer of the cervix during the last twenty years, and quite recently I have seen a painful instance of it which I will briefly relate. A little over a year ago a married woman, 32 years of age, the mother of one child, 8 years of age, which was born after a severe instrumental labor, consulted me for menorrhagia and a painful ovary. On examination she was found to have a badly lacerated cervix, which I urged her to have repaired immediately. It not being convenient to do so then, she asked why it could not wait a year, when it would be more convenient. I replied that it would not only break down her health, but that there was danger of cancer if she waited till she was 45. She went away promising to return in a year. which she did, but when I examined her then I found the everted anterior lip a mass of bleeding, angry-looking granulations. On account of her age I could hardly believe that it was cancer, and I lost two weeks in treating it with soothing applications with very little benefit. I then took her to the Western Hospital for curetting, not having been able to obtain her consent to hysterectomy. When I proceeded to dilate the uterus the anterior lip of the cervix broke easily and came away with the curette. I gave some of the tissue to a pathological friend, who made many sections before he was sure that it was cancer. As she was a resident of New York and had most of her friends there. I sent her to a gynecologist there of world-wide reputation who had many facilities for the care of such a case, which I had not. He kindly took charge of her, but was loath to remove the uterus without first receiving pathological confirmation of our suspicions. It was two months before the pathologist could be sure that it was cancer. but as soon as this was decided my friend removed the uterus and ovaries and tubes. She made a splendid recovery from the operation. but she is doomed to die, as already after three months the disease is recurring in the stump. So that even a woman of 32 with lacerated cervix is not safe from cancer.

Now. with regard to hemorrhage after the menopause, we cannot lay too much stress upon the importance of this as a symptom of cancer, more especially as there is a belief widespread among women that the return of menstruation after the menopause is a matter of congratulation and an evidence of renewed vitality and usefulness. There is no more disastrous idea, and we should do our utmost to controvert it until every woman over 40 shall be filled with apprehension if she menstruates after having gone through the menopause. I consider that this is the only symptom which is present early enough to warn us in time to do anything effective in saving the woman from the dreadful fate overhanging her. When she has pain and a foul-smelling discharge it is too late; when she has the yellow, cachectic appearance of the skin it is more than too late; when she has a profuse watery discharge, even without a bad odor, it is late enough, and so it is with hemorrhage after intercourse. I am frequently asked by medical friends upon whom I am urging these views: "Do you mean to say that you would remove a uterus from a woman of 45 just because she had had several uterine hemorrhages two years after the menopause or because she had a watery discharge?" That is just what I mean to say, and if we wish to save the thousands of lives that are now being lost every year we must adopt an entirely different course from that which has been followed in the past. The plan I advocate gives practically no mortality at the operation and absolutely no ultimate mortality from the disease. The policy of delay which has been followed so long has a high mortality from the operation and holds out little or no hope of ultimate recovery.

Just a word or two about cancer of the breast before closing. My experience in thirty-five or forty cases has been just the same: many cases came too late for any treatment; in others I was obliged to remove not only the whole of the breast, but also the skin covering it, to remove the pectoralis major and minor and every particle of the cellular tissue and glands in the axilla; and not one of these women was alive after two years; most of them died in six to twelve months. The only bright spot in my experience of cancer of the breast is having removed the breast about fifteen times for a small lump which was not fixed and had not yet infected the glands. All these patients are alive and free from recurrence, and some of them have lived now seven years after their operation, although the examination of the growth proved beyond doubt its cancerous nature. Of course I do not wish to detract in the slightest from the value of the thorough operation, but I mean to urge the importance of removing every lump from the breasts of women about 40 as soon as discovered, instead of waiting six months to make sure that it is cancer.

248 BISHOP STREET.

AN OVARIAN SARCOMA DEVELOPING FROM THE THECA EXTERNA OF THE GRAAFIAN FOLLICLE.

BY

W. W. RUSSELL, M.D.,
Associate Professor of Gynecology, Johns Hopkins University,

AND

B. R. SCHENCK, M.D.,
Resident Gynecologist, Johns Hopkins Hospital.

(With five illustrations.)

STATISTICS based on 1,106 cases of malignant tumor of the ovary, gathered from 16 different gynecological clinics, show that about 14 per cent were sarcomata.

During the twelve years in which the gynecological department of the Johns Hopkins Hospital has been open there have been 73 malignant ovarian growths (exclusive of the semi-malignant papillomata), of which 11 have been sarcomatous in structure, or about 15 per cent.

The following case of cystic sarcoma is of considerable interest on account of the unique microscopical findings, from which it is possible to point out the probable genesis of the neoplasm.

Mrs. J. (Gyn. No. 3963), aged 49, was admitted to the service of Dr. Kelly at the Johns Hopkins Hospital on November 16, 1895, complaining of a painful swelling in the lower part of the abdomen.

The family and past histories were excellent.

Menstruation began at about 12 years and was always regular and painless until her forty-second year, when it ceased for a period of nearly two years. She then had a scanty, non-offensive discharge, lasting about three weeks, followed by thirteen months of amenorrhea.

Again there was an apparently normal menstruation, which was also followed by amenorrhea continuing for sixteen months. An offensive brownish discharge then began, accompanied by bearing-down pain in the left lower quadrant of the abdomen.

During the three and one-half years previous to her admission to the hospital there were irregular losses of blood from the uterus, always accompanied by more or less abdominal distress.

The patient had been married twenty-six years and was the mother of four children. The first labor, one year after marriage, was an instrumental one and occasioned a deep perineal tear which had never been repaired. The other confinements were normal and there was no history of puerperal fever.

For several years Mrs. J. had noticed that the abdomen was somewhat swollen, but she had never given this much attention and had not noted the presence of a tumor.

On examination the abdomen was slightly distended and the breathing of the abdominal type. On deep palpation a tumor mass was felt rising as high as the umbilicus. Its mobility was limited, apparently by adhesions. Percussion over the mass gave a dull tympanitic note, while around the tumor was a distinct corona of resonance.

Examination per vaginam revealed an anteposed uterus, freely movable, the tumor mass producing no bulging into the fornices. The right ovary was palpable.

The heart sounds were normal and the lungs clear.

The urinary examination was also negative.

Clinical diagnosis: Adenocystoma of the left ovary, possibly carcinomatous.

Operation.—Dr. Kelly; November 18, 1895; ether anesthesia. An incision 17 centimetres long was made in the median line through moderately thick abdominal walls. The peritoneal cavity was found to contain considerable clotted blood, which was sponged away, exposing an ovarian cyst, springing from the left ovary, adherent in the right flank and right inguinal region. Its walls were black and hemorrhagic. The adhesions on the right side were readily broken by sweeping the hand over the surface of the tumor, the omentum, which was also adherent to the left side of the tumor, ligated off, and the cyst rolled out of the abdomen. It was then discovered that the pedicle was twisted one and one-half times from left to right, thus accounting for the necrotic appearance of the tumor.

The pedicle was then tied off with silk and catgut ligatures.

The patient took ether well from the beginning of the anesthesia, when the pulse was 100 to the minute, strong and regular.

As the last sutures in the incision were being tied the patient suddenly stopped breathing and, despite long-continued artificial respiration and repeated stimulation, died.

The postmortem examination, made by Dr. Simon Flexner,

revealed no metastases.   Death was probably due to changes in
the myocardium and atheroma of the coronary arteries.

Résumé of the Postmortem Protocol.—The body is that of a
well-built, well-nourished woman.   The lips, mucous membrane
of the mouth, and finger tips show a slight cyanosis.   The subcutaneous fat is moderate in amount.

In the middle line of the abdomen is an incision 17 centimetres
in length, closed by silkworm-gut stitches.   On opening the abdomen a small amount of blood is found in the pelvis.

Over an area 12 x 17 centimetres on the parietal peritoneum of
the right side are firm fibrous adhesions, many of which are tied
off with catgut ligatures, while beneath the peritoneum on the
left side are a number of small ecchymoses.

The omentum is delicate, lies across upper coils of intestines,
and its veins are engorged with blood.

The appendix is free, points downward and inward toward the
pelvis, is somewhat shorter than usual, and has a well-marked
mesentery.

The pericardium contains 30 cubic centimetres of clear serous
fluid.   Both layers of the membrane are smooth.

The right side of the heart is collapsed and the left contracted.
The endocardium is smooth and valves are apparently normal.

Pathological Report.— (Gyn. Path. No. 974).   The specimen
consists of an ovarian cyst measuring 22 x 16 x 7.5 centimetres.
Its external surface varies in color from a dark blue to a
reddish brown and is covered by a few vascular adhesions.   Here
and there are numerous small areas of ecchymosis, and just beneath the peritoneum is a network of large branching blood vessels.   Projecting from the surface are many small bosses, varying in diameter from 1 to 5 centimetres.

The tumor is of a semi-solid consistence and its walls in many
places are friable and necrotic.

On section one finds that the specimen is composed, for the
most part, of small cysts, separated by rather firm trabeculæ.
In many places these septa have completely or partially broken
down, forming larger-sized cavities.   These cystic spaces resemble very much corpora lutea, and the whole specimen appears
like a conglomerate mass of these structures.

The outer wall is thin, averaging but 1 millimetre in thickness,
but many of the trabeculæ are much thicker, some reaching 5
centimetres in diameter.   The projecting bosses are seen to be
made up of cysts which project beyond the neighboring cavities.

The internal surface of the cysts presents a varying appearance. In some, particularly the smaller ones, it is smooth and glistening. In others there are small papillary ingrowths covered by a hemorrhagic yellow fibrinous substance. All are filled with a dark-brown mucilaginous fluid which coagulates on exposure to the air.

The tumor is very vascular, many large vessels traversing the septa in all directions.

The portion of the tube present is 9 centimetres long and averages 8 millimetres in diameter. It is free from adhesions and has a patent fimbriated extremity.

The parovarial tubes are well seen and present a normal appearance.

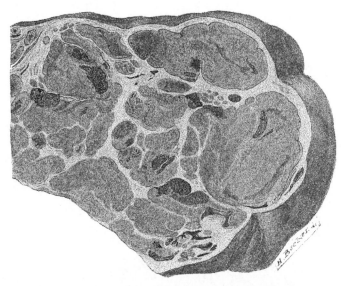

FIG. 1 (natural size).—Cut surface of a portion of the tumor, hardened in Müller's fluid, showing trabeculæ and cysts resembling corpora lutea.

Unfortunately, no sketch was made when the specimen was fresh, but Fig. 1 gives a clear idea of the freshly cut surface of a portion of the hardened preparation.

Many sections were cut from various portions of the tumor. On microscopic examination the majority of these show nothing but large areas of canalized fibrin, together with smaller portions of tissue in which there is so much coagulation necrosis and nuclear fragmentation that the structure of the tissue cannot be made out.

In those parts of the tumor, however, where the necrosis caused by the twisting of the pedicle is least marked, there is a distinct alveolar structure.   The stroma is made up of connective tissue,

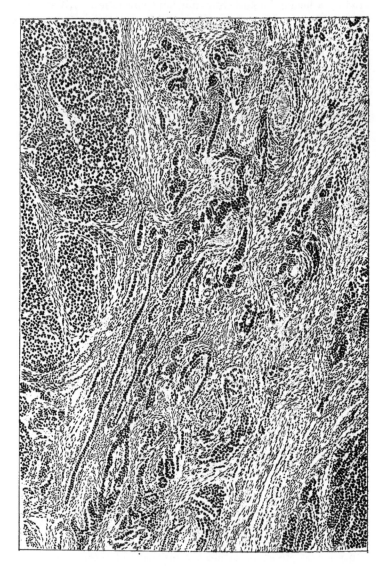

FIG. 2 (× 135).—Section showing the alveolar arrangement of the sarcoma cells, and stroma containing lymph spaces filled with round cells.

the cells of which are spindle-shaped, taking the eosin stain fairly well and presenting long, well-preserved nuclei.

In places this stroma is fairly dense and sends off delicate ramifications which subdivide the tumor mass into alveoli (Fig. 2).

These alveoli are filled by round cells which have an average diameter of 6 to 7 microns. The protoplasm of the cells is generally clear and takes the eosin stain very faintly. The nuclei are relatively large and vesicular in outline, the intensity of the nuclear stain being very variable. In many cells the nucleus is dense and homogeneously stained a dark blue. In others it is

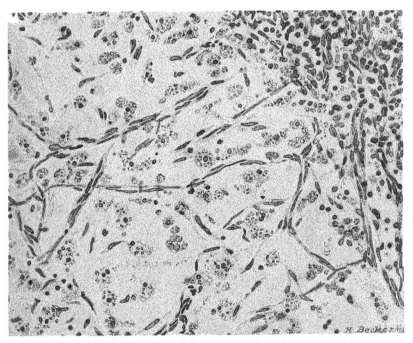

FIG. 3 (× 360).—Section, more highly magnified, showing the round sarcoma cells having relatively large vesicular nuclei, the formation of new capillaries in the stroma, and the large phagocytic cells.

granular and the chromatin network is well seen. Here and there are cells several times larger than the neighboring ones, with large dark nuclei.

Karyokinetic figures are present, but occur in small numbers (Fig. 3).

There is apparently little tendency of the cells to invade the stroma, the alveoli being for the most part sharply circumscribed. Numerous red blood corpuscles are diffused throughout all parts of the specimen.

In some areas the formation of new capillaries is well marked, as is seen in Fig. 3. This also shows numerous large phagocytic cells containing the remains of red blood corpuscles and fragmented nuclei.

So far the description of the specimen might apply to any

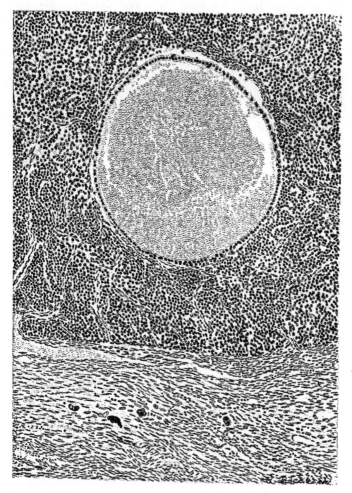

FIG. 4 (× 240).—Section showing a small Graafian follicle surrounded by an alveolus filled with the sarcoma cells.

cystic sarcoma of the round-celled variety having an alveolar arrangement. The peculiarity and the interest in these specimens lie in the fact that the sarcoma cells bear a characteristic relation to the Graafian follicles.

Throughout the sections one sees follicles of various stages, many of them degenerated, but some of them almost perfectly preserved, as seen in Fig. 4.

We have here a small Graafian follicle approximately 0.12 millimetre in diameter. It is filled with red blood corpuscles and lined by an almost perfect layer of large cells with large vesicular nuclei, the cells being characteristic of the granulosa layer. The outer layer of cells, those forming the theca externa, has more or less completely disappeared, and many of them are indistinguishable from the sarcoma cells which everywhere surround the follicle.

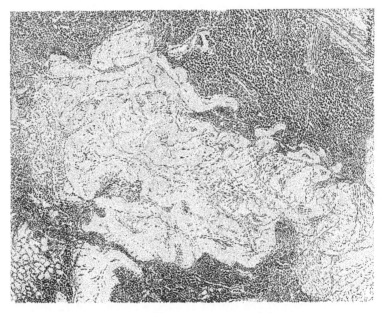

FIG. 5 (× 75).—Section showing hyaline degeneration closely resembling a corpus luteum.

This picture is frequently met with throughout the sections.

Many parts of the tumor show large areas of hyaline degeneration, and in a few places the hyaline material is so arranged that it resembles the remains of a corpus luteum. The most striking of these areas is pictured in Fig. 5.

In the stroma are many blood vessels, a great number of which are of large size. Spaces filled with the sarcoma cells are also seen and may be interpreted as lymphatic spaces into which the cells have grown.

It is probable that malignant connective-tissue tumors may develop from any of the mesoblastic tissue found within the ovary. While most cases undoubtedly have their origin in the stroma cells, as is seen in the usual type of sarcomata, the vessels of the ovary, as of other organs, may also be the starting point of neoplasms, thus producing endo- and peritheliomata of the blood vessels and lymphatics.

There is no reason to suppose that the thecæ of the Graafian follicle may not also be the starting point of such tumors. So far as we have been able to find, however, no such origin has ever been pointed out.

While it is of course impossible to state absolutely what the origin is in this case, it seems probable, from the number of sections showing nests of sarcoma cells grouped about follicles, that the neoplasm has developed from the theca externa of the Graafian follicle.

The very apparent transition from the normal spindle-shaped cells of the outer layer into the fully developed sarcoma cells also supports this view.

REPORT OF A CASE OF EPITHELIOMA OF THE CLITORIS, WITH OPERATION.[1]

BY

CHARLES P. NOBLE, M.D.,

Surgeon-in-Chief, Kensington Hospital for Women,
Philadelphia.

(With one illustration.)

EPITHELIOMA of the clitoris is such a rare condition that the following case is believed to be worthy of report. Mrs. G., aged 65, multipara, consulted me for a tumor of the clitoris. Her general health had been good. Locally she had complained for at least twenty years of pruritus vulvæ. The itching had varied from time to time, but had been very severe for years. She was extremely neurasthenic and very despondent. She had only known of the growth for a short time. Upon examination a distinct tumor of the clitoris was found which was at least half an inch in breadth and thickness, and almost, if not quite, half an

[1]Read before the Section on Gynecology, College of Physicians of Philadelphia, April 17, 1902.

inch in depth.   There were some prolongations of the growth toward the right labium majus.   The skin of the labia majora was
distinctly unhealthy in appearance.   It was edematous, poorly
nourished, its surface macerated, nodular, and covered with
thickened, whitish epithelium.   No enlargement could be made
out in the inguinal glands.   A diagnosis of epithelioma of the
clitoris complicated by long-standing pruritus vulvæ was made
and excision advised.

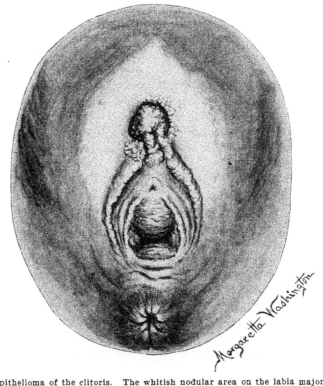

Epithelioma of the clitoris.   The whitish nodular area on the labia majora indicates the inflammatory thickening and the secondary implantation growths.

Owing to the bad prognosis given by standard authorities for
epithelioma of the external genitals, it has long been my intention to apply the principles so well recognized in dealing with
cancer of the breast to operation upon this region when a favorable case should present itself, and on December 13, 1901, the
following operation was performed:

An incision was made from just above the urethra outward and
downward to the labium majus upon each side.   The urethra

was dissected loose from the pubic arch and the incision on each side was made down to the periosteum. From the outer extremity of each incision a second incision was made through the labium majus and extending into the mons Veneris. These two incisions met at a point in the middle line well above the pubic bone. The incisions were carried down to the periosteum of the pubic bones, and the entire tissues of the vestibule, labia majora, and the lower portion of the mons Veneris were removed in one piece. This was done with a sharp knife, dissecting as closely as possible all tissue away from the periosteum. The skin of the outer portion of the labia majora was then separated laterally to a sufficient extent to permit the skin structures to be approximated in the middle line.

The lymphatics from each groin were removed in the following manner: An incision was made from the margin of the wound, over Poupart's ligament, to the anterior superior spine of the ilium. The skin margins of the wound were reflected upward and downward, and then the fatty tissues, including the lymphatics, were removed for a breadth of at least two inches by removing all tissue down to the aponeurosis of the external oblique and the fascia lata. Bleeding points were ligated with catgut as necessary. The extensive wound surfaces were then brought together by sutures.

The convalescence was afebrile. On the fourth day, however, it was observed that the vulvar flaps, particularly upon the left side, were sloughing. A slough, roughly one inch in diameter, formed and separated. Later there was some suppuration in the inguinal wounds; this, however, was clearly due to the sloughing process. The sloughing was due to the poor nutrition of the skin of the flaps, and not to infection. After the slough separated the open wound healed rapidly under the influence of balsam of Peru.

A gratifying feature of the convalescence was the prompt disappearance of the itching which had persisted for twenty years. This feature was borne in mind in performing the operation, and care was taken to cut the ilio-inguinal nerves where they emerge from the external inguinal rings, and also to remove the tissue down to the periosteum over the pubic bones, to cut and remove all branches of the pubic nerves coming up to the vulva from below. The relief from itching has continued, and there has been an entire loss of sensation in the area of the operation.

As the epithelioma was superficial in character, as the operation was a very radical one, and as the report of the pathologist is that the inguinal glands were not involved, the prognosis is good. The principles employed in operating upon this case are to be recommended in dealing with all cases of epithelioma of the external genitals, and there is reason to believe that when this is done the prognosis from epithelioma of the external genitals will become relatively favorable, instead of positively bad as heretofore.

Appended is the report of the pathologist, Dr. Babcock:

"The specimen consists of a portion of the mons Veneris, the upper portions of both labia majora, and the vestibule, with the subcutaneous fascia and fat. It is characterized by a rounded mass with a granular, non-ulcerated surface and a broad pedicle, about 2 centimetres (three-fourths of an inch) in diameter, that projects from the vestibule at the situation of the clitoris for about 1½ centimetres (five-eighths of an inch). The adjacent surfaces of the labia are excoriated and show a number of small, irregular, wart-like growths embedded in and firmly adherent to the skin. Embedded in the fat from the inguinal region are two moderately enlarged lymphatic glands.

"*Microscopy.*—Vertical sections through the tumor of the clitoris, stained and examined under the microscope, show it to be covered by a layer of stratified squamous epithelium. In places this layer is thin or absent. Descending from the surface are large, irregularly rounded columns or masses of characteristic squamous epithelial cells. These invade the deeper layers of the corium, but the subcutaneous fibrous and areolar tissues below are nearly free from invasion. There are numerous epithelial pearls. There is a marked inflammatory reaction throughout the growth, as indicated by areas of intense leucocytic infiltration. Despite the rather superficial character of the invasion, the picture is characteristic of squamous epithelioma. Sections taken from the adjacent wart-like growths upon the labia also reveal a distinct epithelial ingrowth. These growths may be considered as secondary infections from contact. The masses of epithelium have invaded the subcutaneous connective tissues and contain numerous epithelial pearls. There is a marked leucocytic infiltration.

"Examination of the lymphatic glands shows an inflammatory enlargement but no distinct epitheliomatous invasion. The pathological diagnosis is a polypoid epithelioma of the clitoris with implantation growths of the labia majora."

1509 LOCUST STREET.

13

PROPRIETY OF SIMULTANEOUS ATTENDANCE UPON SCARLET FEVER AND OBSTETRICAL CASES.

BY

A. REICH, M.D.,
New York.

THE general practitioner is almost daily confronted with the problem as to what he should do with obstetrical cases while attending infectious diseases. Consulting the literature, we find that Braxton Hicks[1] says "that the puerperal woman, when infected with scarlet fever, develops puerperal fever." The same author is quoted in Playfair's "Midwifery"[2]: "Out of 68 cases of puerperal disease, 37 were distinctly traced to scarlet poison; of these, 20 had the characteristic rash of the disease, but the remaining 17 showed none of the usual symptoms and were not to be distinguished from the so-called puerperal fever. On the theory that it is impossible for the specific contagious disease to be modified by the puerperal state, we have to admit that one physician met with 17 cases of puerperal septicemia in which, by a mere coincidence, the contagion of scarlet fever had been traced, and that the disease nevertheless originated from some other source—a hypothesis so improbable that its mere mention carries its own refutation."

In Olshausen and Veit's book on obstetrics we find that a great deal of attention has been given to a disease called scarlatina puerperalis, which was described as a puerperal septicemia with a scarlet rash.

We meet occasionally with a rash in septicemia and in pyemia. We also know that a puerperal woman may have scarlet fever which runs its natural course, and if it occurs with puerperal fever there is no special effect of one on the other in the majority of cases.

As an illustration of the cases reported as scarlet fever in puerperæ, I cite a case by Fiessinger.[3] Confinement, May 2. On

[1] Transactions of the Obstetrical Society of London, 1871.
[2] American edition.   [3] Gaz. méd. de Paris, 1893, No. 40.

the second day chill and vomiting; no pain in abdomen. The following day, temperature 40.6°C.; tympanites, without pain; intrauterine douche. On the fourth day chill and cold perspiration; temperature 41.5° C.; weak pulse. Eruption like that of measles on backs of hands and forearms, scarlet-like rash on lower extremities and body. Uterine douche. In the evening temperature 37.5° C., pulse 108. Following day, temperature 38.6° C., pulse 116; difficulty in swallowing; redness of pharynx. The eruption became more like that of scarlet fever; temperature 40.4° C., pulse 152. May 5, temperature 39.1° C., pulse 124; exanthem leaving only face free; meteorism disappearing. During the uterine douche a piece of placenta, size of nut, appeared. The days following, temperature 38.8° C. and 38° C. Eruption became paler and the patient was perfectly well on May 8. There was a bran-like desquamation. On the 30th albumin in the urine, which disappeared on milk diet.

This woman was attended by a midwife who had an infected finger; there was also an epidemic of scarlet fever. This case is no doubt one of sepsis from retained placenta, with possible scarlet fever following the infection.

My first experience was with a Swedish woman confined during 1898. On the second day her 8-year-old boy, who slept in his mother's bed, presented an angina and scarlet rash with fever. He was at once transferred to the Willard Parker Hospital, the walls of the room were washed with bichloride of mercury, and the woman made an uninterrupted recovery. Two months later the boy's older sister was taken down with the same disease. Both mother and baby escaped. From November, 1900, until March, 1901, I had occasion to treat 78 cases of scarlet fever in 25 families, with two fatal cases from nephritis. During the same period I attended 40 obstetrical cases; 14 of these were primiparæ and sustained some laceration—one through the sphincter; two had bad lacerations extending along both sulci well up into the vagina; in one a subcutaneous rupture (separation) of the symphysis pubis occurred.

A few cases will show how I was obliged to see these patients.

CASE I.—Incomplete abortion. Scarlet fever of four days' duration. Seen at 4 P.M., and at 7.30 P.M. examination of patient with carefully washed finger in the uterus for retained placenta. Temperature 100°, pulse 86. Slight bleeding. Placenta not removed at urgent request of patient; replaced the retroverted uterus. Ergot and quinine; bichloride douches. Placenta expelled spontaneously the next day. Perfect recovery.

CASE II.—Primipara. Scarlet fever of two days. Seen at 6:30 P.M.; at 8 P.M. examination of primipara. R. O. P. I rotated the posterior fontanelle to the front, and, on account of its tendency to resume its former position, held it there during a few pains. Birth of child in R. O. A. at 3 A.M.; small tear of fourchette granulated. Perfect recovery.

CASE III.—Multipara. Four cases of desquamating scarlet seen during the morning; at 8 P.M. examination of woman. Position R. O. A.; pains very sharp; pendulous abdomen. Applied binder to correct direction of uterus. At 11 P.M. complete dilatation and artificial rupture of membranes. Expulsion of infant at 1 A.M. Normal puerperium.

CASE IV.—Multipara. Same desquamating cases as in previons case, only one day later. Four hours after looking at the scarlet-fever cases, examination of puerpera. L. O. A. Four examinations made. Puerperium normal.

I make it a rule to see the postpartum cases early in the morning and do as little examining as possible. Temperature and pulse are taken daily. The genitals are inspected only for removal of sutures. Fissures of nipples are touched with stick of nitrate of silver and covered with lanolin. Before examining a woman in labor I clean my hands as if for a laparatomy, and also have the vulva washed with soap and water and then with bichloride of mercury. All water used for washing woman after delivery or baby is boiled.

My conclusions from the cases observed are: that, though attending contagious cases, I have succeeded so far in not causing septic infection of the parturient woman; and, from the observations of others, that if the parturient woman is infected with scarlet fever it runs its ordinary course; and that, while scarlet fever and puerperal sepsis may coexist, each runs its distinctive course.[1]

228 WEST THIRTY-FOURTH STREET.

[1]The following letter from one of the medical inspectors of the Department of Health of New York substantiates my conclusions:

MARCH 19, 1902.

DEAR DOCTOR REICH:—During the time which I have been doing Health Department work I have observed thirty or forty women who were confined in the same room and often in the same bed with diphtheria or scarlet-fever cases. I have kept a record of thirteen cases, including the period of the disease to which they were exposed. These cases have never had the slightest sepsis or fever: have gotten up promptly; then the rooms were fumigated. In no case has there been isolation. The women have been attended in confinement by midwives, poor doctors, and good doctors. None of the women have contracted scarlet fever or diphtheria. These cases have all been in tenement houses, filthy, etc. I have seen only one woman who had scarlet fever following confinement. She had it about the third or fourth day. Whether her doctor was attending cases of scarlet fever I do not know. (There was no scarlet in her family.) She did not have sepsis.

The conclusions to be drawn from my experience, and from that of those members of the Health Board staff with whom I have discussed the matter, is that puerperal patients are not unusually susceptible to scarlet fever or diphtheria, the books to the contrary; also, that these women are not rendered any more liable to sepsis. Five of the department inspectors are engaged to a considerable extent in obstetrical or gynecological practice. They assure me they have never had any trouble with their cases traceable to their work with contagious diseases. Personally I have never had any such trouble.

I do not wish to be understood as recommending the simultaneous care of contagious and obstetrical cases, but I believe the danger has been grossly exaggerated. Of course some doctors are filthy and do not understand aseptic or antiseptic principles, and would have sepsis whether they attended contagious cases or not.

You are at perfect liberty to quote any or all of these remarks.

Yours truly,   E. J. GRAFF. JR.

CESAREAN SECTION NECESSITATED BY VENTROSUSPENSION.[1]

BY

ADELAIDE BROWN, M.D.,
San Francisco. Cal.

History.—Mrs. K. P., aged 37 years, came to my office September 26, 1901, well advanced in pregnancy. Last menses had appeared February 1, 1901, so that she was at about the third week of the eighth month, being due November 7-14. Patient had been a delicate woman; operated on in February, 1900, for retroversion of the uterus by some form of ventrosuspension. In the following month, March, 1900, an operation for floating kidney was done. The patient gave the history of a good recovery from both operations, but was never free from abdominal pain. Con-

'Read before the Medical Society of the State of California, April, 1902.

stipation was always marked, menses regular. During her pregnancy nausea was marked in the first three months, and the abdominal pain was quite severe at times, but never enough to make her consult a physician; the pains had grown worse during the last month.

Physical Examination.—Patient sallow; face, hands, and limbs quite edematous; urine normal; heart normal. External examination of the abdomen showed a uterine enlargement very broad and at its highest point reaching one-third the distance from the umbilicus to the ensiform cartilage. Palpation showed the child in a transverse position, head to the right. Fetal heart 124. Pelvic measurements: interspinous, 25 centimetres; intercristal, 29 centimetres; external conjugate, 20 centimetres; bitrochanteric, 32 centimetres.

Internal Examination.—It was impossible to reach the cervix at all; the perineum and the vulva were unusually relaxed, but the vagina was absolutely smooth as far as could be reached.

The suspicion that the fundus was held firmly to the abdominal wall, which was suggested by the low level of the uterine tumor for a Ipara at eight months, was confirmed by the fact that the cervix was drawn up posteriorly out of reach. A second and a third examination showed no change, and I asked for consultation, having told the husband of my patient that the probabilities were very strong that to deliver the child at all a Cesarean section would be necessary. The consultation was set for October 26. On October 24, at 8:30 P.M., the membranes ruptured. I was notified and went to the patient's house, again made a thorough examination, but found the cervix out of reach, though the uterine tumor was much smaller from the loss of liquor amnii.

The patient was removed to the Children's Hospital, and Dr. Von Hoffman met me there in consultation. The patient was anesthetized and prepared for operation. Under anesthesia the cervix could not be palpated. The patient's husband had been consulted and offered, all other things being favorable, the choice of Cesarean versus Porro-Cesarean as the only hope for a living child, and as offering the best prognosis to both mother and child. Cesarean section was recommended, as the pelvis was normal and a second pregnancy in no way fraught with unusual risk to the patient.

Slight labor pains had begun and the child was living at the time of the operation, and the patient in excellent condition. The operation was begun at 12:30 A.M.; the incision, to the left of the former incision, extended from three inches above the umbilicus to the pubes. On opening the peritoneal cavity adhesions were found forming a dense band three inches broad and only long enough to allow with some difficulty the fingers to pass between the uterine and abdominal walls. There were many light adhesions over the uterine wall, and, after freeing these, the band holding down the fundus was ligated in two parts and clamped on the uterine side and cut. The anterior wall of the uterus, thus liberated, rose and occupied the field of the incision. The uterus was then drawn out of the abdominal cavity and anteverted and covered with gauze sponges wrung from hot normal salt solution, while the abdominal wound behind the tumor was closed by silkworm-gut sutures, through and through. The uterus was then incised in the median line, the whole length of the incision being below the point of adhesion between the fundus and anterior abdominal wall, and the child delivered. The child was a male weighing eight and one-half pounds. It was apneic and began to breathe quickly. The placenta followed and its site was to the left and anterior; the child lay as diagnosed, in the right dorso-anterior position. During the uterine evacuation the blood supply was controlled by manual pressure over the uterine and ovarian arteries. Ergot was given by hypodermatic as soon as the child was born.

After sponging out the uterine cavity thoroughly a strip of gauze was passed through the cervix into the vagina and the balance folded back and forth in the uterine cavity. The uterine wall was sutured with silk interrupted sutures passing through the serous and muscular layers. A second row of catgut sutures, double the number, covered in the silk sutures. The uterus was then returned to the abdominal cavity and the abdominal incision closed. Several heavy bands of adhesion between the uterus and intestines were separated during the operation. After six days of normal temperature the patient began to have severe abdominal pains and a rise to 104°, which persisted twenty-four hours and then fell gradually. The abdominal pain was always intestinal in character. The application of ice, etc., necessary to relieve this pain, gave the opportunity for infection of the abdominal wound and two superficial stitch-hole abscesses resulted. The gauze was removed from the uterus gradually, the last at the end of thirty-six hours after operation. The lochial discharge was very scant, amounting in all to less than an ordinary menstruation. The baby was weaned, as the mother's high temperature made lactation very scant. The patient and the baby left the hospital on the thirty-third day after operation, and both have been well since. At a recent examination the uterus was found anteverted, freely movable, and involution completed normally.

This case brings into prominence the serious obstetrical problems developed by surgical advances of gynecology.

Obstetricians are frequently called upon to care for dystocia a result of cervical amputation or of Emmet operations for lacerated cervix. The repair of the perineum by the extensive denudation methods just now in vogue makes moments of intense anxiety to the obstetrician. Such tissue tears readily and heals poorly, and whether to relieve tension by an episeiotomy or not is a very active question.

Again, in pregnancy following the vaginal or abdominal methods for correcting malpositions of the uterus, of which my case is an example, a problem confronts the obstetrician, not of Nature's making. The extensive compilations of cases of ventrosuspension, ventro- and vaginal fixation in which dystocia of varying degrees resulted, can be interpreted in many ways. In 1896 Dr. Charles P. Noble collected 808 cases from American gynecologists, with pregnancy following in 56 cases. Of these, six miscarried, three severe forceps, one Porro-Cesarean with fatal result, one death from uncontrollable vomiting, one death from sepsis, making a total dystocia of 20 per cent and a fatality of 6 per cent.

European statistics collected of 175 pregnancies show 17 miscarriages, 7 premature labors, 133 full-term labors. Of these, 15, or 11 per cent, necessitated operative interference. There were 3 Cesarean sections, of which 2 died. The fetal mortality was not given in any of these cases.

Besides these I have noticed the following cases in reviewing as much literature as I could command. Edebohls reports a case necessitating celiopanhysterectomy; child and mother died. Dickinson: (1) Cesarean section following ventrosuspension; child and mother died; the cervix was found at the third lumbar vertebra at later autopsy. (2) Rupture of the uterus; delivery being impossible, due to a fibroid-like mass formed by the anterior uterine wall and preventing the passage of the head. Dr. X. O. Werder, a Porro-Cesarean; child and mother lived. The operation was done after labor in a IIpara had gone on twenty-one hours with no progress, the cervix remaining very high up. Dr. F. H. Bloomhardt reported, after a labor of four days, an early rupture of the membranes; an examination under anesthetic showed cervix posterior, above pelvic brim. Porro-Cesarean was done; mother and child died. The *Jahresbericht fur Geburtshülfe und Gynäkologie* for 1900 reports one Cesarean section (Case 52) done for threatened uterine rupture due to a ventrally fixed uterus; result not given.

These cases bring out several points in regard to results. The cases necessitating abdominal operations have been largely fatal in results, due to very obvious reasons. Operations have been resorted to too late in the case, and the risk of sepsis has been increased by the exhaustion of the patient and by the previous efforts at delivery by the natural passages.

The cases requiring forceps and version for delivery are generally described as difficult cases. So that fetal mortality must be increased, even under less risk to the mothers.

It is an inevitable conclusion that the perfect method of correction of uterine displacements in the parous woman has not been found in ventral fixation or ventral suspension. An operation which has possibilities which may jeopardize the life of either mother or child has need of searching criticism. The woman facing such an operation has the right of a clear understanding of its risk to her in case of pregnancy. In the light of our present knowledge, in cases where no other course of treatment seems to offer so much as ventral suspension, the patient should be warned of the necessity of careful supervision if pregnancy ensues, that the artificial freeing of the uterus or labor induced before the cervix is drawn too far posteriorly may be done; or, in case the pregnancy is allowed to advance to full term, that she may be delivered by Cesarean or Porro-Cesarean as the operation of selection, rather than of necessity after exhaustion of her vital forces subsequent to a prolonged, ineffectual labor.

1212 SUTTER STREET.

BIBLIOGRAPHY.

NOBLE: Ventrosuspension and its Results in Obstetrics, 1896.

GORDON: European Statistics on Pregnancy Complicated by Ventrosuspension, 1896.

JACOBSON, A. C.: Effects of Ventrofixation and Ventral Suspension on Subsequent Pregnancy and Labor. Report of case. American Medicine, January 21, 1902.

BLOOMHARDT, F. H.: Dystocia Following Ventrofixation. American Medicine, January 21, 1902.

WOODS, R. A.: Ventrosuspension. American Medicine, August 17, 1901.

Jahresbericht für Geburtshülfe und Gynäkologie, 1900. Cesarean section.

TECHNIQUE OF THE DENUDING PLASTIC PERINEUM OPERATIONS.

BY

N. B. ALDRICH, M.D.,
Fall River, Mass.

(With one illustration.)

My excuse for writing this article is that I feel the method of using weighted traction ligatures is a step forward and should supplant the older method which depends upon tenacula.

Take, as an example, the Emmet operation of perineorrhaphy. In denuding, most gynecologists use tenacula to raise the points that are to be denuded to. I have seen so many surgeons lift up a point time and again during an operation, or rather a different point each time by the tenaculum when it should have been the same one, that I have often felt like suggesting the traction loops, but, of course, seldom dared to.

When you use these traction ligatures you have permanent marks, and no need for saying words that are better unsaid. Originally I used two traction ligatures at the upper angles, marking the points I intended to denude to; the other points were picked up as occasion required by tenacula.

Later I tried introducing traction ligatures at five points, namely, the two upper angles, the tip of the tongue piece, and the two outer points in region of the carunculæ myrtiformes. These ligatures were of silk and the two ends of each ligature tied together, making a loop.

I now use silk ligatures introduced at these five points, and sometimes another one in the median line of the skin perineum; the two ends of the silk are clamped together with hemostats.

At the beginning of the operation, before you do anything else, thread a curved needle with a long piece of heavy silk. Introduce the ligature first at the right upper angle, then the left, and then in the median line at the site that is to form the end of the tongue piece. Leave these ligatures six to eight inches long and clip the ends of each with separate hemostats. Next introduce the ligature at the two outer lateral points that are to be denuded to, and cut off these ends two inches long and clip with hemostats.

These ligatures are left and not removed until the operation is completed, when the hemostats are loosened and the thread drawn through and removed. They permanently mark the points we are to denude to, and are a great aid in keeping the parts on the stretch when denuding and in holding them in desired relation

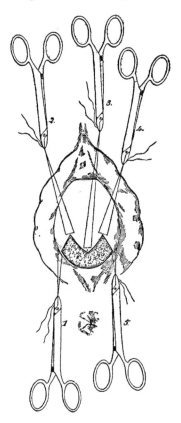

while placing the sutures. In introducing the ligature take quite a bite with the needle, so as to be able to exert traction without having it tear through.

The two short ligatures can be allowed to hang down and are out of the way; the three long ligatures, if they are in the way, can be held up out of the way by simply placing the hemostats on the sterile coverings of the lower abdomen. I find the ligatures with the hemostats attached a great improvement over the simple

traction loops, because the weight of the hemostats holds them
where placed.

Personally I outline the surface to be denuded with the scalpel,
outlining the right lateral half and denuding it before I outline
the left half. While my assistant holds ligatures 1 and 2 taut, I
control ligature 3 with my left hand and proceed to denude from
the median line with scissors. After this the left half is denuded. ligatures 3, 4, and 5 being controlled in order to give the
parts the desired stretch. We are now ready to introduce the
sutures; the ligatures again come into play in holding the parts
in their desired relation while introducing them. Similar traction ligatures introduced into each lip of the cervix are very useful in trachelorrhaphy. Probably the best non-absorbent suture
material we possess is silkworm gut.

The removal of these sutures is a problem that confronts us
later, and to anticipate this is our duty at the time of operation.
These ligatures in the cervix or high up in the vagina are hard to
remove if the ends are cut short, and more than once I have found
it necessary to place patients under chloroform in order to remove the same. One source of discomfort they cause patients
is that the short ends stick into them. If the ends are left
long enough to reach through the vulva, and then bunched,
placing rubber tubing over the same, which is held to them
by a piece of silk tied tightly, the ends will not trouble
the patient. When ready to remove these sutures, cut the
silk, remove the rubber tubing, and apply gentle traction on the
suture, thus raising a loop free from the tissues; then with the
hooked end of Skene's scissors catch the suture, cut it, and remove it by the long end that has been exerting gentle traction.

THE EARLY DIAGNOSIS AND TREATMENT OF HIP DISEASE.[1]

BY

A. R. SHANDS, M.D.,
Washington, D. C.

I SHALL confine my remarks to the two most important features
of hip-joint disease, viz., its early diagnosis and the treatment
in the incipiency of the disease. All who have had to deal with

[1]Read before the Washington Obstetrical and Gynecological Society,
January 3, 1902.

this trouble are fully aware of the great importance of an early diagnosis, for therein rests the only hope of bringing about anything like a fair functional result. This fact is readily appreciated when one remembers that there is tendency to distortion of the limb from the very incipiency of the disease, due to the muscular spasm which is one of the earliest as well as one of the most reliable symptoms.

The prospect that one has to face at the beginning of a case of hip disease is anything but favorable. It is very desirable to be able to foretell the result, but even after a large experience it is hard to approximate the result in any given case, there being so many details in the progress of the case, extending over years, that require not only the closest attention of the surgeon, but the hearty co-operation of the parents, and they often tire of this long course of treatment. It is discouraging, again, for the best one can hope in the severe cases is to have the patient recover with a shortened limb; any other deformity than a short limb is a reflection on the treatment of the surgeon, for all distortion can be either prevented or corrected. One should get good functional results, in the majority of cases, under thorough treatment carried out for a sufficient length of time.

Diagnosis.—It is customary to describe the diagnosis of the three stages of hip disease. This I consider entirely useless, as the time of greatest importance is the first stage, and if the diagnosis were always made in the incipiency the second and third stages would often never be developed, provided, of course, the proper treatment were always carried out. The symptoms to look for in diagnosing an early case of hip disease are as follows:

1. Stiffness of the joint, due to tonic muscular spasm.
2. Attitude of the limb in standing, walking, or lying: either flexion, adduction, or abduction.
3. Lameness.
4. Atrophy.
5. Pain.
6. Swelling.

The above list of symptoms is in the order of their importance, but will vary some according to the stage and activity of the disease. Muscular rigidity of the muscles about the hip is, by far, the most important symptom in the early diagnosis. It is often present in other affections than hip disease. Absence of pain and sensitiveness counts for nothing and atrophy is not character-

istic.   The limp is peculiar, but may be seen in other affections
also.

In manipulating the limb of a young child who is inclined to
resist, great care is necessary to detect the spasm.   Any muscular resistance due to fright will extend to the other joints as well
as the one suspected.   A careful comparison of the motions of
the two limbs will reveal any abnormal resistance.   The limitation of motion will be found to be limited to the extremity of the
normal arc of motion—*i.e.*, flexion, adduction, abduction, and
rotation.   In examining a patient suspected of hip disease
in its incipiency, the patient should have all clothes removed and be placed on a hard surface.   Always begin the examination by manipulating the well limb, carrying it through
all of its normal arcs of motion; this will serve the double purpose of familiarizing yourself with the normal motions of the
hip joint, that you may the more readily detect the limitation
of motion when you come to the diseased limb, and at the same
time will serve to gain the confidence of the patient.   One should
exercise the greatest possible gentleness with the child or the object of the examination will be defeated.

Careful inspection in the early stage will sometimes show fibril-
lary contractions of the muscles of the thigh on any sudden
movement.   In well-developed cases the muscular spasm is often
so marked that it will produce a practical ankylosis.   In such
cases a few whiffs of chloroform will relieve the spasm.   It is
impossible to say just what degree of limitation of motion should
be accepted as evidence of hip disease, but any degree of limitation that has persisted is extremely suspicious.

In considering the second symptom of hip disease—attitude of
the limb—it should be borne in mind that this is due entirely
to the muscular spasm.   The most common attitude is adduction,
which is very often combined with flexion.   Adduction always
gives the leg the appearance of being shortened, and for this
reason the parents always tell you that the lame leg is shorter
than the other.   The anxiety of an intelligent parent can be relieved by explaining the difference between apparent and real
shortening.

About the first symptom noticed by the parent is lameness.
Sometimes this is very slight and often intermittent, but it may
be asserted that no hip disease can be present without it at some
time.   It is an aid to diagnosis only; it cannot be taken as positive evidence without other symptoms.   The lameness in the in-

cipiency of hip disease is generally noticeable in the early part of the day, due to stiffness of the joint from the night's rest, and as the joint is used the lameness passes off. There are often intervals of days, or as much as a week, when there is no lameness, but, as time passes, these intervals will become shorter until there is a daily morning lameness, and still later on this becomes constant. By this time all of the symptoms are so well developed that the diagnosis is very evident.

Atrophy is an early symptom, as a rule, but there are often exceptions. It should be borne in mind that the atrophy is a reflex due to a disturbance of the vaso-motors. This is also caused by the muscular spasm, which deprives the limb of its normal blood supply, hence atrophy takes place from starvation of the tissues and not from disuse.

Pain in the early stage is always located on the inner side of the thigh just above the knee; when it is at the hip it is due either to abscess formation or a nervous hyperesthesia. Night-cries are common in the early stage, and I am convinced they should be given more weight as an early diagnostic symptom than I have ever seen accorded them in any text book. During my service in the Hospital for Ruptured and Crippled, New York, I had an opportunity to observe daily and nightly a large number of these cases, and my attention was often attracted, while passing at night through the wards where over two hundred crippled children were sleeping, probably one-third of them with hip disease in various stages, by the sudden outcries of many. The night-cry is almost always confined to the early or very acute cases. The "night-cry," as all of the early symptoms, is due to muscular spasm. The cry is heard only in the early part of the night, and is due to the fact that when the child goes to sleep the muscular spasm relaxes, which allows a slight involuntary motion of the joint, causing the two inflamed surfaces of the head of the femur and the acetabulum to come together and pain results. Later in the night the child's sleep is more profound from exhaustion and the reflexes are then also asleep and sensation not so acute. In the later stage of the disease the muscular spasm is more intense, which practically produces an immobilization of the joint, thus preventing any involuntary motion of the joint from producing pain.

Swelling is not common in the early stage, unless the course of the disease has been very rapid; and even then it is not very important as a diagnostic symptom, for the diagnosis should be made long before it develops.

In differentiating this disease in the early stage, quite a number of affections at times present themselves for consideration, but only a few of the most important will be considered. The most common one is *contusion* and *sprain*. Here the diagnosis is very easy when there is evidence of violence to the external parts or there is a reliable history of a recent injury; it is not so easy when the contrary is the case and many of the prominent symptoms of early hip disease are present. Usually there is a history of sudden onset of the symptoms—muscular spasm. lameness, distorting of the limb, etc.—while hip disease is very gradual in its onset. When in doubt, put the patient's limb at perfect rest for a few weeks, and if the condition is due to a contusion or sprain the symptoms will rapidly disappear and the patient soon be well. If it should prove to be a case of hip disease. no wiser course could possibly be pursued. The symptoms of sprain always decrease immediately: not so in hip disease.

Rheumatism at times strongly resembles hip disease, but, by close observation of the case for a few days, one should be able to tell the difference. In rheumatism, pain is much more prominent than lameness and muscular spasm; just the opposite in the case of hip disease. The onset of rheumatism is, as a rule. sudden; not so with hip disease. The symptoms in rheumatism will usually subside after use of appropriate drugs; not so in hip disease. Rheumatism rarely affects one joint alone; hip disease in both hips is very rare.

Neurosis of the hip often offers trouble in differential diagnosis. but, as a rule, one who is accustomed to dealing with chronic joint diseases should not have any great trouble in recognizing the nature of the case, for a case of true hip disease has a certain clinical expression that should be recognized, however prominent the nervous phenomena may be. The neurotic case is apt to follow a slight injury very quickly, with symptoms entirely too pronounced to indicate true bone lesion, for, as has been said, the symptoms of hip disease are very gradual in their onset. The remissions of all symptoms in the neurotic case are much more thorough and prolonged than they are in hip disease. The muscular spasm in a neurotic hip will yield very readily to gentle passive motion; in hip disease the least passive motion will cause the muscular spasm to be more intense. There are other troubles that may be confusing in the diagnosis of hip disease—such as infantile paralysis. acute synovitis, bursitis, periostitis. and others—but with close attention to the clinical history and symptoms gross errors in diagnosis should not be made by a close observer.

Treatment.—I regret to say that there has not been a very marked unanimity of opinion on the subject of treatment of hip disease. The surgeons are divided into two grand classes, viz., the conservative and those believing in radical measures; the latter class are the general surgeons, who have never given any special attention to the conservative methods of the orthopedic surgeon. It is the firm conviction of the writer that radical operations in the early stage of hip disease should have no place in the routine treatment of this malady, for statistics have shown beyond all doubt that the conservative methods have brought about far better results, both as to functional results and as to mortality. The bone of contention between these two classes of surgeons is as to the advisability of excision of the head of the femur. It is acknowledged by both that in removing the head of the bone, if the disease can be entirely removed, the patient will make a more rapid recovery; but it must also be acknowledged that in so doing the growth of the femur is checked to a great extent and that a flail limb is the result, which is practically useless for locomotion. On the other hand, it is a well-established fact that there is a tendency to spontaneous recovery in all tubercular bone lesions; this being the case, surely the conservative and expectant method is indicated.

As an evidence that excision of the head of the femur will check the growth of the limb, I refer to the brief history of a case. This boy, at the age of 5 years, had an excision of the hip joint by a surgeon of national reputation. The operation was done in the early stage of the disease, and it is evident that all trace of the disease was removed, as the wound healed by primary union and in a few weeks a cure was the result. At the age of 10 years the boy was measured. He then had six inches of shortening and a perfectly flail limb. At this rate of growth, by the time he is a man the leg will be about one-half as long as its fellow.

My remarks upon treatment will be limited to the early stage before any serious complications have occurred.

The joint should be protected from all jar, exaggerated pressure, or violent motion; therefore the indications in treatment are to furnish *fixation, extension,* and *protection;* to benefit the patient's health in every possible way; to prevent and correct deformity and to meet such complications as may arise. The

14

treatment should be so adapted that it can be continued not only through the acute stage, but through the entire convalescence until'the joint is able to stand without injury from the jars incident to locomotion. It matters little what means are used to meet the indications above mentioned. Muscular spasm is undoubtedly Nature's effort to produce immobilization of the joint to relieve the pain; therefore one should do for Nature what she is trying to do for herself and thereby relieve her of the strain incident to her efforts.

By far the most perfect mechanical means of immobilizing the hip joint is the plaster-of-Paris spica; this method fulfils all three of the indications above mentioned—fixation, extension, and protection—when properly applied. If distortion is present it should be corrected before the plaster-of-Paris is applied. If the contraction is not very intense the deformity can be corrected by gentle traction as the dressing is applied, without an anesthetic; if this cannot be done an anesthetic should be used. If the contraction is of long standing the tendons at fault should be cut subcutaneously before applying the dressing. The joint should be thus protected until all tendency to muscular spasm has subsided, which occurs very rapidly under the perfect rest thus afforded. No rule can be laid down as to the length of time the plaster should be kept on. This will depend upon the severity of the disease and the perfection of immobilization. Generally speaking, it will be necessary to keep the plaster on from three to six months, but in very severe cases it often has to be worn for a year or more. After the plaster is left off the ambulatory brace should be applied. It is worse than useless to apply a brace until the spasm has subsided.

Two questions now arise: 1. When shall the brace be applied? 2. How long shall it be worn? It should not be applied until the muscular spasm has been sufficiently overcome to prevent a recurrence of the deformity, so that the traction exerted by the brace shall be in line with the correct position of the leg; and it should be continued just as long as there is any evidence that the disease remains be the time one year or five. Gibney says that the joint should be protected first, last, and all of the time against trauma, from accidents without or from muscular spasm induced reflexly by the disease itself.

There are several hip braces in use. The best one is that which will afford the best protection to the joint and furnish traction sufficient to prevent the occurrence of deformity during the convalescence.

ESSENTIAL OR TOXEMIC DROPSY IN CHILDREN.[1]

BY

GEORGE N. ACKER, M.D.,
Washington, D. C.

In pediatric practice cases are met with which occasion much difficulty in diagnosis, for they present all the general appearances of renal disease. There are swelling of the extremities, puffiness of the face and edema of the skin, but rarely dropsy within the serous cavities. When the exciting cause of the anasarca is sought for little of a positive nature can be ascertained. The examination of the urine is negative and thus the kidneys can be eliminated as the cause of the trouble; for though cases of Bright's disease without albuminuria have been reported, a careful microscopical examination of the urine will always reveal some disease of the kidneys, especially in those cases where there is extensive dropsy. The heart and lungs are also found, as a rule, to be in good condition. Thus the organs which are usually at fault when there is dropsy cannot be charged with the causation of this symptom.

This form of dropsy has been described under the terms essential, toxemic, or idiopathic dropsy. W. P. Herringham[2] gives an excellent account of this disease and considers fully its etiology. The following illustrative cases have come under my observation during the past year:

CASE I.—C. S., male, white, 6 months old, was admitted to the Children's Hospital August 28, 1901.

Family History.—Mother living, very nervous and not in good general health. Father dead; cause unknown. No other children. No tubercular or specific history obtainable.

Previous History.—Labor normal. Breast-fed only during first few days, then given at varying intervals cow's milk, condensed milk, and Mellin's food. Though seemingly a very

[1]Read before the Washington Obstetrical and Gynecological Society, February 21, 1902.

[2]Pediatrics, November 1, 1901.

healthy child, has always been predisposed to gastro-intestinal disorders. Has had none of the diseases of childhood.

Present Illness.--For the past two weeks bowels have been loose; stools loose and undigested. Five days ago first noticed edema of the face and extremities.

Present Condition.—The child is very fretful and restless, tossing limbs about and crying out. Lies on back. Face swollen, eyelids swollen, giving a puffed appearance to face. The extremities are very much swollen and, with the skin of the entire body, pits on pressure. The skin is shining, smooth, and pale. Hair scanty and harsh. The glandular system is normal. The muscular system is poorly developed and adipose tissue lacking. The respiratory system is normal, there being only a few râles. Thirty-two respirations to the minute. The second pulmonic sound is accentuated and the pulse 120 per minute, small, soft, and compressible. Temperature 97.4° F.

Digestive System.--Mucous membrane of mouth pale. Tongue coated. No teeth. Takes food poorly and frequently vomits. Stools frequent, green, and undigested, with mucus and curds. Strains constantly. Liver and spleen normal. Slight abdominal distension. Nervous system normal.

Genito-Urinary System.—Passed a normal quantity of urine which was free from albumin and casts. The weight is eleven pounds two ounces. The child was placed upon the following mixture, of which six ounces were given every three hours: Milk one-third, sterile water two-thirds, lime water two teaspoonfuls. A warm bath was ordered, and small doses of sweet spirits of nitre were given every two hours.

On September 2 the milk was increased to one-half, and half a drachm of sugar of milk was added, and on September 5 barley water was used in place of sterile water. The child lost weight during the first few days, but the general condition improved, the stools becoming less frequent and digested, the gastric symptoms disappearing and the anasarca rapidly diminishing. The color of the skin and mucous surfaces improved. The child became quiet and appeared satisfied. September 16: The anasarca has disappeared. The bowels are regular and stools well digested.

The patient made an uneventful recovery and was discharged October 2, 1901. The temperature was normal during the attack. The pulse ranged from 100 to 130 and respirations from

23 to 36. He gained about a pound. When seen recently he had gained in weight and was healthy.

CASE II.—G. C., æt. 5 years, male, white, entered the hospital November 19, 1900.

Family History.—Father died of pulmonary tuberculosis. Mother for the last four months has had general anasarca of unknown origin. Three other children living, all in perfect health. Tubercular history on both paternal and maternal sides.

Previous History.—Has had none of the ordinary diseases of childhood and has always been healthy. About six weeks ago had severe attacks of some gastro-intestinal disturbance. He received no treatment, but condition has since much improved. The family has just moved from Virginia, where they lived in the plainest way and often exposed to cold and wet. The cellar of the house was constantly filled with water.

Present Illness.—About three weeks ago, following an attack of diarrhea, first noticed edema of face and eyes, rapidly spreading to entire body. Has some fever. Appetite has been good and bowels regular. The urine scanty and high-colored.

Present Condition.—Skin smooth and pale. The cellular tissue of the entire body is edematous and pits on pressure. The child is very listless, dull, and anemic. Gastric and intestinal digestion good. All the systems are normal. Repeated examinations of the urine were made with negative results. December 1: The anasarca almost gone, only slight edema beneath the eyes. The temperature remained normal until December 1, when it rose to 101° F., and during the next nine days remained up with marked remissions, the highest point being 105.2° F. It then declined by lysis. During this time the liver began to enlarge, the lower border being felt about one and one-half inches above and to the left of the umbilicus. The stools were white and there was slight icterus. The blood examinations were negative for malaria and typhoid. The diazo-reaction was also negative. The liver gradually became reduced until it was of normal size, about January 4, and the child was discharged cured March 1, 1901.

CASE III.—B. C., æt. 3 months, female, white, entered the hospital September 19, 1901. Family history good.

Previous History.—Labor normal. Breast-fed only two days, then on modified cow's milk, but also given Mellin's food and malted milk in addition. Has had none of the diseases of childhood, but has never been healthy, often having gastro-intestinal disorders.

Present History.—Four weeks ago became ill with vomiting, diarrhea, and slight fever. Since then has had four or five green, undigested stools daily and has lost much flesh.

Present Condition.—Child appears small for age. Weight 8 pounds 6 ounces. Very restless, cries constantly, and appears in pain. Keeps limbs flexed. Is much emaciated. The skin is dry, harsh, pale, and flabby. No glandular enlargements. The respiratory and circulatory systems are normal. The pulse is 124, small and of low tension. Temperature 96° F. on admission.

Digestive System.—Tongue coated. Appetite poor. Vomits frequently. Six to ten loose, undigested, greenish stools in twenty-four hours. Liver and spleen normal and the abdomen distended with gas. Passes a sufficient quantity of pale urine. The child was first placed upon albumen water, followed by modified milk. The intestinal condition improved slightly at times, though patient suffered several acute exacerbations, during which time the temperature would rise and remain high until the bowels were flushed out and diet modified. Stools would improve in character and lessen in number during the intervals of improvement. Two grains of phosphate of soda were given at each feeding, with good results when the stools lacked color. During the course of the sickness the weight of the child fluctuated, there being no regular gain. Food was frequently regurgitated.

December 12: The temperature, which had been normal, rose to 104.4° F. in the morning and the child became very restless. There had been four watery, greenish stools in twenty-four hours. December 13: Temperature lower. Slight edema of the eyelids noticed, and on the 14th there was edema of the hands and feet. The edema became general on the 15th. The examination of the urine was negative. The edema gradually disappeared, and when the child died from weakness, on December 21, it could hardly be noticed.

CASE IV.—H. E., æt. 9 months, male, white, entered the hospital November 27, 1901. Family history negative.

Previous History.—Weaned at the third month. Since then he has been brought to the Children's Hospital four times for medical treatment, three times for gastro-intestinal disorders and the fourth time for croupous pneumonia with delayed resolution and termination by lysis, but with perfect recovery. Recurrence of the intestinal disturbances found to be due to unhygienic surroundings and improperly modified milk.

Present Illness.—During past ten days has had diarrhea. Stools loose, watery, and very offensive, containing much mucus. Vomits all nourishment given. Three days ago the condition became much worse, the stools increasing in number and containing blood.

Present Condition.—General condition good. Has eight teeth and weighs fourteen pounds four and one-half ounces. Sleeps fairly well. The above condition continued with slight improvement in stools. The temperature was irregular, reaching, when intestinal symptoms became aggravated, 102.6° F., then falling to normal. Albumen water was given for twenty-four hours and afterward milk mixture, though feeding proved very unsatisfactory. It was frequently necessary to stop milk and resort to albumen water and broth. The child steadily lost weight. He strained at stools and had prolapsus ani.

December 17: First noticed slight puffiness under eyes. The child was cross and fretful. There were nine loose, greenish stools with mucus and blood. Temperature 99.2° F., respiration 29, pulse 108.

On the 18th the dropsy had extended to the hands, feet, and legs, which pitted on pressure. Hands and feet cold and blue. Face swollen. The child is anemic and waxy in color. The fontanelle is sunken. The urine was pale, alkaline, containing no albumin or sugar; microscopical examination negative. Several examinations were made. The edema gradually improved until December 26, when it had disappeared. Skin harsh and dry. Very emaciated. The stools continued bad and the child grew weaker. The temperature was irregular. January 1, 1902, large ecchymotic spots appeared upon the chest, abdomen, and extremities. Weight ten pounds. The child's condition became worse, and he died January 6.

In all these cases the dropsy took place in children who had suffered for some time from gastro-intestinal disease, being in poor physical condition and worn out by the drain upon the system before dropsy appeared. It will be noted that in the third and fourth cases the edema disappeared before death, though there were no heavy sweats or unusual action of the bowels to account for the removal of the fluid.

I have never seen this form of dropsy occurring as a primary disease, but always secondary to gastro-intestinal disorders. and, as far as my observation goes, it cannot be described as an independent disease.

The question of greatest interest in regard to this condition relates to the etiology. The dropsy appears first in the face and then extends to the extremities and body, as in kidney disease. The postmortem examinations do not assist us in arriving at the cause, for, from the reports of those who have written upon the subject, no constant lesions have been found and the alterations in the kidneys have not been of such a nature as to point to these organs as having anything to do with the production of the disease. I regret that autopsies were not permitted to be held in the fatal cases reported by me, but from the number of urinary examinations made I can assert that the kidneys were free from disease.

Such writers as Holt, Ashby, and Bristowe hold that anemia will account for the dropsy. Holt says: "Dropsy is not infrequent in infants in simple anemia due to an impoverishment of the blood, especially in the red cells, with a corresponding diminution in the specific gravity and the amount of hemoglobin. There is an insufficient production of blood in consequence of deficient food or interference with the absorption of food, and there can be an increased drain or destruction of blood, as in exhausting diseases." As a rule it is found in anemic and rundown children, yet we often see severe cases of anemia without anasarca. Therefore there must be some other factor besides the anemia to cause the dropsy. In my last two cases the edema came on late in the disease and the fluid was absorbed some days before the death of the patient. Now, if the cause of the dropsy was the anemic state of the patients, this should have increased as the children became weaker; yet the contrary was the case.

This has been called toxemic dropsy because it is supposed that there is a toxic poison which produces the edema. This poison, I think, arises in the intestines and the dropsy is due to the action of the agent upon the capillaries. If there is not a toxic agent, there must be some chemical alteration of the blood which causes the serum to transude into the tissues.

No symptoms can be ascribed to the dropsy, for it does not appear to modify the regular disease in the course of which it appears. There was fever in all but one of my cases, and this would argue against feeble circulation being the cause of the disease, for in this case there would be a lowering of the body temperature. While the prognosis is unfavorable, the disease is not necessarily fatal.

The treatment must be directed to the condition which is at the root of the trouble. It will be in the main dietetic. Strict attention to the food supply, and measures directed to keeping the alimentary canal in good condition, with remedies which will tone up the system, will fulfil all the indications.

TRANSACTIONS OF THE SECTION ON GYNECOLOGY OF THE COLLEGE OF PHYSICIANS OF PHILADELPHIA.

Stated Meeting, April 17, 1902.

GEORGE ERETY SHOEMAKER, M.D., *in the Chair.*

DR. R. P. McREYNOLDS presented

A CASE OF ELEPHANTIASIS OF THE VULVA.

When I first thought of reporting this case I was under the impression that elephantiasis was a disease rarely seen in this country; but on looking over the literature I am afraid (since there have been so many cases reported) that I shall have nothing new or even interesting to report to the members of the Section.

Miss F. was admitted to the Presbyterian Hospital July 29, 1901, and, through the kindness of Dr. Willard, came under my care. The points of interest in her history are: White girl, aged 23, single. Mother, father, and one sister died of consumption. Since she was 12 years old she has had enlarged glands in the neck, which are probably tubercular. Her menstrual periods have been very irregular—amenorrhea frequently for months at a time. When 19 years old she noticed a small red papule around the vulva; this gradually increased in size and began to discharge a white fluid (probably lymph). In January, 1901, she was admitted to the St. Agnes Hospital, diagnosis of elephantiasis made, and a large mass excised from both labia majora. Soon after recovering from the operation her left ankle began to swell, and this has gradually extended up to the knee.

On admission to the Presbyterian Hospital, seven months after the operation, the left leg and foot were one-half as large again as the right one, and the skin here hard and bluish-white in color. The labia contained the scar from the operation, but were not markedly enlarged. . The examination of the rest of the body (including an examination of the blood) was negative. She was placed in bed and for three months given the most careful medical treatment. During this time her leg improved but little; much to my surprise, the right labia majora and minora, the clitoris and tissues around and above it, began to rapidly enlarge. On November 14, 1901, she was etherized and an incision made down through the whole length of the right labia majora and a lot of hard, dense connective tissue dissected away. She was discharged from the hospital December 23, 1901. She had recovered nicely from the operation and the vulva presented a much more normal appearance: the leg had improved somewhat. I believe, however, that there will be a recurrence of growth about the vulva, and that if she uses the leg it will get gradually and progressively worse. The pathological diagnosis of the tissue removed was fibrolipoma with marked hypertrophy of the skin.

I think this case represents the type of elephantiasis generally seen in this country; the filaria sanguinis hominis is not, as a rule, found in the blood, and the disease is not of the same gravity and the parts affected do not assume the same proportions as when seen in tropical and Eastern countries.

The etiology of the disease is obscure, but it is said to generally attack those who are physically weak, poorly nourished, and who live with unhygienic surroundings. I have been able to find no mention of tuberculosis *per se* as a cause of the disease, yet it seems to me that in this case it might be a predisposing factor. On the other hand. syphilis is said to sometimes cause it, and the rule is given by some writers to always give a course of antisyphilitic treatment before resorting to any operative procedure.

In order to cure the enlargement of the leg it has been proposed to ligate the femoral artery. This has been done a number of times and the success following the operation seems to justify it. I fail to see just how it works, yet. if it is true, from a clinical standpoint I do not see why ligating both internal pudic arteries would not cause the enlargement to disappear from in and around the vulva. If there is a recurrence in the case reported I hope to have an opportunity to try this treatment, and, should the leg continue to increase in size, shall advocate ligating the femoral artery in the apex of Scarpa's triangle.

Dr. JOHN C. DA COSTA.—I would like to ask the age of the woman. how long before the doctor saw her had the disease existed, also whether filaria were found in the blood examinations. I ask regarding the filaria because I know of a case in Reading of a woman who had not been out of this State, and yet the filaria were found in the blood. We see a great many cases of elephantiasis confined to the vulva, but few in which it extends to the leg. Was it simply on the leg of the corresponding side, or on both?

Dr. GEORGE E. SHOEMAKER.—It seems to me that if the chief seat of the disease is in the vulva there would be little gained from ligating the femoral artery, as it could only affect a portion of the distribution of the disease. As I remember the case, the involvement of the leg by elephantiasis proper, as distinguished from edema or infiltration of some other type, was not marked. Might the condition not have been caused by thrombosis?

Dr. McREYNOLDS (closing).—In answer to Dr. Da Costa, I would say that the woman was 23 years of age when I saw her, and she had had the disease from the time she was 19 years of age. The blood examinations were made during the day and the filariæ were not noticed. We regret that we did not have examinations made at night, when possibly they would have been found. The growth was confined to one leg, the left.

In reply to Dr. Shoemaker, the hardness of the leg was marked, and not edematous as seen in cardiac failure and other diseases. Thrombosis might have been a probable cause.

DR. JOHN C. DA COSTA.—If I may be allowed to speak a second time, I would say that the fact of the blood examinations not having been made at night may account for the filaria not being found, as it is not, as a rule, found during the day when the patient is up and about, except in the diurnal form. It is ordinarily found in greatest numbers about 12 to 1 o'clock at night, three or four hours after the patient has lain down. If the doctor can see the case again, I would suggest that examinations be made at night. We know how prone the filariæ are to abound in the scrotum of the male, where they often appear first, and why not in the vulva of women? I would be glad to know the result of any examinations that may be made of the blood at night. I have been particularly interested in the cases because of their rarity. There have been but five reported in Pennsylvania, and my son has seen all of them. Two of them were patients of Dr. Henry, one, in the Pennsylvania Hospital, a patient of Dr. Gibbons. one was in Reading, and the fifth in the German Hospital.

DR. GEORGE ERETY SHOEMAKER read a paper on

APPENDICITIS BY CONTIGUITY.

The specimen here shown illustrates in a striking manner the fact, familiar to gynecologists, that one of the common causes of appendicitis in women is primary disease in some other organ, usually the ovary or tube. Appendicitis independent of disease of other organs of course occurs in women, though less frequently than in men. Difference in habits of life, lessened exposure to the mechanical and climatic causes of appendicitis, with probably some influence due to a difference of diet, work in this direction. If one reviews his experience and observations in the wards of a general hospital, for example, while cases of pelvic inflammation from all causes are relatively more common in women than in men, the number of cases of primary appendicitis in women with no tubal involvement is comparatively small. Certainly in the experience of the writer this has been the case. If an operator is looking for appendicitis, is in the habit of operating for appendicitis frequently and for pelvic disease of other types but seldom, especially if in the presence of acute right-sided inflammation he cuts down upon the appendix without making a previous careful bimanual examination of tubes, ovaries, and uterus, he may, it is true, find an inflamed appendix; but if the investigation be stopped there—and if the incision be small it very frequently does stop there—this operator may, even after operation, consider a case of combined disease to be one of appendicitis only. The position of the writer is this, that in all cases a combined involvement must be expected and looked for. No case of abdominal section for tubal and ovarian disease or for tumors is complete unless the appendix is examined through the wound and, if not found normal. removed. Likewise the condition of the right tube and ovary should always receive careful investigation before and during operation. otherwise the operation in a considerable proportion of cases will fail to cure the patient. When both tube and appendix are at fault the incision through the right rectus muscle will reach both conditions.

The patient from whom these specimens were removed was a girl of 19 years from Shamokin, Pa., who. unknown to her friends, had led an immoral life and had contracted gonorrhea. This had run an extremely mild course as far as external symptoms were concerned, and at the time of coming under observation for an attack of severe right-sided pain there were absolutely no clinical symptoms of gonorrhea present, though microscopically and by culture the gonococcus was demonstrated in mucus from the neighborhood of the external urethral meatus. The leucocyte count was not positive in indication, but suggested pus. Clubbed, contorted. closed tubes. each three-fourths of an inch in diameter, were removed through an incision in the right rectus muscle. They contained pus. The left ovary was removed. as it contained a hematogenous cyst and appeared badly involved by subacute inflammation. The right ovary was allowed to remain. A small abscess was dissected out of the uterine fundus one inch from the cornu.

The appendix was long. dipping into the pelvis. It was adherent to the right tube and presented the following condition: Length, four inches. More firm than normal throughout. but not macroscopically showing serious disease except for an inch from the tip; here the entire organ was swollen to three or four times the diameter of the remainder of the organ, the walls were dark red, softened. and showed extensive inflammation but no perforation. On section the walls were seen to be about five-sixteenths of an inch in thickness. while no extensive destruction had occurred even in the mucous membrane, which showed purplish hemorrhagic infarcts. In other words, though extensive inflammatory changes have occurred, they have proceeded from without inward and not from within outward.

The girl recovered. In this case the symptoms of tubal and ovarian disease were not marked and her menstrual history was not far from normal. The chief symptom was severe recurrent pain in the right lower. quadrant. and had the ordinary rapid appendicitis operation been done through a short incision and an appendix such as this delivered, it would have been easy to overlook the real condition and attribute to adhesions any hardening felt through the wound. The demonstration of the gonococcus determines the origin of the whole process.

DR. GEORGE M. BOYD.—I feel that Dr. Shoemaker's paper is of interest in that it brings up the importance of studying more closely than heretofore cases of inflammation about the appendages. It would seem that in many cases of appendical involvement the trouble primarily was in the tube or ovary. It has been my custom for a number of years, in cases in which the pain seemed referable to the appendix and to the tubes as well, to make a median incision and explore not only the region of the appendix, but also the pelvis on that side, inspecting the tube and ovary. I have in mind several cases where the operator, because of symptoms referable to the appendix, has made the lateral incision, finding the appendix in some cases diseased and in other cases no trouble. A second operation has revealed tubal or ovarian abscess. In one case an incision was made over the region of the appendix, a healthy appendix brought into view and removed. The incision was closed, but the patient's symptoms did not improve. A short time afterward a second incision was made per vaginam, opening up a pelvic abscess.

DR. JOHN C. DA COSTA.—If examination was not made for the gonococcus, I take it that there is nothing but surmise in concluding that the inflammation started from the tubes.

DR. SHOEMAKER.—The specimen in the dried state does not show as distinctly as in the fresh state the apparent direction which the inflammation has taken. The mucous membrane in that early stage of inflammation showed the familiar appearance. It was the outer coats of the appendix which made up most of the swelling.

DR. DA COSTA.—I hope Dr. Shoemaker has made sections from the appendix. They would have determined the origin of the inflammation. We have all seen cases in which the appendix has been fastened to the uterus.

DR. SHOEMAKER.—The proportion is small compared with the number of cases of pelvic diseases we meet with which we have to operate upon.

DR. DA COSTA.—I am getting doubtful about a good many cases originating from the tube and ovary, because I have removed appendices which were fast to either ovary, tube, or uterus, that appeared healthy except for the adhesion. I think the suggestion of Dr. Shoemaker, of examining the appendix in every case of celiotomy, a very good one. I have made it a rule in celiotomies to examine the contents of the abdomen, and do not satisfy myself with a two-inch incision. I make the incision long enough to insert my hand and bring up the appendix, and then examine the liver and kidneys.

DR. CHARLES P. NOBLE presented

TWO CASES OF DECIDUOMA MALIGNUM [1]

and

[1]Will appear in the September issue of this JOURNAL.

A CASE OF EPITHELIOMA -OF THE CLITORIS.[1]

DR. R. P. McREYNOLDS.—I would like to ask Dr. Noble if there was any microscopical examination of the uterus after it was removed.

DR. GEORGE ERETY SHOEMAKER.—I would like to ask whether the flaps consisted of anything but the skin.

DR. NOBLE.—I first cut away the tumor, and the labium was then separated on each side enough to let it come together. I fancy that the skin and some of the flaps were separated from the subjacent fat. Incision was made through the fatty layer.

DR. GEORGE E. SHOEMAKER.—The point to which I had reference was to account for the sloughing. If the flap were made very thin, with no fat under the skin, it would suffer from lack of nutrition and not from any inherent disease.

DR. R. P. McREYNOLDS.—I would like to ask Dr. Noble if the glands in the groin were enlarged, or if they were removed simply as a prophylactic measure. In epithelioma in various parts of the body the glands are not always involved. In epithelioma about the face it seems sufficient to remove the tumor with the skin around it.

DR. NOBLE (closing).—The literature of the subject shows that heretofore the prognosis of epithelioma of the external genitals has been very bad, almost, if not all, cases dying of secondary invasion. Owing to this fact I long ago determined to employ a radical operation whenever a suitable case of epithelioma of the vulva or external genitals should present itself. The other cases of epithelioma of the external genitals which have come under my observation have all been hopeless when first seen.

DR. GEORGE M. BOYD exhibited

A DICEPHALIC MONSTER.[2]

TRANSACTIONS OF THE
NEW YORK OBSTETRICAL SOCIETY.

Stated Meeting, April 8, 1902.

The President, MALCOLM McLEAN, M.D., *in the Chair.*

SPECIMEN OF ECTOPIC PREGNANCY (TUBAL ABORTION) WITH THE FETUS IN THE UNRUPTURED MEMBRANES.

DR. HOWARD C. TAYLOR.—The history of the case is as follows: The patient was admitted to the Roosevelt Hospital March 9,

[1]See original article, p. 190.
[2]Report will appear in full in a later issue of this JOURNAL.

1902. She is 32 years old and had one child twelve years ago; no miscarriages. The last regular menstruation previous to her admission to the hospital was from February 8 to 15. This menstruation was regular as to time, duration, and amount. Four days later, February 19, the patient began again to flow and continned to do so moderately until admitted to the hospital on March 9. No special pain. The patient had enlarged and tender breasts, nausea, and was positive she had been and was pregnant. On examination the uterus was found to be slightly enlarged, but no mass was detected in either side. The diagnosis was made of early miscarriage and the uterus curetted. Under ether a small, movable mass on the right side was detected and the possibility of the case being one of ectopic pregnancy was considered. The patient was kept under observation in the hospital and ultimately the diagnosis of ectopic pregnancy made beyond reasonable doubt, on the following signs: the examination of the curettings showed no signs of uterine pregnancy, though the woman was sure she had been pregnant and had positive signs in the breasts; the presence of an indefinite change in the feeling of the mass on the right side, though there had been no special increase in size; the constantly increasing anemia, as shown by the blood count, the hemoglobin reaching 50 per cent and the red corpuscles 3,250,000.

At the second operation, March 24, a small amount of blood was found in the peritoneal cavity. The right ovary was much enlarged and cystic and the right tube was unruptured, its outer end distended and occupied by the fetal sac. The fetal sac was partly in the tube and partly against the pelvic wall. The case has had an uneventful recovery, though still in the hospital.

Dr. Le Roy Broun.—This specimen is unusual. Equally so are the reports of two cases at a meeting of the Woman's Hospital Society, one report by Dr. Aspell, the other by Dr. Baker. of Boston. In Dr. Aspell's case the diagnosis of ruptured ectopic gestation was made; the patient, however, refused operation. Death followed; the postmortem examination revealed that the blood in the peritoneal cavity had come, not from the ruptured tube, but from a rupture of a vessel on the side of the tube, and that the tube itself or the sac had not ruptured. Dr. Baker reported a similar case having occurred in his practice some years previous. In his case the tube was not ruptured; the blood, however, was seen to be coming from the fimbriated extremity of the tube.

RETROPERITONEAL ECHINOCOCCUS CYST.

Dr. Howard C. Taylor.—The patient was admitted to the Roosevelt Hospital in May, 1893, with an abdominal tumor which was removed by Dr. Tuttle and proved to be an echinococcus cyst of the omentum. The recovery was uncomplicated.

The patient was again admitted to the hospital in August, 1893, with an abdominal tumor in the region of the spleen extending four inches below the free border of the ribs. At the operation Dr. Cragin exposed the tumor by an incision at the outer border of the rectus muscle, and the diagnosis of an echinococcus cyst of the spleen was made. The wound was packed to allow the formation of adhesions to shut off the peritoneal cavity, and the cyst was not opened until four days later. At this time eight ounces of daughter cysts were evacuated and they continued to be discharged from the wound for some months afterward. The patient left the hospital in January, 1894, with a sinus persisting, which subsequently closed and has given the patient no further trouble.

The patient was admitted to the hospital the third time in September, 1901, with a tumor about five inches in diameter, so situated that the diagnosis was made of intraligamentous cyst. At the operation I found the tumor situated behind the peritoneum and to the right of the rectum and entirely independent of the uterus and its appendages. The tumor was enucleated without difficulty, though the cyst was ruptured in doing so, and the divided edges of the peritoneum brought together with catgut, leaving a clean peritoneal surface. The tumor proved to be an echinococcus cyst which had developed behind the peritoneum.

The patient is a seamstress, 40 years old, born in Ireland, and has lived in Brooklyn or its vicinity since she was 18 years of age. I examined the patient about sixteen months after the last operation and could detect no evidence of a return of the disease.

VESICAL CALCULUS.

DR. EGBERT H. GRANDIN.—I wish to present a vesical calculus which I removed a few weeks ago by vaginal cystotomy. I show the specimen because in my experience calculi in the female bladder are rare. This is only the second that I can recall. The first I saw three years ago, and it had as its nucleus a silkworm-gut suture which had not been removed after the repair of a vesico-vaginal fistula. As a rule, in women a foreign body of some kind is found as the nucleus of a calculus.

DR. ABRAM BROTHERS.—I have also seen one case which was directly of kidney origin. The patient passed through an attack of kidney colic, and, under cystoscopic examination, a small calculus was noted at the mouth of the ureter. Later this patient passed the calculus.

DR. LE ROY BROUN.—Does Dr. Grandin mean to say that all calculi have some foreign nuclei about which accumulations must form?

DR. GRANDIN.—I naturally exclude those calculi that are passed from the ureter. In the vast majority of cases calculi that are formed in the bladder have some nuclei. During an experience of twenty-two years I have seen but two cases, and one had a nucleus. The other will be examined, and I believe that the consensus of opinion among those present here to-night will bear me out in this statement as to the nucleus in a calculus primary in the bladder.

Dr. Broun.—I removed one from the urethra which entirely blocked it. The urethra was opened to accomplish its removal: it was too large to be passed without operative assistance.

Dr. Malcolm McLean.—It is a well-recognized fact that idiopathic calculi requiring removal by operation, occurring in women, are rare, but the last woman that I operated upon was such a one; there was no nucleus from foreign substance.

CHOLESTEATOMA OF THE MESENTERY.

Dr. Egbert H. Grandin.—The patient was brought to my office for diagnosis as to the nature of an abdominal tumor which her family physician had detected. Upon opening the abdomen I was unable at first to locate the tumor. After suspension of the uterus to the parietal peritoneum and doing an appendectomy, I made further search, and, after enlarging the incision, brought the jejunum into view and enucleated this specimen. It resembles a hen's egg, is about four inches in diameter, and on section its walls are about one-eighth of an inch thick, very hard, and the specimen contained material which resembles somewhat the yolk of a decomposed egg. I should like to have the specimen sent to the official pathologist for his opinion.

Dr. S. W. Bandler.—On this question I have had experience, personally, only in the reading of the literature, and I think that what Dr. Grandin has stated covers the possibilities fully. It has impressed me, from a casual observation, that this might belong to the division of dermoid cysts coming under the head of cholesteatomata. As regards the etiology of such a tumor situated in the mesentery, embryological development renders it so readily possible that the wonder is that not more such tumors are developed instead of so few.

SPECIMENS FROM THREE RECENT CASES OF EARLY ECTOPIC GESTATION.

Dr. Abram Brothers.—As is the case with most of the members of this Society, it occasionally happens to me that groups of the same kind of cases run together. Thus, within the past month I have operated upon three cases of early ectopic gestation, two of them within a few days of each other, and, as each presented different varieties, I thought it would be of interest to bring the specimens.

Case I.—This specimen shows the fetus and ovum intact. It was neither a case of ruptured nor of unruptured tube, nor of a tubal abortion, although the abdominal cavity was full of blood and the pulseless patient was operated upon in a state of profound collapse. Dr. Bandler, who has been kind enough to carefully examine all of my recent specimens, tells me that the chorionic villi had simply grown through and perforated the peritoneal coat of the tube and caused the fearful hemorrhage.

15

Case II.—This specimen illustrates an unruptured tubal pregnancy. A little clotted blood had escaped into the peritoneal cavity, after which the fimbriated end of the tube became agglutinated. The little sausage-shaped tumor has been hardened and the transverse sections simply show a large intratubal clot. Ordinarily, from macroscopical examinations and appearances, this might be pronounced to be a simple hematosalpinx. The microscopic examination, however, has shown the presence of chorionic villi. It is interesting to note that the ovary removed with the tube does not show a corpus luteum, which corresponds with my statement, made on a former occasion in connection with other specimens, that the ovum frequently is derived from the opposite ovary through transperitoneal migration.

Case III.—This specimen illustrates the well-known form of ruptured tubal pregnancy. On the upper surface of the tube is a ragged gash, about one-half an inch long, from which the adjacent ball of blood escaped. This large clot, as well as the edges of the rupture, shows the presence of chorionic villi. The accompanying ovary, removed with the tube, shows very beautifully the corpus luteum.

I wish to accentuate this fact, that the largest hemorrhages that we see in the early cases of ectopic gestation may not come from true rupture, but from the outgrowth of the chorionic villi.

DR. BANDLER.—The point that Dr. Brothers mentions is of interest. I have seen several cases where it was macroscopically impossible to understand how so much blood could have entered the peritoneal cavity; it could not have entered through the closed abdominal opening nor through any evident point of rupture. Yet, when examined microscopically, only two, three, or half a dozen villi were found to have perforated the peritoneal covering. Not alone the ends of the villi but the placental sea or intervillous space was involved and enough blood thus entered the peritoneal cavity to produce symptoms of a profound intraperitoneal hemorrhage. Openings only microscopical in character may close, and it may be that for days or weeks the patient may go without further bleeding, and then another perforation occurs at the same or at another point. This process is of the greatest interest in this specimen.

COLON BACILLUS INFECTION OF THE FEMALE GENITAL AND URINARY SYSTEMS.

DR. ALBERT H. ELY.—Although much attention has been given, by the bacteriologists and those engaged as clinicians in general medicine and surgical work, to the study of this variety of bacteria, we cannot but feel the results thus far obtained have been less definite than is desired. That the results have been less definite is undoubtedly due to the great frequency with which we observe this bacillus in many different types and locations of pathologic processes. That lesions by reason of continuity of anatomical parts to the habitat of the bacillus coli communis show their presence in such frequency, is but natural, but what most demands consideration is, *what* factors cause these bacilli to vary so much in their pyogenic action. The virulency of the infection from the colon bacilli seems in most cases to depend upon their associate pyogenic organisms, for we find the colon bacilli present in great numbers in the urine without at times giving any symptoms.

Again, when the other pyogenic organisms have disappeared, the colon bacillus will remain as *the* organism which produces a most intractable type of disease. Hence we conclude that a suitable nidus is necessary for their propagation and action which give us the clinical symptoms of infection and disease of the tissue. Many of the cases which are designated as autoinfection, sapremia, and septic intoxication may be due, in a measure, to infection from the colon bacillus, and can be illustrated by cultures taken from what appears, and the later process shows, to be a mild degree of wound infection. These cases are observed in celiotomy wounds, especially where there has been trauma of the intestines during the process of abdominal operations. Analogy is drawn, also, to those cases which show a mild form of the infection coming on after sixty hours from the time of normal labor, especially where opportunity is so advantageously given for the infection direct from the feces.

From these mild forms of infection we pass to those severe types as illustrated in the most pronounced degree of infection, where the colon bacilli are found associated with streptococci and staphylococci pyogenic organisms, only that the proportion between the number and virulence of the organisms shows that it is the colon bacilli that have played the chief rôle in causing the fatal peritonitis and abscesses, such as nephritic, hepatic, and subphrenic. To illustrate the normal type of pelvic inflammation followed by evident colon infection, as shown by frequent cultures, the following case is presented:

Case I.—Mrs. L.; 34; married four years; sterile. Curettage with divulsion was performed in the general operating room of one of the large hospitals. No untoward symptoms developed until the fourth day, when a slight rise of temperature was noted and a distinct local tenderness of the pelvic tissues and the first symptoms of a mild grade of cystitis, as shown by frequent micturition with slight degree of vesical tenesmus. Under mild treatment employed for the pelvic inflammation, this quickly subsided, but the cystitis continued to increase in severity, although irrigations of the bladder were made to remedy this trouble, together with the usual measures for sterilizing the urine, especially the employment of urotropin. The cystitis continuing for ten days, cystoscopic examination was then made and a marked hyperemia of the trigonum was discovered and treatment by local applications instituted. This was continued for some time and was productive of good results in so far that the symptoms of vesical tenesmus disappeared, and yet the colon bacillus was found in the urine in large numbers. Desiring to leave the hospital, she passed from observation for six months. when she again returned, and at this time (seven months from the time of the original curettage) examination showed no lesion of the pelvic organs, but a very pronounced type of cystitis, and now for the first time quantities of pus were passed containing the typical bacilli of pyogenic infection. There had been, for a short time previous to readmission to the hospital, evidences of a general septic infection, as shown by irregular temperature, accelerated pulse, and sweating. By cystoscopic examination the greater part of the lower zone of the bladder, including a very marked area of inflammation about the mouth of the left ureter, was observed. Fearing that by ureteral catheterization further infection might result, this was not employed, but it was found by the use of the Kelly speculum, arranged to obtain the urine as excreted from either ureter, that the urine obtained from the right ureter was clear and failed to show pathogenic organisms, while that of the left was loaded with them. The diagnosis of pyelonephritis of the left kidney was then made. Measures were employed for the next ten days to improve this condition, without relief of the symptoms of the general infection, and recourse was then had to nephrotomy, which was successfully performed on the left kidney, and, except for a slight wound infection, a progressive but very gradual improvement of the bladder occurred and complete recovery took place.

Case II.—H. C., aged 9. First came under my observation during the summer in the country, where I was called to see the child, who was suffering at that time with what appeared to be a mild form of gastro-enteritis. The measures employed to relieve this condition were apparently effective and after a few days the child seemed well. The following week I was again called to see the child, who at this time gave all the symptoms of a typical colitis, frequent stools with large quantities of mucus and some blood. No examinations were made of the stools, but colon irrigation was employed and again the symptoms disappeared so far as the colitis was concerned, but the child now located a pain above the pubes with pain radiating down the right thigh. The urine now for the first time became thick and the symptoms of some vesical tenesmus with frequent micturition were presented. The highest temperature was 100.2°, pulse 94; no pain or rigidity of the rectus muscle was observed on the right side. This condition continued for thirty-six hours without any special pain, yet the thought that he might have a case of appendicitis was considered. Consultation with the family physician, Dr. G. B. Brewer, resulted in the belief that it was a case of appendicitis and operation for that lesion was accordingly performed. A long appendix, gangrenous for a quarter of its distal extremity and firmly attached to the pelvic floor and adherent to the right tube, was removed without special difficulty. The abdominal wound was closed, except for a long cigarette drain carried to the pelvic floor, and this was allowed to remain *in situ* until the fourth day, when it was removed. Following that removal the temperature and pulse, which before had been normal, gave evidences of a septic condition. The wound was now thoroughly explored and absolutely nothing was found indicating infection at that place.

The child gradually became more profoundly septic, and on the seventh day it was noticed that the hepatic area was enlarged and the diagnosis of a subphrenic abscess was made. The leucocytes at this time had increased from 14,000 to 36,000. Operation for draining the abscess was performed by excision of the ninth rib, and following the location by aspiration of the abscess; drainage was introduced and the contents of a large abscess of a most fetid character were evacuated. The child never rallied from the operation and died that night. This case, in my opinion, was one of mixed infection, with the colon bacillus as the most important of the pathogenic organisms.

Case III.—The third and last case which I present is that with the following history: Miss K. M. C., aged 26; family history good, and except for occasional attacks of supposed intestinal indigestion, probably reattacks of mild catarrhal appendicitis, no other symptoms were given until she began, two years prior to coming under my observation, to have symptoms referable to bladder trouble. At that time there was a slight hematuria and frequent micturition. Being then in England, she consulted medical aid and the family was informed that she was suffering from tuberculosis of the bladder and a bad prognosis was made. She returned to America and passed the following year without any special increase in symptoms referable to the bladder, and, except for the occasional attacks of hematuria and the necessity to frequently urinate, she enjoyed fairly good health and engaged in her usual amusements and recreation, including horseback riding. In July, summer of 1900, after an unusually long sea-bath, taken just prior to the time of her expected menses, she became suddenly quite ill, suffering from general abdominal pain, and the bladder symptoms became very pronounced. It was at this time that I first saw her, and found on examination an hypertrophied, retroverted, and firmly fixed uterus, with exudates in the left broad ligament. The menstruation became established twenty-four hours after she first came under my observation, and was accompanied with marked dysmenorrhea lasting for three days. At this time there was temperature of 101.5°, pulse 110, and a leucocyte count of 11,000. She referred some pain to the region of the appendix and there was a rigidity of the right rectus. Treatment for this condition was employed, but without any result, and she became gradually more septic and the leucocytes increased to 16,000. Examination per vaginam now revealed a boggy mass in Douglas' cul-de-sac. This was incised and drainage established, which for the following four days gave great relief of all septic symptoms. On the fifth day after the vaginal incision she again gave symptoms of recurring sepsis, and it was decided, after consultation with Dr. W. C. Bull, to perform abdominal section with the idea of thorough exploration of the abdominal and pelvic viscera, and, if necessary, to establish drainage from any focus of septic inflammation that might be above with the drainage which had been made per vaginam. A distinct abscess cavity was found about the caput coli containing typical fetid pus associated with lesions of this type. A second abscess cavity was also found involving the left ovary and tube. Large drainage tubes were inserted into these abscess cavities and also brought out through the vaginal incision. For nine weeks the patient continued to progressively improve and the sinuses had now entirely closed. During all this time the bladder had been a source of great annoyance, and, although efforts had been made by frequent irrigation to improve this condition, the distressing symptoms of painful and frequent micturition continued. The urine was filled with pyogenic organisms which seemed to vary in their type. At one time, when it was evident there were large quantities of pus, the streptococci and staphylococci were present in great quantity, but always large colonies of colon bacilli were found. At this time the first satisfactory cystoscopic examination was made, and it was found that almost the entire bladder mucosa had been denuded, and on the left side, about a half-inch below the entrance of the left ureter, was located a distinct depression. The patient was now seen by Dr. Howard A. Kelly, of Baltimore, who on examination pronounced the pelvic organs in a remarkably healthy condition, considering the virulent septic process which had taken place in and adjacent to them. On cystoscopic examination he confirmed the diagnosis of a most virulent type of cystitis, and, from cultures made, found the colon bacilli in great numbers, and stated that there was a sinus which communicated with the left side of the bladder upward and had undoubtedly been a fistulous track connecting a left tubo-ovarian abscess with the bladder. On his advice the bladder was drained by vesico-vaginal incision for three months, during all of which time topical applications were made to the interior of the bladder, and a gradual and continual improvement occurred, such as warranted the closure of the vesico-vaginal fistula. For the past six months there has been progressive increase of bladder capacity, and instead of being compelled to urinate always as often as once each hour or each hour and a half, she now goes four hours, and the capacity was increased from one or two ounces to six or eight ounces. The interior of the bladder now is normal, except for a slight grade of trigonitis; there is no other pathological condition.

This case illustrates the virulence and persistence of the colon bacillus infection; also how much more active these bacilli become when, as above stated, a suitable nidus for their propagation is afforded.

It is my desire that the presentation of these cases shall serve to remind members of the Society of experiences which they have had with colon bacilli infection, and warrant me in deducing the following conclusions:

1. That there exists as much necessity for thorough cleansing and rendering as aseptic as possible the rectum and colon as the field of operation, especially when that operation is performed per vaginam; that, in all cases of election, the routine treatment of mild mercurial catharsis, followed by a saline and irrigation of the colon with salt or boracic acid solution, should be employed.

2. Again to reiterate a warning that best results can be obtained when the intestines receive the minimum degree of trauma from handling, and especially the absence of careless use of retractors, where, for cosmetic effects or fear of hernia, too small incisions are made to permit of operation by sight rather than by touch.

DR. BROTHERS.—During my work at the Post-Graduate Hospital several years ago I had a series of pus cases, which I had operated upon, examined microscopically, and I must say that those cases in which we found the colon bacillus were very much in the minority; I do not recall any case in which the colon bacilli were the only bacteriological elements present. The gonococci were the most frequent and then the streptococci and staphylococci. The colon bacilli were exceptionally rare. In one case, unfortunately, the pus was not examined; it was in connection with a fibroid ovary. The case was presented to the gentlemen of the class for examination prior to operation, and, as the result of manipulation, pelvic inflammation occurred. Abscess formed which was operated with the fibroid tumor; colon bacilli were present, as shown from the intense fecal odor given the pus.

DR. GRANDIN.—I should like to ask Dr. Ely what topical application was made in the last case reported.

DR. ELY.—Ten per cent ichthyol in lubrichondrin as prepared by Van Horne. This was not so painful as was the application when some other solvent, as water, was used.

DR. BROUN.—How much was used at a time?

DR. ELY.—This patient could not stand, without much pain, more than one-half to two ounces; gradually this was increased to seven or eight ounces when solutions were employed to distend the bladder. But better results were obtained with the use of the Clark balloon, which, when inflated, brings every part of the mucosa in contact with the ichthyol applied to the surface of the balloon.

DR. BROUN.—That coincides with an experience I had at the Woman's Hospital, where we used ichthyol in watery solution and good results were obtained; a ten per cent solution was employed. I think, too, that the solution as made by Dr. Ely adheres better than the watery one.

DR. ELY.—I am surprised to hear what Dr. Brothers has said,

for I am sure, if an examination had been made for the different pathogenic organisms, the frequency of the colon bacilli would have been very great. If they are found, as reported by bacteriologists, even in arthritic joints, then the point I want to bring out is, *why* do they vary so much in intensity and intractability?

TRANSACTIONS OF THE WOMAN'S HOSPITAL SOCIETY.

Meeting of April 22, 1902.

The Vice-President, JAMES N. WEST, M.D., *in the Chair.*

DR. LE ROY BROUN reported for DR. CLEMENT CLEVELAND

I. A CASE OF LARGE OVARIAN CYST.

DR. BROUN.—This specimen is presented for Dr. Cleveland, who is not present. It is shown on account of the size and the difficulty attending its removal. Years ago it was no uncommon occurrence to see ovarian cysts of enormous size, but with the increased knowledge of later years their removal is always accomplished early. The solid portion of this tumor, as shown, weighs twenty-five pounds. Four gallons of fluid were evacuated at the time of operation, giving the actual weight of the tumor removed as at least sixty-five pounds.

A week before the operation Dr. Cleveland removed two gallons of fluid in order to relieve dyspnea. The cyst was unilocular, densely adherent to the parietal peritoneum, from which it was separated with difficulty. At the base of the cyst was a large, solid mass wedged into the pelvis, and to dislodge it required considerable strength. The left ovary was also the seat of a cyst of about eight inches in diameter, also containing much solid material.

The patient is doing well, as far as the temperature, pulse, and respiration show. A peculiar complication, however, is a marked edema of the face and a frequent occurrence of mental aberration. Both of these symptoms appeared since the operation. I do not regard these conditions as connected with a kidney lesion, since she is passing twenty ounces of urine with ten grains of urea to the ounce. She is on infusion of digitalis and nitroglycerin. I would like Dr. Janvrin to express an opinion as to the cause of this mental condition.

The patient now, three weeks after the operation, is well, the above-mentioned symptoms having subsided gradually.

DR. JOSEPH E. JANVRIN.—The specimens themselves are very interesting from the fact that there is so much solid tissue in both. However, considering the amount of fluid in the large sac, the amount of solid tissue is perhaps not disproportionate compared with what we find in smaller cysts.

As to the character of the tissue, I hardly think there is anything malignant about it. I think, if there were, the patient would have presented not only the ordinary symptoms of which Dr. Broun has spoken—extreme exhaustion, etc.—but a good deal of cachexia in appearance, which she did not have. I think, when examined, it will be found not to be malignant.

The case reminds me of one I operated on in my sanitarium seven years ago. It was almost a fac-simile of this, though it was larger. I knew, from examination, the patient had an immense ovarian cyst and some smaller ones; I knew also there was a fibroid condition of the uterus—at least I thought so before operating. She came from the northern part of the State and was in excellent condition, about 46 years of age. I removed a large ovarian tumor; the amount of fluid from the large cyst weighed eighty-seven pounds. Then lower down, at its base, connected with the uterus, quite an amount of solid material, one-fourth as much as in Dr. Cleveland's specimen, was present. In addition to this large tumor on the right side there was also a small one on the left side, which I removed, and then, on account of the fibroid, I went on and removed the uterus, as Dr. Cleveland did in this case, except that I made a total ablation down through the vagina. The combined weight of the whole of the uterus and tumors was some ninety-three pounds. It was the largest I ever removed. The recovery was perfect. No temperature—never above 99°. She was a big, strong, robust woman. In three weeks she went home.

I suppose the combined weight of this specimen, all told, is about seventy-five pounds.

Dr. Cleveland.—As to the pathological condition, my impression was, when I looked at the large papillomatous growths (one very near the diaphragm, the other low in the pelvis), that they might be in the beginning stage of malignant papilloma. Possibly we shall find it to be so on microscopic examination. This tumor had been in the woman's body for over ten years. She had been seen by several gentlemen and operation had been advised against. One of the most interesting features of the case was the very firm adhesion to the peritoneal peritoneum at every point. In consequence I had the greatest difficulty in enucleating the mass from the abdominal cavity, and particularly so that portion which lodged in the pelvis. The second tumor was isolated and pediculated and very easily removed. The first tumor was the most adherent one removed totally that I have ever seen. The woman has done very well, as Dr. Broun said.

Dr. E. L'H. McGinnis.—Was there no previous history of brain symptoms—mind-wandering?

Dr. Cleveland.—A history of coma at one time was given, said to be due to the condition of the kidneys.

DR. McGINNIS.—I wondered if that could account for her being flighty at times, following the operation.

DR. CLEVELAND.—I suppose that would be the explanation.

II. LAPARATOMY WITH FAILURE OF WOUND TO UNITE, AND FINALLY A COMPLETE SEPARATION OF ALL THE LAYERS OF THE ABDOMINAL WOUND AFTER REMOVAL OF THE STITCHES ON THE EIGHTH DAY.

DR. BROUN.—The second case of Dr. Cleveland's showed a most interesting and unusual condition. Some twelve days ago Dr. Cleveland had occasion to remove a very adherent double pyosalpinx, and he did a supravaginal hysterectomy, establishing drainage posteriorly. On account of the poor condition of the patient the abdomen was closed with through-and-through sutures. Each alternate suture embraced only the skin and fascia.

The sutures were taken out at the usual time, the morning of the eighth day. She had no temperature, but had an obstinate cough during the convalescence. On the afternoon of the eighth day the house surgeon reported that the entire abdominal wound gaped. The wound was finally sutured layer by layer. She has had no temperature since the closing of the wound, a week ago to-morrow morning. This morning the wound was examined and found sloughing. As far as we know, there is no history of syphilis.

DR. WEST.—The breaking open of the wound without the presence of pus is very interesting. I remember a case which occurred several years ago in the Woman's Hospital. The patient was supposed to have peritonitis which was expected to be fatal. The stitches were removed a little ahead of the usual time. She had typhoid fever—showed symptoms the second day; the wound broke open very deep, to the peritoneum.

DR. CLEVELAND.—I have seen one or two cases where the wound has broken open after the removal of stitches at the usual time. A number of years ago I removed a fibroid by supravaginal method, taking out the stitches on the eighth day; the wound opened down to the peritoneum. The wound healed by granulation. A very good line of union resulted, almost as good as after taking stitches. It was like union by first intention. In this case which Dr. Broun reported for me to-night I feel pretty well convinced there is a constitutional taint. She is on mixed treatment now.

DISCUSSION ON CERTAIN STEPS IN CELIOTOMY.

DR. WEST.—First, as to abdominal incisions, there is a great variety in the way of length and character, from the straight median incision to the cross incision and turning up a flap.

DR. BROUN.—We are all pretty well united in this, that the median line of incision of the abdomen is the most favorable one. I am convinced that it is much to the patient's benefit that the incision should be of sufficient length to enable the surgeon to work with ease. If the case is one of pyosalpinx or fibroid tumor, the length of the incision should be such as to enable the operator to work by sight. The attempt to do such an operation through small incisions can only increase the difficulty of the operation and be a detriment to the patient. It is the habit of some to enter the abdomen a little to the right or left of the median line, in order to go through the rectus muscle. This has certain advantages, especially in the final closing of the wound, since each layer can be approximated accurately.

In closing the wound I prefer coaptating each layer separately, chromicized catgut being used for the fascia. To take off tension from these sutures caused by vomiting, it is my custom to place two or more silkworm-gut retaining sutures through all layers (excepting the peritoneum). These sutures can be removed after vomiting has ceased.

Dr. E. E. Tull.—I always feel that the abdominal incision is a very important part of the operation, from the infection point of view. I try, in making incisions, to make a clean cut. I invariably, before going into the abdomen, pick up the abdominal wall and measure its thickness, and keep some sort of record as to how long it takes to go into the abdominal cavity. It should not take more than one minute or one and one-half minutes to go through the anterior abdominal wall.

It is much more convenient to cut from below upward. We have a fixed point below; we must go as near the pubis as possible, but we can extend as far as we please. From above we do not know how large an opening we may require; we limit the incision. If we start from below upward it can be extended *ad libitum.*

As to going to one side of the median line, I do believe we get better union if we go to one side or the other, and have muscle to cut through. In pyosalpinx or where pus is more or less likely to be spilt, I would rather have fascia in contact with it than the raw edge of the muscle.

In regard to the use of retractors in opening the abdominal wall, I think that the use of this instrument is fruitful in producing abscesses and giving trouble. I have known of several such cases within the last seven or eight years. I think we can get along without retractors.

The incision should be clean cut, generally in the median line; if we have pus to deal with the incision should certainly be in the median line. If we have a definite condition in the centre of the abdominal cavity, without pus, we may select a muscle. I think the incision should be very concise and clean.

Dr. Cleveland.—In regard to whether it is better to go directly through muscles or to take advantage of the separation of the muscles, I am not absolutely clear myself. I have always been in the habit of finding the spot where muscles separate and drawing them apart with my fingers, and going in in that way.

Several times I have gone through the muscles. I cannot see any particular advantage in that method. I cannot make up my mind that there is really any.

In sewing up layer by layer, if you know the spot where the edge of the muscle should be stitched to the other side, it is very easy to stitch it to that spot.

I was surprised at what Dr. Tull said as to retractors. I have used them all my life. I can see no contraindication. I cannot see how their use might lead to abscess. Of course in a pus case it is important that great care should be taken to keep the abdominal wall covered with gauze.

DR. TULL.—I mean simply that retractors give rise to trauma.

DR. CLEVELAND.—I always use retractors. I cannot see that they bruise the tissues enough to produce injury such as you mention.

DR. JANVRIN.—I would like to ask Dr. Tull for an explanation. If he goes directly through in making abdominal section, he does not pick up the tissues and peritoneum separately, as is frequently done. I find it absolutely necessary to do so in many cases where there are adhesions to the anterior wall of the tumor or of the bladder. If I understand Dr. Tull aright, he said he would trim off the sides of the cut afterward.

DR. TULL.—I mean in approximating several layers, ragged edges may be made; if so, I am very careful to trim them off.

DR. JANVRIN.—That would not militate against slowness in making the abdominal incision and so avoid going into the bladder where adhesions were suspected, and you thought it best to pick up the tissues slowly and so avoid injury to the intestines or bladder, especially in cases of hernia.

DR. TULL.—In hernia, as a rule, I make the first incision down to the peritoneum. That means I do not have one layer at one angle and another at another angle. I pick up what the thickness is, one or one and one-half inches, and protect the point of the knife for that length. I never cut the intestine in my life.

DR. CLEVELAND.—I would like to emphasize what Dr. Tull said about the point of beginning the incision. I always stand on the patient's left side and cut from the pubis upward, for the very reason he states. If you make a short incision you know where to begin below and can limit it at the umbilicus, if you choose. That is a very important point and I would like to emphasize it.

DR. WEST.—I believe that the length of the incision is an extremely important factor with the patient. I have seen incisions which varied between the extremely long one, extending from the umbilicus to the pubis, for simple ovariotomy, and the one that was only two inches long and the attempt made to remove a pus tube. The latter is extremely dangerous. The question is not settled. Some men prefer very short incisions, others very long ones. It is a question of judgment. In slight operations, as for chronic oöphoritis, a very short incision—one and one-half inches—is sufficient. For the dissection of pus tubes, where one should have his eyes upon the work he is doing, to have an incision of sufficient length is of great importance. In pyosalpinx an incision from three to four or four and one-half inches in length is required. In hysterorrhaphy an incision of one or one and one-half inches will suffice.

Another factor enters into this question, namely, hernia. An extremely long incision is much more injurious to the abdominal wall than a short one. I have known of men who operated for simple ovaritis and made an incision from the umbilicus to the pubis, followed by abscesses and ventral hernia. The operation could have been done through a two-inch incision with probably much less danger of hernia. The less the length of the incision, the less shock; the less to sew, the more time saved. One must not attempt to use a small incision for a pus case or where a tumor has to be dragged out.

METHODS OF CARING FOR AND PROTECTING INTESTINES DURING OPERATION.

DR. WEST.—I think if there is one aspect more important than another in performing celiotomy, it is that of the care of the intestines, and the subject is so large one hardly knows where to begin it. It is easier to care for the intestines with a small abdominal opening. There are times when large incisions are necessary, and where the intestines must be exposed and must themselves be operated upon.

I think that, in the first place, we may consider that aspect of the case which involves the handling or moving of the intestines about. It has been my experience and observation that if the intestines are dragged upon the shock produced is more profound. This should always be avoided. The mesentery should not be stretched, as the effect on the sympathetic system is bad. In such manipulations a condition of shock has been produced where death has followed. Whether the bowel is to be sutured or handled otherwise, let us not drag on them. Do the work with the intestines lying loosely under the hand, not dragging upon the mesentery.

Second, protection of the intestines. They are near the seat of the great blood supply, sympathetic nerve supply, and should not be exposed to the air more than is necessary. This can be accomplished, when exposing is necessary, by keeping them covered with warm towels moistened with saline solution. The best protection is in the abdomen, covered with omentum, kept warm, and covered with normal secretions.

When separating adhesions, if we rupture pus tubes or pus accumulations of any kind, and get the intestines soiled, the chances are very great for fatal peritonitis. It is of the greatest importance possible that we should prevent such infection of the intestines. I believe a ruptured intestine should be at once sewed up. Intestinal adhesions are always to be feared, and some patients have especial tendencies toward their formation. A great deal of thought and experimentation has been given to the subject, but no satisfactory conclusion, so far as I know, has been reached in regard to preventing adhesions. Dr. Morris has been carrying on some interesting experiments, using aristol. He gives the intestines a good coating of aristol. Some writers advocate the practice of filling the abdomen with normal saline solution. This is not satisfactory; it does not prevent intestinal adhesions. I operated upon two cases and filled the abdomen with normal saline solution, and the adhesions occurred again as badly as before operation. Dr. Morris is now experimenting with sterilized animal peritoneum. He prepares the peritoneum of the ox, which will at once adhere to a denuded surface when placed upon it, the opposite side forming a glistening, non-adhesive membrane. What the outcome will be we do not know. He is to present a paper shortly upon that subject.

Dr. Broun.—I agree with Dr. West that there is nothing on the line of our abdominal work which demands closer attention than the protection of the intestines. My belief is that the protection of the intestines should chiefly be done at the commencement of the operation. That is, when the abdomen is opened the intestines should be gotten as completely out of the way as possible, so that the field of operation, whether for pus tubes or pyosalpinx, cancerous uterus or otherwise, will practically be extraperitoneal so far as the intestines are concerned—entirely cut off from the intestinal mass. It is our custom at the Woman's Hospital to use the regulation abdominal pads, eight inches square, with long tape attached. To prevent their adhering to the intestine they are moistened with salt solution. The patient is put in extreme Trendelenburg position: if no adhesions exist the intestines at once gravitate toward the diaphragm. We usually put in eight or nine, sometimes ten, abdominal pads, and cover the intestines thoroughly, so that if there should be any escape of fluid it will be met by the pads and not soil the coils of the intestines. Where dense adhesions exist and we fear the spilling of pus, the patient is put in extreme Trendelenburg position to get the intestines as far back as they will go. Pads are put over them, special attention being paid to the sides where there are least adhesions, so that any escape of pus or fluid must necessarily fall against the pads as the operator begins to separate the adhesions. As he gets down closer to the mass he is followed by his assistant, who keeps the pads well applied. As the adhesions are separated and the intestines liberated they are pushed back and covered with fresh pads, if necessary. Although I know that after the removal of these inflammatory masses, pus tubes, etc., in a large majority of cases their contents are sterile, it adds to the operator's discomfort to soil the intestines with escaping fluids, and greatly to his comfort not to do so.

If we have pus to deal with, the assistant slips pads over each side of the edge of the abdominal wound underneath the retractors, and any spilled pus does not come in contact with the wall but with the pad that lies against it. No intestines get out and none are exposed. As little dragging as possible is done. By keeping the intestines covered in that way, if pus be spilled no flushing out is necessary; dry pads are placed in after touching up the soiled field with peroxide. After the pelvis is cleared, soiled pads are taken out, fresh ones put in, and we change our gloves. We know that in a large majority of cases the pus is sterile, yet it is comfortable to feel that in all human probability we have not soiled the intestines with pus. The results are excellent.

DR. J. DOUGAL BISSELL presented a paper on

CLOSURE OF THE ABDOMINAL INCISION.

Permit me to say a word, first, in regard to the opening of the abdomen. I prefer the median incision, chiefly for the reason that the abdominal walls are more easily retracted and manipulation within facilitated when the incision is along the linea alba. The length of the incision should depend upon the extent of work to be accomplished. I had promised to prepare a paper for this Society, to be read next fall, and had selected as my subject for that occasion the one you have assigned me for this evening; being thus anticipated, I shall be brief in my remarks, reserving for the future a more detailed description. The methods of closing the abdominal incision are numerous; that which is used by the majority of operators may be described as a "through-and-through" method, the suture, silkworm-gut or silver, being passed through skin, fat, fascia, muscle, and peritoneum. A modification of this method. introduced by Dr. Waldo and used now by many, consists in omitting alternately the fascia. Rapidity is the chief advantage in these methods. The layer-by-layer suturing is being more commonly used and is the method I personally prefer. Every method has its successes and failures, but these successes and failures depend, to a very great extent, upon the precision of the operator. My objection to the "through-and-through" method is that it is difficult to regulate the tension of the sutures; often traction is too great, the circulation is thus impaired, and the tissues break down. Stitch abscesses are a very common sequel to this method. Until within the past year it had been the custom on our service at the Woman's Hospital to close the incision by suturing separately each layer and passing two silkworm-gut sutures entirely through the abdominal wall for the purpose of relieving strain upon the sutures which unite the separate layers. It was our habit to use chromicized catgut for fascia. We repeatedly found abscesses in the angles of the wounds. On two occasions the incision broke down its entire length, leaving only the peritoneum intact. We attributed the cause of the breaking down of the wound to chromic gut; this gut was examined, but pronounced free from microscopic life, which led us to conclude that the chromium itself, being a chemical irritant, was in excess in the strands of gut used and was the probable cause of tissue destruction. Last summer I abandoned altogether the chromic gut, also the silkworm gut, substituting for these plain catgut, adopting the following method: Two or three No. 3 catgut sutures are first passed through fascia, muscle, peritoneum on one side, peritoneum, muscle, fascia on the other, which, when tied, act as supporting sutures to those uniting the peritoneum and fascia. The peritoneum is closed with No. 1 catgut, the fascia with No. 2, and the skin with black silk. Our successes have been most gratifying, and I hope to report results more fully at another time.

DR. SHAILER.—Dr. Bissell has spoken of two ways of closing wounds, with silkworm and catgut. Wounds may be closed another way: Starting at the deep fascia, passing silkworm gut down through the peritoneum and through the opposite edge of peritoneum, then passing through deep fascia, crossing the ends and passing them through the skin, making a figure-of-eight suture. That brings in approximation the several layers better than anything I have seen in the way of using silkworm gut.

In regard to the failure of union in Dr. Cleveland's case: In one case I saw, the ovary and tubes had been removed in a very virulent form of pyosalpinx. The woman died at about the end of a week. We found, just before she died, pus pouring out and the intestines exposed in different areas along the incision. In one section the peritoneum would be closed, and in another open. A virulent microbic infection had destroyed the whole abdominal incision. I have also seen cases where through-and-through sutures had been used—eighteen silver wires in an incision of about four inches in length. All but about one inch of the incision had burst open at the end of two weeks when the silver wires were removed.

DR. CLEVELAND.—I think the point Dr. Bissell brings out with regard to the chromium retained in catgut a very good one. At his suggestion the chemists Van Horne & Co., who have established a reputation for their excellent preparations, examined the catgut. They found that some of the larger sizes did contain the chromium, and I believe they have now succeeded in getting rid of all of it. They do not state how, but I imagine it is by very thorough washing of the catgut. I believe the catgut they have produced of late is not open to the same objection as formerly.

At one time I had a passion for the figure-of-eight suture. I felt that I must use it frequently. I thought once it was a very good method—did for several years, but I have abandoned it for no particular reason. I think it a very good way, a little more difficult, possibly, than the ordinary method. I used it continually with silkworm gut.

In regard to the case of breaking open of the wound, it is the first case I have ever seen of complete separation of all the layers, peritoneum, fascia, and integument. In this case the accident occurred, and the following morning the patient was put under ether. I found what proved to be edematous intestine with the peritoneal edges attached all along the line. It was remarkable how firmly the peritoneum was attached to the intestine in such a short time. I had some difficulty in separating it. The wound must have been thoroughly cleaned, as no peritonitis followed. The peritoneum was not infected in the slightest degree. Why I should have pus after the secondary closure is a mystery. There was none in the first place.

DR. JANVRIN.—I would like to speak in favor of silver wire in closing abdominal wounds. I find any approximation used to bring peritoneum together sufficient. to hold it. There is no strain upon the peritoneum, as I understand it, because it is such elastic tissue. I have used catgut for the peritoneum itself. and then other sutures, as Dr. Bissell and others have mentioned. I believe there is no strain at any time upon the peritoneum itself.

I have tried chromicized catgut, silkworm gut, etc., but have got back, within the last five or six years, absolutely to the use of the through-and-through silver-wire suture. In putting it in I always pass my needle through the skin about one-third of an inch from the edge. I invariably carry the needle point outward, so as to take a good hold upon the muscle, carry it down through the fascia, and then simply catch the peritoneum. Then carrying it through from inside cut and making a reverse, the result is that I have a perfect loop. Every suture is applied in that way. When the surfaces are brought together and sutures tightened, I always resort to the practice Dr. Emmet taught us of shouldering the sutures. I take the tenaculum and lift the loop and twist a little more; consequently, as I believe, there is not too much traction upon the sutures, the walls are approximated, and I very rarely see any abscesses whatever. Too much stricture is not put upon the stitches, just sufficient strength and power to hold the surfaces together in a looped form, and they are held perfectly. Enough tension is put upon them so that muscle and fascia are brought together properly, but not sufficient to cause any undue tension which might lead to the formation of abscesses. I have used silver wire almost invariably for the past five or six years; once, for a period of two or three years, I resorted to other methods. I had always used the silver wire before this for at least twenty years, and, after trying the catgut and silkworm gut for two or three years, I returned to the silver wire, applied as before described.

DR. LANGSTAFF.—I notice, in the drawing Dr. Bissell showed us. that the stitch which includes skin and fat runs very superficially to the surface of the cut. I think when tied it would make a pocket in the tissues there. I believe it should be made

16

with a full curved needle, to include a great deal of tissue as in the perineum; then you will eliminate the dead spaces and press the tissues more firmly together. Not only that, if you put in a superficial stitch which runs close to the cut surface, you produce greater strangulation of the vessels. The more superficial the stitches, the more are required and the greater the strangulation of vessels. The Hagedorn needle is something like a small tenotomy knife. You take a deep stitch and you do not know how many vessels you catch in its passage through the tissues. The incision is closed up by the tension of the stitch, and that prevents the escape of blood on the surface. In that way you do not know how much blood escapes in the tissues below. I think these conditions will often explain the suture abscesses which form.

DR. BROUN.—The impression produced upon the minds of those present would be that we are in the habit of having abscesses at the Woman's Hospital. It is the rarest thing. When they do occur we want to know the cause.

DR. WEST.—In regard to finding free chromium, etc., I think we used some chromicized gut at the Woman's Hospital. In all the winter's work there has been but one abscess in the service of Dr. Bache Emmet in these closings of celiotomy wounds; we constantly use the chromic gut. We had one abscess last summer; in one year's work, two abscesses, which I consider an excessive number in that service. We ought not to have more than one in a couple of years. We have used chromicized gut, closed the peritoneum with fine catgut, fascia with medium-sized chromium gut, and skin with silk.

Official transactions.   H. GRAD, *Editor.*

TRANSACTIONS OF THE
CHICAGO GYNECOLOGICAL SOCIETY.

Meeting of February 21, 1902.

The President, LESTER E. FRANKENTHAL, M.D., *in the Chair.*

UREMIA IN PREGNANCY.

DR. FRANKENTHAL.—I desire to briefly report the case of a multipara who was delivered some six years ago. At that time no urinalysis was made. The woman is the wife of a lawyer, a remarkably bright man, who of his own accord, after her delivery, concluded that there must be something wrong with his wife because her extremities were so badly swollen. This case occurred in the Northwest of our country, and my interne obtained this history after her admission to hospital: Three weeks before her first confinement, six years ago, she noticed a swelling of the feet and legs. She had at that time suffered from occipital headaches, but manifested no other symptoms. She had an easy confinement which lasted but two hours. One week later the headaches returned, particularly in the back of the head. This continued for five months, during which time the pains became at times more severe and were distinctly remittent. It was seven months before the swelling in the feet and legs decreased and she was well again. During that time, at the instigation of the husband, her urine was examined and found to contain large quantities of albumin. At the expiration of eight months the albumin had disappeared entirely from the urine. A few years after that she had a miscarriage. I saw the patient a week ago, and the history given at that time was the following: A week previous to my seeing her she suffered from a severe toothache, and her family physician administered chloroform and the tooth was extracted. Two days after the extraction of the tooth there was general edema of the body, and upon examination of the urine large quantities of albumin were found. She was then in her thirty-first week of pregnancy. The physician asked me to see the patient at that time. She was taken to the hospital and kept on a milk diet, given sweat baths, bowels attended to, etc., etc.; and while the albumin decreased somewhat in quantity at the expiration of three or four days, the decrease was so little that I felt the woman's kidneys would be permanently impaired if pregnancy were to continue, especially if so slight an insult as the administration of the chloroform could provoke another attack of nephritis; and inasmuch as we would have to wait at least eight more weeks before the expiration of her pregnancy, I deemed it advisable to bring on labor.

I put in several Barnes' bags of the largest size, tied them to the bed, intending to make slow dilatation, but each and every one broke after being attached for five or six minutes. I finally put in Champetier de Ribes' bag and made steady traction for about thirty to forty minutes, when the os was sufficiently well dilated for me to feel that her labor would have to continue; it was then not larger than two inches in diameter. I left the patient long enough to take some supper, and in my absence the physician, who was likewise in attendance, ruptured the bag of waters, thinking the os completely dilated. It was one of those conical bags of waters that we find in breech presentations. After my return I found an incomplete breech presentation, with the os no more dilated than when I left. She gave birth to a dead child, life having ceased during the delivery.

The most interesting feature of this case is the urinalyses, which show speedy improvement after the delivery of the child. The woman is making an uninterrupted recovery. The edema has disappeared; the headaches have gone, also the epigastric pain, and the chronic uremic restlessness has disappeared, so that I am in hopes of her having in time a completely restored kidney.

DR. GUSTAV KOLISCHER.—I desire to speak of only one point in connection with this case, as Dr. Frankenthal has already stated that I indorsed his opinion of inducing labor in his case. It is the experience of the last two years that, in all cases where we want to dilate the cervix rapidly or within a short time, it is better to use a non-elastic colpeurynter for two reasons. Elastic colpeurynters are hard to keep in good shape; they become brittle and break easily, and if you pull hard, or the cervix is rigid, as is usually the case, the colpeurynter, if it does not burst, becomes stretched out to the shape of a sausage and slips. So it is better, in case one desires rapid dilatation, to use one of the French colpeurynters. They do not give way and they do not become brittle.

DR. ALEXANDER HUGH FERGUSON.—I would like to ask Dr. Frankenthal whether he has noticed, in his practice in this line. the effect, in bringing on labor, on the secretion of urine and the amount of urea during that time; whether the amount of urea was increased or decreased, or whether the amount of urine was decreased or increased.

DR. FRANKENTHAL.—I believe that our clinical estimate of the amount of urea secreted by a patient is simply a fake, because we have hardly any right to estimate the amount of urea secreted by a patient when we do not know the amount of nitrogenous food taken by the patient, likewise the amount of sweating, the bowel movement, etc. All these things have an important bearing on the amount of urea, and unless we are accurate in one instance we have no right to make deductions in the other. In pregnant patients of whose cases I have kept careful records of urinalyses, say ten to fifteen times through pregnancy, I have found that the patient's urea varies anywhere from one-half per cent to 2.2 per cent all through pregnancy, whether we take fresh specimens or twenty-four-hour specimens, and I do not find that the induction of labor has any instantaneous appreciable effect on the amount of urea excreted by those patients.

DR. ALEXANDER HUGH FERGUSON read a report on

UTERINE SUSPENSION PER VAGINAM.

During the last three years indications presented themselves in a limited number of cases to suspend the uterus to the anterior abdominal wall and fasten it in the same position of slight anterior flexion that is obtained by the Kelly method through an abdominal incision. It is simply Kelly's suspension without his technique. The indications for it are the same, the same objections obtain, and the results cannot be different.

By this method the objectionable scar on the abdomen is obviated. I perform it when I am not allowed to open the abdomen above the pubes and do my operation of "anterior transplantation of the round ligaments," and also when Webster's operation is not feasible through the vagina.

Operation.—Perform anterior colpotomy; turn the uterus out

(Fig. 1) ; fasten a long double suture of No. 1 chromoform catgut to the posterior surface of the fundus of the uterus, and pass a narrow-bladed knife through the abdominal wall at the suprapubic fold without penetrating the peritoneum; insert a sound (Fig. 2) into the bladder and with it push that viscus to one side and down, so as not to receive injury. Now pass a long, curved, blunt-pointed needle through the abdominal puncture and pierce the peritoneum between two fingers of the left hand that have

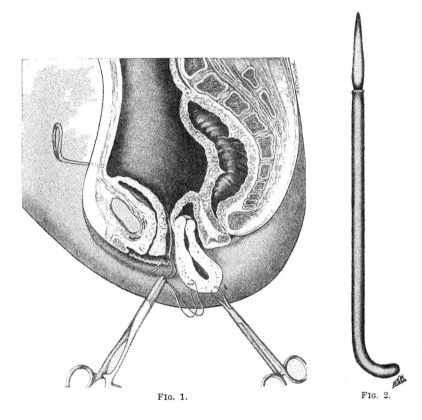

FIG. 1.   FIG. 2.

been inserted through the vaginal incision to the anterior abdominal wall where the needle penetrates. The fingers feel the bladder and serve as an additional guide to protect it. The needle is allowed to pass behind the bladder and come out through the vagina by way of the colpotomy incision. Thread the needle (Fig. 1) and withdraw it through the abdominal puncture, then make traction on the catgut suture until the uterus is brought to its normal position (Fig. 3).

One strand is threaded into an ordinary curved surgical needle and a bite taken of the linea alba, the needle emerging through a second small puncture in the skin; then the other strand is similarly dealt with, the suture tied, and the uterus is held suspended. A horsehair suture closes each puncture in the skin and a collodion dressing seals them up. Two or three sutures are inserted in the vaginal vault to close the wound there, the vagina is packed with gauze, and the operation is completed.

Should omentum or intestines show in the vaginal wound or come in contact with the seat of operation, then the patient is

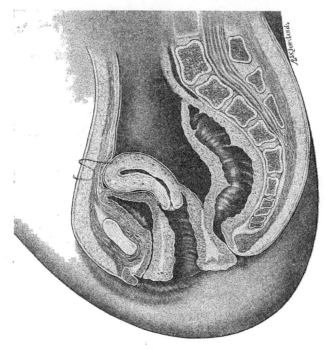

FIG. 3.

placed in the Trendelenburg position, when they at once recede out of the way.

I have performed this operation thirteen times successfully without an accident. In eight cases the uterus was simply retro-displaced; one of these has since borne a child. In two cases conservative work was done on cystic ovaries and the ovaries suspended in place by shortening the utero-ovarian ligaments. These are symptomatically cured, but have not become pregnant. In the remaining three cases the tubes and ovaries were removed for chronic inflammation and the displaced womb suspended.

Dr. Ferguson also reported

THREE CASES OF ACUTE GASTRECTASIA, TWO FOLLOWING OPERATIONS.

Acute dilatation of the stomach causing pyloric obstruction is rare. Works on medicine make slight reference to it, and surgical text books make no mention.

Case I.—J. P., 24 years of age, was referred to me by Dr. Bacon and sent to the Post-Graduate Hospital in June, 1895. He was complaining of repeated attacks of pain in the right iliac region, these becoming more frequent and severe. The pain be-

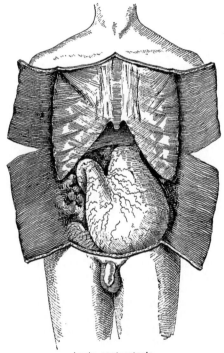

Acute gastrectasia.

came nearly constant. In short, he had a clear clinical history of chronic appendicitis, which proved to be so by operation. It was an easy case to operate upon. The appendix was not adherent, it was enlarged toward its distal end, had two strictures in it, and contained three gallstones. The abdomen was closed without drainage and the young man placed in bed. He vomited once or twice on the operating table, but he was free from it for three hours after the operation. Then vomiting set in, in a mild manner and without distress. Day by day he became worse. No bile or intestinal contents in the matter vomited. Consultation was called on the fifth day. Then he was bloated over the entire abdomen, pulse rapid and weak, skin cold, temperature normal. He died on the eighth day. A complete postmortem of the chest and abdomen was performed. The organs were normal except the stomach.

The seat of the operation upon the appendix was in a perfect state. The stomach literally filled the abdomen and extended into the pelvis (see illustration). The pylorus was completely obstructed on account of being acutely bent. The pyloric end of the stomach was greatly thickened and congested. A sketch was taken of it, as here presented.

Case II.—In July, 1897, Dr. G. G. Burdick called me to the Chicago Charity Hospital to see a case of supposed intestinal obstruction. He was 24 years old, a healthy laborer. He complained of abdominal distress, a sore sense of fulness, constant vomiting, great thirst, general prostration, and increasing tympany of the abdomen. The illness was of three days' duration and attributed to overeating. On the fourth day of July he ate corned beef, cabbage, carrots, etc., to an enormous extent, and even before he left the dinner table he felt the distress and in a few minutes began to vomit. For twenty-four hours he suffered, but a doctor was not called till the next day.

The vomiting, etc., became alarming and he was sent to the hospital. A physical examination revealed an alarming condition. Pulse 120, rapid and weak, sighing respirations, temperature subnormal, restless, eyes sunken, cold perspiration over his body, and extremities cold. Everything he swallowed was soon rejected. The vomited material was from the stomach alone. It contained no bile nor intestinal contents. Stomach tympany extended below the umbilicus and succussion could be elicited. Acute dilatation of the stomach was recognized and treated by washing out the distended organ. I have no note of the quantity of liquid material removed by the first passing of the stomach tube, but it was several quarts.

At the end of a week he left the hospital, able to take his food by the stomach. Three months later he was in normal health.

Case III.—Mr. C. H. R., aged 43 years, patient of Drs. Cotton and C. H. Andersen, entered the Chicago Hospital on June 5, 1901. He was complaining of colicky pains in the region of the appendix, tenderness on pressure, the presence of a tumor, constipation, and losing flesh and strength. Trouble began four or five years previously in the form of attacks of pain in the right iliac region. Since that time he has had a clinical history of chronic catarrhal recurrent appendicitis. The last attack of this nature he had a temperature of 102°, two weeks before entering the hospital, and a mass in the iliac region was detected for the first time.

Physical examination revealed a mass in right iliac region about two and one-half inches in diameter, firm, hard, and tender. Right iliac region below the mass was quite tympanic, while

above it there was flatness. Upon listening with stethoscope the
noise of gas rushing through a narrow opening could be heard.
Diagnosis: Probably carcinoma of the cecum. Operation advised.

Operation.—The next day I removed entire cecum, about two
and one-half inches of ileum, and four or five inches of ascending
colon. Made an anastomosis between small to large bowel, end to
side, with Murphy button; closed the abdomen. Specimen removed was cancerous in character, with pathologic stricture large
enough to admit the end of an artery forceps. A couple of cancerous lymphatic glands were removed. Patient stood the operation well.

After-Treatment.—For the first two days after the operation
patient vomited not more frequently than is often met with after
such an operation. His pulse and temperature remained normal.
On the third day the vomiting became very distressing and frequent, even though nothing was allowed by the mouth. On the
morning of the fourth day the stomach extended below the umbilicus and was considerably larger than on the previous day.
Diagnosis of acute gastrectasia was made, in which Drs. Cotton
and Andersen agreed. Several quarts of stomach contents were
siphoned off. Stomach was washed out with salt solution at
temperature of 120° at once and afterward every four hours.
Large doses of strychnine sulphate were given every four hours.

Next day he was so improved that the stomach-washing was
stopped. Small portions of hot water were allowed to be swallowed. In the afternoon the vomiting returned and the stomach
dilated as before, and in order to avoid the use of the stomach
tube he rolled over the edge of the bed and pushed his fingers
into his throat. For the next forty-eight hours he repeated this
several times to cause vomiting, in order to relieve the distress
caused by the dilatation of the stomach. Nothing was given by
the mouth during this time. On the seventh day he was able to
take liquid diet, after which he rapidly improved.

DR. GUSTAV KOLISCHER.—I would like to ask Dr. Ferguson
what he does with the peritoneum between the bladder and uterus
after the uterus is replaced.

DR. FERGUSON.—I simply close the cul-de-sac with tier stitches.

DR. KOLISCHER.—In discussing abdominal or vaginal operations for displacement of the uterus there will always be great
diversity of opinion. If one prefers to make the vaginal operation, he does it for two reasons: First, the operation is considerably less dangerous, and the uterus is not so exposed as it is
in abdominal operations. Second, the uterus is placed in a
physiological position; it is not dragged out of the minor pelvis,
and it should be able to become pregnant without any interference by adhesions. If we pull the uterus down we expose it and
we lose the advantages of the vaginal operation. These advantages are only to be had, first, if we do not expose the uterus;
second, if the uterus is not fastened in an unphysiological posi-

tion. When the uterus is fastened with the fundus to the abdominal wall low down, the development of the uterus during
pregnancy will be at the expense of the posterior wall only. This
is a condition which is most dreaded in all methods of fixation of
the uterus. There are cases on record where, during the performance of version, such uteri ruptured. The uterus, when
held in such a position, causes serious disturbance in the bladder which, as a rule, is not reported. You will find ultimately
that there is not a patient, who has undergone abdominal fixation of the uterus or an extreme Alexander operation, who does
not suffer from serious disturbances of the bladder which cannot
be relieved or cured. I cannot see any good reason for suspending or fixing a uterus to the abdominal wall in the way Dr.
Ferguson does it. We lose all the advantages of the vaginal
operation by so doing, and I do not believe it is possible to control what we are doing high up inside the abdominal cavity
through the vagina. We are fortunate if we can see what we
are doing with the appendages in vaginal operations. That is
the strongest objection, so far as the technique is concerned. I
do not believe such an operation is justifiable. If we make an
abdominal fixation at all of the uterus—and I do not approve of
it—we have to make an abdominal incision.

Dr. T. J. Watkins.—The operation described by Dr. Ferguson
of fixation of the uterus reminds me of one which was reported
by a New York surgeon some five or six years ago. He did his
operation very much as Dr. Ferguson does, with the exception
that he made a vaginal incision posterior to the cervix and then
carried sutures up through the abdominal wall. I would hesitate to do this operation for fear of injury of the bladder and
intestines.

I do not know how Dr. Ferguson can tell when the knife gets
to the peritoneum, and how he can be sure that the puncture does
not go through the peritoneum. Considering the number of bad
results of abdominal fixation of the uterus, I have come to fear
very much all methods of fixing the uterus to the abdominal wall.
Although I have done a large number of abdominal suspension
operations, hereafter my abdominal operations for retroflexion
will shorten the round ligaments or suture the broad ligaments
in such a way as to hold the uterus forward. Fixation of the
uterus to the abdominal wall has caused quite a large number of
cases of intestinal obstruction. I believe the uterus fixed to the
abdominal wall is in an abnormal position. It is not normal for
the uterus to be fixed up so high, which causes the same circulatory disturbances as prolapse of the uterus.

I fail to see the use of Dr. Ferguson's attempt to carry the
bladder to one side with a staff, because I believe the bladder is
attached to both sides of the pelvis.

Dr. Albert Goldspohn.—It pleases me to see the ingenuity
displayed by Dr. Ferguson in connection with this operation,
and I can see how it can be safely done. But I would second the

objections raised by Dr. Kolischer and Dr. Watkins, that fixation of the uterus to the abdominal wall means drawing the uterus out of the pelvis into the abdomen, where it does not belong. And supposing that it were a legitimate and desirable object to attach or approximate the uterus to the abdominal wall, and that we could do it safely and avoid the greater scar on the abdomen, etc., so that there would be some more practical reason for this technique, even then I must declare that I am sorry to see Dr. Ferguson retrograding in his principles; for a few years ago we could give him credit for devising a procedure that is of considerable merit, namely, suspending the uterus, not by improvised, or so-called artificial, ligaments, but by actual ligaments, viz., drawing the round ligaments into the abdominal wall. This was first suggested by Dr. Carl Beck, of New York, some ten years ago, and published in the *Centralblatt für Chirurgie*. He did it with one ligament only. But what are the comparative merits of an actual ligament, a structure that is made of uterine muscle extended into the form of a ligament? The actual ligament can and does participate in the evolution or growth, and in the involution or contraction, which the uterus undergoes during gestation and after labor. When such a thing is available, what shall we think if a man goes to work and fixes a uterus, after the idea of Kelly, with a junction or a band wholly pathological in nature, and whose strength or tenure of service is beyond the knowledge and power of any operator to certainly determine? When we consider the general principle that we cannot do any operating without slight infection making its way into our work, which may not change the clinical course at all, but it makes a big difference in the amount of round-cell infiltration that occurs in order to overcome the infection. This round-cell infiltration ends in connective-tissue formation, and I may get in that way a strong structure when I am doing my level best to make only a weak one. Let me illustrate this point:

I had a case of pus tube on one side which I removed by abdominal section and shortened the round ligaments by loop formation for the heavy retroverted uterus. Then I thought it would be safer if I added to the round-ligament shortening a slight supravesical fixation by a little sero-serous junction. If the woman became pregnant, this could not hold anything, I felt sure. It would give way. Well, the woman became infected during the year following that operation, and I had a pus tube to deal with on the other side and a diseased uterus. I then did a vaginal hysterectomy, and, much to my surprise, when I had everything free I could not get the uterus out of the abdomen down into the vagina. There were two strong cords, like lead pencils, extending upward from the fundus—structures of such strength that I could not sever them with blunt dissection. I had to catch them in forceps, ligate them, and cut them off. These large bands would have caused disaster in case of pregnancy, and they resulted from a little auxiliary sero-serous attachment which I had made of the serous covering of the uterus to the peritoneum above the bladder, thinking they would be as harmless as anything could be. I did not expect it to hold. I thought it would guide the heavy body of the uterus forward, and it would be more successful cure of the displacement than to depend upon loop formation of the round ligament alone. This case impressed upon my mind a fact which every one must recognize, namely, that we are not able to control the strength of the structures that we mean to construct. If we intend to make them strong we may constrict the necessary circulation in suturing the part and obtain a weak structure. We are dealing blindly with serious things. The fruit of our labor may be a disaster without our knowledge and in spite of our best efforts. Kelly in no case can say how long a period will elapse before his peritoneal ligament will stretch an inch or a foot; and certainly it can never retract after stretching. Therefore, if I were to draw the uterus up and attach it to the abdominal wall, instead of drawing the stitches through the fundus or back of the uterus, as Dr. Ferguson does, why not put the loops around the round ligaments and draw them up? It seems to me that would be a rational procedure. But even this method of approximating the uterus to the abdominal wall is eligible for retroversion or prolapse of the uterus only in the cases that require a regular abdominal section for other more serious lesions. In cases that present no such graver disorders as pus somewhere or larger neoplasms, the retroversion or descensus should be corrected by shortening the round ligaments either via their natural channels or by way of the vagina, if pregnancy is possible.

DR. O. BEVERLY CAMPBELL (by invitation).—With reference to the operation described by Dr. Ferguson, I have seen him perform it once and it was certainly very easily executed by him. I believe any competent gynecologist could perform this operation without any danger of transfixing or doing injury to the bowel. In a few instances where one decides to do a ventrosuspension this method would certainly be practical, and I can see no objections to it.

I do not understand the position taken by Dr. Kolischer in regard to the criticism that he has made concerning Dr. Ferguson doing his operation through the vagina. If I understood him rightly, he said that the aim of the vaginal operation was lost sight of when the uterus was turned down into the vagina. I do not know how much can be accomplished through an anterior vaginal incision without delivering the fundus of the uterus into the vagina. I am not skilful enough to deliver badly adherent ovaries and tubes into the vagina through an anterior vaginal incision so that I can operate upon them without first bringing down the uterus. I do not know of anything of consequence that can be accomplished through an anterior vaginal incision without delivering the fundus into the vagina, except vesical suspension and vaginofixation. Vaginofixation is not practised very much in this country, although it is still practised in Germany and England. Strange to say, the objections that are raised by the men who shorten the round ligaments in this country are not realized in the countries mentioned. When I was with Prof. Martin in 1899 he informed me that he had had no unsatisfactory results in his practice, although Dr. Ries, in a recent conversation I had with him, told me that he had seen unfavorable reports from Martin's work, as regards subsequent labor. The objections to vesical suspension are that it is not permanent in its results, that the uterus will again become retrodisplaced, such recurrences being quite frequent. Dr. Goldspohn tells us of encountering fibrous cords in a case upon which at a former time he had done vesical suspension, the formation of which must be the exception rather than the rule, else the results of vesical suspension would prove more permanent.

I do not believe that I can agree with Dr. Kolischer concerning the operation of shortening the round ligaments through the vagina. I do not believe that Ries' method, or any of the methods, except in simple cases, can be scientifically performed through the vagina. It is very difficult to do the Ries operation through the vagina, but it is quite easy of accomplishment through the suprapubic incision. I have an operation somewhat similar to that of Dr. Ries, of invaginating the round ligaments beneath the peritoneal covering of the uterus. I have on several occasions found it extremely difficult, after shortening the ligaments, to return the uterus into the pelvis. I do not doubt that Dr. Ries has met with the same difficulty in practising his method. The question of operative methods for the correction of retrodisplacements is a large one, and I am not satisfied, so far as I am personally concerned, as to any single method to apply to all cases. When we have considerable pathology in the pelvis, a retrodisplaced adherent uterus with adherent ovaries and tubes, I do not believe any of the round-ligament operations will prove efficient. I am inclined to favor ventrosuspension under such circumstances. It might be suggested that where the ovaries and tubes are so markedly affected, the selection of a method whereby the inflamed appendages could be successfully treated should be our first aim, the treatment of the retrodisplacement being a secondary consideration. Where the retrodisplaced uterus is markedly adherent there is frequently pathology in the adnexa, and I claim that there is no method of treating the retrodisplacement that is scientific unless it gives access to the pelvis either through an abdominal or vaginal incision. In cases of retrodisplacement with pronounced inflammation in the adnexa, the abdominal method is superior to the vaginal, permitting of better and more conservative work being done, the vaginal route being applicable to simple cases.

Now, as regards ventrosuspension, which is considered so unscientific by the gentlemen who have brought forward a round-ligament operation of their own, I have seen very good results from it—as good as, if not better than, from any other method of correcting retrodisplacement. The statement has been made that the uterus is in an unphysiological position when fastened in the manner described by Dr. Ferguson. We certainly know that the uterus will not remain as it is temporarily fastened. Ferguson's operation is practically a Kelly's suspension, and, as has been demonstrated by Kelly, after a very short period of time a ligament forms which allows the uterus to assume a nearly normal position. Many of you will recall the report of Noble in which he gives a tabulated list of all the available cases of ventrosuspension that had been performed up to the time of the report, showing that the only hindrances to confinement were in the early cases of Kelly—cases in which a ventrofixation rather than a suspension had been performed. I have confined twenty-five women, largely from my individual practice, upon whom a ventrosuspension had been made, the time ranging all the way from six months to two and three years after operation, and I did not find it necessary to use instruments in a single instance.

DR. GUSTAV KOLISCHER.—I hope Dr. Campbell will understand me this time. I stated that Dr. Ferguson lost sight of the advantages of the vaginal operation by resorting to the method he had described. We do the vaginal operation, first, because it is less dangerous than abdominal section; second, because in vaginal operations for fixing the uterus we place it in a physiological position; third, we do not perform the vaginal operation because we do not want to do an abdominal section.

So far as Dr. Campbell's statement is concerned that it is impossible to do any conservative work on the ovaries and tubes, that it is impossible to bring the ovaries and tubes into view without pulling down the uterus, I will invite him to witness this operation, which can be done by anybody who is conversant with the method. It is unnecessary to pull the uterus down in order to have the appendages in sight; did he never hear about turning the uterus on one edge?

If Dr. Campbell tells us that in twenty-five cases of women upon whom he operated and did ventrosuspension all became pregnant, and that he never met with an obstetric accident, then I am inclined to think that, if one has such a large number of pregnant women after performing ventrosuspension, he has operated on some of those women without the real indication, thus gaining his rather unique statistics.

DR. EMIL RIES.—Dr. Campbell referred to Martin's operation and his results. The statistics of which I reminded him are published by Rieck in the *Monatsschrift für Geburtshülfe und Gynäkologie,* July and August, 1901. These statistics of Martin's cases contain the remote results. There are two periods of Martin's operation—one which he calls the older operation, and another period which he calls the new operation. The new operation is one of the low or middle fixations; the old operation is the well-known vaginal fixation, with high fixation. With the old operation he has had some poor results, such as disturbances during labor, difficulty attending delivery; in one case Cesarean section was performed and the woman died. With the new operation no bad results are reported. But the new operation is so new that it is difficult to say whether there will or will not be any bad results. So much for Martin's statistics. I think Dr. Campbell out-Martins Martin.

Then Dr. Campbell proceeds to discuss the operation I have devised and recommended, and refers to it as being practically the same as his operation, of which he reported some eighteen or twenty cases before the Western Surgical and Gynecological Association in St. Paul last year. I am astonished to hear him say now that this method is dangerous and bloody, hard to perform and unsafe. I am sure, if the operation were as dangerous and bloody as he has pictured it, I would have desisted in performing it long ago; but the fact is, I have not desisted from doing the operation, as I devised it, and I find it neither bloody nor dangerous nor particularly hard to perform. The fact that I do not do vaginal operations for retroflexions of the uterus every day, or twice or three times a week, is explained by the fact that I do not do operations for retroversion or retrodeviation in general in cases of freely movable uteri without pathological conditions of the appendages. I am very much of the opinion that freely movable uteri can be safely let alone and do not need any operative treatment.

Dr. Campbell has informed us that he has found it very hard to return the uterus into the abdomen after he had put the ligaments under the surface of the uterus. I am glad he made that statement, because now I know why he claims this operation as his own. In this one point his operation differs from mine, but in all other respects I cannot see any difference. The fact that he puts the ligaments under the surface of the uterus, while the uterus is turned down into the vagina, explains why he finds it difficult to put the uterus back again. In the method which I am using the uterus is pushed back into the abdomen, if it has been delivered into the vagina, before the ligaments are pulled through the tunnel. Of course there is no difficulty in replacing the uterus as long as the ligaments are not pulled through the tunnel. It is well known that in shortening the ligaments through the vagina it is not always necessary to pull down the uterus into the vagina.

Even for the treatment of the appendages it is by no means always necessary to pull the uterus down into the vagina. The procedure described by Dr. Kolischer is well known. Dr. Campbell is not aware of the fact that ventrofixation is generally considered a dangerous operation. He will find some reports in medical literature which will satisfy his scientific curiosity. The results of ventrofixation in a large percentage of cases are unfavorable, not only if the women become pregnant, but without pregnancy. Cases of disturbance of the bladder and of strangu-

lation of the bowel have been reported as following ventrofixation; not to mention disturbances in subsequent labors, which
are quite numerous and very considerable.

DR. O. BEVERLY CAMPBELL.—The statistics quoted by Dr. Ries
in regard to ventrosuspension, I suppose, came from Germany.
In Hart and Barbour's work on gynecology you will find the percentages of hindrances to confinement from the various operative
procedures for the correction of retrodeviations about as follows:
ventrosuspension, ten per cent; vaginofixation, fifteen per cent:
Alexander's operation, four per cent.

Now, I do not know that the operation of ventrosuspension is
altogether obsolete, or that the profession, especially in America,
have for scientific reasons ceased to perform it. I am still of
the opinion that it is often the very best method of correcting
retrodisplacement, and while, under usual conditions, a round-
ligament operation is to be preferred, especially during the childbearing period, yet ventrosuspension will always be accorded a
place as a rational procedure. In regard to the rather suggestive
criticism of Dr. Kolischer regarding the number of cases of confinement following ventrosuspension, largely from my own practice, it might be well to call to his attention that I have been doing abdominal and gynecological work for over twelve years, and
have been doing ventrosuspension for at least eight years. I
have not operated in a single case where I did not find sufficient
pathology in the pelvis to warrant operative procedure. In two
cases out of the twenty-five I had removed an ovary and tube.
In some of the cases the uterus was freed of adhesions, conservative work done upon the ovaries and tubes. I do not consider
that this is such a very large number as the gentleman has intended to have you infer, covering a period of eight years. I am
quite sure that I can substantiate the correctness of my claim.

DR. A. GOLDSPOHN.—As a matter of explanation to Dr. Campbell, I believe he understood me to say that I regarded vesical
fixation of the uterus as objectionable because it produced bands.
That was not my statement at all, because this is an unusual occurrence, and the reason I mentioned it at all is because it illustrates very well the principle that we cannot govern the strength
or the size of artificial ligaments, make them up of whatever tissue
we will. The fact is that vesical fixation is one of the flimsiest
operations for holding a retroverted uterus that can be performed. He made the statement that vaginal fixation of the
uterus was a regular procedure in Germany. I must deny that
statement most emphatically, because the German literature of
the last three years will show any man who will go over this
ground that there are only two men who, because they introduced
the operation, are like drowning men hanging to a cord desper-
ately, struggling against giving it up, and these men are Mackenrodt and Dührssen, of Berlin. Besides these two men no German has advocated vesical fixation of the uterus in women who
can still become pregnant, and ventrofixation is almost as wholly

given up in Germany. This principle of real ligaments is well recognized, almost universally, and the round ligaments are therefore the only available means. And the only difference of opinion is as to which is the better way of dealing with them. So far as uncomplicated cases of retroversion in reproductive women are concerned, if surgery is needed the Alexander operation is now chosen in the majority of the German university clinics.

DR. FERGUSON.—I plead guilty of doing ventrofixations, but while I think the operation is a good one, I do not think it is ideal. When I get into the pelvis and remove a good share of the ovaries, when I find it necessary to remove the tubes to the cornu of the uterus, the best thing to do is to take a strong stitch and pass it through the back of the uterus, bringing the uterus well under the edge of the pubes, which I do, with a stitch turned a good half-inch behind the fundus, with the uterus reasonably bent upon its anterior position, and then passing the finger on the side, watching the amount of gaping, putting in one or two little sutures on each side to the peritoneal surface of the bladder, so as not to leave a place for the bowel to get in. Some of you will say I am going to have trouble with the bladder in those cases. Of course my patients may have trouble without my knowing it, but I know a number of women in this city for whom I have operated in the manner described, and whose friends I meet right along, who talk to me about their ailments, but not one has trouble with the bladder. I have never had a case of obstruction of the bowel.

With regard to uterine suspension, uterine fixation, and vaginal work generally, I must say a few words. First, I want to correct my friend Dr. Goldspohn for saying that I have retrograded in my work. At the Denver meeting of the American Medical Association I presented a preliminary report on anterior transplantation of the round ligaments—an operation which I am doing now every chance I get in preference to all others. It is easy to perform. There is little or no danger connected with it when it is done by a careful operator. Dr. Kolischer says that this operation is not easy to perform. I have no doubt he could do it to-morrow, if need be. By means of a retractor you can see the interior of the abdominal wall, and, if the vagina is roomy, through that incision you can introduce your whole hand, if necessary, but two fingers are just as good. I am astonished to hear able gynecologists say they are afraid of turning the uterus out. It can be done in dealing with pathological conditions of the tubes and of the ovaries. It is true the work can be accomplished without that, but I believe it is better to turn the uterus out; then you can determine the exact condition of the posterior wall itself. It is better to get the fingers behind the fundus and feel whether it is normal or not. I recommended the operation to Dr. Kelly, and he adheres to it in the majority of cases. I have never performed the operation described by Webster a short time ago, of cutting the proximal end of the two round liga-

17

ments, putting them through the broad ligaments, lapping them behind the posterior fundus of the uterus; but I regard it as the best operation that has been brought forward, because I believe it will hold the uterus in its position. It appears to me to be the most surgical of any procedure that has been performed upon the round ligaments.

I am not an advocate of Kelly's operation. When I have a case and prefer a suspension to any of the round-ligament operations through the vagina, then I do this, and I can do it in half the time that you can do any round-ligament operation

TRANSACTIONS OF THE WASHINGTON OBSTETRICAL AND GYNECOLOGICAL SOCIETY.

Meeting of January 3, 1902.

The President, G. WYTHE COOK, M.D., *in the Chair.*

DR. A. R. SHANDS read a paper entitled

THE EARLY DIAGNOSIS AND TREATMENT OF HIP-JOINT DISEASE IN CHILDREN.[1]

Meeting of January 17, 1902.

The Vice-President, JOHN F. MORAN, M.D., *in the Chair.*

DR. I. S. STONE presented a

CALCULUS FROM THE URETER

of a woman 45 years of age. She had been treated for appendicitis. There was no history of renal colic and the diagnosis was not made until after the abdomen was opened. The appendix was found to be normal, but the kidney was enlarged. Following down the ureter the stone was found just behind the broad ligament. He packed about with gauze and opened the ureter over the stone; a small quantity of urine escaped. The ureter was easily closed with sutures and a drainage tube was inserted. The house physician drew off about a drachm of fluid after twenty-four hours; this he thought serum and not urine. She is now well.

DR. E. E. BALLOCH asked if a very little urine in the abdomen does any harm.

DR. STONE had never seen any ill results.

DR. J. W. BOVÉE said if the slit is made in the long axis of the ureter it will close without sutures, though there is no objection

[1]See original article, p. 204.

to sutures. The wound in the ureter should be kept away from the abdominal cavity, and the peritoneum should be closed over the ureter and drainage made with gauze through the vagina. There is danger from leakage if the urine contains pathological organisms. Normal urine in the abdominal cavity, in small quantities, except under rare conditions, is harmless. Kelly acknowledges that with his wax-tipped bougie he may sometimes fail to detect a stone in the ureter. The detecting of a stone in the ureter is pretty work, and the suturing of the ureter is very delicate surgery. There are three natural constrictions in the ureter for the calculus to pass; the one interfering the most is where the ureter crosses the iliac artery.

DR. JOSEPH TABER JOHNSON read a paper entitled

THE CHOICE OF OPERATIONS FOR THE RELIEF OF RETRODISPLACE-
MENTS OF THE UTERUS.[1]

DR. J. W. BOVÉE said the causes of retrodisplacements are weakening of the supports and increase of weight. The condition in multiparæ and virgins should be considered separately. The special reason of displacement in the virgin is faulty ligamentation or some accident or injury. In almost all there is a marked nervous element which may have antedated or followed the condition. In multiparæ the cause is the trauma of childbirth and lacerations of the parts. These two classes can be better treated by means other than ventral suspension. The anterior vaginal wall may be too short and the utero-sacral ligaments attached too high on the uterus, so that the cervix is allowed to go under the pubes, and the fundus, exposed to the intra-abdominal pressure, is retroverted. This is the trouble with Alexander's operation, which pulls the fundus forward, the faulty ligamentation remaining. There are cases where the utero-sacral ligaments are torn in labor. The broad ligaments may support the uterus somewhat, but the round ligaments very little, curving around in the arc of a circle; when tension is made they straighten. Their function is to pull the uterus forward after a full bladder is emptied. Ventral suspension is not reliable for cases of retroversion due to faulty ligamentation. There are not two ligaments formed between the abdominal wall and the uterus in ventral suspension, but one. He has seen the uterus fail to come back to place after delivery and has seen it fail in virgins. A virgin with a retroversion from a nervous retention of urine he taught to catheterize herself and she was cured. Ventral fixation should not be done unless the patient cannot bear children. He does a ventral fixation sometimes after a double oöphorectomy. The Alexander operation was originally devised for normal uteri. The surgical treatment for retroversion should apply to the lower supports. He cuts loose the anterior vaginal wall and attaches it to the uterus higher up; the utero-sacral ligaments are shortened next and attached lower;

[1]See original article, June JOURNAL, p. 818.

thus the leverage is changed and the uterus is kept in place by the abdominal viscera. The shortening of the utero-sacral ligaments can be done through the vagina or abdomen.

It is advisable after the abdominal operation to insert a retroversion pessary to lift up the posterior vaginal wall to support the uterus while the ligaments are mending. All other needful operations should be done—perineorrhaphy, trachelorrhaphy, curettage, etc.

Dr. I. S. Stone was not aware of any accident following his cases done by the Kelly method. Whatever else Kelly has done for women, his ventral suspension stands paramount. Catheterization of the ureter has not benefited so many.

Meeting of February 7, 1902.

The President, G. Wythe Cook, M.D., *in the Chair.*

Dr. J. Wesley Bovée read a paper entitled

THREATENED TUBAL ABORTION, WITH REPORT OF A CASE.[1]

Dr. J. T. Johnson said not many tubal abortions are diagnosed so early. Tait and Price were not sure, formerly, until after rupture and abdominal symptoms. Now we can make the diagnosis just as we do of pyosalpinx, and the point is that operation should be done at once, as in malignant disease or placenta previa.

Dr. J. T. Winter read a paper entitled

SELF-ABUSE IN INFANCY AND CHILDHOOD.[2]

Dr. S. S. Adams disagreed with the essayist as to masturbation causing epilepsy, but felt that a certain neurosis caused the two, no local cause being present. The saddest cases are seen in the hospitals. It is very unsatisfactory to treat in girls. No two children manifest the same methods. He reported a case of a girl 6 years old in whom he was able to make a diagnosis by staying at the house and observing the child for a time. Some children sit on the corner of a chair and wriggle. Boys get the hand in the napkin and tickle the parts. One child in a hospital will teach it to all the others, and he does not admit them if he knows it. He thought it unjust to brand every child with an acne as a masturbator. If the child has a long prepuce, circumcision should be done; but sometimes it fails. Corporal punishment does no good. You should get the mother to get the confidence of the child and appeal to its moral sensibility; also to carefully watch it, and, when it is seen going off by itself, to interest it in something.

Dr. T. C. Smith thought there is always some abnormal de-

[1]See original article, June JOURNAL, p. 841.
[2]See original article, June JOURNAL, p. 828.

velopment of the genital organs—a long prepuce in males and an adherent prepuce in females, circumscision should be done in the former and the adhesions liberated in the latter.

DR. W· S. BOWEN reported the case of a child 3½ years old. It was an only child of extremely neurotic parents. The nurse was of excellent character. The mother had never heard of masturbation and thought the child had nervous attacks. If the child was approached at the time of a paroxysm it became very angry and would throw things. There was nothing abnormal about the genitals. Talking, threats, and cod-liver oil did no good. He finally took the child into a room and showed it a large knife, and told it he would cut it with the knife if it ever masturbated again. It stopped immediately. Another case after circumcision would tear out the stitches in its effort to get at the parts.

DR. J. T. KELLEY spoke of children learning the habit by being kept in school too long without emptying the bladder. He also said that children are little animals and that in serious conditions like masturbation they could be better brought to understand by some proper punishment than by appealing to their moral sensibility, of which the average child has very little at this age.

DR. ADAMS said in his cases there was no abnormal development of the genitals. He thought very young children could be taught the difference between right and wrong. He was inclined to think that the cure in Dr. Bowen's case was due to the building up of the child's constitution.

———

Meeting of February 21, 1902.

The President, G. WYTHE COOK, M.D., *in the Chair.*

DR. I. S. STONE showed a

TUBO-OVARIAN ABSCESS AND FIBROIDS

removed from a widow 47 years of age. The illness began five months ago with pain in the pelvis and left side. There were very dense adhesions of the tumor to the intestines. The operation lasted two hours and thirty minutes. To combat shock he used salt solution, one pint under each breast and filled the rectum. At night he put three pints into the cephalic vein; two pints brought the pulse up to normal pressure.

DR. J. W. BOVÉE showed a

KIDNEY AND URETER.

The patient was 28 years old and there was a history of renal colic for three years. Pus was found in the urine at times. He incised the kidney, removed some pus and a calculus, and drained. Three months after the wound still discharged and he removed the kidney and ureter postperitoneally, the ureter down to the bladder. This is the only case on record where the whole ureter has been removed by a lumbar incision. The incision was fourteen inches long.

Dr. G. N. Acker read a paper entitled

ESSENTIAL OR TOXEMIC DROPSY IN CHILDREN.[1]

TRANSACTIONS OF THE
AMERICAN GYNECOLOGICAL SOCIETY.[2]

Proceedings of the Twenty-seventh Annual Meeting, held at Atlantic City, N. J., 1902.

Second Day—Morning Session.

A FURTHER CONTRIBUTION TO THE STUDY AND PRACTICAL SIGNIFICANCE OF LACTATION ATROPHY OF THE UTERUS.

In a paper on this subject, the author, Dr. Hiram N. Vineberg, of New York, said that although the writer six years ago drew the attention of the profession in this country to lactation atrophy, the subject had not yet received the consideration here that it deserved, as was evidenced by the literature and the recent text books on obstetrics. It was a physiological process accompanying lactation, with or without amenorrhea, the atrophy or superinvolution being temporary only, the return to the normal size being in some cases dependent upon the cessation of lactation. In others, again, the regeneration of the uterine tissue occurred while lactation was still going on. It was not to be confounded with what was commonly known in this country as hyperinvolution, which was usually permanent in its character, although in some rare cases it terminated in this form. While the author had seen during his ten years' service at the dispensary over 500 cases of lactation atrophy, he had not met with more than 20 cases of permanent hyperinvolution.

When the atrophy was slight, and was manifest only by a thinning of the uterine walls, it was known as eccentric atrophy; when it was more marked, as was evidenced by a marked diminution in the size of the uterus, the term concentric atrophy was employed. The cervix usually participated in the atrophic process, but the ovaries did not as a rule. The hyperinvolution or atrophy was fully established between the eighth and twelfth weeks, and persisted for a variable period in different nursing women, its persistence usually being dependent upon the continuance of lactation. Anemia did not play an important rôle in the causation of the condition, as had been stated by some

[1]See original article, p. 211.
[2]Continued from p. 103, July Journal.

writers, notably Engström. The author had the blood examined in a series of cases, and he found that the degree of atrophy bore no relation to the diminished number of red blood cells and to the lowered percentage of hemoglobin. Cases with the smallest uteri had the largest number of red blood cells and the highest percentage of hemoglobin.

Hyperinvolution might occur independently of lactation, as shown by Hansen and P. Müller. Most writers hitherto had concerned themselves chiefly in showing that lactation atrophy was not an injurious condition and that it seldom led to permanent atrophy. But the writer drew attention to its decidedly beneficial effects upon the uterus in bringing about a normal hyperinvolution. Women, therefore, who nursed their babies were rarely the victims of subinvolution, with its usual sequel, chronic metritis—one of the most unsatisfactory and rebellious conditions to treat. When, as was usually the case among the better classes, the mother was unable or disinclined to nurse her baby, it was the duty of the attending obstetrician to keep the parturient under observation and treatment until nearly the same degree of hyperinvolution was established as obtained in lactation. This period would seldom be less than eight weeks and frequently would extend to three months. Unfortunately, the importance of this desideratum was not very generally recognized. The accoucheur rarely considered it necessary to examine the parturient after the second or third week.

In conclusion, the writer directed attention to a peculiar circumstance, that in the class of women from whom he had drawn his material in dispensary practice uterine cancer was exceedingly rare. From the fifteen hundred to sixteen hundred new patients he saw yearly, not more than one or two were the victims of cancer of the uterus. He thought one would expect almost the opposite if improper attendance during the puerperium and lacerations of the cervix played any rôle in the causation of that dread disease. He asked the question whether the circumstance that these women were shielded, in a great measure, against the occurrence of chronic metritis rendered them less susceptible to the development of uterine cancer.

DR. A. LAPTHORN SMITH, of Montreal, said he did not think it was right to limit the time of lactation to six or seven months, because he had known women who had been either pregnant or nursing for about thirty years of their lives and they were very healthy. He had heard of many other women in the practice of his colleagues in Montreal who had had the same experience. He thought it was a mistake to tell a woman to stop nursing at seven months. There was a close connection between the breasts and the uterus. Every physician who had been engaged in general practice knew from experience that a woman would feel her uterus contract every time the baby began nursing at the breast. The uterus was sympathetic. These contractions might be such as to cut off the supply of blood to the parts. He had noticed in a number of such cases that the uterus was smaller than usual. He did not consider it an abnormality, but a natural condition.

Dr. Egbert H. Grandin, of New York, criticised the term lactation atrophy as used by the essayist, saying it was a bad one. Atrophy conveyed the idea of degeneration. The uterus did not degenerate, but simply returned approximately to its normal size, particularly in women who nursed their babies, while it remained subinvoluted in women who did not do so. He thought the importance of lactation was being forgotten by the better class of women, as well as by a great many physicians. Not many weeks ago a female agent drifted into his office and asked him if he had ever used maternal milk. "Yes," he replied, "in my infancy." "Oh," she said, "I don't mean that kind of milk; I mean the kind of milk which the company I represent has put on the market." He said to her: "Where do you keep your herd of mothers?" She replied: "We modify our milk so that it is as good as, if not better than, mother's milk." He thought the tendency of the times was to eliminate woman as a nursing animal, and to substitute the preparations of the pharmaceutical chemist or the products of firms who go into the modified-milk business.

Dr. Robert A. Murray, of New York, considered lactation atrophy to be a physiological process. He suggested that the term atrophy be changed and the condition called involution, because in reality it was not an atrophy. If it were an atrophy and the tissue were destroyed, pregnancy would not follow. He made this plea, that wherever we had any condition preventing a woman from nursing through the whole time, the physician should insist, if at all consistent with perfect health and safety, that for two months, at least, she should nurse her baby, because it was physiological in bringing about involution.

Dr. Vineberg, in closing, said that Dr. Smith had misunderstood him when he said that he objected to women nursing their babies for more than six or seven months. Most of the patients he had observed nursed their babies from one pregnancy to the other, under favorable conditions. As to the terms atrophy and hyperinvolution, he had used them synonymously in his paper, but, if we were to be accurate, the process of involution was a distinct atrophy. If we had an organ that was seven or eight centimetres in depth, and it decreased five or six centimetres, there must be atrophy and absorption of the tissue. The researches of Sänger and others had shown that there was a distinct atrophy of the muscular tissue of the uterus, and he could not think of any other term which would apply more accurately.

THE RELATIVE ADVANTAGES OF THE COMPLETE AND PARTIAL HYSTERECTOMY.

Dr. E. E. Montgomery, of Philadelphia, in a paper on this subject, spoke of the difficulty the present student had in appreciating the slow process of development in the operation of hysterectomy, whether partial or complete. The procedure, as perfected by Goffe and Baer, marked an epoch in the progress of partial hysterectomy. For the complete operation he advocated the Doyen procedure as the one most desirable. He preferred panhysterectomy to the partial operation, for the reasons that it was more expeditious, rendered hemostasis more secure, and decreased the danger from sepsis by removing any dead space in which fluids could accumulate and become infected. The cervix retained by the former method was not always free from danger from subsequent degenerative processes.

DR. CHARLES P. NOBLE, of Philadelphia, believed that in performing hysterectomy it was safer to remove the cervix. With reference to the results of the originator of the particular operation advocated by Dr. Montgomery, the mortality was bad. The speaker was told in Europe this year that of ten exhibition operations which he (Doyen) had done at various times, eight of the patients bled to death, a ninth died of tetanus, and one recovered. He had seen the operation done a good many times, and there was no doubt one could remove the tumor with fair rapidity. There was no doubt that, by good method, a simple tumor could be removed rapidly where it could be easily delivered. It was only by hurrying the steps in the technique that time was saved. His experience in watching men use rapid methods was that, while they started promptly, they were slow in finishing their operations, and both in this country and in Europe, in watching operators work, it had been his observation that it took them about an hour to complete the operation. The only real claim for not favoring total hysterectomy was that cancer had been known to develop in the cervix when it was left. After having done three or four hundred hysterectomies, he had never seen cancer of the cervix except in one case, and in this it was present before operation.

DR. E. W. CUSHING, of Boston, said that he had tried nearly every method of total removal of the cervix, and he did not believe the operation could be done as quickly as by cutting the cervix across. The cervix had a certain physiological function of its own that was of value, and this was ground enough for leaving it in all young women, and was much more important than the ultimate chance of its becoming the seat of malignant disease. If it ever did so it could be taken out.

DR. A. PALMER DUDLEY, of New York, had seen the operation performed by Doyen last summer. He designated it as ''scientific butchery'' and protested against the use of such a method. While the operation could be quickly performed, the patient was strung up in the Trendelenburg position like a sheep and almost disembowelled. The case he saw was one of simple epithelioma of the cervix; the uterus was perfectly movable; an incision was made from the pubic bone to about two inches above the umbilicus; the tendinous attachments of the two recti muscles were severed and drawn apart, and the woman's abdomen had been opened sufficiently to introduce a man's head of large size. True, the operation was quickly and skilfully performed, but imagine the condition of that woman after she recovered from such an operation as that!

He saw another case operated upon by another surgeon the same morning, in which the same method was used, and with the delivery of the uterus four inches of the sigmoid flexure of the colon at the same time. There was rapid excision, and the result was a colotomy. The case was a simple epithelioma of the cervix. For his part, he came home to denounce the operation.

Dr. Philander A. Harris, of Paterson, N. J., said with reference to the removal of the cervix, when there were no indications present of disease of the cervix, when it seemed to be of normal size as to length and general conformation, he would do a supravaginal amputation for myoma or fibroma of the uterus. Unless there was some reason for believing that there was disease of the cervix, he would leave it in position. It was better for the integrity of the vagina to leave the cervix.

Dr. Joseph E. Janvrin, of New York, thought the matter resolved itself into the two operations the essayist had described, namely, supravaginal amputation and total extirpation. In all cases of fibroma or myoma of the uterus where there was unmistakably no disease of the cervix, and where there was sufficient cervical tissue remaining to form a stump, it had been his practice to do such an operation rather than remove the entire cervix. In all other instances in which there was a possibility of disease occurring afterward in the cervix, it had been his practice always to remove the entire organ. From a somewhat extensive experience in the treatment of cancer of the uterus, he had been led to the conclusion that, unless there were actual ocular evidences of cancerous degeneration in the cervix, or evidence furnished by the microscope that the cervix was involved, he would not operate, but he thought that in all cases where the cervix was implicated total extirpation was demanded.

Dr. Matthew D. Mann, of Buffalo, said that the decision in the matter of whether to take out the cervix or not depended upon two or three points. First, was there more danger of cancerous degeneration of the cervix afterward? For his own part, he thought there was, but others denied that there was any particular danger, and the number of cases in their experience was small. Personally, he had seen three cases of cancerous degeneration of the cervix after supravaginal hysterectomy. If there was a real danger the cervix should not be left. Others maintained that its removal added materially to the risk of the operation. If that be the case, then probably the dangers of taking out the cervix were greater than those in connection with leaving it. He would say that there was danger of degeneration afterward if the cervix was left, and if it did not make any difference in the result at the time of the operation, it would be better for the woman to remove the cervix. Another advantage in removing the cervix was that it made drainage. Everybody who left the cervix in these cases knew that if any blood collected in the peritoneal flaps over the cervix there was a rise of temperature until that blood had been discharged from the cervix. He had dilated the cervix in some cases to allow the infected blood to escape, after which the temperature had declined and everything went on right. This was entirely obviated by removing the cervix. If the vagina was thoroughly cleaned before operation and kept packed with iodoform gauze, there was no danger of infection extending to the broad ligaments and peritoneal cavity. He used to leave the cervix entirely, but the more work he did, and the more experience he had, the more convinced was he that the proper thing to do was to remove the cervix, particularly if the woman had borne children and if there were any laceration or disease of the cervix. The sum total of lives in the cases operated on would be materially increased if the cervix was removed in every case.

DR. JOSEPH E. JANVRIN, of New York, stated that his own personal experience had been that in some cases there was a collection of pus on top of the cervix under the peritoneum. He had seen two such cases in the hands of professional friends, but he thought it was a rather uncommon accident. In such cases there was no difficulty whatever in dilating the cervix and letting the pus out. One should thoroughly convince himself whether the cervix was sound and healthy or not. If healthy it should be left; if diseased it should be removed.

DR. CLEMENT CLEVELAND, of New York, said it was formerly his practice for many years to remove the uterus entirely for fibromata. He did so chiefly because he felt that drainage was absolutely necessary. At that time he used either silk or catgut ligatures. Silk he believed to be the best material until he succeeded in getting a catgut which was rendered absolutely sterile by cumol, and then he had perfect confidence in it. It was chiefly for that reason he did total hysterectomy. Since he had been able to sterilize perfectly catgut by means of cumol, he found he was doing more supravaginal operations, leaving the cervix where it was healthy. As to the danger of leaving blood above the cervix underneath the peritoneal flap, and possible sepsis occurring afterward, he thought this could be obviated by the layer suture of the cervix. He never performed a supravaginal hysterectomy without sewing up the cervix completely from the bottom with one or two layers of catgut. His own preference to-day was for the supravaginal method, and he did it unless there was positive indication for the removal of the cervix.

As to chromicized gut, he had never used it inside the peritoneal cavity, because he did not see the need of it. Ordinary catgut sterilized by cumol was entirely satisfactory. Moreover, the examination of chromicized gut recently had shown in a good many instances the presence of free chromin, which was more or less an irritant and produced more or less sloughing. Careful washing of the catgut would remove the chromin.

Dr. J. Riddle Goffe, of New York, said the essayist had done him the honor to refer to what he had contributed toward this method of leaving the cervix, covering it with peritoneal flaps. He still continued to use this method in preference to doing total hysterectomy. He believed the shortening of the operation was a great consideration, that there was less shock, less danger of immediate hemorrhage at the time of the operation, and that convalescence was more prompt and smoother in those cases where the cervix was left.

Another consideration was that operations for the removal of fibroid tumors of the uterus were done upon rather young women, much younger than those upon whom operations were performed for cancer, such as hysterectomy. It was important in young patients that the vagina should retain its size and formation, length, etc., and where the cervix was left it was better nourished, and atrophy took place more slowly than where the cervix had been removed. With these considerations, in addition to those presented, it was the better plan to leave the cervix rather than to do total hysterectomy.

Dr. William H. Baker, of Boston, thought the length of the operation and the condition of the patient should be considered in connection with total removal. Sometimes the uterus was drawn up and the cervix was of such length that it required considerable dissection to remove the latter, and a prolonged operation might be fraught with some consequence. In such cases there would be no question as to the advantage of supravaginal amputation; but in cases of suppurative disease of the tubes and ovaries there could be no longer any question in regard to supravaginal amputation. The whole uterus should be removed; and instead of establishing free drainage from above, it should be effected through the vagina.

Dr. I. S. Stone, of Washington, D. C., said he had found carcinoma of the cervix in only one instance. This was a sarcoma really, associated with a tumor, and fortunately it was discovered in time and examined before the patient left the hospital. The cervix was subsequently removed and recovery followed. In looking over his operative work in the last few years, including that done with the angiotribe, two deaths were vividly in his mind owing to the use of silk resulting in suppuration, embolism, and sudden death. This occurred about 1897 or 1898, so that he discarded the use of silk and had adopted the angiotribe with excellent results.

Dr. Charles P. Noble, of Philadelphia, did not recall ever having seen a case of infection from an infected blood clot after a supravaginal amputation; nor had he seen it after hysterectomy for pus cases, so that he thought that with the improved technique, as contrasted with what it was ten years ago, this was very largely an imaginary complication, and he did not believe it would occur to-day. He had used cumol catgut and had not had any trouble with it. No one need be afraid to use catgut on account of hemorrhage.

Dr. Francis H. Davenport, of Boston, felt that the occurrence of suppuration from infected blood clot in the flaps could be avoided by improved technique. He thought the mistake was often made of making the peritoneal flaps too large. It was hardly necessary to strip off the peritoneum, either anteriorly or posteriorly, to any great extent, in carrying the incision from one side of the uterus to the other. His practice was to loosen it slightly, cut out the uterine body, leaving a wedge-shaped portion, and, in passing sutures, to include not only peritoneum but a certain portion of the uterine structure as well, and by a running and over-and-over suture to approximate the edges.

Dr. J. M. Baldy, of Philadelphia, stated, as to the operation of choice in cases of cancer or tuberculosis, that complete removal of the cervix was a necessity, and in no instance where hysterectomy had been done by this method had he seen suppuration in the stump. He had seen operators leave the peritoneal surfaces open. Formerly this was a comparatively common practice. Cases of suppuration had been reported following this method. A great many used interrupted sutures; and after the use of a suture of that character, unless the spaces were closed, he could readily see how there might be an accumulation of pus under the flap. With a running suture, such as he used, there was no possibility of these flaps being left long enough to cause any trouble.

He always examined the cervix, and had never seen it fail to atrophy at the menopause. The objection brought forward by Dr. Goffe was a crying reason for leaving the cervix. One could not take it out without shortening the vagina an inch and a half, and this, in an unmarried woman, was a serious thing.

Dr. Edwin B. Cragin, of New York, said it seemed a simpler operation to leave than to remove the cervix, for the reason that the vagina was more natural. He had no doubt that most gynecologists would leave the cervix, unless there was distinct evidence, on inspection, of malignant disease.

Dr. A. Palmer Dudley, of New York, referred to one practical point in regard to the use of catgut in hysterectomy or any form of operation. He was constantly called upon to lecture his nurses and assistants on account of one great fault. Catgut was twisted when it came out of the glass, and the party who handled it would almost invariably strip it through the fingers to get the kinks out, thus infecting it.

Dr. Montgomery, in closing the discussion, said he would not condemn the operation of Doyen on the evidence that had been presented by Dr. Noble. The report that Doyen had lost nine cases out of ten by this method was incorrect. There was no reason why such a great mortality should occur from this operation; nor was he so rabid as not to yield to any one in his admiration and appreciation of the work that had been done by American surgeons. Again, he was not so rabid a protectionist that he could not appreciate the work and methods of Europeans, nor did he believe in the principle that we should claim everything and not give credit to others. He did not believe that the retention of the cervix had much influence upon the subsequent nutrition of the vagina. When the cervix was left and the uterine ligaments were tight, it received its nutrition from the vaginal branches, and it was consequently a parasite in the vagina rather than a support to its subsequent nutrition. He did not believe the vagina was shortened to any degree by the removal of the cervix. Speaking of degeneration of the cervix, he thought it was a matter of very slight importance. He had seen but one case in which he thought it was necessary to operate upon the cervix subsequent to the removal of the uterus by a supravaginal operation. He had seen the occurrence of a collection of infected blood above the cervix, necessitating measures to evacuate it. But this was absolutely avoided by the complete operation.

(To be Concluded.)

BRIEF OF CURRENT LITERATURE.

OBSTETRICS.

Cardiac Disease in Pregnancy.—Robert Jardine *(Jour. Obst. and Gyn. of the Br. Emp.,* Apr.) reports 13 cases of cardiac disease in pregnancy, selected to represent the different lesions as far as possible. The death rate of this condition is given by most authors as about 50 per cent. Jardine has had only one death in his cases. Pure mitral stenosis is the most deadly of all the lesions. The danger lies in the engorgement and paralysis of the right side of the heart during the third stage of labor, when a large amount of blood must necessarily be returned to the right side of the heart from the diminished circulation in the uterine vessels. When mitral stenosis exists, free bleeding should be allowed in the third stage. Next in seriousness comes aortic incompetence. Mitral incompetence is not so serious unless very marked. If a woman has suffered from failure of compensation at any time, no matter what the lesion is, or if the lesion is mitral stenosis, aortic incompetence, or incompetence and stenosis combined, she should be advised against marriage. Pregnant cardiac cases must be kept at perfect rest and every effort must be made to strengthen and relieve the heart. The bowels must be kept clear, the kidneys stimulated, the lungs relieved, and cardiac tonics freely given. In bad cases premature labor is apt to occur. The results from induced labor are very bad, and Jardine is inclined to question the propriety of doing the operation. In bad cases he advises the induction of abortion before the fourth month. When labor begins a large dose of strophanthus or digitalis should be given. As soon as the os is fully dilated labor should be terminated. The patient should never be allowed to bear down. If the cervix is rigid it should be incised. These patients take chloroform well and it should always be used in bad cases. During the third stage the uterus should be allowed to relax and bleeding be encouraged. Ergot is therefore contraindicated. Nursing should be prohibited, as it tends to have a bad effect on the heart.

Etiology of Eclampsia.—The experimental studies of Blumreich and Zuntz (*Arch. f. Gyn.*, Bd. lxv., H. 3) were directed toward determining the relative irritability of the motor centres in pregnant and unimpregnated rabbits when acted upon by toxic substances. For these experiments they employed 8 pregnant and 13 non-pregnant rabbits for trephining and placing kreatin upon the brain, and 5 pregnant and 8 non-pregnant for injection of a solution of the same substance into the carotid artery. Convulsions occurred in all the pregnant animals, but were absent in over one-third of the unimpregnated of the first series and in all but one of the second. The writer believes that this sensibility to kreatin of the motor centres of rabbits during pregnancy is of significance in connection with eclampsia. It explains for him why such convulsive disorders as tetany and chorea are associated with pregnancy in women.

General Peritonitis during Pregnancy.—Katz (*Comptes Rendus de la Soc. d'Obst., de Gyn. et de Ped. de Paris,* Mar.) describes a case of acute general peritonitis of unknown origin occurring in a woman who had finished eight and one-half months of a normal pregnancy. The woman died after Cesarean section, performed after an exploratory laparatomy to determine the cause of the severe abdominal symptoms. No cause for the peritonitis could be discovered in the woman's history. Autopsy showed a primary general peritonitis, which is supposed to have been due to intestinal paralysis from pressure of the gravid uterus, with bacterial emigration from the damaged intestine.

Menstruation during Pregnancy.—Lop (*Soc. Obst. de France,* ix. session) describes what appears, from the result of palpation and subsequent events, to have been an interstitial molar pregnancy. The discovery was made during a curettage for repeated hemorrhages, followed by tamponade. Three days later the tampon was removed and a mole expelled. Menstruation had occurred at regular intervals during the ten weeks of this pregnancy.

Postpartum Pelvic Arthritis.—According to V. Van Hassel (*Bull. de la Soc. Belge de Gyn. et d'Obst.,* t. xii., No. 6) the physiological modifications in the texture and mobility of the pelvic articulations during pregnancy diminish their power of resistance, so that they may become diseased on account of abnormal mechanical distension or infection. The writer has found these complications only in cases with a flat pelvis or perineal tears. In the first class the anterior ligaments of the sacro-iliac synchondroses are over-stretched by the head at the brim. In the second class there is a local infection, often causing infiltration of the parametrium, and leading to fever and pain in the pelvic joints. This pain may be protracted and severe enough to confine the patient to bed, and is liable to be mistaken for sciatica, inflammation of the hip joint or psoas magnus, appendicitis, etc. Examination of the pubic symphysis is easy. For the sacro-iliac the writer advises placing the hands over the joints, while the pubic bones are grasped through the overlying soft parts by an assistant and separated forcibly. Palpation of their anterior surfaces through the vagina elicits pain and a sensation of periarticular infiltration. The prognosis is good, but treatment must be long continued. Four cases are reported, the treatment of which consisted in antisepsis of the genital tract. immobilization of the joints by a firm pelvic bandage, and sodium salicylate internally for the relief of pain.

Double Pregnancy in Double Uterus.—In an VIIIpara, 34 years of age, seen by Treub *(Soc. Obst. de France,* ix. session), both halves of a double uterus were pregnant. During labor their contraction was sometimes simultaneous; at others they contracted successively. One child was finally delivered by forceps; the other had not been born when the case was reported.

Charles W. Doughtie *(Phil. Med. Jour.,* Apr. 19) reports a case of twin pregnancy in a uterus bipartitus. The woman went on until the fifth month, when she aborted. Each compartment contained a complete pregnancy, child, sac, and cord. The patient had twice previously aborted twins.

Precocious Conception.—James Milner *(Lancet,* June 7) cites a case of labor at full term in a girl 14 years and 6 weeks old. The delivery was at full term and the child alive. The labor pains were very mild and delivery easy. As yet the patient has no hair on the pubes. Menstruation started at 12½ years.

Quintuplets.—The case is reported by M. S. Sato and M. N. Sato *(Sei-i-Kwai Med. Jour.,* Mar. 31). The mother was a Japanese farmer's wife, 37 years old. She had had eight normal labors. A paternal cousin and her daughter had given birth to twins, but there was no other hereditary history of multiple conception. During the present pregnancy the abdomen had been unusually large, there had been marked edema of the lower extremities after the middle of pregnancy, and fetal movements seemed less active. She was not examined until the time of labor, which occurred at eight months. When first seen the first child was half delivered, and within half an hour all had been born. The first child was born surrounded by membranes; after rupturing the membrane of the second, this one was delivered four minutes later. In another five minutes the third child was born, followed by the common placenta of the first and second. In five minutes more the fourth child was delivered by the breech and the common placenta of the third and fourth discharged. Abdominal examination showed the presence of a fifth child, which was then delivered with assistance, followed by its single placenta. The children were all feeble and evidently premature. They died on the third and fourth days. The first, third, and fifth were males; the second and fourth, females.

Effect of Sugar on Labor.—Keim and Lehmann *(Soc. Obst. de France,* ix. session) hold that sugar is not an oxytocic but an actual muscular tonic. It will not initiate labor, but will stimulate the uterine as well as other muscles after labor has begun.

Effect of Spinal Anesthesia on Uterine Contractility.—Fifteen experimental subarachnoid injections of cocaine in the rabbit, goat, sheep, bitch, and cow, and one observation in the case of woman, have led J. Audebert (Toulouse, Imprimerie M. Cléder, 1902) to very different conclusions from those drawn from what he characterizes as the two isolated cases of Doléris. He believes that these injections do not exert a manifest action upon uterine contractility, and are, at least, not an efficacious means of inducing labor. They do not appear to interfere with the normal course of labor. For these reasons Audebert does not regard pregnancy as a contraindication to spinal anesthesia. The most suggestive results obtained were in the first four experiments, in which a rabbit received, between the twentieth and twenty-seventh days of pregnancy, six subarachnoid injections of cocaine without influencing the usual course of gestation.

One Hundred Cases of Abortion.—These 100 abortions were treated by Dr. Blondel *(Bull. de la Soc. d'Obst. de Paris,* Mar. 20). Although many of the cases were severely infected, none were lost. In view of the uncertainty as to the means by which an abortion has been induced, he would treat all cases suspected of being criminal radically as follows: digital curettage if large fragments are left in the uterus, instrumental curettage, swabbing with creosote and glycerin 1 in 3, injection of tincture of iodine, and drainage with gauze saturated with ichthyol and glycerin 1 in 10.

Significance of Pulse and Temperature in the Puerperium.—C. Daniel *(Ann. de Gyn. et d'Obst.,* May) gives a paper containing typical pulse and temperature charts of various infections and other complications of the puerperium, and draws the well-known conclusion that they are of great value in the diagnosis of such accidents, particularly when associated with physical examination.

Infectious Utero-ovarian Thrombosis.—The case reported by L. Hoche *(Ann. de Gyn. et d'Obst.,* May) is one of unusually extensive thrombosis. Abortion occurred at four months, nom-

18

inally after a fall. The placenta was retained and symptoms of
sepsis followed. Entering the maternity hospital, this was removed and temporary improvement resulted from intrauterine
douches. Six days after admission there were violent lumbar
pains. This is supposed to be the indication of the beginning
of the thrombosis in the inferior vena cava. Death did not occur, however, for a month, during which time there were signs
of extension of the thrombus. Autopsy showed that the process
beginning in the uterine veins extended to the utero-ovarian
plexus, then to the inferior vena cava, right auricle, right
ventricle, and pulmonary artery. It had also extended to the
vaginal plexus, iliac veins, right renal and hepatic veins. The
bacteriological exciting cause could not be absolutely determined, but the organisms isolated resembled gonococci very
closely.

Suppression of Urine Following Labor.—R. G. McKerron
(Jour. Obst. and Gyn. of Br. Emp., Apr.) believes the most important factors in the causation of this condition are: A pathological condition of the kidneys resulting from pregnancy, but
in some cases dependent on a pre-existing defect of the organs,.
congenital or acquired; a neurotic temperament; shock incident
to an undue rapidity of labor or arising from excessive pain.
The treatment of suppression of urine after labor does not differ from that of the same condition apart from pregnancy. In
addition to the usual measures, rectal injections of saline solution will be found of value. Opium should be withheld in all
cases where anuria is to be feared. Treatment should be instituted without delay.

Superstitions Connected with Placenta and Cord.—L.
Bouchacourt *(L'Obst.,* May 15) has compiled a number of interesting superstitions connected by different races with the
placenta and umbilical cord. The placenta has been used as
an ingredient of a vaginal suppository to aid conception; as
an abdominal poultice to hasten delivery; applied, when fresh,
to the face to remove freckles; applied to the abdomen of a
feeble or apparently still-born child as a restorative, or boiled
in wine or water for the same purpose. For the same purpose
the child has been exposed to the smoke of the burning cord
and placenta. A further use of the placenta has been the removal of birthmarks. Many superstitions are also connected
with the umbilical cord, some races preserving it in the dried
state and carrying it throughout life. The paper also describes
the customs of various nations in connection with the final disposal of the placenta, which in one locality is supposed to im-
part to the soil where it is buried the power to render fertile the
women who tread upon it, hence it is buried in a much-fre-
quented path.

Symphyseotomy.—P. Zweifel *(Cent. f. Gyn.,* No. 13) has
found that the postoperative period is always febrile when the
symphyseotomy wound is entirely closed or even drained above

the symphysis. Noting the good results in an apparently unfavorable case with a wound extending into the vagina, he now drains all symphyseotomy wounds from behind by such an incision reaching into the vagina. In five cases the healing has been rapid. When the condition of the vagina is such as to make it unfit to communicate with the symphyseotomy wound, he carries the drain out through one of the labia majora.

Gangrene of the Nipples.—Ralph Vincent *(Lancet,* Apr. 5) reports a case of gangrene of both nipples in a primigravida. Five days after delivery the nipples were excoriated. They were thoroughly dusted with orthoform. This treatment was continued for some days. On the thirteenth day the whole of the front of the chest was covered by a rash, both nipples were excoriated, and the skin was edematous and very tender. On the sixteenth day the nipples were grayish-black and loss of sensation in the left nipple occurred. By the twentieth day both nipples had separated. The progress of healing was uneventful. The milk ducts were not obliterated, and if the patient becomes pregnant again she can nurse by means of a shield. Probably the orthoform was the primary cause of the gangrene.

GYNECOLOGY AND ABDOMINAL SURGERY.

Spinal Anesthesia.—Socrate Tsakona *(Gaz. de Gyn.,* Apr. 15) is one of the enthusiastic advocates of anesthetization by subarachnoid injection of cocaine. He has employed the method in 120 operative cases, both gynecological and general surgical. According to his statement the Athenian surgeons have collectively performed 350 operations with this form of anesthesia without a single death or serious accident. The points which he emphasizes are the material of the needle, which should be platinum in order to avoid the possibility of a sudden movement of the patient breaking it; rapidity of operation, especially in abdominal cases, as vomiting, which would interfere seriously in such a case, rarely begins under ten to twenty minutes after the injection; and, finally, the age of the solution employed. In his last cases he has used a solution which had been kept for from twenty to thirty days, and had been sterilized only at the time of making. With this solution he noted no vomiting or fever.

Morphine after Abdominal Section.—L. H. Dunning *(Jour. Am. Med Assoc.,* Apr. 12) believes the routine use of morphine or other preparations of opium after abdominal section is to be condemned. The serious after-effects of morphine may be largely overcome by the drinking of liberal quantities of water before the operation and the rectal injection of a pint of normal salt solution immediately after the operation. In persistent vomiting not due to sepsis or peritonitis, small doses of morphine hypodermatically not infrequently afford relief. In secondary shock due to fright or over-anxiety, morphine in small doses is often a potent remedy.

Suprapubic Abdominal Incisions.—Berthold Daniel *(Cent. f. Gyn.,* No. 15) reports favorably upon Pfannenstiel's transverse suprapubic incision for laparatomy. It had been used in Pro-chownik's clinic in 15 cases during the year 1900, including 7 cases of suppurative disease of the appendages, 1 of uterine fibroid, 5 of retroflexion of the uterus, and 2 of ovarian cyst. In all cases in which primary union took place there had been no occurrence of hernia after periods varying from twelve to twenty-one months.

R. v. Fellenberg (ibid.) warmly advocates Küstner's curved suprapubic incision, chiefly on account of the cosmetic effect, the scar lying in the fold existing in fat persons above the mons Veneris or covered by hair. The results were also favorable. In 70 cases primary union was secured in 54. Hematoma was noted in 15. The smallest proportion of these occurred in cases in which drainage was employed, for which reason Fellenberg favors drainage of the wound for twenty-four hours. No hernia formed in any of the 70 cases.

Ovarian Cyst.—F. W. N. Haultain *(Jour. Obst. and Gyn. of the Br. Emp.,* Apr.) reports a case of expulsion of a dermoid ovarian cyst through the vagina during labor. The cyst was about the size of a small cocoanut. It was forced through the posterior wall of the vagina and was removed during the second stage of labor, coming away while the patient was being ex-amined. The child was delivered by forceps without trouble. The rent in the vagina was packed with iodoform gauze. Patient made an uninterrupted recovery. Haultain suggests that on recognition of the condition the alternative methods of simple reposition, vaginal ovariotomy, and reposition with subsequent early ovariotomy should be carefully weighed. Where condi-tions admit of vaginal ovariotomy he is inclined to advise this method. Should reposition have been successfully performed, subsequent removal of the tumor within twenty-four hours seems a good method of treatment when the surroundings permit.

Conservative Operative Treatment of Old Puerperal Uterine Inversions.—In the April number of this JOURNAL (p. 602) was given an abstract of the treatment of inversion of the uterus advised by Oui. The present paper *(Ann. de Gyn. et d'Obst.,* Apr.) is devoted to a detailed description of conservative oper-ative measures, both abdominal and vaginal. Of these he favors anterior colpo-hysterotomy. The only objection to this oper-ation which he can find is the possibility of injuring the bladder; but he regards this as very remote, as in cases of chronic in-version of the uterus the bladder is usually entirely separated from that organ. The uterus is drawn down and a large trans-verse incision made in the anterior vaginal wall just above the cervix. After examination to determine that the bladder and intestine will not be injured, the entire anterior uterine wall is opened longitudinally and in the median line. With the thumbs on its posterior surface and index fingers on the borders of the incision, the uterus is reinverted. The uterine wound is then closed by interrupted catgut sutures through all layers except the mucosa, with intervening catgut sutures through peritoneum and superficial muscular fibres. The fundus is then pushed through the vaginal incision until entirely within the abdomen. The cervix and vaginal wound are then closed with catgut, a gauze drain being left in the latter for three days, and the vagina tamponed.

Vulvar Lymphangiectases.—The case reported, together with the four other recorded European cases, furnishes H. Duret *(Jour. des Sci. méd. de Lille,* May 10 and 17) with the material for a paper on lymphangiectases. His patient was a pale, emaciated girl of 17, with hypertrophy, edema, and redness of the labia majora, from which exuded a profuse sero-purulent liquid. This condition extended to each inguinal region and above the anterior superior spines. Since the age of 11 she had had an irregular swelling of the left labium majus, which had become red and painful within fifteen days. After incision large quantities of lymph were discharged. This continued for some days. Each time the cut edges became agglutinated the temperature rose. The cachexia and anemia increased. After several months the inflammatory appearance and symptoms disappeared under tonic treatment, and the affected region showed a large number of hemispherical vesicles easily emptied by pressure and giving issue to lymph when opened, while the upper part of the labia and the anterior commissure were covered with papillomatous growths. Five months after admission the skin remained simply thickened, while the papillomatous growths had become merely warty elevations. Duret's conclusions are that certain native cases of lymphangiectasis occur which are not due to the filaria sanguinis hominis, but are the result of obstruction to the lymphatic circulation by obliterating adeno-lymphangitis, caused by other organisms, especially the streptococci. The dilatations may occupy the ganglia and afferent vessels, the large lymphatic trunks, and the lymphatic reticulum of the skin, constituting respectively adeno-lymphocele, lymphatic varix, and varix of the skin. Varices of the cutaneous lymphatic network are most common on the lower extremities and external genitals and are accompanied by edema of the skin. They appear as the vesicles described above. The lymph flow when they are opened may cause severe cachexia. The vulvar lymphangiectases occur as clear vesicles or papillomatous vegetations as in the author's case.

Treatment of Recto-perineal Fistula.—Gérard Marchant *(Presse méd.,* Mar. 15) employed the following method for the closure of a recto-perineal fistula through which the rectal mucosa prolapsed. The fistula was presumably the result of an infected suture from a rectocele operation. After dilatation of the anus the mucosa was everted and amputated circularly one-half centimetre above the anus. The mucous membrane was freed around the perineal portion of the fistula and drawn down through the anus. A circular amputation of the rectum just above the rectal opening of the fistula removed all the damaged portion, and the part above this incision was drawn down and sutured to the narrow collar left at the anus. The perineal opening was freshened and then closed with sutures. The result was all that could be desired.

Treatment of Pyelitis.—In connection with the report of the removal of a large vesical calculus from a woman, Graefe *(Cent. f. Gyn.,* No. 13) reports two cases of pyelitis successfully treated by the internal administration of methylene blue.

Ovarian Hematoma Complicating Uterine Fibroids.— Lauwers *(Bull. de la Soc. Belge de Gyn. et d'.Obst.,* t. xii., No. 6) calls attention to a complication of uterine fibroids which is not mentioned in several leading modern text books. In 150 operations for fibroids he encountered 11 cases with hematoma of the ovary and one with hematosalpinx. In 10 cases the ovarian hematoma was bilateral.

Cystopexy.—A cystocele being formed by prolapse of the base of the bladder, Umberto Chiaventone *(Ann. de Gyn. et d'Obst.,* May) prefers to approach through the abdomen in order to attack that portion of the organ. The operation, which is described at great length, consists simply in an abdominal incision and a transverse incision of the vesico-uterine cul-de-sac, through which the bladder is stripped off down to the level at which the ureters enter the bladder. At this level the connective-tissue attachment of the bladder, which has been loose above, suddenly becomes dense and firm. The base of the bladder is then sutured to the anterior wall of the uterus; the utero-vesical peritoneum is reunited; and the uterus is fixed by hysteropexy or intraperitoneal shortening of the round ligaments, according to the degree of prolapse. The abdominal wound is then closed.

Inheritance of Hypospadias and Pseudohermaphroditism.— F. Neugebauer *(Monats. f. Geb. u. Gyn.,* Bd. xv., H. 3) has collected the histories of 39 cases, 37 of masculine hypospadias or pseudohermaphroditism and 2 of feminine pseudohermaphroditism. In 26 of these the individual had previously been supposed to be of the opposite sex. In 20 cases hypospadias was transmitted from father to son, or to the second generation through a normal father, or through the mother. The frequency of hypospadias is shown by Rennes' figures of 10 cases in 3,000 French recruits and Bouisson's one in 300 venereal cases. That it is not necessarily the cause of sterility is shown by a case with a separation of the halves of the penis to the extent of 5 centimetres, in which a condom with the top removed permitted repeated fruitful intercourse. Associated developmental or functional testicular disturbance often causes sterility.

DISEASES OF CHILDREN.

The After-History of the Children born of Insane Mothers.—
An editorial *(Med. Press and Circular,* Mar. 28, 1902) calls attention to the statistics collected by A. F. Tredgold. The conclusions drawn therefrom are that (1) the mental and physical condition of the child is in nowise influenced by the mere fact of the mother being insane during pregnancy; (2) neither is the condition of the child influenced by the variety of the insanity, the duration of the attack, or the age of the mother, nor even directly by the number of attacks from which the mother may have suffered; but that (3) *this condition is directly dependent upon the presence or absence of morbid hereditary influences.*

Bright's Disease in Children.—Henry Ashby *(Practitioner,* Dec., 1901) says that it is hardly necessary to remark that the systematic examination of the urine of sick infants and children is just as important as the examination of the urine of adults, and that unless such systematic examinations are made renal complications will certainly be overlooked. The common type of nephritis in childhood is the acute or subacute type of inflammation, with exudation of blood and fibrin which more or less choke the tubules, and the urine in consequence is dark in color and albuminous. Chronic nephritis is much less common, and is usually the result of repeated subacute attacks. There is also the septic form, which differs from those already described in that the inflammation is local rather than general, while the chief feature is an exudation of leucocytes from the vessels, and there are often minute points of suppuration; and reference must also be made to the toxic degeneration changes which are associated with the acute febrile disorders, more especially diphtheria, though these can hardly be classed with nephritis. In 3,000 cases of scarlet fever that have been under the writer's care in the fever ward of the Manchester Children's Hospital, nephritis supervened in from six to seven per cent of them. Acute nephritis in rare instances is a sequel of certain other specific diseases besides scarlet fever. It is comparatively common for it to occur without any history being obtainable of some previous acute disorder. In these primary cases the onset is often insidious, and it may happen that no previous examination of the urine has been made till the puffy white face suggests kidney disease. It is this insidious type which is met with in children under 2 years of age when it is not scarlatinal. Very little can be said about the treatment of nephritis which is not the common property of every text book—there is unfortunately no drug known that in any way modifies or checks inflammatory or degenerative changes in the kidneys. Fortunately recovery from scarlatinal nephritis is usually complete and permanent if the patient is placed under favorable conditions, though in some instances it may be prolonged and tedious. After the acute process is over small quantities of albumin may from time to time be detected in the urine, especially if the patient is allowed to get up and go about.   During the acute stage there can be no two opinions with regard to the importance of keeping the patient in a horizontal position, clothed in flannel, and surrounded by blankets, with perhaps several rubber hot-water bottles in the bed.   For the first two days or weeks a diet consisting of from one to two pints of milk in the twenty-four hours, freely diluted with warm barley water or some thin gruel, should be given.   Warm baths are beneficial, and should, of course, be brought to the bedside of the patient.   Excessive purgation is to be avoided, unless there are symptoms of uremia.   When the acute stage is over a more liberal diet may be allowed: eggs, toast, cooked vegetables, and rice pudding are allowable, while meat and meat extracts are best avoided until the kidneys are on full work again.   In the more severe cases, when there is much edema, scanty urine, and perhaps troublesome uremic vomiting, treatment becomes a much more serious problem.   Hot-air or vapor baths act on the skin much more powerfully than simple warm baths, but even these at times will fail to make the patient sweat freely.   Pilocarpine and jaborandi are apt to depress; smart purgation with calomel and euonymin will be necessary if the vomiting is troublesome.   Diureties are mostly disappointing, the best, perhaps, being the citrate of caffeine.   Digitalis and strychnine should be given if there is any evidence of cardiac dilatation or a failing heart. Chloroform is useful to check the violence of uremic convulsions, and injections of morphia (one-twentieth to one-tenth grain) may be safely given, the danger of this drug in kidney disease having been greatly exaggerated by some writers.   In chronic nephritis, when there is albuminuria and no acute or subacute symptoms, the great thing is to place the patient under the most favorable life conditions. Too much bed and indoor life is a mistake, and no good can come of long periods of a purely milk diet. A varied diet must be prescribed, consisting in the main of vegetables, eggs, and milk, and an out-of-doors life in a warm climate.

Diphtheria.—John H. McCollom (*Providence Med. Jour.*, July, 1902) says that when one sees a patient with membrane covering the tonsils and uvula, profuse sanious discharge from the nose, spots of ecchymosis on the body and extremities, cold, clammy hands and feet, a feeble pulse and the nauseous odor of diphtheria, and finds that after the administration of 10,000 units of antitoxin in two doses the condition of the patient improves slightly, that after 10,000 units more have been given there is a marked abatement in the severity of the symptoms, that when an additional 10,000 units have been given the patient is apparently out of danger and eventually recovers, one must believe in the curative power of antitoxin.   When one sees a patient in whom the intubation tube has repeatedly been clogged, when the hopeless condition of the patient changes for the better after the administration of 50,000 units, one cannot help but be convinced of the importance of giving large doses of antitoxin in the severe and apparently hopeless cases. From a comparison of the health reports of Boston before and after the introduction of the antidiphtheritic serum, from a comparison of the health reports of other cities, from a study of hospital reports, from a clinical observation of 10,526 cases of diphtheria, the following conclusions are justifiable: 1. That the ratio of mortality of diphtheria per 10,000 of the living was very high in Boston previous to 1895. 2. That the ratio of mortality per 10,000 has been very materially reduced since the introduction of antitoxin. 3. That the percentage of mortality in the South Department is lower than that of any of the hospitals taken for comparison. 4. That since larger doses of antitoxin have been given the death rate has been materially reduced, this reduction having occurred in the apparently moribund cases. 5. That no injurious effect has followed the use of the serum. 6. That to arrive at the most satisfactory results in the treatment of diph-theria, antitoxin should be given at the earliest possible moment in the course of the disease.

Diphtheria Treated with Massive Doses of Antitoxin.—L. G. Le Beuf (*New Orleans Med. and Surg. Jour.*, June, 1902) reports the case of a child of 3 years suffering from laryngeal diphtheria. He had profound dyspnea, pulse was 144, temperature 100°, respiration 32. He was injected in the lumbar region with 3,000 units of antitoxin March 6 at 4 P.M. March 7 he was in much the same condition, but with a little less abdominal tirage. On this day he received three injections of 3,000 units each, making a total of 12,000 units in less than thirty-two hours. During this time the child was apparently *in extremis* and the injections were given as a last resource. The next day the child was much better and expectorated, after a most violent strangulation fit of coughing, a nearly perfect cast of his pharynx and larynx, with three long, flat, grayish digitations at the bottom, no doubt part of some larger bronchial casts also. The child also swallowed a large piece of membrane. Immediately after this his condition improved. Another injection of 3,000 units was made, to be positive of getting every particle of exudate out of the throat. After all this dosage the only reaction which took place was a profuse diaphoresis. Calomel in one-tenth grain doses was given for catharsis and as an intestinal asepssis. March 11 and 12 the heart beat was still intermittent, but after that it became normal, and the child recovered completely. The author says that undoubtedly when aseptic methods are used and a good serum employed we have an agent which causes very little re-action and seems to work the greatest good when administered most fearlessly. It is believed, to explain this benignity, that antitoxin enters directly into combination with the specific toxin it is to neutralize. Hence it is made to combat it without danger to the patient, because probably a neutral salt is found in the system. McCollom, of Boston, has repeated 4,000 units until 80,000 and 100,000 have been given, especially in the infantile

paralysis following diphtheria.   In severe cases he does not
believe there is any way of estimating the amount of toxins
generated by the exudate, hence his conclusion is to go on administering it until the membranes are shrivelled and the improvement of the patient tells when to stop.

Diphtheria of the Conjunctiva Treated by Antitoxin.—L.
Emmett Holt *(Arch. of Ped.,* May, 1902) gives the following
report of a case: The patient, an infant 6 months old, was admitted to the New York Foundling Hospital May 18, 1901,
without any history. Examination showed swelling and redness
of the right eye, especially of the upper lid, to such a degree
that the child was unable to open it. On everting the lid a
thick, yellowish-gray patch of pseudo-membrane was seen upon
the conjunctiva, covering about one-half of the lid. This membrane was very adherent. There was evidence of considerable
conjunctivitis and the cornea was slightly cloudy. There was
no membrane in the throat or elsewhere, and the general symptoms were those of moderate prostration, temperature 102°. A
fresh smear and afterward a culture from the conjunctiva
showed diphtheria bacilli in numbers, and 2,400 units of antitoxin were administered. Ice compresses were applied and a
solution of atropine dropped into the eye. The progress of the
case was rapid and uneventful. In twenty-four hours the temperature had fallen to 100⅘°, and in forty-eight hours to normal. Improvement in the eye began almost immediately, and
in twenty-four hours a very decided change was seen. On the
third day the swelling had so far diminished that the child
could open the eye and the membrane was nearly gone. It did
not disappear entirely until the sixth day. Diphtheria bacilli
were found by cultures as late as the seventh day, but on the
tenth day the eye was entirely well. No more convincing demonstration of the value of antitoxin can be found than in cases
like this, which formerly, under any treatment known, almost
invariably went on from bad to worse, ending in the destruction
of the eye.

The Etiology of Hodgkin's Disease.—John M. Dodson *(Pediatrics,* April 15, 1902) reports a case as his contribution to the
discussion of the tubercular origin of this disease. There was a
general enlargement of all the superficial glands of the neck,
varying in size from that of a large filbert to a hen's egg. The
glands were not in the least tender, even on firm pressure, nor
was there any evidence of inflammatory process about them.
There was no indication of pressure on the vessels, nerves, or
other structures of the neck; no enlargement of the axillary, inguinal, or abdominal glands could be detected. The spleen was
not palpable; temperature 99°, pulse 100. There was at no time
pronounced leucocytosis. A diagnosis of lymphadenitis was
made, probably of tubercular origin, though the possibility of
Hodgkin's disease was noted. A small gland was removed, but
careful examination failed to show any of the usual appearances

of a tubercular process, and carefully stained sections showed no bacilli. The failure of tuberculin tests previously made, and the result of the microscopic examination of the gland removed, seemed to warrant the exclusion of tuberculosis, and the case was considered to be one of Hodgkin's disease. The patient was placed on Fowler's solution, in increasing doses, and at his last appearance there was a noticeable diminution in the size of the gland. It may be objected in this case that the diagnosis of a chronic lymphadenitis cannot be excluded, but the writer thinks that the apparent absence of any antecedent affection of the throat, of pain and tenderness in the glands, of periadenitis, or of any tendency to suppuration, and, finally, a characteristic appearance of the gland removed for examination, speak strongly against such an opinion. This case seems, therefore, to have been one of Hodgkin's disease, not of tubercular origin. That this disease is of infectious origin is extremely probable, but the infectious agent is as yet unknown to us, though doubtless cases of tubercular and syphilitic disease of the lymphatics may simulate it closely and may have been mistaken therefor. In case of doubt as to the tubercular character of the disease, tuberculin should be carefully and thoroughly tried, and, this failing, one of the glands or a portion of one should be removed, carefully examined for the presence of tubercular lesions and of bacilli, and then emulsified with sterile water and inoculated into guinea-pigs.

Inheritance of Recurrent Attacks of Jaundice and of Abdominal Crisis with Hepato-Splenomegaly.—Thomas Barlow and H. Batty Shaw *(Med. Press and Circular,* May 28, 1902) report cases in mother and son. The special points to be noted are: 1. The chronicity of the affection, lasting in the son at least fourteen years and being probably congenital, and in the mother for a much longer period. 2. The occurrence of indolent ulcers in both cases. 3. The fact that the jaundice is always slightly present and undergoes periodic intensification, and is then associated with pain in the spleen or the liver, or both. 4. The mother's would appear to be a case of Hannot's cirrhosis of the liver, while her son's cannot but be considered as an earlier incomplete stage, possibly of the same malady. 5. Finally, attention is called to the extremely guarded prognostic view to be held in such cases. Mrs. W. has grown to maturity and has had several children, and but for the disturbance caused by the periodical attacks of jaundice and abdominal pains is able to enjoy life.

The Importance of Rickets in Girls from an Obstetrical Standpoint.—C. S. Bacon *(Clin. Rev.,* April, 1902) describes two cases which illustrate the importance of rickets in girls, on account of the serious pelvic deformities resulting and causing obstetrical complications during the childbearing period. While these results of rickets manifest themselves in adult life, the disease is one of infancy. From a study of a limited number of cases in private and dispensary practice, the author would be inclined to state that nearly one-half of all pelvic contractions are caused by rickets. From the report of others this ratio would be too high. We are still considerably in the dark concerning the etiology of this disease. There is no agreement as to the kind of food that is essential to proper development of the body, and to the lack of which rickets may be ascribed. The natural attempt, in the early study of the disease, to attribute it to deficiency in the lime salts has been generally abandoned, because such a deficiency in the food could not be demonstrated. Zweifel contends for the importance of sodium chloride; Christopher finds fat generally lacking. Animals are made rachitic by withholding various food elements, as proteid meat in the case of dogs. A question of very grave importance is that of early diagnosis. There are unfortunately no marked signs which call the attention of the parents of the child to the fact that an important disease is developing. The earliest sign of the disease is probably the beading in the fourth, fifth, and sixth ribs. As a rule, the next deformity to show in the long bones is in the lower ends of the radius and ulna. About the same time comes the thickening of the bosses of the parietal and frontal bones of the skull. Theoretically two things are important in the treatment of rickets in its acute stage. One is control of the disease process as soon as possible, and the other is the care of the child to prevent the pelvic deformity. The disease process is fortunately generally corrected by proper dietetic and hygienic management. If there be a gastro-intestinal infection, which is not infrequently the case, its correction is of course the first thing to be attended to. Not infrequently we find that the child is on a starvation diet of diluted milk. There seems to be a widespread fear among physicians that fat will injure a baby's digestion. The writer has sometimes found nursing children rachitic, and in all of these cases there was an abnormally low proportion of fat in the mother's milk. It is a pretty general rule that a child with rickets will improve with a considerable addition of fat to its diet. Infants may be given diluted cream, while older children should be encouraged to eat plenty of good fresh butter. In the case of nursing children two or three feedings of diluted cream should be introduced among the nursings. In all cases cod-liver oil has an unusually good influence, and not only makes the cure quicker, but in many cases seems to be a necessity. Is it possible to do anything to prevent the development of a pelvic deformity in a rickety girl? So far as the author can learn, the orthopedists have not considered this phase of the subject of rickets. Yet, instead of being a rare deformity, it is probably one of the most common. If anything can be done for the rachitic girl to save her one or two centimetres in the conjugata vera, it is well worth the effort. Of course we can attempt to keep the child lying down, but that is difficult in the case of an otherwise healthy child. Whether it is possible or practicable to devise any kind of an apparatus to relieve the trunk pressure on the sacrum must be left to the orthopedist to decide.

Intussusception in Children.—R. Hamilton Russell *(Inter. Med. Jour.,* March 20, 1902) used to attempt to secure reduction by water pressure, but, having become convinced that it is not possible to be certain that reduction has taken place, he now subjects every case to immediate operation as soon as the diagnosis is made. He says, however, that water pressure is sometimes perfectly efficient, and it seems as if there ought to be a sphere of usefulness for it. A surgeon can hardly perform abdominal section on an infant away in the country with little or no assistance, while he can use water pressure quite easily. He is inclined to think that the majority of cases that are diagnosed within a very few hours may be reduced by water pressure, and where the obstacles to operation are great the chance of the lesser procedure proving effective should be offered. The compressing agent should be the weight of a column of water not more than two feet in height. All kinds of inflators are forbidden as being dangerous to the integrity of the bowel. The apparatus employed should be a funnel with a long soft-rubber tube attached. The tube will be gradually introduced higher and higher into the bowel as the water flows in; return of the water by the side of the tube will be prevented by compression of the nates around the tube. At first only a relatively small amount of water can be introduced; and this amount should be noted, as it will be a measure of the extent of large bowel unoccupied by the intussusception. As this latter becomes gradually reduced the quantity of water that passes in will gradually increase; after four or five minutes the bowel should be allowed to empty itself, and examination of the abdomen be made in order to ascertain what alteration, if any, has taken place in the size and position of the tumor. If the tumor is still present, although much reduced, the procedure should be repeated; if no alteration can be detected, any further attempt to achieve the desired object by this means will be fruitless. During the proceeding the child should be well anesthetized, with the buttocks well raised and the legs held up by an assistant. With respect to the technique of the operation, the first question is as to the site of the incision. The writer has always operated in the median line, and he thinks the best incision to be about two and a half inches in length, with about one-third of its length above the umbilicus and passing to the left of that structure. As soon as the abdomen is opened a loop of stout silk should be passed through the whole thickness of the abdominal wall on either side; the tumor is then felt for and gently coaxed out of the abdominal wound. Reduction should now be effected on much the same principle that we reduce a strangulated hernia. The intussuscipiens is grasped with the left hand, and the finger tips of the right hand are applied to the apex of the intussusceptum, pressing it steadily backward. Reduction having been effected, the sides of the opening are lifted well up by means of the silk tenacula; the small intestine is gently returned first, and finally the cecum and large intestine. The abdominal wound is then closed by interrupted sutures of catgut or silk, which pass through the whole thickness of the musculature and peritoneum; the skin is sutured separately. The wound is then sealed with gauze and collodion in two portions, above and below the umbilicus respectively. A dry covering of gauze and wool is then bandaged on over all and the operation is completed. It is constantly asserted that infants stand an operation very badly, that they are unable to bear a prolonged operation, and that rapidity in operating is of the first importance. The author considers that gentleness and care in the handling are of more importance than mere rapidity. He has seen an infant die within an hour after its return to bed, having sunk into fatal collapse under the hands of an operator who studied rapidity a little too much and gentleness just a shade too little. In intussusception, as in other forms of intestinal obstruction, early diagnosis is everything.

Gangrenous Intussusception in a Child Four Years Old; Intestinal Resection; Recovery.—Charles N. Dowd *(Annals of Surgery,* July, 1902) reports the case of a child who showed in a most exaggerated degree the symptoms of prolonged intestinal obstruction, viz., constipation, persistent vomiting of intestinal contents, tympanites, emaciation, the retention of a good temperature, and a fairly good pulse. Laparatomy showed that there was an intussusception about the middle of the ileum, about two and a half inches long. The intestine below this was empty. On gentle manipulation an opening appeared through the intestinal wall, which was gangrenous at the site of intussusception. The intussusception, two or three inches of intestine at each end of it, and a gangrenous piece of the mesentery were excised. Much gas escaped from the upper intestinal end, also intestinal contents; after this the coils of intestines which had been so greatly distended, and which had been kept in hot, moist towels, could be returned into the abdomen. The intestine about the excised portion was washed repeatedly in warm saline solution. A circular enterorrhaphy was then done. The first row of stitches passed through all the layers of the intestine and brought the peritoneal surfaces into close apposition at the margin. At the mesenteric border they were so placed as to obliterate the dead space there and hold broad peritoneal surfaces together, well supported by intestinal wall. A second row of Cushing stitches was then taken outside of this, and this was in certain places reinforced by a third tier of similar stitches. The intestine was then returned into the abdomen and thorough irrigation with hot saline solution given. The abdominal incision was closed with tier sutures. The child made an excellent and uneventful recovery. The author says that the case suggests several topics which are important in the management of irreducible intussusception. He calls attention to only two: 1. Intestinal resection versus the making of an artificial anus. 2. The method of uniting the ends of the resected intestine. As to the first, he says that in consideration of the reports (which he submits), and which were many of them made before intestinal resection was practised as successfully as it is now, one hardly feels justified in making an artificial anus in gangrenous intussusception. As to the method of uniting the ends of the resected intestine, the author reviews the various ones in use and declares his preference for an end-to-end suture with an inner row of stitches through all the layers of the intestine and an outer row through the outer layers. This was the method used in the case described, and, although it was independently worked out, it possesses the essential elements of the method of Frank. Taking into consideration all the possibilities of error in statistics which are taken from various operators instead of from a single institution, we may feel that the results are favorable to the use of through-and-through stitches. Most surgeons, however, do not feel it safe to leave such a row of stitches without reinforcing them by a second row of superficial ones. When so reinforced any infection which might follow the stitch is much more likely to work its way on to the lumen of the intestine along the thread than to push the peritoneal adhesions apart and force its way into the peritoneum. The time consumed in applying these two rows of stitches differs little from that required for the application of a Murphy button. The suturing can be completed in fifteen minutes without hurrying.

ITEM.

The American Association of Obstetricians and Gynecologists will hold its fifteenth annual meeting in the Convention Hall of the Hotel Raleigh, Washington, D. C., Tuesday, Wednesday, and Thursday, September 16, 17, and 18, 1902, under the presidency of Dr. Edwin Ricketts, of Cincinnati. All physicians, and especially those in Washington and vicinity, are most cordially invited to the scientific sessions.

The following-named papers have been offered: 1. President's address, Edwin Ricketts, Cincinnati. 2. Normal saline solutions during abdominal operations, William H. Humiston, Cleveland. 3. Further notes on ovarian transplantation, Robert T. Morris, New York. 4. Surgery of the ileo-cecal valve, N. Stone Scott, Cleveland. 5. Ice following abdominal sections, Frank F. Simpson, Pittsburg. 6. Etiology and prophylaxis of traumatism of the female pelvic tract following labor, E. J. Ill, Newark. 7. Pelvic disease in the unmarried, C. L. Bonifield, Cincinnati. 8. Report of a few cases of operation for peritoneal tuberculosis, with remarks, Rufus B. Hall, Cincinnati. 9. Suppression of urine as a post-operative condition, T. J. Crofford, Memphis.   10. Occipito-posterior positions, J. M. Duff, Pittsburg.   11. Intestinal anastomosis, J. A. Lyons, Chicago.   12. Retained placenta due to uterine fibroids, with cases, M. A. Tate, Cincinnati.   13. Hydramnion, with report of a case, E. F. Fish, Milwaukee. 14. (a) Personal experiences in the use of the angiotribe; (b) Two fatal cases of tetanus following abdominal section, Walter B. Dorsett, St. Louis.   15. A second contribution to the treatment of gastric ulcer, Henry Howitt, Guelph.   16. Hemorrhagic cysto-sarcomata of the ovary; their infectious character, J. B. Murphy, Chicago.   17. General consideration of drainage in abdominal and pelvic surgery, Joseph Price, Philadelphia. 18. Surgical relations that the appendix region or zone bears to pelvic suppuration and operative complications, Joseph Price, Philadelphia.   19. Infantile intestinal diverticula, Joel W. Hyde, Brooklyn.   20. Myomectomy vs. hysterectomy, C. C. Frederick, Buffalo.   21. Anterior transplantation of the round ligaments for uterine displacements, A. H. Ferguson, Chicago. 22. The cases of peritonitis which recover after operation, William E. B. Davis, Birmingham.   23. Dystocia following ventrofixation of the uterus, William H. Wenning, Cincinnati. 24. Surgery of the ureters, C. R. Dudley, St. Louis.   25. Curettage in streptococcus infection of the uterus, D. Tod Gilliam, Columbus.   26. A new operation for displaced kidney, with report of cases, Charles A. L. Reed, Cincinnati.   27. Cancer of the large intestines, with special reference to Mikulicz's method of resection, M. Stamm, Fremont, O.   28. A short review of the advances made in intestinal surgery, James F. W. Ross, Toronto. 29. Ectopic pregnancy, H. D. Ingraham, Buffalo.   30. Unusual cases of appendicitis, Miles F. Porter, Fort Wayne.   31. Pelvic abscess and its treatment, H. E. Hayd, Buffalo.   32. Abdominal section during pregnancy, J. H. Carstens, Detroit.   33. Ruptured pus tubes, Charles G. Cumston, Boston.   34. Title to be announced, H. O. Pantzer, Indianapolis.   35. Gastrectomy, with report of two cases, A. Vander Veer, Albany.   36. Four cases illustrating the difficulties of diagnosticating appendicitis, William Wotkyns Seymour, Troy.   37. The vaginal route for operations on the uterus and appendages, with cases, Joseph H. Branham, Baltimore.   38. The management of cases of emergency arising from rupture in ectopic pregnancy, A. P. Clarke, Cambridge.   39. Some unsettled questions in the surgery of the appendix, John Young Brown, Jr., St. Louis.   40. Deciduoma malignum, with report of a case, L. S. McMurtry, Louisville. 41. Relationship of the colon to abdominal tumors, James F. Baldwin, Columbus.   42. Some problems in exploratory laparatomy, Walter B. Chase, New York.   43. Title to be announced, L. H. Dunning, Indianapolis.   44. Extirpation of the gall bladder through the lumbar incision, with report of a case, W. P. Manton, Detroit.

THE AMERICAN

JOURNAL OF OBSTETRICS

AND

DISEASES OF WOMEN AND CHILDREN.

VOL. XLVI.   SEPTEMBER, 1902.   No. 3.

ORIGINAL COMMUNICATIONS.

TWO CASES OF DECIDUOMA MALIGNUM.[1]

BY

CHARLES P. NOBLE, M.D.,

Surgeon-in-Chief, Kensington Hospital for Women,
Philadelphia.

(With plate and two illustrations.)

THE two cases of deciduoma malignum herewith reported have each certain points of interest and are reported as a contribution to the study of this subject. The first case was operated upon in 1893 and is apparently the earliest operation in this country. The real nature of the growth was not recognized, however, until shortly before the second patient was operated upon, in November, 1900.

CASE I.—Mrs. K., aged 30, has had two children and one miscarriage. The miscarriage occurred between the births of the two children. The youngest child is aged 30 months. She is quite anemic and feeble, and consulted me because of almost constant uterine hemorrhages. The general history presented nothing of interest, she having had no general disease except malaria. Her menstrual history was normal until September,

[1] Read before the Section on Gynecology, College of Physicians of Philadelphia, April 17, 1902.

19

1892, ten months before presenting herself and twenty months after the birth of her youngest child. During the last ten months she has had almost constant hemorrhage from the uterus. Examination showed that the uterus was much enlarged, suggesting either a small fibroid or malignant disease of the corpus.

Curettage was performed June 23, 1893, in the Kensington Hospital for Women, and a large amount of necrotic tissue was removed. Influenced by the teachings then current, a clinical diagnosis of sarcoma was made. Under similar conditions to-

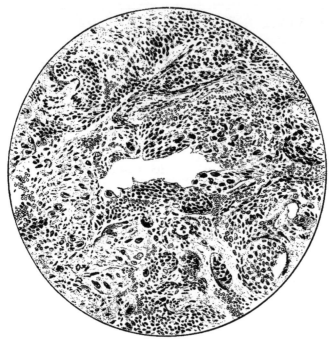

CASE I.—Syncytioma malignum. ' Section consists chiefly of syncytial cells with erythrocytic infiltration.

day a clinical diagnosis of carcinoma of the corpus would be made. The scrapings were referred to Dr. Joseph McFarland, pathologist to the hospital, who reported that the case was probably one of necrosis of a submucous fibroid. The pathologist's report not being received promptly, and having no question that the case was one of malignant tumor, the uterus was removed by a vaginal hysterectomy June 28. The patient made a good recovery from the operation and remained well until November, 1893. At that time I saw her; found her in bed with evidences of consolidation in the right lung and with effusion in one pleura. Several small tumors were present—one under the skin of the breast, another under the skin of the loin, and a third under the skin of the thigh. The patient died in December, 1893.

The extirpated uterus was preserved in Müller's fluid and was referred to Dr. McFarland for examination. He reported that the case was one of sarcoma (endothelioma) of the uterus,[1] deciduoma being practically unknown in this country at that time.

Just before the specimen from the second operation was examined a slide from this older case was accidentally re-examined and a diagnosis of deciduoma malignum made.[2]

This case is of interest, first, as being apparently the first one operated upon in the United States, and, second, because of the long time which had elapsed (about twenty months, the longest recorded time) between the date of the last puerperium and the appearance of hemorrhage from the uterus, this being the first sign of the presence of the new growth.[3] Thirty months had

[1]Medical News, December 8, 1894.

[2]Philadelphia Medical Journal, December 22, 1900.

[3]The following table from Ladinski, "Deciduoma Malignum," THE AMERICAN JOURNAL OF OBSTETRICS, April, 1902, shows the recorded time between the termination of pregnancy and the beginning of symptoms from the deciduoma malignum:

APPEARANCE OF THE DISEASE AFTER TERMINATION OF PREGNANCY.

	After Mole.	After Abortion.	After Labor at Term.
1 week	15 cases	10 cases	9 cases
2 weeks..........	1 case	3 "	0 "
3 "	0 cases	1 case	5 "
4 "	13 "	12 cases	5 "
5 "	1 case	0 "	1 case
6	2 cases	3 "	0 cases
7	1 case	0 "	1 case
8 "	2 cases	1 case	4 cases
9 "	0 "	0 cases	1 case
10	0 "	0 "	0 cases
12	1 case	5 "	2 "
16 "	1 "	0 "	0 "
6 months........	4 cases	2 "	1 case
7 "	0 "	1 case	0 cases
9 "	1 case	0 cases	0 "
10	1 "	1 case	0 "
20	1 "	1 "	0 "
	44 cases.	40 cases.	29 cases.
Average	8 weeks.	7 weeks.	5 weeks.

elapsed between the delivery and the operation, which is the extreme.

CASE II.—Mrs. D., aged 24, has had two pregnancies. The first ended in miscarriage at the fourth month in November, 1899, and the second at the sixth week, August 15, 1900. The patient's

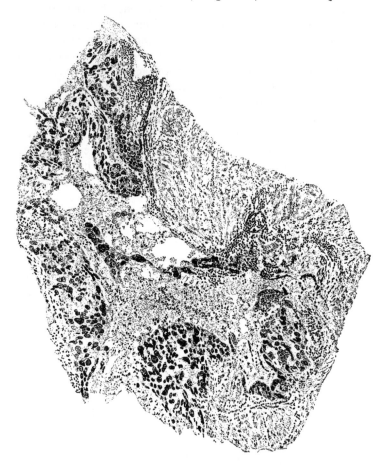

CASE II.—Syncytioma malignum. Section of infiltrated uterine wall showing masses of syncytial cells, collections of lymphoid cells, and degenerating thrombi.

general history presented nothing of interest. Her menstrual history was normal from the age of 13 to 23. During the past year menstruation has been irregular, appearing in from three to six weeks. The duration of the flow has been seven days. There has been marked pain for one week before and also during the

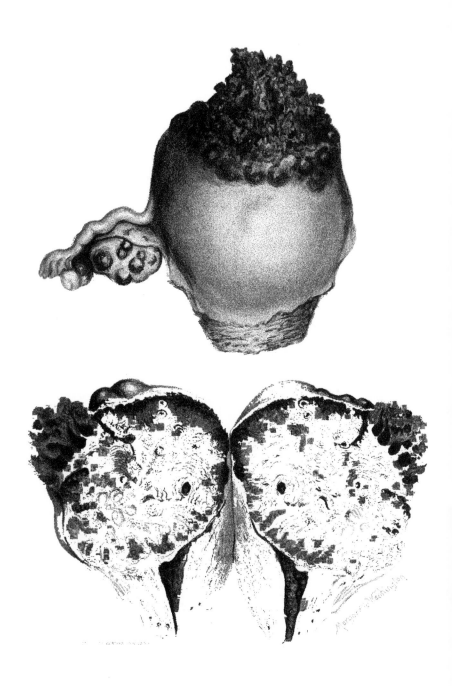

DECIDUOMA MALIGNUM. Noble

flow. Since the last miscarriage, August 15, 1900, the flow has been constant. It was profuse during the first two weeks and has varied since that date.

The patient was admitted to the Kensington Hospital for Women November 14, 1900. Examination showed a normal vagina and cervix. A tumor connected with the cervix filled the pelvis. The tumor had the general characteristics of a fibroid, but was notably softer than the average fibroid. A diagnosis of fibroid tumor was made and hysterectomy advised, and performed November 17. When the abdomen was opened it was evident that we had to deal with a malignant tumor of the fundus. The tumor filled the pelvis, was of dark-bluish, mottled appearance, looking much like a hematocele covered by membrane. The omentum was adherent to the bladder, and apparently the tumor had penetrated both the omentum and the bladder. A diagnosis of deciduoma malignum was at once made from the history and the appearance of the tumor. In attempting to separate the bladder from the tumor the finger pushed through the very soft structure of the tumor, and a definite amount of tumor substance was left upon the fundus of the bladder. It was believed that the malignant growth had involved the bladder and that its complete extirpation would necessitate the removal of a large portion of that viscus. As the patient's feeble condition did not warrant such an extensive operation, this was not attempted. A supravaginal hysterectomy was performed, with the view that the case was a hopeless one from the standpoint of radical cure. Gauze drainage was employed. Convalescence was febrile until the sixth day, after which it was uninterrupted.

February 12, 1901, or about three months later, the patient had regained the appearance of health and expressed herself as feeling well. Upon pelvic examination the vagina was found normal; a distinct mass could be palpated upon the bladder wall where the portion of the tumor had been left at the operation. March 26, 1902, or a little more than sixteen months after the operation, the patient was again seen. She presented every evidence of good health and expressed herself as being quite well. A careful examination failed to show any evidence of malignant disease in any portion of the body. The mass which had been felt on the bladder at the preceding examination had disappeared. The vagina, bladder, and broad ligaments were entirely normal to touch. A small ventral hernia is developing as a result of the gauze drainage.

The case of Mrs. D. is of interest because of her apparent recovery from what appeared to be, at the date of the operation, a
hopeless situation on account of the involvement not only of the
uterus itself, but of the bladder and omentum, and this in spite
of the fact that, owing to her condition, it was impossible to extirpate the involved portion of the bladder. It is entirely possible that the malignant mass was merely adherent to the bladder
and had not penetrated the bladder walls, and the pathologist's
report indicates that this portion of the growth was necrotic;
but even upon this hypothesis it is of special interest as showing
the apparent disappearance of the mass of malignant tissue firmly attached to, even if not penetrating, the bladder. The further
history of this patient will be watched with interest and reported
upon at a later date.

The pathological report upon Case 2 was made by Dr. W.
Wayne Babcock, pathologist to the hospital, and the following
pathological reports have been furnished by him:

"*Case I.*—Sections from this specimen which, through the
courtesy of Dr. McFarland, I have had the privilege of examining, show a picture closely simulating that described in the second
case.   There are large masses of fused cells of the syncytial
type with hyaline protoplasm and large, irregular, and at times
multiple nuclei, together with collections of smaller cells of the
lymphoid type, and degenerating blood clot.

"In the early description of this growth[1] it was described as a
sarcomatous or endotheliomatous degeneration of a fibroid tumor,
but the restudy of these old sections made entirely through the
growth gives no evidence that the fibromuscular tissue present is
more than that which would have accompanied the growth of the
syncytial tumor.   It is believed, therefore, that this is a primary
syncytioma malignum in a uterus not the seat of any other
tumor.

"The growth measures 3 or 4 millimetres in diameter, and the
invasion is much less marked than that which occurred in the
second case.

"*Case II.*—The submitted specimens consist of a uterus amputated through the cervix, containing a uterine tumor, together
with the uterine appendages.   The uterus measures 9 centimetres
(3½ inches) in diameter, 8 centimetres (3¼ inches) antero-
posteriorly, and is 11½ centimetres (4½ inches) in length.   It
is globular in shape from the presence of a new growth, the bulk

[1] Medical News, December 8, 1894.

of which lies above the level of the attachments of the round ligaments. Above this level the peritoneal surface is irregularly convoluted and shows distended and arborescent blood vessels. Over the anterior upper portion of the fundus a neoplastic mass has perforated the peritoneal surface over an area measuring 7 by 5½ centimetres (2¾ by 2¼ inches). This marks the point of attachment to the bladder wall when the uterus was *in situ*. The projecting mass is deep red in color, irregular and friable. In other areas over the fundus the nodular mass seems nearly to have penetrated the peritoneal coat. For the most part the peritoneal surface is smooth, and below the level of the round ligaments shows no abnormality.

"The section through the cervix shows no evidences of disease. The ovaries and tubes are free from grave lesion. The former are slightly enlarged, have a cicatricial surface, and contain small, clear fluid cysts. The fimbriæ of the tubes are free from adhesions, and there are a few minute pediculated cysts attached to the walls of both tubes. The tubes are not enlarged and show no gross evidences of old or recent inflammatory condition.

"On sectioning the uterus in the antero-posterior plane it is found to consist chiefly of a dark-reddish, rounded, hemorrhagic growth measuring 8½ centimetres (3⅜ inches) in breadth, 8 centimetres (3⅛ inches) in thickness, and 7½ centimetres (3 inches) in a vertical direction. Posteriorly and below lie the displaced and distorted uterine cavity and the rather attenuated posterior uterine wall. Superiorly and anteriorly there is little remaining of the uterine wall except the peritoneal coat, which has been destroyed where the tumor has perforated. Laterally there is a layer of muscular tissue from a few millimetres (one-twelfth inch) to 1½ centimetres (one-half inch) in thickness.

"The tumor resembles a mass of coagulated blood, showing narrow, indistinct bands, apparently of connective tissue, which curve in various directions. In consistence it is soft and friable, and is fairly well circumscribed, but not encapsulated. It is in contact with the uterine mucosa, but apparently has not invaded the uterine cavity. The uterine cavity is small and flattened, and contains a moderate quantity of coagulated blood. Below the tumor the cervical canal is dilated, measuring 1 centimetre in diameter, and is also filled with coagulated blood. It tapers gradually to the usual size at the plane of amputation.

"Microscopic sections were taken from the centre and various portions of the periphery of the tumor, and from portions of the uterine wall and cervix, and were stained by thionin and by hematoxylin and eosin.

"1· From the centre of the tumor the mass was found to consist chiefly of a network resembling coagulated fibrin, the fibrils of which entangled red blood corpuscles in various stages of dissolution, and numerous polymorphonuclear leucocytes. Besides this there are numerous irregular areas taking the eosin stain, but too necrotic to show cellular structure.

"2. Sections taken from the periphery of the growth show an organized structure for only a few millimetres from the periphery, the tissue within this line being almost entirely necrotic or consisting of fibrin and infiltrated blood cells. At the periphery irregular masses of large cells are found infiltrating the muscular wall of the uterus and apparently lying in distended uterine sinuses. These cells contain one or several oval, rounded or irregular, or more frequently fusiform, nuclei. In certain of the cells karyokinetic figures are present. The nuclei are of various sizes. The surrounding protoplasm is finely granular, large in amount, and there is no distinct cell wall, so that when massed together the demarcation between adjoining cells is not perceptible. Adjoining these cells, and frequently infiltrating between the muscular fibres, are much smaller cells with small, regular, rounded nuclei encircled by a narrow band of protoplasm. These are not universally present and are not nearly as conspicuous as the larger cells. The uninvaded portions of the uterine muscle show sinuses and blood vessels distended by blood. Invasion by small lymphoid cells seems to precede that of the larger cells. As one recedes from the periphery, masses of the larger cells are found embedded in the fibrin and amid collections of red corpuscles. There is only a moderate infiltration of polymorphonuclear leucocytes.

"3· *Section from the mucous membrane of the cervix uteri.* The epithelial lining of the cervical mucosa is absent and apparently has been removed by the curette. There is a slight hyperplasia of the uterine glands, and in some of these a tendency to a desquamative catarrhal process is indicated by the loosened cells and the granular débris found filling the cavity. About a few of the glands there is an infiltration of small cells of the lymphoid type.

"The pathological diagnosis is syncytioma malignum of the corpus uteri."

1509 LOCUST STREET.

SPINAL ANESTHESIA.[1]

BY

SAMUEL L. WEBER, M.D.,

Attending Surgeon, Cook County Hospital,
Chicago, Ill.

THIS method of inducing anesthesia has been in practical use about three years. It has so far been employed in between three and four thousand cases and has therefore passed the strictly experimental stage. The time has arrived to form conclusions as to its scope and usefulness. It has been most generally used in France and the United States. Though its practical application originated in Germany, the Germans are taking to it but charily, and the English hardly at all. Tuffier, of France, has used it the greatest number of times. I employed it first in February, 1900, and have had, so far, an experience of about 150 cases. Although my impressions on the scope, value, and contraindications of subarachnoid anesthesia are still in the formative period, I have arrived at certain more or less definite opinions on the subject, and these I propose to state in this paper. I shall divide the subject into a number of divisions and discuss each under its heading.

TECHNIQUE. (a) *Site of Injection.*—The site in general use is between the fourth and fifth lumbar vertebræ. This can be found by taking a line connecting the crests of the iliac bones. The spinous process of the fourth lumbar vertebra can be felt in the median line of the body near this line. The needle is inserted about one-half inch to one or the other side and a little below the tip of this spinous process. It is pushed in a little upward and inward. If the interspace is not found at once, the needle is withdrawn somewhat and again pushed in at a slightly different angle. An experience of half a dozen lumbar punctures, either for diagnosis (Quincke's) or anesthesia, will teach one to penetrate the spinal canal readily where there is no marked deformity of the vertebræ. As soon as the subarachnoid space has been penetrated, the cerebro-spinal fluid begins to drip from the needle. The barrel of the syringe is now promptly attached

[1]Read before the Chicago Gynecological Society, April 18, 1902.

to the needle and the cocaine is injected. The injection is made slowly, and, when finished, the needle is suddenly withdrawn and the puncture wound sealed with collodion and cotton. That all this should be done under strictest asepsis is understood.

(b) *Position of the Patient.*—The injection can be made with the patient in the sitting or the recumbent position. It is more readily made, however, when the patient is sitting. In either position the patient must be made to arch his back as much as possible, so as to increase the size of the vertebral interspace.

(c) *The Instrument.*—Any hypodermatic syringe barrel may be used, but the needle must connect with it without a screw arrangement. The needle itself must be one made for this operation; it should be about three and one-half inches long, fairly stout, and with a very short bevel.

(d) *Preparation of the Cocaine.*—This is of importance. I have the druggist prepare, in as cleanly a manner as possible, a solution containing two per cent cocaine hydrochlorate, two per cent boric acid, and two per cent antipyrin. The solution is put up in one-ounce bottles with glass stoppers. This solution after forty-eight hours I consider sterile, and it keeps. I have used some made up three months before and it was as active as though just prepared. Boiling the solution spoils it, as cocaine is thereby broken up, partially or wholly. Pasteurization has the serious defect that it takes too long to prepare the cocaine solution. Both boiling and pasteurization have the fatal defect that the cocaine solution so prepared will not keep. A cocaine solution for spinal cocainization is needed at once. There is no time to pasteurize it. Prepared as I have described, the solution is always ready and sterile. I have had no experience with eucaine or with tropacocaine. The reports from those who have used them have not been so far encouraging enough to induce me to use either in preference to cocaine.

THE ANESTHESIA.—The anesthesia comes on very rapidly; in from three to ten minutes it is sufficient to begin the operation. Ten to fifteen minims of the solution are used. The anesthesia extends upward and is usually complete up to the level of the iliac crests; generally it extends higher, rarely to the level of the neck, and occasionally it is complete. In one of my cases I could have operated on the head. As a rule it tapers off above the waist line. The duration of the anesthesia is usually about one hour; sometimes only half an hour. Sometimes it lasts an hour and a half, and occasionally longer. When the anesthesia begins to disappear it does so very slowly, and the regions usually most sensitive regain their sensibility first. These irregularities in the extent and duration of the analgesia do not depend definitely upon the dose of cocaine injected, but upon personal idiosyncrasy. In this area of anesthesia, after cutaneous sensibility has disappeared, there is gradual abolition of the senses of temperature and pressure. The applications of heat and cold call forth only the sense of contact, which in some cases also disappears. Tickling of the soles of the feet may be perceived. but the usual reflex is not called forth. The sensation in the deeper tissues, muscles, bones, etc., is abolished in direct proportion to the insensibility of the skin. As the anesthesia passes away sensibility to touch reappears, then the senses of pressure and temperature, and lastly that of pain. Visceral sensibility is never wholly abolished, though it is more or less diminished, during cocaine anesthesia.

Failure to obtain anesthesia may be caused as follows:

(*a*) Most often by the use of a decomposed cocaine solution, one that has been boiled or one that has stood a long time without a preservative.

(*b*) In some cases the operator has been unable to penetrate the spinal canal. This has never happened to me. In rare cases this may be due to deformity of the spinal column at this point, but usually simply to lack of experience.

(c) The solution of cocaine is not injected into the subarachnoid space. This is due to faulty technique caused by unfamiliarity with the method. One can be sure of injecting the cocaine solution into the subarachnoid space only if the needle has penetrated it and not passed beyond it. One knows that the needle is in the subarachnoid space only when the cerebro-spinal fluid is dripping from the needle. The injection must be made only while this is taking place.

(*d*) In some cases the packing of the barrel of the syringe was defective, so that nearly all the cocaine solution dribbled outside instead of going into the subarachnoid space.

PHYSIOLOGICAL EFFECT OF COCAINE.—The physiological effect of cocaine must be understood by those who use this method of inducing anesthesia. This must be considered under three different headings: (1) The local effect when injected subcutaneously or painted upon mucous membranes; (2) the systemic effect; and (3) the effect when injected into the subarachnoid space. The local effect when injected subcutaneously or painted upon mucous membranes is too well known to need description. The general physiological action can be epitomized as follows: On the heart its action is similar to that of atropine. It lessens the vagus control of the heart in proportion to the size of the dose, so that central or reflex stimulation of the vagus becomes less and less effectual in controlling and slowing the action of the heart. The heart, as a result, in proportion to the size of the dose of cocaine, beats faster and not quite so steadily and forcibly. The blood pressure is slightly raised by an ordinary dose and gradually falls after a large dose. The most marked effect in the circulatory system is that shown by Dr. Crile on the splanchnic area. Causes which ordinarily produce congestion of the blood vessels of the abdominal viscera do not do so in an animal under the influence of cocaine. Ordinarily, in an animal, severe injuries, shock, exposure and handling of the intestines produce engorgement of the blood vessels of the mesentery and intestines; if the animal is under a moderate systemic effect of cocaine, congestion does not follow such stimulation. Small doses have no effect on the respiration; large doses produce less frequent and shallower breathing. There is no influence on the kidneys. Clinical evidence shows that cocaine produces a tonic contraction of the uterine muscle.

When injected into the subarachnoid space wholly different actions are induced. We get two sets of effects: one, the action on the nerve trunks and roots in the cauda equina and even higher up within the membranes of the spinal cord; and the second, the possible action on the medullary centres. The latter must be carefully considered. The anesthesia is produced by the cocaine solution which bathes the sensory nerve roots within the envelopes of the spinal cord. A sufficient quantity of cocaine must be injected to produce surgical anesthesia. The nerves usually affected are only those comprising the cauda equina. It is here that the cocaine is injected. As is shown by experiment, it diffuses rapidly upward in the cerebro-spinal fluid within the subarachnoid space. The higher it diffuses, however, the more diluted the cocaine solution becomes and therefore the less energetic its action. The sensory nerve roots higher up are therefore anesthetized later and less completely, and the anesthesia in their area disappears earliest. The area of anesthesia and its duration is not, as might be supposed, dependent on the quantity of cocaine injected, but seems to depend on personal idiosyncrasy of the patient toward the drug.

On the medulla the cocaine solution acts on its three vital centres. It depresses these in proportion to the quantity of cocaine which reaches the medulla. An ordinary dose, injected into the subarachnoid space for purposes of anesthesia, is, unless great idiosyncrasy to the drug exists, too small to depress these centres to an extent at all dangerous. In the vast majority of cases there is scarcely any appreciable depression of the cardiac, respiratory, or vasomotor centres; occasionally the respiration is somewhat shallow and labored. I have operated on several patients during shock from severe injury or severe hemorrhage, whose pulse was wretched. In none of these was it observed that the pulse became any poorer during the spinal anesthesia. Some persons are, however, abnormally sensitive to the action of cocaine, as is shown by delirium or by more or less depression of one or the other three vital centres in the medulla. This is the uncontrollable factor in spinal anesthesia. It is possible that even a normal dose of cocaine injected into the subarachnoid space may produce alarming depression of the respiratory or cardiac centres. Death is possible from this cause.

DISAGREEABLE ACCOMPANYING OR AFTER EFFECTS.—(a) *Parasthesiæ* occur in the beginning of the anesthesia. These are neither annoying to the patient nor are they of long duration.

(b) *Nausea* occurs in about half of all cases. This varies in intensity in different patients. The nausea is accompanied by pallor, feebleness of pulse, rapid respiration, and sweating. Usually vomiting occurs during the early part of the nausea. The nausea and retching come on within five minutes of the injection and continue five to fifteen minutes, then gradually abate in severity. With the disappearance of the nausea the pulse improves, the color returns, and the sweating ceases. I have had no case in which the nausea was alarming or of long duration.

(c) *Headache* occurs in about one in five patients. It comes on usually at the end of the anesthesia or some time later. It lasts hours and varies much in intensity. It, as well as the fever, undoubtedly is caused by the meningeal irritation which the cocaine produces as a foreign ingredient in the cerebro-spinal fluid.

(d) *Fever.*—A rise in temperature happened in about one in ten of my patients. It comes on some hours after the injection, and in none of my cases did it give rise to a mistake in diagnosis or cause any alarm. It lasts but a short time—in none of my cases longer than twenty-four hours.

(e) *Delirium.*—In one of my cases the patient had a mild

talkative delirium which lasted during the whole operation and a little while after, altogether about two hours. Fifteen minims of a two per cent solution were injected. The delirium was such as is occasionally seen when cocaine is injected subcutaneously.

(*f*) *Deaths.*—I have had no deaths, nor any case in which the patient presented during or at any time after the injection alarming symptoms. The latest digest reports, under the heading of spinal anesthesia, eleven deaths. Of these Tuffier has had five. These five all occurred early in his work with subarachnoid anesthesia. He himself attributes none to the cocaine itself. No cases have been reported in this country, although the procedure has probably been employed here as often as in all other countries combined. I do not wish to underrate the import of these eleven deaths, but I have carefully read the brief reports of these, and am not satisfied that any are the immediate result of cocaine. They have not deterred me from continuing the use of this method of anesthesia. However, death from cocaine is a possibility to be reckoned on, and, until a safer drug is found, this will be the great factor limiting the use of spinal anesthesia. If the heart muscle is in good condition, this danger is very remote indeed. Almost all deaths so far reported have been in patients who were in such a condition that death would very likely have followed the operation under any anesthetic. The mortality of cocaine subarachnoid anesthesia can only be determined by many more cases.

OPERATIONS FOR WHICH SPINAL ANESTHESIA MAY BE USED. (*a*) *For all Operations on the Limbs.*—I have done almost every kind of operation on the lower extremities under spinal anesthesia—incisions of phlegmonous inflammations, amputations, ligations, exsections, operations for compound fractures, for osteomyelitis, wiring of bones, etc. In all of these the anesthesia was ample and sufficiently sustained.

(*b*) *For All Operations on the Perineum,* in both male and female subjects, spinal anesthesia is ample and ideal. This includes hemorrhoids and fistula in ano, operations upon the vulva and female urethra, external and internal urethrotomy in the male, incisions for urinary extravasation, etc. I would not hesitate to do a prostatectomy under such anesthesia.

(*c*) *All Groin Operations,* such as herniotomies, Alexander's operation, removal of inguinal glands, incisions, varicocele, castrations, etc., are all easily done under spinal anesthesia.

(*d*) *Vaginal Work.*—Plastic work on the cervix, vagina, and perineum and curettages are easily done under this anesthesia; so are incisions for the purpose of draining pelvic abscesses.

(e) Vaginal Hysterectomy and Adnexa Operations through the Vagina.—These can be done in an emergency under spinal anesthesia, but, as a rule, general anesthesia is preferable. In the majority of cases spinal anesthesia is ample for this work, but frequently handling the adnexa and intestines (in cases of adhesions) is sufficiently painful to the patient to make her restless in her already irksome position, so that she draws herself up and moves about, making it difficult for the operator to do good work; besides, anesthesia so high up may not last long enough in case the operation lasts much over half an hour.

(f) Bladder Operations can all be done under spinal anesthesia without any trouble.

(g) Intra-abdominal Work.—From choice I would do no intra-abdominal operation under spinal anesthesia. The objections are many. The anesthesia may not be ample so high up, or it may not last long enough to complete the operation. If nausea and vomiting occur, they will cause protrusion of the bowels and perhaps serious interference with the operation. The patient may contract the abdominal walls at the wrong time, and it is difficult to maintain the Trendelenburg position. Still, all of these annoyances are only possibilities, so that if, for reasons I shall state later, general anesthesia is contraindicated or impossible to give, all intra-abdominal operations may very well be done under spinal anesthesia. It has been employed in a very large number of laparatomies.

(h) In Obstetrics.—I think that spinal anesthesia will in the future find its most extended use in obstetrical work. It has been given in two or three hundred cases, either for the purpose of lessening the suffering of the second stage of labor or to produce anesthesia for the purpose of performing obstetric operations. I have used it only for the latter purpose. We must consider these two indications for spinal anesthesia in obstetrics separately. I have had no experience in giving subarachnoid cocaine injections for the purpose of lessening or preventing the pain of the second stage of labor. If this could be done safely, it would at once place cocaine anesthesia as one of the greatest advances in the obstetric art; remembering that it is not followed, as is chloroform anesthesia, by a tendency to uterine hemorrhage. There is, however, a very serious objection to this method which precludes it from a routine use for this purpose.

We can never tell how long the second stage of labor is going to last. The anesthesia from cocaine lasts but an hour or so, and in the great majority of cases a second and even a third cocaine injection will be necessary. Although there is very little risk from the quantity of cocaine injected in one dose, the danger of cocaine poisoning is exceedingly great if two or three doses are injected in rapid succession.

The great value of subarachnoid cocainization in obstetrics is for the purpose of inducing anesthesia for obstetrical manipulations and operations, and its value lies in the fact that any of these operations may be done under it without the aid of trained assistance. In city practice among wealthy patients this is of no importance. In obstetric practice among the poor and in the country the conditions are lamentably different. Among the poor neither the patient nor the obstetrician can afford to call in an anesthetizer to give chloroform or a trained nurse to assist. In the country it is very frequently impossible to procure an anesthetizer in time. An obstetrical operation must be done at once, and most of them are done without anesthesia for these reasons. Some obstetrical operations absolutely require anesthesia, and all can be done better with the patient anesthetized, as this allows deliberation, exactitude, thoroughness, and stricter asepsis. With this method of anesthesia the obstetrician requires no assistant.

(*i*) *Occasional Operations* higher up on the body can be done under spinal anesthesia. Excision of ribs, empyema operations, amputation of the breasts, operations on the arm, tumors of the neck, and even a goitre operation, have been done under such anesthesia. All such high operations are, however, as yet in the nature of curiosities rather than regular procedures.

In all operations spinal anesthesia, of course, comes into competition with ether and chloroform narcosis. The question arises what, in a particular case, should induce the surgeon to use one or the other method of anesthesia. To answer this question has been the object of this paper. In no case in which it is practicable and safe to give ether or chloroform would I use subarachnoid cocainization. In my opinion, in the present state of our experience with spinal anesthesia, there is no even choice between the two methods of anesthesia. It is only in a case in which it would be dangerous, impracticable, or impossible to employ general anesthesia that I would use spinal anesthesia. When this is conceded, we can study the merits and demerits of spinal anesthesia so as to form a general idea when this is preferable in a given case.

MERITS COMPARED WITH GENERAL ANESTHETICS. *(a) It Saves Assistants.*—It thereby enlarges the scope of work by the surgeon alone or by the surgeon and one assistant. Compound fractures of the leg, strangulated hernias, severe injuries of the lower half of the body, even ruptured tubal pregnancies, intestinal obstruction, intestinal perforations and appendical abscesses, can be attended to by the surgeon alone when no trained assistance is available. In the army during the time of great engagements there are always too few surgeons and trained surgical assistants. This adds largely to the horrors of the battle and to the suffering of the wounded. Surgical work is hurriedly and unskilfully done and asepsis is imperfect; the wounded must wait long for their turns, and many die who might have survived had their injuries been more promptly or more skilfully cared for. With spinal cocainization the operator can dispense with at least one assistant—the anesthetizer. Many of the operations on the lower half of the body could be done by one surgeon alone. It needs but little imagination to realize what a boon this method becomes under such conditions.

(b) Kidney Disease is no contraindication to cocaine anesthesia. Quite a large number of deaths occur from acute suppression of urine following ether narcosis; some have followed chloroform narcosis. In the case of a patient whose kidneys are diseased and in whom we may reasonably fear such an acute suppression of urine, cocainization of the spinal cord becomes the method of choice, provided, of course, that the operation is on the lower half of the body and cannot be done under local anesthesia.

(c) Acute or Chronic Bronchitis, or any other acute or chronic disease of the lungs or obstruction of the air passages, makes ether and chloroform, especially the former, risky. A large number of broncho and lobar pneumonias, many of which have resulted in death, have followed ether narcosis, and not a few have followed chloroform. There is always an element of danger in administering a general anesthetic to a patient suffering from adenoid growths, nasal obstructions of any kind, or chronic nasopharyngitis. Partial asphyxia during the operation and postoperative broncho-pneumonia are always possibilities. In all patients in whom these troubles exist, and in whom the surgeon may reasonably fear these consequences from general narcosis,

20

cocaine anesthesia may be given if the operation is on the lower half of the body and if it cannot be done with local anesthesia.

(d) *In Myocardial Disease* spinal anesthesia offers no advantage over ether narcosis in the matter of safety. Most of the deaths from spinal anesthesia have been in patients suffering from degeneration of the heart muscle and the arterial system. It is only when the myocarditis is associated with lung or kidney disease that we may hope for greater safety in spinal anesthesia.

(e) *Old Topers.*—Frequently general anesthesia cannot be induced in old hard drinkers. No amount of ether or chloroform carries them beyond the stage of excitement. Spinal anesthesia is the only resource in these cases.

(f) Occasionally general anesthesia cannot be induced for some unknown cause. I have had two such experiences within a short time. One was a girl of 18 whom I wished to anesthetize for an operation on the lower jaw. I gave her almost an ounce of chloroform and could not carry her beyond the stage of excitement. The other was a woman of 30 in labor for the fifth time. Two of her former accouchements were followed by puerperal insanity. With a transverse presentation and a tightly contracted uterus a version was imperative. The physician who was called to take care of her after the midwife had abandoned the case called help, and they proceeded to give chloroform. They could not bring her beyond the stage of excitement. I was called and performed the version and extraction promptly and painlessly under spinal anesthesia. Frequently the insane cannot be anesthetized with ether or chloroform. In all such cases spinal anesthesia is our only resource, at present, for large operations on the lower half of the body.

(g) Patients suffering from shock or hemorrhage, or from both, combined, bear ether and chloroform badly. These general anesthetics lower the body temperature, which is already subnormal, thereby diminishing the vital resistance; they depress the heart and circulation still farther and increase the disposition to bronchitis or pneumonia. If the operation is one that can be done under spinal anesthesia, this should be employed. These patients are indifferent to operating-room sights. If nausea is not present —and it very seldom is in patients under the influence of pain or of shock—they may even be given nourishment and hot drinks during the operation. Nausea and vomiting very seldom follow spinal anesthesia induced in patients who at the time are in pain, excitement, or in shock. It therefore seldom follows spinal anesthesia in obstetrical work. The fact that nourishment may be given to patients during the operation and immediately afterward may be of great importance in weak patients, such as those under consideration.

OBJECTIONABLE FEATURES OF SUBARACHNOID COCAINIZATION. (a) *Fussiness of the Injection.*—It is more fussy, more complicated, and requires, superficially considered, more experience and skill to give spinal than general anesthesia. There is always a remote possibility that by a sudden movement of the patient the needle may be broken off. There is always a possibility that the cocaine solution is not active, either because it was not a reliable drug or that it became decomposed by boiling or standing. The needle may drop to the floor and so necessitate a wait of some minutes for resterilization; the packing of the barrel may leak and the cocaine not reach the subarachnoid space. Every detail of the injection must be carried out with the strictest aseptic precaution.

(b) The Nausea and Vomiting, with pallor and depression, which occur in about one-half of all cases, are positive annoyances both to the patient and the operator. It is not alarming in character and can frighten only an operator unfamiliar with spinal anesthesia. After having an experience of half a dozen or so of such nauseas, the operator views them with the same absence of alarm that he views the choking and cyanosis which so frequently occur in the early stages of ether narcosis. The headache and fever following some cases might possibly be mistaken in some cases for beginning sepsis.

(c) The Patient is Conscious during the Operation. While in some cases, as during an obstetrical or a hernia operation, and occasionally in some others, this may be an aid to the surgeon, in the vast majority of cases it is a nuisance. It is the feature of spinal anesthesia that I most dislike. It bars much clinical work. It makes it difficult during an operation to discuss etiology, pathology, and prognosis. It is on this account not a practical anesthetic for children. The child, being conscious, sees and hears things which occasionally frighten it into a condition of terror that makes it almost impossible to go on with the operation. As a rule chronic invalids among children, especially those who have become accustomed to white-gowned doctors and operating-room paraphernalia, are much less apt to be frightened when operated upon under spinal anesthesia. Hysterical and nervous women are the worst to operate on under spinal

anesthesia. They should never be subjected to the ordeal. It is no little strain on the mental balance of such a patient to be conscious and know that, for instance, her abdomen is open and her insides are being handled. Even on better-controlled minds the mental strain, from the sight of instruments and the realization that they are being used on them, must be great. Permanent neurasthenia may date from such an operation. I must repeat what I have said: that even nervously disposed patients bear such sights and experiences with indifference when they are in great pain or suffering from shock. The consciousness of the patient is therefore no bar to the use of spinal anesthesia in obstetrical work and in emergency surgery.

(d) The Mortality.—It is impossible, in consideration of the comparatively limited experience with spinal anesthesia, to state this in figures. The number of deaths reported so far have been large for the number of times this method has been used, but the method is as yet in its infancy. Inexperience no doubt has had something to do with some of these deaths, the size of dose has not been stated in each case, and, above all, spinal anesthesia has been used for many operations on feeble, diseased, and old patients who would have given a high mortality under general anesthesia, and who, in fact, were given spinal anesthesia for that very reason. An abnormal sensitiveness to the action of cocaine is the only cause of death. How frequently such idiosyncrasy exists is not known. We must not overlook the fact that it is in these old, feeble, and diseased patients that the mortality from ether and chloroform is very high. The ordinary text-book mortality statistics of 1 in 3,000 for chloroform and 1 in 15,000 for ether are wholly fallacious for this class of patients. Those are the statistics for deaths on the table, but do not include the deaths from urinary suppression and from the various forms of pneumonia which occur some days after the ether or chloroform narcosis and are directly due to the narcosis. And, further, the great fact remains that these deaths, if indeed they were due to the spinal anesthesia, were deaths from cocaine and not due to the method of administration. It remains only to discover a substitute for cocaine, a drug which shall produce local anesthesia like that of cocaine, and shall not have that selective poisonous action on the vital centres in the medulla. There is nothing impossible in this and we can look for an early discovery of such a drug.

MAMMARY SUBSTANCE IN UTERINE FIBROIDS.[1]

BY

H. W. CROUSE, M.D.,
Victoria, Texas.

IN presenting mammary substance for the treatment of uterine fibroids, I realize that many points will be brought forward difficult of explanation. The many remedial agents derived from glands of the sheep, hog, and goat have created a new medicinal group, known as orrotherapy. It is necessary to review the history of the use of these agents by the medical world, to consider by what train of thought each has been adopted, which in proper sequence leads us to consider their actions, their chemical properties, and, finally, their clinical results, before deciding to accept them as new medicinal recruits.

Brown-Séquard, when bringing before the medical world his testicular fluid, stated that all the organs of the body contributed to make perfect blood, that each yielded a secretion which contributed its quota, and that all made perfect. If one is deficient in secretion, the contribution to the blood is deficient to that extent. A clever chain of scientific thought started with Schiff, 1859, who first removed the thyroid in animals. This was repeated by Reverdin, 1882, and Kocher, 1883, and gave a clinical condition known as operative myxedema. Further experiments by Schiff, 1884, Buchner, 1890, and others upon myxedematous animals showed that the various conditions resulting from thyroidectomy could be improved or completely overcome by implanting the thyroid gland of a healthy animal under the skin or within the peritoneum of the one void of a thyroid gland. George B. Murray, 1891, using these experiments as his base, injected a glycerinated extract of sheep thyroid into men suffering from myxedema, with startling curative results. Shober, in 1898, in a paper on the use of mammary substance in uterine fibroid, recalls an interesting historical fact mentioned by Pliny, that it was a common custom among the Greeks and Romans to

[1]Read before the Gynecological Section of the Texas State Medical Association, May 8, 1902.

use the testicles of donkeys in impotency; also that he, Shober, had been told by a trustworthy African explorer that even to this day certain obscure tribes in the interior of Africa practise a disgustingly inhuman cannibalistic operation upon slaves and captives for the same condition. R. B. Bell, of Glasgow, in a paper read before the British Gynecological Society, May 14, 1896, states that he was led, through the knowledge of the embryonic origin from the epiblast of the thyroid gland, the known remedial effects of thyroid medication upon the diseased epithelium in the skin manifestations of myxedema and psoriasis, and the cessation of metrorrhagia in myxedema, to use thyroid gland in the treatment of two cases of cervical epithelioma with good results. Bell further mentions Jouan's attention being called to its effects upon the uterine fibroid, by noticing a case he was treating for myxedema, suffering at the same time with a fibroid which extended two inches above the navel, and which at the expiration of a year had been reduced to one inch above the pubes. This observation, together with those of Bouilly, Tuffier, Gunnard, Pieque, and Block that thyroid hypertrophy frequently underwent retrogression in pregnant women, and that thyroid tumors would at times disappear or at least diminish after extirpation of pelvic organs, led him to study the seeming essential relationship existing between the various organs. He noticed the metastatic involvement of the testicles, and at times the ovaries, in mumps; the synchronous changes in the mammary glands and genitals at puberty, in pregnancy and lactation, and evolved his theory "that when local disease commences in an individual the organ which it takes possession of must have departed from a healthy standard prior to this, and that the weakened organ may have been influenced by a morbid or functionally altered state of an organ in close physiological relationship with it." This was the proper theoretical deduction to make preceding clinical proof. Waller, mentioned by Stehman, reasoning along the same line, stated that this metastatic involvement of related glands proved that "the waste of one organ serves as the raw material for another ,and that this interorganic relation plays an important part in general metabolism." The question promptly arises, how? Some suppose that the secretion of these special organs affects nutrition by removing toxic substances which result from tissue waste (Schafer); that, for example, one of the functions of the ovary is to eliminate organic toxins through the menstrual flow (Spillman and Etienne); that the secretion of the thyroid favors uric acid excretion and thus increases nitrogenous denutrition (Vos, Gara, Isai); while others maintain that general nutrition, and more especially the central nervous system, is affected by this glandular secretion entering the blood (Howell).

Taking these points into consideration, along with the knowledge that in the phenomena of orrotherapy we are dealing with substances derived from the great group of racemose glands, which vary not only in size but also in the character of the secretions yielded by each and their physiological significance, and we unconsciously enter the study of the pathological phenomena of involvement of various glands, and investigate whether a relationship may be proved or disproved to exist between certain of them. Every physician of experience can recall a metastatic involvement of the testicle, and at times of the ovary, in parotitis; each one utilizes in diagnosing pregnancy the accompanying mammary-gland phenomena; each is familiar with these gland changes at puberty and during lactation, the stimulation of the sexual sense by the manipulation of the nipple, and the erection of the nipple during sexual excitement. Pathology has proved the synchronous enlargement of the thymus gland and pituitary bodies with thyroid hypertrophy. Bell has used the observations of Bouilly, Tuffier, Gunnard, Pieque, and Block concerning thyroidal change during pregnancy and after removal of the uterus and adnexa. Hulde has proved in the study of suprarenal-gland removal that the thymus and spleen become enlarged. Shober mentions the induction of uterine contractions by the nursing of the child during the first few days of the puerperium. Pain in the mammary gland previous to menstruation has been noticed by Stehman during thyroidal therapy. Hertoghe found that thyroid gland given by mouth increased the quantity but not the quality of milk; also that nursing women suffering with diminution of lacteal secretion synchronous with the appearance of menstruation had the secretion restored by the use of thyroid gland. One of my fibroid cases, taking the mammary gland, complained, on increase of dose, of sensitiveness of the nipples and mammary tenderness. Pathology also recognizes the involvement of the pancreas in diabetes, etc.

As to the nature of the secretion of the various glands now being used medicinally, Murray in his Goulstonian Lecture No. 1, in speaking of the formation and absorption of the thyroid se-

cretion, describes the two cells occupying the alveolus as the chief
cell and the colloid; he states that a large nucleus is contained
in the former, and that colloid matter is formed in the latter.
The colloid, he says, is a true epithelial cell which secretes in two
ways—either in droplets in the cells with gradual extrusion into
the lumen of the alveolus, or by breaking-down of whole cells and
discharge in the colloid substance of the matter they help form.
In the first the cell continues to secrete; in the other, after being
destroyed its position is taken by a reserve cell. Owing to the
ductless condition of the thyroid the secretion of the cells can
escape in only two ways—by lymphatics or veins. By the
lymphatics is the most frequent route, as King and Horsley
found by pressure upon the gland that the colloid matter could
be squeezed from the acini into the interacinous lymphatics,
where it could be seen by means of the microscope. Hurthle believes that the secretion escapes into the interalveolar spaces
through weakened wall of alveoli, by intercellular spaces, and
by rupture. There it comes in contact with lymph which bathes
alveolar cells, to be discharged into the blood stream in the in-
nominate vein and so distributed to the entire economy. Early
thought the thyroid secreted a mucoid substance, the retention
of which led to an accumulation of mucin in the body and produced cutaneous swelling in myxedema. Investigation has
shown that colloid contains no mucin. Accurate information as
to the true nature of this substance is scarce, but most have considered the proteids to be the important and active constituent of
it. Nolkin considers this thyroproteid, a substance that behaved
like an enzyme. Gourley found that a nucleo-proteid was the
only proteid to be secured from colloid in quantity that contained phosphorus. Baumaine and Roos found it contained
iodine in an organic compound with proteid, and named it thyroidin; Hutchins, that two proteids exist in the gland, a nucleo-
albumin which is contained in the epithelial cells, and a colloid
material which fills the acini. The gastric secretion splits up the
secretion of a gland into two parts, one of which is proteid and
contains a small amount of iodine, having but slight physiological action; the other, non-proteid, contains more iodine and all
the phosphorus of original colloid, and is more active in relieving
symptoms caused by loss of the gland than is the proteid. As
to the substances contained in the mammary gland, Sturrock, of
Edinburgh, says that there is nucleo-proteid in the cells of the
mammary gland which is of a highly complex constitution, con-

taining a carbohydrate and a proteid radical. The suprarenal has been difficult to investigate as to the nature of the substance secreted by it and useful as a therapeutic agent. Auld states that it is an alkaloid; Abel confirms this opinion and he and Crawford call the separated principle "epinephrin"; Takamine, an alkaloid, adrenalin. The nature of the secretions of the testicles, of the thymus, and of the pituitary bodies has been but indifferently studied, and their principles, in consequence, unnamed and unrecognized. Among another group of these glands, substances long familiar present themselves, such as the bile, the enzymes of the spleen, pepsin, pancreatin, etc.

So step by step we are driven to the conclusion that we have in all glands, with or without ducts, not alone an excretion, as ova in ovaries, semen in the testicles, milk in the mammary gland, pancreatic juice in the pancreas, etc., but also an internal or circulatory secretion which enters the system through the circulation, modifying nutrition (Spillman and Etienne). Does all this not lead one to believe that mayhap there lies within the epithelial cells an inherent egotistical principle which was demonstrated by Vaughn and McClintock (Ernst[1]) to be a nuclein substance derived from the cells of the various glands, borne in the circulation partly in solution and partly in the form of multinuclear white corpuscles, the so-called phagocytes? In presenting this point further it is but necessary to continue with Vaughn, who believes that the nuclein passes from the cell into solution, but is unable to say whether this process is due to the breaking-down of the cell or to its active secretion. The word nuclein is used in the broad sense, including the nucleo-acid and nucleo-albumins.

The next feature of the study of these remedies, naturally, should be their physiological effects. THYROID GLAND study has demonstrated its principle to be a powerful lymphatic stimulant, utricular gland stimulant, muscle contractor, blood oxidizer (Whitney), capillary constrictor; an inducer of tachycardia, headache, tremors, gouty and rheumatic pains, general debility, persistent vomiting, and profuse diarrhea. The tachycardia with its dyspnea is fatal at times (Polk). Cunningham considers the unfortunate symptoms to be produced by decomposed animal matter in the thyroid mixture, and not by the essential thyroid secretion—in other words, by ptomaines and leucomaines.

PAROTID GLAND.—The special agent it contains has not as yet

[1]Twentieth Century Practice of Medicine, vol. xx.

been separated, it being, according to Shober, an absorbent, an anodyne, seemingly confining itself to the pathological conditions of the ovaries, governed by the following states: so-called ovarian neuralgia or dysmenorrhea unassociated with extensive pelvic inflammation; enlarged, tender, prolapsed ovaries, pain occurring a day or two before the period and during its first day or two. According to Jack, "it is the best remedy yet brought out in the treatment of dysmenorrhea, relieving, as it does, the aches and pains of ovaritis, and improving nutrition. Pelvic exudates soften and are often absorbed. Menstruation becomes regular, and less in amount when excessive, and shorter in duration. The headaches and nervousness so often accompanying the cases are, as a rule, cured; health and spirits revive, and, indeed, its action here can be denominated nothing less than specific."

MAMMARY GLAND.—Clinically it has been proved to be a muscular stimulant, a nerve sedative, a general reconstructor, when a systemic depravity is induced by a uterine degeneration, as found in myoma, myofibroma, and subinvolution; a substance with no depressing effects, or detrimental symptoms outside of the contractile pains induced in a fibroid when the maximum dose is given. Sturrock states that its action is due to a nuclein base which is not excreted, but seems to remain in the gland, probably in the nuclei of the cells as active agents in the formation of more mother substance. These may possibly contain the active principle when the gland is medicinally employed. "The *modus operandi* of thyroid and mammary glands in controlling hemorrhage seems entirely different—thyroid, an epithelium, utricular gland, and lymphatic stimulant and blood oxidizer; mammary gland acts on uterine muscles, either primarily or through nerve supply, increasing contractile power, thus diminishing blood supply to endometrium and body of tumor" (Shober).

OVARIAN SUBSTANCE.—Is mainly used in ovarian insufficiency, as after double oöphorectomy, with infantile ovaries, and like conditions inducing amenorrhea. Chrobak found that by implanting ovarian tissue under the skin or within the peritoneum in a case subjected to double oöphorectomy, benefit to the nervous symptoms of an operative menopause would be secured. I have found it beneficial administered in the form of the substance by mouth, controlling markedly the nervous phenomena of complete hysterectomy. Jack says: "Ovarian extract is indicated in all cases of menopausal nervous symptoms, or when for any reason it is desirable to increase the flow from the uterus. It is now known almost beyond doubt that the ovary has, besides its function of ovulation, another almost as important, that of internal secretion, and that, like the thyroid, it secretes an active oxidizing agent, spermin, that aids in the metabolism of the blood.   Marked decrease in the elimination of phosphates has been observed after ovariotomy.   I have taken,'' says he, ''this as a hint and administered ovarian extract in all cases of ovarian disease presenting constantly this symptom, and I have as yet to be disappointed in the results.''

SUPRARENAL GLAND.—The active principle has been separated by Abel and named epinephrin.   Furth has separated an agent which he calls suprarenin.   Takamine has isolated one, named by him adrenalin.   Epinephrin and suprarenin are claimed by Reichert to be contaminated, while adrenalin, he says, is pure. Its principal physiological effects have been found to be as follows:

(a) The Pulse is Retarded.   By vagus stimulation (Schafer, Oliver, Cushing).

(b) The Force of the Systole is Increased.   By stimulation of the cardiac muscles (Schafer, Cushing).   By stimulation of the cardiac motor ganglia (Gottlieb).

(c) The Blood Pressure is Elevated Secondary to Arterial Constriction.—By peripheral action (vasomotor) (Schafer).   By peripheral action (on capillary muscular fibre) (Shoemaker, Cushing).   By central action (Cushing).

(d) Tissues are Blanched (Mucous Membrane, Peritoneum, Skin).   By peripheral action (vasomotor or capillary muscular stimulation) (various observers).

THYMUS EXTRACT.—No practical investigation has as yet been made as to the nature of the substance or its active agent, and but little is known except that its physiological effect is to reduce thyroid hypertrophy, as in goitre.

TESTICULAR SUBSTANCE.—Outside of the Brown-Séquard investigation of the studies of Claude-Bernard, nothing further has been learned.   It has been used in impotency.

The following cases of the use of mammary-gland extract have been reported: Bell, in May, 1898, reported 4 cases treated with this substance, all of whom were under 35, so the influence of the menopause should be eliminated.   The length of treatment varied from two to four months.   The form of the gland principle was the elixir and platinoids.   Of the elixir, one drachm was given three times a day; of the platinoids, ten grains per day. The results were brilliant. In one illustrative case a fibroid tumor the size of a seven months' fetus was reduced one-fourth as a result of six weeks' treatment, and ceased to cause any trouble. Another case—a small fibroid on the anterior uterine wall, which had caused marked metrorrhagia resulting in decided anemia—at the conclusion of eight weeks' treatment with ten grains of the platinoids daily, showed disappearance of the anemic condition, restoration of general health, and absence of metrorrhagia. Two cases of menorrhagia accompanied by dysmenorrhea, fibroids absent, subinvolution present, were seemingly cured by the mammary gland.

J. B. Shober, of Philadelphia, who was the first to utilize the mammary and parotid glands in this country, reports 9 cases. The length of treatment varied from two to fifteen months; the ages of the patients were from 24 to 37 years—mean average below 35. Five were colored. Size of tumor, as in Case 1, perpendicular measurement, 7½ inches; lateral, 10½ inches; girth, 37 inches; height, 2 inches above navel—an immovable, globular, impacted fibroid. At the expiration of fifteen months, girth, 30 inches; perpendicular measurement, 5½ inches; lateral measurement, 8½ inches. Flow formerly profuse, with clots and dysmenorrhea, duration six to ten days; at the time of report flow regular, three days, amount normal, no clots, no pain, general health greatly improved. His examinations were always made with the patient under ether before treatment was commenced. In all, the general health markedly improved; the dysmenorrhea, clots, metrorrhagia, and menorrhagia were controlled; the flow became painless and normal. Of the extract and desiccated gland from fifteen to thirty grains were given three times a day.

W. R. Pryor, of New York, called my attention to the use of mammary substance two years ago in the handling of Case 1. In this connection he lauded very highly its effects, and stated, if I remember rightly, that he had utilized and was still observing the treatment of 33 cases of uterine fibroid with it. His results, he informed me, were more than encouraging.

As to my personal cases, inclusive of the one watched for Dr. Pryor:

CASE I.—Mrs. F., æt. 32, IIpara. Subperitoneal myofibromata located on the posterior uterine wall close to the internal os; largest was of the size of a small lemon; the other, of a walnut. Tumors found at accouchement. Case later examined by Pryor. Curetted; given mammary substance, five grains three times a day. Metrorrhagia ceased. No flow during lactation. Tumor not examined. Treatment was periodical; cessation of lactation, metrorrhagia recommenced, with dysmenorrhea and clots. Mammary substance, five grains three times a day, was given for six weeks. Metrorrhagia ceased and the general condition improved; no dysmenorrhea or clots; length of flow, four days. Treatment was continued two months. The patient again became pregnant and it was stopped. At the fourth month of pregnancy the tumors were found increased in size, the largest 3 by 6 inches. The patient said a rapid growth had occurred during pregnancy, according to her sensations. Successful vaginal myomectomy by Pryor.

CASE II.—Miss B., single, æt. 32, had noticed a growth for two years. Examination, January, 1901, showed a subperitoneal fibroid connected with the left cornu, size three by four inches, globular; metrorrhagia, dysmenorrhea, and anemia. Curettement was refused. Given Blaud's mass and mammary substance, five-grain tablet three times a day. At the sixth week reported last period as seven days long; few clots; dysmenorrhea markedly improved, general condition also improved; able to work. At the end of the fourth month reported good general health, five periods lasting three to four days, with no clots or dysmenorrhea. Tumor nodular, reduced to half original size. Mammary substance continued. Seen recently, but not examined, patient's false modesty forbidding. She reported perfect health, periods normal, dysmenorrhea absent. Mammary gland taken two weeks in the month.

CASE III.—Mrs. D., æt. 39, IVpara, had had profuse menstruation for years, gradually extending into metrorrhagia and menorrhagia, with dysmenorrhea. Saw her in a profuse hemorrhage, exsanguinated. Tampon, ice to abdomen, atropia, ergot and stypticin by mouth, together with quiet. Bleeding was controlled in two days to a show only. Examination one week later showed uterus nodular from multiplicity of fibroids, varying from mere nodules to those the size of a large walnut. Vaginal hysterectomy was advised and refused. Gave mammary substance, five grains three times a day for three months. Metrorrhagia, menorrhagia, dysmenorrhea, and general condition all gradually improved, until at the end of the third month periods were normal. Never able to secure second examination.

Cases IV. and V.—Both single, æt. 25 and 28, gave histories of metrorrhagia for one and two and one-half years, respectively, with dysmenorrhea and debility. No examination permitted. Gave mammary substance, five grains three times a day. Symptoms improved. Lost track of cases.

Case VI.—Mrs. L., æt. 49, gave history January 19; 1902. First knowledge of fibroid 1890. Metrorrhagia marked; debility; dysmenorrhea. Periods gradually increased until they lasted two weeks, profuse, with clots. In 1892 was curetted, with improvement. In 1893 relief temporary. In 1894 consulted several eminent gynecologists; radical operation advised against. In 1897 metrorrhagia was so severe as to demand packing twice, and the patient so weak that months were required for recovery. In 1901, while in Canada, severe hemorrhage demanded packing. Menstruation after that was irregular, the flow being excessive, every two or three weeks. In December, 1901, there was a very severe hemorrhage. January 19, 1902, examination showed several fibromyomata, of the size of a small walnut to that of a small orange, situated subperitoneally and located laterally, one on the posterior wall low down. Mammary substance, five grains three times a day, given for six weeks. After a week's intermission, resumed treatment with six grains three times a day. On April 9, when this history was written, she was still taking the same dose. Results: no flow for three and one-half months; a slight show once or twice. Since taking the mammary substance the nipples have become sensitive, indicating that the mammary glands are affected by this substance.

In reviewing these cases there are five features that stand out prominently: Mammary substance will control menorrhagia, metrorrhagia, and dysmenorrhea; will improve the general condition; and in properly selected cases of uterine fibroid where the myomatous feature predominates, will reduce the size of the growth.

In presenting a new remedy, or an old one in a new rôle, it is essential to compare it with others, already accepted, in order to determine its true worth. We have in the medicinal handling of uterine fibroid several remedies, used for years, whose shortcomings are well understood. I will tabulate briefly their pernicious influences, together with their companion remedy, and request you to recall the points needed to round them out in their complete physiological rôles.

Ergot.—Fails in about 50 per cent of cases to arrest menorrhagia, and, when successful, is so at the expense of the general health. Induces gastro-intestinal irritation and cardiac and general muscular degeneration.

Hydrastin.—Beneficial when used briefly. Persisted in, is a gastro-intestinal irritant and induces constipation.

Stypticin.—Brief use beneficial, same results as with hydrastin when long continued.

Oleum Erigerontis.—Can be employed only when no irritation exists; attacks the kidneys, as does its colleague, turpentine, when used persistently.

Belladonna and Atropine.—Used briefly, results in menorrhagia and metrorrhagia are brilliant; persisted in it produces the conditions which it first corrects. Is a cerebral irritant.

Thyroid Gland.—Causes tachycardia and dyspnea to a dangerous extent at times; also gastric irritation, with profuse diarrhea.

Bromides.—Induce bromism.

Digitalis.—As an adjuvant to ergot, results are fair; alone, it fails to control.

Electricity has given but slight results, and then only when used as a caustic. The indications for its use are the same as for curettage. It is dangerous, does not stop growth, and induces peritoneal adhesions, rendering subsequent operation difficult.

Curettage.—Involves anesthesia and invasion of the uterine cavity, not once but repeatedly, and is the ideal light operative course preceding the use of mammary substance.

Ligation of Uterine Artery.—Is an operative procedure, and is still in the balance, experience being rather against than for it.

Removal of Ovaries is a capital operative procedure, and suggests the question whether, when doing a laparatomy, it would not be best to do a radical operation, *i.e.*, hysterectomy.

Myomectomy for either submucous or subperitoneal fibroids and *total extirpation* are strictly operative methods and should not be compared when considering medical treatment.

Mammary Substance.—No deleterious effects have yet been noticed, except contractile pains in the tumor when given in maximum doses. This symptom promptly subsides when the remedy is stopped or the dosage reduced.

Through the medium of two letters, one from the introducer of mammary substance to the notice of the medical profession of America—Dr. John B. Shober, of Philadelphia—the other from

Prof. W. R. Pryor, of New York, I wish to illustrate the type of cases in which the gland substance has been of benefit and those in which it has failed:

1731 PINE STREET, PHILADELPHIA,
April 6, 1902.

H. W. CROUSE, M.D., *Victoria, Texas.*

My dear Doctor:—In reply to your letter of March 30, requesting information in regard to the value of mammary-gland substance in cases of uterine fibroid, I beg to refer you to the enclosed reprints of two articles which I published about two years ago.

I am still using the substance with satisfaction, and have nothing new to add except that it has been found of positive value in a few cases of the vomiting of pregnancy.

I employ a tablet of desiccated mammary gland of sheep; each tablet contains two grains of the desiccated powder, which represent twenty grains of the fresh gland. One or two tablets three times daily with food should be taken for periods of weeks or months, depending upon the nature of the case. The mammary gland is said to contain certain nuclein bases which are not excreted, but seem to remain in the gland, probably in the nuclei of the cells, as active agents in the formation of more mother substance (Sturrock, *Brit. Med. Jour.,* September 17, 1898, p. 776). These bases probably contain the active principle upon which depends, in a measure, the normal metabolism of the uterus, and upon them may depend the value of the substance as a therapeutic agent. Preparations of mammary gland, when fed to women, seem to stimulate the uterine muscle, increasing its contractile power, thus diminishing the blood supply to the organ. I have used it with benefit in the following classes of cases:

1. In uterine fibroids it controls menorrhagia and metrorrhagia, relieves pain and dysmenorrhea, and in some cases diminishes the size of the growths. Personally, I believe in radical operation for most uterine fibroids, especially as they are usually complicated by adnexal disease and many by degenerative changes in the tumors. In cases, however, which did not call for immediate operation, and in others when it was refused, I found mammary-gland substance of decided value. In cases characterized by marked anemia, I think I have placed my patients in better condition to stand the operation by controlling the bleeding for several months or until the hemoglobin percentage and blood count showed a positive improvement.

I am not prepared to make any positive statement in regard to the absorption of fibroid nodules under this treatment. Two cases, however, who had been under my treatment with mammary-gland substance for two years, in both of whom a fibroid nodule the size of an egg could be felt before treatment was begun, and in both of whom the diagnosis was confirmed by my colleague, Dr. J. M. Baldy, came to operation on account of adnexal disease. In both the uterus was fibrous (small interstitial fibroids), but the nodules which we thought we felt two years before had disappeared. The personal equation comes in here. We may have been mistaken. What we thought were fibroid nodules may have been enlarged ovaries or thickened tubes.

I have had two cases of large submucous fibroids with uterine cavities measuring about six inches, in which the mammary gland failed to control the profuse hemorrhage. This, however, was to be expected.

2. In subinvolution following miscarriage or labor, mammary-gland feeding controls the bleeding and rapidly restores the uterus to its normal size.

3. In menorrhagia due to congestion or relaxation I have had very satisfactory results. I have not found the treatment applicable in cases complicated by exudate or structural disease of the ovaries or tubes.

4. In the vomiting of pregnancy it has in three cases given almost immediate relief when all other measures failed.

In one case, when the treatment was stopped the vomiting returned and could be controlled only by returning to the drug.

In conclusion, I would say that I have entirely abandoned the use of ergot, in the class of cases outlined above, and I believe that the obstetrician would find mammary-gland substance more valuable than ergot at the termination of labor.

Hoping to hear from you again, I am,

Very truly yours,

JOHN B. SHOBER.

Dr. Pryor states:

April 9, 1902.

My experience with mammary extract is as follows: Where the tumors are submucous, intramural, or even subperitoneal, yet distinctly sessile, I find the mammary extract of distinct advantage in causing a reduction of the tumor mass, no matter how large it may be; *provided* the growth does not spring from the region of the cervix, is not retroperitoneal, and is not intraligamentous. I have also found that pedunculated fibroids are not influenced by the extract. The medical treatment has its happiest effect when preceded by curettage. We are having prepared here a preparation of thyroid extract which is still more efficacious, and which has not the disagreeable influence upon the bowels and heart which the old thyroid had. Not the least attractive feature about this medical treatment of fibroid tumors is that it may succeed in reducing the mass from a size demanding laparatomy to one admitting of the vaginal operation.

Yours very sincerely, etc.,

W. R. PRYOR.

In conclusion, then, we have in mammary feeding an agent of proved worth in the medicinal handling of uterine fibroids. The

21

nearer the type of tumor approaches the pure myoma, the better the results in arresting the growth; the more nearly the tumor assumes the fibromyomatous form, the more beneficial has the gland been in controlling the metrorrhagia. It has been proved of positive value in a few cases of vomiting of pregnancy, also of marked worth in subinvolution following confinement, and in all these types of cases it has been practically innocuous. We have dealt with the subject of the medicinal use of the various organs called the group of racemose glands, their chemical and physiological findings, and have thereby derived a comparative idea of the various agents concerned in orrotherapy. We cannot but feel that they are brilliant though mysterious, beneficial though empirical.

A DICEPHALIC MONSTER OBSTRUCTING LABOR.[1]

BY

G. M. BOYD, M.D.,
Physician to the Philadelphia Lying-in Charity,
Philadelphia.

(With three illustrations.)

THE dicephalic monster is of sufficient rarity to merit a brief report of the case and description of the specimen.

May 14, 1901, Dr. C. H. Gubbins, of Philadelphia, asked me to see with him in consultation a patient who had been a long time in labor. She gave the following history. A negress, aged 21 years and a primipara, had been in labor already more than one day without any appreciable advance of the presenting part. The patient's general condition was good. The pelvis was only slightly below the normal in size. The head, which was in a posterior position, was dipping into the inlet of the pelvis, indicating that there existed no great disproportion between the pelvic canal and the fetal ovoid.

On palpating the abdomen the uterus was found to be irregular in shape, suggesting a fibroid tumor or ovarian cyst complicating pregnancy. Anticipating the necessity for some obstetric oper-

[1] Read before the Section on Gynecology, College of Physicians of Philadelphia, April 17, 1902.

ation, we immediately sent her to the hospital. The history, as taken from the hospital notes, is as follows:

"Philadelphia Lying-in Charity. Case No. 2985. Patient has been in labor forty hours. The abdomen is large, fetal heart not heard. The cervix is dilated to the size of a silver dollar and the membranes are ruptured. The presenting part is now found well engaged, with the occiput posterior.

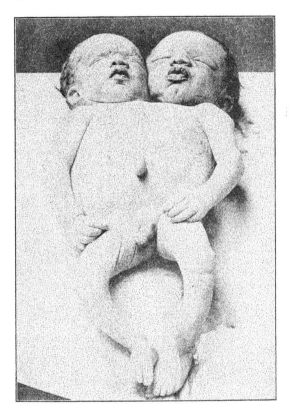

FIG. 1.

"Without suspecting so unusual a monster, an attempt was made to deliver with axis-traction forceps. The forceps application was easily made, but traction failed to advance the presenting part. The forceps was now removed and a manual exploration of the uterus made. A second head was found attached to the single trunk. As the patient's condition did not warrant abdominal section, the uterus was emptied by first decapitating the head engaged, then performing podalic version. Fig. 3 .shows the position of the child. The puerperium was normal and the patient left the hospital in good condition.''

Description of Monster.—Autopsy made by Dr. F. J. Kalteyer, pathologist to the institution: The body is that of a well-nourished male fetal monster. Its weight is 8½ pounds; length, 19½ inches; circumference of chest, 10 inches. The left head is

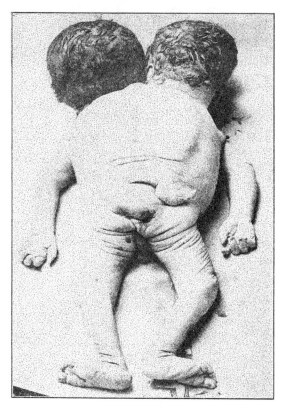

FIG. 2.

slightly larger than the right, the trauma of labor explaining this inequality. Both heads are well formed. The arms and hands are normal, as are both lower extremities, with the exception of a green-stick fracture of the left femur. There exist two anal orifices. One and a half inches above the anus is seen a cord-like extremity 3½ inches long. It is divided into four parts. The proximal and middle parts are of equal length, separated by a narrow constriction. The distal portion is 1⅛ inches in length. The second portion from the proximal end is the largest. It is one-quarter inch in thickness and apparently contains bony structures. The umbilical cord is normal.

Thoracic Cavity.—Two hearts in one pericardial sac are seen. There are two aortæ and pulmonary arteries; two lungs, each trachea dividing into a right and left bronchus. The *left heart* contains two openings in ventricular septum (one under the aortic valve). The mitral valve of the left heart has three cusps. The left pulmonary vein is normal. The pulmonary artery di-

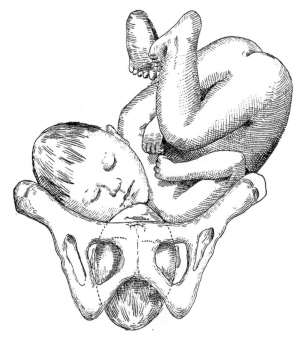

FIG. 3.

vides into two parts, one going to the right and one to the left lung. Tricuspid valve of left heart normal. Left heart has two auricles. *Right heart:* Stenosis of right pulmonary artery; right pulmonary vein normal; one opening in interventricular septum. Two spinal columns. The ribs are apparently joined by bony union, esophagus on both right and left sides. Thoracic aortæ on each side. Double urachus. Urethra patulous. Pelvis single, with distinct saccule on either side. Two ascending colons running parallel.

PUERPERAL AND GESTATIONAL PARALYSES.[1]

BY

CHARLES J. ALDRICH, M.D.,

Lecturer on Clinical Neurology and Anatomy of the Nervous System, College of
Physicians and Surgeons; Neurologist to the Cleveland General Hospital
and Dispensary; Neurologist to the Cleveland City Hospital,
Cleveland, Ohio.

VARIOUS forms of paralyses may appear during gestation or complicate any part of the puerperal period. Writers have usually described these nervous affections as puerperal. It is obvious, however, that, both for convenience and accuracy, they should be considered apart. Hence in the following discussion all paralyses occurring in the gestational period will be called gestational paralyses, and all appearing during labor or the lying-in period puerperal paralyses. Hysterical paralysis may occur in any form, and at any time during gestation or the puerperium, but will not be considered in this connection.

GESTATIONAL PARALYSIS may be due either to a central or a peripheral lesion.

Central Paralyses (Gestational).—Hemiplegia from central lesion is rather common in pregnancy; it may be the result of a cerebral hemorrhage, or less commonly from embolism; it is also said to rarely occur from cerebral anemia. In grave renal lesions complicating pregnancy, uremia has been known to produce cerebral paralysis without discernible lesion. Cerebral monoplegias have been reported, but are rare indeed.

Paraplegia of spinal origin may also complicate gestation; literature shows, however, that its occurrence is extremely infrequent.

Peripheral Paralyses (Gestational).—Peripheral paralyses occurring during pregnancy are neural in origin and are either *toxic* or *traumatic*.

The *toxic* varieties of gestational neuritis usually appear in women who have come to confinement weakened and cachectic

Read before the Ohio State Medical Association, May, 1902.

from some unusual drain upon nutrition, most frequently from prolonged and intractable vomiting.

The following report is typical of this form of neuritis; the case was exhibited to the Cuyahoga County Medical Society but a short time since:

Mrs. F. K., aged 27, a widow with three healthy children, the eldest of which is 6 years and the youngest about 10 months. She has not been very strong since her marriage. She has never lost any children nor has she had any miscarriages. Her husband died on September 16, 1901, of acute tuberculosis. Careful examination reveals neither pulmonary nor cardiac disease in our patient.

During all of her pregnancies she has been very sick at the stomach and vomited continually from the second month until her accouchement. During the latter months of her last pregnancy she suffered from considerable swelling and much pain in her legs, and states that they felt numb, powerless, and heavy; her arms, however, were strong. This weakness, powerlessness, and numb feeling in her legs became more marked just previous to her delivery. Immediately after the birth of the child her legs became very painful and tender to touch. After the usual stay in bed she attempted to get up, but found that, although the swelling had disappeared, the legs were weak and numb. This weakness and numbness was particularly marked in the right leg. She now states that when she attempts to go up-stairs her feet feel heavy, and if she does not watch where she is going her toes catch in the carpet. Her legs are so weak and her ataxia so great that she cannot go up-stairs unless there is a baluster for support, nor can she walk in the dark. She is not constipated and her sphincters are intact. She has no headache or backache, nor any affection except her inability to walk and the numbness in her feet and legs.

Examination.—She is intelligent, of medium height, and thin to emaciation. The heart, lungs, abdominal and pelvic organs appear normal. There are no ocular affections nor any weakness or paralysis of any muscle or group of muscles in the face or upper extremities. Tendon reflexes in the upper extremities are quite indistinct. The tongue is protruded straight; the labio-nasal fold is deepest on the right. The left pupil is larger than the right, both react promptly to light and accommodation; the palpebral apertures are equal; the discs and fields are normal, but a fine lateral nystagmus is present.

She walks with a distinctly ataxic gait, and marked foot drop is present on the right side.' She cannot stand with her eyes closed; in fact, she stands poorly with them open. Both knee jerks are absent; front tap and Achilles jerk are also absent; plantar reflexes are absent; gluteal and abdominal reflexes are present. A well-defined anesthesia of the sole of the right foot and toes is demonstrable. There appears to be a distinct atrophy of the intrinsic muscles of the feet, which is most noticeable in the right foot, and there is evidently some atrophy of the anterior tibial and peroneal groups, most marked, however, on the right side.

Her sense of localization is not good. She thinks I am touching the great toe when, in fact, I am extending the foot strongly. On the anterior aspect of the left tibia is considerable periosteal thickening which looks very much like a specific periostitis, although all other evidences and history of specific disease are entirely wanting.

Vinay[1] has reported a very similar case which is well worthy of brief abstract: During the first months of pregnancy the patient lost a great deal of blood and during the latter months suffered from hyperemesis, so that she came to confinement in a cachectic state. During the last two months of pregnancy she complained of paresthesiæ of the extremities and of pains and weakness in the legs. On the third day after delivery she had a chill with fever which lasted only forty-eight hours; on the fourth day she noticed that there was marked loss of power in all the extremities. This rapidly increased until she was almost completely paralyzed. About six weeks after confinement she began to improve and four months from that time had fully recovered.

In some of these forms of neuritis it has been assumed, and with good reason, that circulating in the mother's blood is some unknown toxic agent which has a selective affinity for the nerves.

That something besides a cachexia or nutritional failure exists which conduces to the production of gestational neuritis the two cases reported by Elder appear conclusive. Both women were normal, neither being cachectic, anemic, nor exhausted. In each, symptoms appeared at about the sixth month, and consisted of tingling and paresthesia, chiefly in the hands, but in one of the cases it was also in the feet. Sensation in both cases was lessened to some extent, but there was little or no muscular paralysis. All other known causes of neuritis could be excluded. After delivery recovery immediately began and proceeded rapidly, one recovering in four or five weeks, and the other in about four months. Elder[2] takes the absence of hyperemesis, weakness, and cachexia, which are usually characteristics in most cases of gestational neuritis, as evidence that they are not necessarily concomitants, but expresses the opinion, which I believe to be well founded, that some toxin is elaborated within the body of the mother or child which has a selective toxic effect upon the nerve tissues of the pregnant woman. Windscheit[3] states that the etiology of these rare cases is unknown, but they are supposed to be due to the action of some poison circulating in the blood. The clinical picture is usually that of a pure form of motor neuritis. No special nerve seems to be selected. Usually there is a gradual development of the motor weakness of the extremities, pain is infrequently complained of, but slight sensory changes may be present. The muscles usually atrophy and show the reaction of degeneration. Other trophic changes have been observed to occur.

Solowjeff[4] and Polk[5] have reported fatal cases of peripheral neuritis occurring in pregnancy, and, since most of these cases quickly recover when the uterus is emptied, one should be prepared to induce labor if there be indications of progressive and violent neural inflammation. Eulenberg induced labor in his most severe case in order to save life.

The following personal observation possesses features varying so much from the preceding cases, but strong with suggestions of a cause similar to that which Elder assumes in his case, that a brief abstract will be of value:

Mrs. F., aged 36, family history good; has one daughter aged 17 years. She became pregnant in the early part of 1892. She worried very much about her condition and became quite melancholic over the fact that she should have another child when she had a daughter nearly grown up, and that it would also prevent her from attending the World's Fair at Chicago. She visited the Fair while she was in her seventh month, and while there noticed a beginning weakness and numbness of the legs. This grew worse, until she was able to be on her feet only a part of the day. She returned home and was confined nearly three weeks before her expected time. Her labor and puerperium were normal. The weakness increased ·in her lower extremities and was accompanied by some slight loss of sensation, considerable aching pains, and a very marked amount of ataxia. All of her symptoms were distinctly those of a neuritis. Dr. J. H. Lowman concurred in the diagnosis of a gestational neuritis. She has made a partial recovery, but still suffers some weakness and ataxia.

Since this form of neural inflammation usually terminates at birth, is it not possible that we have some toxemia as a result of the metabolic changes incident to the relations existing between mother and unborn child? Is it not possible that the neuritis is a direct result of poisoning from the blood laden with effete matter from the failure of the established ratio between production and elimination of the poisonous emanations of the two individual organisms?

Study of the literature of gestational and puerperal neuritis shows that many of the reported cases begin during gestation and become complete only after labor—truly gestational, but entitled to be considered as transitional forms.

Traumatic Neuritis (Gestational).—Traumatic gestational neuritis has been assumed to exist by some authorities, and examination of the literature seems to afford grounds for their claims. In placing it in this classification I wish to state the belief that some of these cases are ischemic paralyses due to the pressure of the fetal parts upon the vessels of the mother, or a pressure neuritis caused by an edema of the nerve sheaths produced by disturbance of the pelvic circulation.

It is a well-recognized fact that a mixed nerve may temporarily lose its power to conduct motor impulses from having its nutrition disturbed by any cause which either deprives it of blood or unduly congests its delicate elements. The same effeet may supervene from the elastic and slowly developed pressure of exudations into contiguous tissues or even into the nerve sheath, or from simple elongation of the nerve by stretching. If, however, the pressure remains too long or becomes too great, or the anemia or congestion continues too long, inflammation and degeneration of the nervous tissues will occur, with final involvement of the sensory power of the nerves, and paralysis of more permanent character supervene.

Since the days of Albrecht von Haller[6] it has been known that the interruption of the blood supply of the lower extremities would cause them to become paralyzed and stiff. Later the great Volkmann[7] called the attention of the surgeons of the world to the fact that rigidity and stiffness with contracture of the muscles not infrequently followed too tight bandaging, and conclusively demonstrated that it was not pressure upon the nerve trunks, but the direct result of interference with the blood supply, that produced what is now called ischemic paralysis.

It is the belief of the writer that some of the transient paralyses which have been noted to complicate gestation and to follow labor, and have been formerly ascribed to reflex, dynamic, and other fanciful causes, were due to an ischemic paralysis which was produced by interference with the circulation from too long lodgment of the head in the inferior strait, the pelvis being either too small or misshapen, or containing a head whose proportions were too great, particularly in certain diameters; or perhaps the gravid uterus exerted too much pressure upon the large arterial trunks above the brim of the pelvis or upon arteries pursuing an unusual and anomalous course.

This view will probably explain some of the accounts of transient paraplegias which followed labor and recovered in two or three days. The disturbed circulation of the lower limbs incident to pregnancy is more likely the cause of the muscular cramps which precede and accompany labor than pressure upon the nerves, since it is a well-recognized fact that the portion of the sacral plexus which goes to the formation of the external popliteal or peroneal nerve is more likely to be affected than the nerve supply of the calf muscles, which are well known to be most frequently the seat of cramps both before and during labor.

It is the opinion of the writer that some of the reported cases of isolated paralysis of the nerves of the upper extremities immediately following labor may have been due to stretching the nerve by ill-directed muscular effort during the agonies of travail, or faulty position of the member while under anesthesia.

I recall a case of pain, loss of power, and formication occurring in the distribution of the ulnar nerve, which immediately followed a severe but normal labor in a very excitable and muscular woman. This nerve lesion was thought to be due to pulling on some upright rods in the bed above her shoulders, thus exercising considerable tension upon the branches of the brachial plexus.

PUERPERAL PARALYSES.—All those paralyses occurring during labor or in the lying-in will be classed under this general head.

As in the paralyses of gestation, the paralyses of the puerperium may be divided into central and peripheral.

Central Paralyses (Puerperal).—Hemiplegia complicating or following labor is not particularly uncommon and the prognosis is usually good.   I recall a patient who was confined by Dr. H. J. Lee, of Cleveland, who some hours after labor developed a slight paralysis of the right side, with considerable loss of speech, who, however, made a perfect recovery in less than eighteen months. The lesion was undoubtedly embolic, probably originating from the dislodgment of a small bit of fibrin or a fragment of a clot of blood from one of the uterine sinuses.   While embolism is the most usual cause of cerebral palsies in the puerperal period, yet the occurrence of hemorrhage as the result of the hydremia of pregnancy has been recorded.

Cerebral monoplegias from like causes may occur, but examination of the literature shows them to be so excessively infrequent as to suggest a coincidence rather than a complication.

It is also stated that a transient puerperal paraplegia due to exhaustion of the centres of the cord may occur.   I have never met with such a case, from which all the organic and hysterical elements could be confidently excluded, that was not directly ascribable to a disturbance of the circulation of the lower extremities.

Mills[8] reports a case of paralysis of both legs which followed soon after labor and which was due to a transverse myelitis.   In the septic conditions which complicate the puerperium the occurrence of a septic myelitis is not only possible but has been observed.   Handford[9] has reported a case which is evidently a diffuse myelitis resulting from puerperal sepsis.

Peripheral Paralyses (Puerperal).—The peripheral paralyses which occur during labor and the lying-in period are neural in origin and for convenience of discussion may be divided into two classes which will to some extent indicate their cause— *traumatic* and *non-traumatic.*   Traumatic is used in relation to the nerve tissue alone, and not in reference to the traumatisms of other tissues during labor, which open them to a septic inflammation and thus by a traumatism produce septic neuritis.

Non-traumatic neuritis (puerperal).   The non-traumatic forms of puerperal neuritis are either (1) *septic* or (2) *non-septic.*

(a) Any nerve of the body may be inflamed during a septic puerperium.   Instances of neuritis of the median, ulnar, and

facial nerves have been recorded as occurring as a result of puer-peral sepsis.

(b) Cases of extensive polyneuritis have been observed to complicate or follow a septic lying-in period.

Both of these forms undoubtedly depend upon a true degen-eration of the nervous tissue itself or septic inflammation of the perineurium. Quite a large percentage of the cases are paraplegic in distribution. They are undoubtedly examples of the ordinary septicemic neuritis, and literature contains not a few classical examples. The following case, quoted from Rey-nolds,[10] affords an apt example:

"*Chronic Pyemia Following Labor; Atrophic Paralysis of Both Legs; Gradual Recovery.*—Mrs. H. was quite well until her first child was born, in 1892, when she was 18 years of age. The confinement took place in a Manchester hospital and she told me that shortly afterward she was very ill and was operated on for a 'liver abscess.' She was then removed to the Manchester Royal Infirmary, and I am informed by one of the late resident surgi-cal officers that she was found to be suffering from chronic pyemia and paralysis of the legs. She was removed to the work-house, and came under my care early in 1893 in the Manchester Workhouse Infirmary. She was then suffering from total atro-phie paralysis of both lower extremities, with contractures of the knees; there was absence of knee jerks, but the arms and sen-sation were unaffected. She was treated by massage and was discharged much improved in eighteen months. At the present time (June, 1897) she is practically well and can do all her ordi-nary housework. She walks a little lamely because of the rigid contracture of all the joints of the toes into the soles of the feet, but all other muscles of the lower extremities are normal and well nourished. There was no previous history of alcoholism."

There occasionally occur examples of puerperal neuritis in women who have suffered no traumatism at labor nor have had any septic symptoms. That they should be regarded as non-traumatic and non-septic is proved by the occurrence of similar cases previous to labor. These cases were first described by Moebius[11] and later by other observers, especially Eulenberg,[12] who distinguished two forms:

(1) *A localized form,* in which only one or two nerves are affected—in the *arm type,* the median and ulnar; in the *leg type,* the crural. Other isolated nerves have been found affected, even

the optic nerve. Pain, sensory or-circulatory disturbances are exceptional, but atrophy of the muscles and reaction of degeneration commonly takes place. While many of these cases recover, there are not a few of them which remain permanently crippled.

(2) *A generalized form*, in which there is widespread neural inflammation which may take the ascending type and closely resemble Landry's paralysis. The cranial nerves have been observed to be affected in these cases, and death result from involvement of the respiratory nerves.

While some of these cases, as has been stated, present isolated neuritis, others widespread neural degeneration, yet they rarely develop the severe and rapid forms which are met with as a result of sepsis or other infections provocative of high fever and constitutional disturbance commonly noted in the so-called neuritis of infections.

Every grade of this form of neuritis may be met with, from a transient tingling, numbness, and weakness in the distribution of a single nerve to widespread paralysis with consequent atrophy, contractures, and permanent disability.

A recurrent type of neuritis has been noted to appear after each labor. The following case, reported by Rhein,[13] is of this type:

The patient was a healthy woman who, after a normal first labor, began to suffer pain and numbness over the flexor surface of the left forearm. Weakness of the flexor muscles soon manifested itself. This condition remained with little change until after her second uncomplicated labor, when the symptoms and disability became more intense. Finally, after a third normal labor, the other arm became the seat of a like trouble and the left arm grew still worse. Examination revealed inability to raise the hand to the head; flexion of the fingers weak; slight loss of sensation over the flexor surface of the forearms; atrophy of the intrinsic hand muscles; nerve trunks not tender to pressure.

Traumatic neuritis (puerperal). The most frequent and most important varieties of puerperal neuritis are those which are traumatic in origin and either the direct result from injuries received by the nerve itself or from pressure exerted by exudations into contiguous tissues, thereby producing a temporary interference with its normal conductivity from a disturbance of its molecular continuity rather than an actual disintegration of its elements.

For a clearer conception of this subject these traumatic varieties of neuritis are best considered under two separate heads: (1) those which are strictly contusional in origin, and (2) those due to pressure from exudations, which exudations may be septic or non-septic in origin.

The following case will serve to introduce us to a study of a form of neuritis which I believe to be of contusional origin and directly ascribable to the wounding of a part of the sacral plexus by the forceps or parts of the child during labor. The case was referred to me by Dr. Geib, of Cleveland:

Mrs. L. C. W., aged 28, after a normal pregnancy came to confinement November 9, 1900. After fifteen hours of labor, was delivered with forceps by Dr. W., without the aid of anesthetics, a slight laceration resulting. *Immediately after the application of the instrument she felt a sensation of weakness and paralysis in the right leg and thigh.* Following her delivery the leg remained powerless, became cold and numb, with considerable loss of sensation below the knee. She suffered but little pain, except in the hips and back. The control of the urinary sphincters was lost for a time and is still weakened. The anal sphincters were not affected. She had no chills nor did any fever develop during her lying-in period. Although the left leg felt cold, numb, and powerless, it has never been very sore nor tender to touch, and she has suffered but little pain except when she attempted to walk. She was on crutches for over three months. Dr. Geib first saw the case about eight weeks after the confinement, and, recognizing its peculiar features, very kindly referred it to me for examination.

Examination.--The patient is under-sized and the pelvic diameters are all under normal. She walks with a slight limp. The right leg is found to be cold, but little discolored. The patient states that the toenails on the right foot do not grow as rapidly as on the left. The shin line is very plainly seen on the right leg, revealing the fact that the anterior tibial and peroneal groups are considerably atrophied. The extensor hallucis, extensor pollicis, extensor brevis, and minimi digiti are intact.

The calf muscles are strong and not wasted. The knee jerks on both sides are equal and active; Achilles jerk is marked on the left, but faint on right; no ankle clonus on either side; front tap present on the left, absent on the right. Three and one-half inches below the patella the right leg measures 10¼ inches, the left 10¾ inches; five inches below the patella the right leg measures 10 inches, the left 10½ inches; seven inches below the patella the right leg measures 8½ inches, the left 8 inches. Measurement of the forearms shows that the left is one-half inch smaller than the right. The patient being right-handed, these measurements show the loss of nearly an inch in circumference of the right leg. The peroneus longus contracts very slightly to a powerful faradic current, but no contraction of the tibialis anticus can be secured. To the galvanic current both peronei and tibialis anticus show the reaction of degeneration, which is particularly marked in the latter. There is slight loss of sensation on the dorsum of the foot, which continues up the outside and anterior aspect of the right leg and corresponds to the cutaneous distribution of the external popliteal nerve.

This case is so typical of a form of paralysis which occurs in the distribution of the peroneal nerve following labor, and of traumatic origin, that I will give a brief recapitulation of two similar cases which I have previously reported:[14]

CASE II. *Prolonged Severe Labor Terminated by Forceps; Right Peroneal Paralysis, Anesthesia, Paresthesia, and Neuritis; Recovery from Neuritis and Sensory Disturbances, but Persistence of Paralysis and Atrophy.*—Mrs. L., aged 26; long severe labor; forceps and chloroform. The morning after delivery had much pain in the right leg and hip, with inability to lift that member. All of her symptoms increased in severity, accompanied by all the distressing symptoms of a severe neuritis. The pain was manifested entirely in the distribution of the external popliteal nerve. Some anesthesia was present on the dorsum of the foot and toes. Eighteen months later the patient was examined and there was found considerable loss of volume in the right anterior tibial and peroneal groups.

CASE III. *Prolonged Labor; Instrumental Delivery; Severe Left Peroneal Neuritis with Paralysis and Atrophy; Limited Loss of Tactile Sensation; Slow Recovery, with Weakness and Atrophy of the Anterior Tibial Persisting.*—Mrs. E., primipara, aged 30; small woman with contracted pelvis. Labor severe, fourteen hours in duration; terminated with forceps and chloroform. In the evening her accoucheur was sent for on account of severe pain in the left hip and leg. also numbness and tingling on the outer and anterior aspect of the right leg.   There was also loss of power.   The following week the sensory paralysis remained about the same, but 'the motor symptoms increased until her leg was practically useless.   She suffered no chills nor rise of temperature, nor could a pelvic exudate be demonstrated. Twenty-two days following her labor I examined the patient and found no evidence of pelvic mischief, except the exquisite tenderness of the pelvic nerves.   Quantitative and qualitative changes to the galvanic current were present in all the muscles supplied by the peroneal nerve.   Examination disclosed inability to dorsally flex the foot or extend the toes.   She could depress the outer border of the foot, but could not draw it up.   There was loss of tactile sense on the dorsum of the foot and lower part of the outer and posterior aspect of the calf.   Atrophy supervened, but she finally made a good recovery.   This patient has had two children since this case was reported, both of them being much smaller children, and in each instance she has suffered a repetition of this attack, but much less severe than the first.

The following case of extensive paralysis from injury to the sacral plexus during an ill-conducted forceps delivery was seen with Dr. R. E. Skeel, September 5, 1899:

Mrs. P., aged 30, an under-sized woman with small conjugate diameter.   Has been married nine years and has had two children.   One boy, now aged 6 years, was born after a severe labor with aid of forceps—a very small child, weighing but three pounds.   She states that she suffered a phlegmasia alba dolens during her lying-in period.   Her second pregnancy was normal and she came to confinement February 25, 1899.   She was in labor thirty-six hours, during which her pains were strong.   Her physician then applied forceps, which she and her husband state was kept on for a period of three hours without result; no anesthetic was administered.   The forceps was then removed and after an interval of three hours was reapplied, and after another three hours of active traction, during which but little chloroform was given, she was delivered of a dead child whose head was lacerated by the forceps and the under jaw broken.   Evidence does not show that the child was large.   Immediately after her delivery it was found that the sphincters of the bladder were paralyzed, and she also experienced difficulty in securing a movement of the bowels.   Her greatest suffering, however, was from pain about the hips and pelvis extending down to the posterior

22

portion of the legs; there was also a burning pain and loss of sensation on the outside and anterior aspect of each leg and dorsum of the foot. The limbs were swollen, cold, and useless. Nothing would control the pain and she became a morphine *habitué*. About three months later she came under the care of Dr. Skeel, to whose courtesy I am indebted for the privilege of examining the case.

I found her lying in bed with marked contractures and considerable atrophy of the hamstring muscles, which was most marked on the right side; complete paralysis and wasting of the anterior tibial and peroneal groups on either side; the sphincter control had been regained. There was some numbness and tingling in the legs and feet. A complete foot drop was present on each side. Pelvic examination revealed great tenderness in the region of the sacral plexus, and a separation of the symphysis pubis sufficient to allow the finger to drop between the ununited ends. Involution had taken place; no evidence of pelvic exudate could be detected. This case was extremely interesting from a number of standpoints, but the greatest interest to me was the paralysis, atrophy, and loss of sensation, most marked in the distribution of the external popliteal nerves.

That the paralysis in these cases is due to an actual contusion of some part of the sacral plexus during labor seems to me to require no further demonstration. When we take into consideration the very sudden onset of the paralysis with all the characteristics of a neuritis, the distribution and course of the disability, it is impossible to conceive of any other hypothesis that is adequate to explain its development. Indeed, the not infrequent occurrence of this particular type of paralysis following labor presupposes a common origin and one intimately related to the physiological process of parturition. Being a sequence to difficult labor causes us to immediately suspect mechanical injury to some of the component or contributing parts of the sacral plexus within the pelvis, and a resulting descending neuritis of those nerve fibres which ultimately emerge from the great sciatic to form the external popliteal or peroneal nerve. In order to appreciate the mechanism of the injury it is necessary to refer briefly to the anatomy of the parts.

You will recall that part of the fibres from the fourth and all of the fibres of the fifth lumbar segments unite to form the lumbosacral cord, which passes downward winding over the sharp angle of the linea innominata into the pelvis, where it contributes to the formation of the sacral plexus. Since from the apex of the sacral plexus arises the great sciatic, from which the peroneal or external popliteal nerve is given off, and since the sacral plexus is formed by the junction of the first, second, third, and part of the fourth sacral nerves with the lumbo-sacral cord, it follows that any injury to the lumbo-sacral cord will result in damage to some of the branches of the great sciatic.

Rarely the lumbo-sacral cord fails to join the plexus, but continues as a separate trunk down alongside the great sciatic to become the peroneal nerve without any plexal connection. Mills,[15] Le Febre,[16] and others have shown that the fibres which mainly compose this lumbo-sacral nerve preserve their identity and are given off as the external popliteal or peroneal nerve. From these facts Hünermann[17] was led to believe that this form of leg paralysis was caused from injury to the lumbo-sacral cord, and believed that the contributing causes were (a) an abnormal position of the nerve, (b) a lack of proportion between the head and the pelvis, (c) a faulty position, (d) or careless instrumentation.

Bardeen,[18] after a study of two hundred dissections, found that "the common formation of the external popliteal nerve is from the fourth and fifth lumbar and the first and second sacral nerves (60.5 per cent). The common formation of the internal popliteal nerve is from the fourth and fifth lumbar and the first three sacral nerves (64.5 per cent)."

In view of the fact that these cases present a paralysis so sharply delimited to the distribution of the external popliteal without injury to the internal popliteal renders their explanation not as simple as it appears, and, as Thompson suggests, Hünermann certainly fails to explain its occurrence as completely as science demands.

Thompson[19] quotes Bardeen, who has suggested a possible explanation which the former puts into the following words: "The upper roots of the sacral plexus do not lie upon the pyriform muscle, but against the bony wall of the pelvis, and are thus exposed to injury from pressure during certain difficult labors. It is the dorsal offsets of these roots which lie against the bone and which receive the chief injury. The external popliteal nerve is made up from these dorsal offsets, and therefore the paralysis is chiefly localized in the distribution of this nerve." I think that this is on the whole the most scientific explanation of the action of traumatic force in producing this form of neuritis.

We have yet to consider those cases which occur from a slowly developing pressure from exudation, which certainly must be looked upon as traumatic in origin. These cases possess considerable interest and may result from septic or non-septic exudates. As an instance of a pressure paralysis from a septic exudate, the following case was recorded by Hervieux[20] more than twenty-five years ago, and is a thoroughly scientific contribution, and, considering the time of its report, stamps the reporter as a man of great scientific attainments and powers of observation:

A healthy woman of 19 years experienced a natural delivery. On the sixth day pelvic pains, fetid lochia, and fever announced the onset of puerperal infection. The septic condition was marked two days later by a dry tongue, rapid pulse, insomnia, pains in the abdomen, and a typhoidal aspect of the face. On the thirteenth day there appeared loss of power in the legs. At this time she had great fever, pulse 128, rapid respiration, distended abdomen, abundant lochia, and an erythematous rash. Later pain developed in the left iliac fossa and meteorism, pulse and temperature remained high, patient exhibited a dry tongue, loss of power and profuse perspirations. On the sixteenth day it was noted that she was unable to lift the lower limbs; there was no anesthesia nor involvement of the upper limbs. Tenderness and phlegmonous indurations could be demonstrated in the left iliac fossa; they seemed to be in relation with the adnexa at the left of the uterus. Under blistering and Neapolitan ointment she improved, and as her general condition mended power began to return in the legs; the pelvic indurations were gradually absorbed, but the patient continued to complain of vague pains in her thighs. At the end of two months the pelvic indurations had disappeared, she had regained the use of her limbs, and was discharged from the hospital in a good way to recovery.

This is an apt illustration of septic infection producing metritis and pelvic cellulitis marked by large exudates which evidently involved the nerve trunks, producing a paralysis entirely by pressure. That we may thus confidently assert its origin is further shown by the fact that the motor nerves were principally involved, the only sensory symptoms being the neuralgic pains;

and, moreover, the recovery occupied a space of time too short·
to admit of a complete regeneration of the nerve tissues.

Paralysis following the peroneal distribution occasionally develops several days after labor, sometimes occupying a week before it is fully evolved, oftentimes presenting no evidence of
sepsis, and examination reveals little or no sign of pelvic exudation. Mills,[21] Dercum,[22] Sinkler,[23] and others have reported
such cases. The following is an abridged report of the first of a
series of cases reported by me in 1899.[24]

*Prolonged Labor; Right Peroneal Paralysis and Neuritis with
Extension to the Other Side; Slow Recovery from Neuritis, but
Persistence of Some Atrophy and Paralysis.*—Mrs. T., large, robust woman; second marriage; by first husband had one small
child, whose delivery was easy and normal. Second husband is
a large man, and by him this was her first pregnancy, which had
been uneventful. Her labor lasted ten hours, during which she
was in almost continuous pain, but terminated naturally, the child
weighing nearly twelve pounds. Three days after confinement
severe pains began in thé right groin and hip, extending down
to the foot and toes, which were found to be slightly swollen and
sensitive to touch; loss of power was apparent. No intrapelvic
exudation or inflammation could be detected; lochia were normal;
temperature raised 1.5° F.; no chills. During this time she was
under the care of Dr. Walker, of Carleton, Ohio, who states that
she had much pain in the groin and leg. No anesthesiæ were
present, but a distressing burning sensation was felt on the outside of the right calf, the dorsum of the foot and toes. About
five days later she had a similar but much less severe pain in the
same region of the left leg and foot. There was no loss of sensation on either side; legs were sensitive to handling, considerable
loss of power in both, but most marked on the right. In eight
weeks she walked without assistance, and in two and one-half
months the sensory disturbance had disappeared. Three months
later atrophy was present in the anterior tibial and peronei of the
right leg.

Winckel[25] states that even such slight pelvic exudations as
accompany phlebitis may compress the nerves, and, still more
important, small extravasations into the nerve sheaths may occur.
Hünermann[26] refers to a case of severe sacral neuralgia where
an autopsy disclosed numerous thrombotic veins in the pelvis, one

of which lay alongside of the sciatic, to which it was bound by inflammatory deposits.

612 Prospect street.

BIBLIOGRAPHY.

1. Vinay: Rev. de Méd., 1895, No. 5.

2. Elder: Lancet, July 25, 1896.

3. Windscheit: Sammlung zwangloser Abhandlungen aus dem Gebiete der Frauenheilkunde u. Geburtshülfe, v. Max Graefe, Bd. ii., 1899.

4. Solowjeff: Med. Oboz., 1892, tome xxxviii., p. 11, cited by Vinay and Stembo.

5. Polk: New York Medical Record, 1890.

6. Von Haller: Lausanne, 1766, p. 544.

7. Volkmann: Contributions to Surgery, p. 219.

8. Mills: University Medical Magazine, May, 1893.

9. Handford: British Medical Journal, November 28, 1891, vol. ii., p. 1144.

10. Reynolds: British Medical Journal, October 16, 1897, p. 1081.

11. Moebius: Münchener med. Wochenschrift, 1887, Nos. 8 and 9.

12. Eulenberg: Deutsch. med. Wochenschrift, 1895, Nos. 8 and 9.

13. Rhein: University Medical Magazine, February, 1897.

14. Aldrich: American Gynecological and Obstetrical Journal, August, 1899.

15. Mills: Ibid.

16. Le Febre: Quoted by Mills, University Medical Magazine, May, 1893.

17. Hünermann: Archiv. für Gynäkologie, Berlin, 1892, vol. xlii., part 3.

18. Bardeen: Quoted by Thompson, Johns Hopkins Hospital Bulletin, November, 1900.

19. Thompson: Johns Hopkins Hospital Bulletin, November, 1900.

20. Hervieux: Traité des Maladies puerpérales, Paris, 1870.

21. Mills: Ibid.

22. Dercum: Recorded in Discussion of Mills' paper, University Medical Magazine, May, 1893.

23. Sinkler: Recorded in Discussion of Mills' paper, University Medical Magazine, May, 1893.

24. Aldrich: Ibid.

25. Winckel: A Text Book of Obstetrics, translated by J. Clifton Edgar, A.M., M.D., 1890.

26. Hünermann: Ibid.

OTHER REFERENCES.

Bernhardt: Deutsch. med. Woch., 1894, p. 935.

Lever: Guy's Hospital Reports, 1847: Disorders of the Nervous System Associated with Pregnancy and Parturition.

Whitfield: Lancet, March 30, 1889: Peripheral Neuritis due to the Vomiting of Pregnancy.

Ramskill: Obstetrical Journal, Great Britain, 1880, vol. viii., p. 678.

Jolly: Archiv. für Psychiatrie, Band xvi., Heft 3.

BIANCHI: Des Paralysies traumatiques des Membres inférieurs chez les Nouvelles Accouchées, Paris, 1867.

DONATH: Pest. med. chirurg. Presse, December 16, 1900.

DESNOS JOFFROY AND PINARD: Bulletin de l'Académie Royale de Médecine, 1889, tome xxi., p. 44.

WELCH, J. C.: Medical News, October 19, 1895.

ROBERTS, LOYD: Lancet, 1880, vol. i., p. 54.

ADAMS: Lancet, 1880, vol. ii., p. 699.

VINAY: Nouvelles Archives d'Obstétrique et de Gynécologie, 1895, p. 463.

KORSAKOFF AND SERBSKI: Arch. f. Psych., Bd. xxiii., Heft 1.

STEMBO: Deutsch. med. Woch., 1895, p. 461.

MADER: Wiener klin. Woch., Band viii., Nos. 30 and 31, 1895.

LINDEMANN: Centralbl. für allgemein. Pathol., 1892, August 20.

MADER: Neurolog. Centralbl., 1895, p. 871.

LEYDEN: Charité Annalen, 1862.

LLOYD: Twentieth Century Practice of Medicine, vol. xi., 1897, pp. 303-327.

WICHMANN: Die Rückenmarksnerven u. ihre Segmentbezüge. Berlin, 1900. Verlag v. Otto Salle.

MOEBIUS: Ueber Neuritis puerperalis, Münchener med. Woch., xxxiv, 1897, 9; Beiträge zur Lehre v. der Neuritis puerperalis, Münchener med. Woch., xxxvii., 1890, p. 14; Weitere Fälle von Neuritis puerperalis, Münchener med. Woch., xxxix., 1892, p. 45; Collected in Neurologische Beiträge, iv. Heft.

HUBER, W.: Zur Prophylaxe der Neuritis puerperalis. Monatsschr. Geburtshülfe u. Gynäk., Bd. ix., 1899, Heft 4, p. 487.

BAYLE: Jour. de Méd. de Paris, February 25, 1897.

WHAT ARE THE KNOWN FACTS ABOUT FOLLICULAR CYSTIC DEGENERATION OF THE OVARIES?[1]

BY

A. GOLDSPOHN, M.S., M.D.,

Professor of Gynecology, Post-Graduate Medical School; Attending Gynecologist to the German, the Post-Graduate, and the Charity Hospitals, Chicago.

WITH the volume that medical literature is assuming on many subjects, a review of what others have wrought and thought, or what they are now thinking on some given subject, is sometimes much needed, especially if it has some important practical bearing. And when, as in this instance, that which is known has been practically misrepresented, a correct understanding of the thing is needed before adding much that is new.

[1] Read before the Chicago Gynecological Society, May 16, 1902.

According to Waldeyer's[1] recent and most authentic work upon the anatomy of the pelvis, the normal Graafian follicles are vesicular bodies varying in size from that of a poppy-seed to that of a pea. They are situated normally in the cortical layer of the ovary, which is from 2 to 3 millimetres thick. The larger and more superficial ones gently protrude from the general surface of the ovary, beneath a thin vascular layer and the surface epithelium, through which they appear as clear or translucent vesicles. The smaller ones have a less distinguishable envelope, do not contain fluid, and are known as primordial follicles. The larger, or Graafian follicles proper, have a double coat: a more dense theca externa composed of lamellated connective tissue, like the membrana propria of the tubuli seminales, and a more areolar and vascular inner layer of connective tissue containing numerous peculiar large cells which have many nuclei ("granula") and show a yellowish tinge when fully developed. This envelope is lined with the membrana granulosa, composed of low columnar epithelium resting upon a structureless basal membrane, and arranged mostly in a single layer, except where it gives rise to the cumulus oöphorus (conus proligerus) which holds the ovum, that is in size about equal to a grain of sand. The larger portion of the Graafian follicle contains a clear albuminous fluid. This fluid originates, according to Wendeler,[2] Luschka, Waldeyer, Flemming, Schottländer, and others, from fluid transuded from the surrounding vessels and from transformation and disintegration of follicle cells.

In 1855 Rokitansky[3] minutely described a cyst of the size of a child's head from the right ovary, and one of the size of a fist from the left ovary of the same case. These were simple serous cysts without any evidences of proliferation. They were associated with numerous smaller follicle cysts that were located in adjoining remnants of ovary, and, by encroaching upon each other, had assumed irregular shapes. Of these, those that were enlarged only to the size of a bean contained a degenerated ovule, mostly without a germinal vesicle, and a broken-down membrana granulosa in most cases. This demonstration by Rokitansky has been accepted as proving the origin of simple cysts from degenerated Graafian-follicle cysts, by nearly all writers on the subject except Nagel[4] and Von Kahlden,[5] the latter regarding them as of adenomatous origin. Ritchie and Webb[6] also early described an analogous case. Virchow[7] defined the pathological anatomy of these follicle cysts, which are not neoplasms, in 1865 as follows: "The characteristic feature of the true follicle hydrops is that in the beginning of its formation, at least, an ovum is found in the fluid, because the formation occurs thus: that a larger quantity of albuminous watery but not mucoid fluid accumulates in a Graafian follicle that usually contains a cell mass, an ovum, and a membrana granulosa. Later on the ovum dies. One can clearly see how it disintegrates. First its protoplasmic mass becomes a softer substance, which is easily divided and is finally completely dissolved. Then there is merely a serous sac left. Occasionally this cystoid degeneration occurs in a solitary follicle; and, in the main, it can be accepted that unilocular hydrops of the ovary is of follicular origin. But I have shown that not a few ovarian dropsies which are multilocular in the beginning, secondarily coalesce and form a single sac." Förster[8] describes the same condition and ascribes it to trophic changes or inflammatory processes in the ovary. These hydropic Graafian follicles, when they become enlarged to more than from 1 to 1½ centimetres approximately in diameter, are regarded as retention cysts by a very large majority of pathologic anatomists, including Klob,[9] Birch-Hirschfeld,[10] Ziegler,[11] Orth,[12] Hektoen-Riesman,[13] and others, and by nearly all gynecologists, in the sense that their physiologic rupture or opening has been prevented and that they have also not disappeared by normal atrophy. The prevented opening and discharge of their contents is accounted for (a) by thickening of the follicle walls, (b) thickening or greater density of the tunica albuginea of the ovary, (c) pseudo-membranous exudate upon the surface of the ovary. These factors are made quite obvious by the evidences of chronic inflammation which the ovarian stroma so frequently presents generally, or in proximity to these small cysts and by evidences of previous peritonitis. But the initial edema is also attributed to trophic changes such as result from varicosity of the ovary, which has frequently been seen by several investigators. Several authors think it may be due to lack of intensity of the menstrual congestion. Among the long array of practical gynecologists who have professed and defended these views since 1887 and 1888, and who hold that the condition is certainly not an innocent one and sometimes at least requires treatment—among this number Schröder,[14] Olshausen,[15] and Hegar[16] (as far as I know) had declared themselves, also, previous to that time. Nevertheless in those years one dissenting voice arose, but it did not sound very long. William Nagel,[17] an assistant of Gusserow in the Berlin Charité, appears to have had some preconceived ideas that he was too anxious to prove. And, judging also from the quite general and severe criticism which he aroused, he attempted to do it by the use of bad logic, irrational ideas in pathology, and rather violent construction of other men's observations. But he failed and has not attempted, in reply to much adverse criticism since then, to urge his views as to the origin and possible evil clinical bearing of ovarian follicle cysts. But his work on the embryology and normal histology of the ovary is duly credited.

Nagel's argument is as follows :

I. The ovum originates from the membrana granulosa, therefore the latter cannot undergo degeneration before the former does; and that, therefore, if the ovum is still healthy, it is a proof that the whole Graafian follicle is healthy. The fallacy of this is shown by Bulius[17] and by Bollenhagen,[18] who, each in more extensive investigation, found that the membrana granulosa had degenerated first, quite as often as the ovum began to do so; that both must be taken into account; further, that degeneration is gradual and may for a time be limited to a part of the epithelium. And they both charge Nagel with the fallacy of concluding that because he found some follicles healthy (as he says), therefore all the follicles in the same and in other ovaries were also healthy.

As to this finding of healthy ova in these hydropic follicles not all investigators are so positive. Von Kahlden examined both ovaries of 16 such cases and did not find them in any of them, notwithstanding the greatest care to harden the entire contents of the follicles before making sections. Again, Pettipierre[19] very carefully examined 23 ovaries that were removed from 12 patients for ovarian and other neuralgias and nervous symptoms, chiefly to ascertain in how many of them he could find in Graafian follicles granulosa cells that had penetrated or were embedded in the ovum. He found this phenomenon of degeneration in 22 follicles contained in 12 of the 23 ovaries examined. He says it was found mostly in the smaller of the readily visible follicles, and was accompanied by a marked state of disintegration of the membrana granulosa. And he says that this evidence of death in the latter is probably a necessary antecedent for the migration of granulosa cells into the ova. For us it is significant that these processes of decay were found chiefly in the *smaller* follicles.

II. Nagel found in Graafian follicles some larger protoplasmic cells that he interpreted as nourishing cells *(Nährzellen)* of the follicle fluid; and he then jumped to the wild conclusion that this liquid which is found in the Graafian follicle could be formed only from the epithelial cellular contents of the follicle. Then, if the membrana granulosa and the other cells within the follicle were disintegrated or dissolved, no more follicle fluid could be formed; the follicle must undergo atrophy and could not give rise to an accumulation of fluid or form a cyst. And if this be so, then the simple serous follicle cysts, from about a pigeon's egg to a hen's egg in size, which he admits to be of not infrequent occurrence, must (by exclusion) be formed from corpora lutea, although only the smallest ones show remnants of lutein cells and although he found only 2 cases that did. The erroneousness of this play of imagination is mentioned by several of his critics. For it is generally accepted that the follicle fluid is formed partly from disintegration of its epithelial cells and partly by transudation of serum from the blood vessels, particularly from the veins that abound around these hydropic follicles, according to Von Kahlden; and from this abundant source fluid enough is derived to fill and to distend the follicle sacs into simple cysts when their ova and epithelial contents have perished. But they rarely become much larger than an orange. As a reason for this Pfannenstiel[20] says that with the greater distension of the walls of the sacs the pressure gradually reduces the blood vessels in them, and the cysts then become stationary.

III. While Nagel admits that these hydropic follicle cysts exist, he alone contends that they have no epithelial lining and that they must come from corpora lutea that have no lining to give them. But nearly all of the investigators who have followed him say that they mostly do have a lining of low columnar epithelium, and that its absence in any given case is due to its detachment or loss during preparation; that it is the preserved or somewhat transformed membrana granulosa of the former Graafian follicle. And that these simple cysts which contain an albuminous but rarely a colored fluid, without pseudomucin, and which rarely exceed the size of a fist, and are called "cystoma simplex serosum" by Pfannenstiel, do originate from hydropic Graafian follicles is conceded by all who speak about it, except Nagel and Von Kahlden. But the latter, a pathologic anatomist, while recognizing the anatomical condition and its name, "hydropic follicles," denies the retention-cyst theory and construes these cysts as adenomata in origin, or as having had an adenomatous intervening stage; and holds that their lack of the signs of proliferation which characterize the true adenomata is due to an early arrest of connective-tissue proliferation in and about their walls.

Thus all the peculiar tenets of William Nagel on this subject have been refuted promptly and some years ago. And as no one, not even he himself, has appeared since then in their defence, there is no foundation in recorded facts for the assertion made by Emil Ries[21]: "That all those little cysts that are punctured and scraped and cauterized are normal follicles, a trifle enlarged; and the microscope reveals a perfectly normal ovum in each one."

The normal status of this subject, as far as it is understood, is probably best judged from the opinions of able and mature practical gynecologists who have both the allied anatomical knowledge and extended clinical experience in the subject. And the men of that class who have written upon this subject during the last ten years, as Von Winckel,[22] Fehling,[23] Fritsch,[24] Pfannenstiel, Gebhard,[25] Hofmeier,[26] Howard Kelly,[27] August Martin,[28] and others, agree quite uniformly as to the retention-cyst theory and recognize the condition as mostly the result of inflammatory processes, evidences of which are usually present in other parts of the ovary or in its surroundings. Some regard it as due to trophic changes induced by venous hyperemia in a prolapsed ovary, mostly in conjunction with uterine displacements. The writer called attention to "The Fate of the Ovaries in Connection with Retroversion of the Uterus," nearly five years ago. All of these authors agree that these follicle cysts and cysts formed in corpora lutea sometimes require surgical treatment, chiefly as an auxiliary feature in connection with correction or relief of other more pronounced disorders in these parts. The indication for such treatment is decided not merely by the mere feature of the size of the follicle, whether it be two or four centimetres in diameter, but largely by its probable liability to rupture, and by the degree and nature of abnormal changes in the remainder of the ovary or in other parts of the internal generative organs, and by the age of the patient.

1. In ovarian cystic tumors of any kind, if they cause no symptoms—which is often the case with the smaller cystic adenomata (true neoplasms)—and are not large enough to do harm by crowding upon the adjacent organs, I do not propose an

operation unless something else in the abdomen or pelvis requires surgical treatment; and sometimes I do not inform the patients about the cyst being there, unless it becomes deleterious later on.

2. With the patient in dorsal recumbency and with the abdominal recti muscles relaxed by tilting the pelvis upward so as to reduce the distance from the symphysis pubis to the sternum, with all constricting apparel unfastened, and with the intestines and bladder empty, ovaries that are the seat of follicular cystic degeneration can be diagnosed quite generally in bimanual palpation, by their usually somewhat increased size, by the globular contour of a part of or the entire ovary, and by their tenderness. Sometimes these follicle cysts rupture during this palpation, usually with some improvement in symptoms; but in my observation they have generally refilled inside of two months, with return of the symptoms.

3. Ovaries, of no matter what size, I make *a prime object* of treatment only when they cause symptoms and are proved to do so by observing that bimanual palpation, as above mentioned, directly excites or increases the pain that is ascribed to them. And they become with me the chief object of *surgical* treatment only when, in addition, they have attained at least the size of a hen's egg by cystic degeneration or abscess formation, and otherwise only after rational general and local medical treatment has been fairly made use of and proved to be ineffectual.

4. Solely as an *auxiliary or incidental* object of surgical treatment, and without incurring any greater surgical risk, in younger and middle-aged women I also resect follicle cysts whose diameter exceeds the thickness of the remainder of the ovary itself (the measure also stated by August Martin), for it is only rational to assume that in such a distended follicle the feature of abnormal retention must be present, and that the development of a deleterious cyst is far more likely than the supervention of a normal corpus luteum. Smaller follicle cysts I enucleate or excise—rarely cauterize—only when they are under a thickened and dense tunica albuginea or are discovered abnormally located deep in the vascular zone of the ovary, so that the prospective normal discharge of their contents will be impeded.

5. Many of these hydropic follicle cysts cause no symptoms and are therefore, at the period of examination at least, without clinical dignity. But that a majority of those that are discovered in women who come for an examination cause either local

or referred pain or figure in the disturbed function of some other organ, is equally certain.

In scores of cases I have been able to observe the following succession of events:

(a) Bimanual examination or compression of an ovary, directly exciting or aggravating a pain, mostly in the inguinal region, or loin, or hip, or in a limited intercostal area of the same side, and much more frequently on the left than the right side.

(b) Removal of one or more of these follicle cysts by exsection and closure of the gap.* Sometimes also an incidental improvement in the location of the ovary, as when operating for retroversion of the uterus.

(c) An immediate, occasionally a gradual, but permanent cessation of the pain. These events, occurring in the same succession in, say, seventy-five similar cases, must have more than the mere post-hoc relation to each other in the majority of cases. Nor can the results be accounted for, among sensible men, by the old platitude of the mere suggestive effect of an operation.

REFERENCES.

1. WALDEYER: Das Becken, S. 509, 1899.
2. WENDELER: Die Krankheiten d. Eierstocke v. i. Halfte. Aug. Martin, S. 56.
3. ROKITANSKY: Wochenblatt d. Zeitschrift d. Gesel. d. Aerzte zu Wien, 1855, p. i.
4. NAGEL, W.: Archiv. f. Gyn., Bd. xxxi., S. 327, 1887; Archiv. f. Gyn., Bd. xxxiii., S. 1, 1888.
5. VON KAHLDEN: Beiträge z. pathol. Anatomie u. allgem. Pathologie, Band xxii., Heft 1, S. 1.
6. RITCHIE AND WEBB: Spencer Wells, Med. Times and Gazette, Aug. 6, 1864.
7. VIRCHOW: Die Krankhaften Geschwülste, Bd. i., S. 260.
8. FÖRSTER: Handbuch d. pathologischen Anatomie.
9. KLOB, J. M.: Pathol. d. weiblichen Sexualorgane, Wien, S. 377, 1864.
10. BIRCH-HIRSCHFELD: Pathol. Anatomie, ii. Aufl., S. 759, 1882.
11. ZIEGLER: Pathol. Anatomie, iv. Aufl., S. 924, 1886.
12. ORTH: Lehrbuch d. speciel. patholog. Anatomie, Bd. ii., Abt. i., S. 564, 1893.
13. HEKTOEN AND RIESMAN: American Text Book of Pathology, 1901, p. 1066.
14. SCHRÖDER: Krankheiten d. weibl. Geschlechtsorgane, vii. Aufl., S. 377, 1886.

*For technique and remote results see Journal American Medical Association, August 24, 1901, and THE AMERICAN JOURNAL OF OBSTETRICS, vol. xliv., No. 5, 1901.

15. OLSHAUSEN: Die Krankheiten d. Ovarien. Deutsche Chir., Lief. 58, S. 48, 1886.

16. HEGAR: Operative Gynecology, iii. Aufl., S. 368, 1886.

17. BULIUS: Hegar's Festschrift, 1889, S. 187. Also, Zeitschrift f. Geb. u. Gyn., Bd. xxiii., S. 358.

18. BOLLENHAGEN: Zeitschrift f. Geb. u. Gyn., Bd. xliii., S. 90.

19. PETTIPIERRE: Archiv. f. Gyn., Bd. xxxv., S. 460, 1889.

20. PFANNENSTIEL: Veit's Handbuch d. Gyn., Bd. iii., S. 291 u. 310.

21. RIES: Jour. Amer. Med. Association, Aug. 17, 1901, p. 438.

22. VON WINCKEL: Lehrbuch d. Frauenkrankheiten, ii. Aufl., p. 626.

23. FEHLING: Lehrbuch d. Frauenkrankheiten, 1893.

24. FRITSCH: Die Krankheiten d. Frauen, vi. Aufl., S. 414.

25. GEBHARD: Pathol. Anatomie d. weiblichen Sexualorgane, S. 311, 1899.

26. HOFMEIER: Handbuch d. Krankheiten d. weiblichen Geschlechtsorgane v. Carl Schröder, xii. Aufl., S. 460, 1898.

27. KELLY: Operative Gynecology, vol. ii., p. 177.

28. MARTIN, AUGUST: Die Krankheiten d. Eierstocke, i. Halfte, S. 243.

29. GOLDSPOHN: AMERICAN JOURNAL OF OBSTETRICS, vol. xxxvi., No. 4, 1897.

FETAL MORTALITY IN INDUCED LABOR.

BY

WARREN R. GILMAN, M.D.,
Worcester, Mass.

THIS case is reported for the purpose of putting on record the unsatisfactory result of an induced labor.

Mrs. B., born in England thirty-three years ago; height, 4 feet 10 inches; weight, 180 pounds. The development of bones is everywhere symmetrical and she is active and healthy. Her first labor, four years ago, was tedious and was terminated by a forceps operation; the baby was still-born. Her second confinement occurred in December, 1900. The head did not engage and podalic version was done; the delivery of the head was difficult and the child was still-born. The physicians who attended her in her confinements were men of experience and acknowledged skill in obstetrical work, but forceps in the first instance and version in the second failed to deliver a live child. In each case she was subjected to a prolonged obstetrical operation involving an appreciable amount of danger to the integrity of the genital canal.

She came to me when about four months advanced in her third

pregnancy. Measurements of the pelvis were as follows: Crests, 27.3 centimetres (10¾ inches); spines, 24.8 centimetres (9¾ inches); external conjugate, 19.7 centimetres (7¾ inches); oblique conjugate, 9.5 centimetres (3¾ inches); true conjugate, 8 centimetres (3⅛ inches).

Soon after her second confinement she had been told that it would be impossible for her to give birth to a living child. When she became pregnant for the third time she consulted two nurses whom she knew and from them obtained a vivid impression of the danger of Cesarean section. As the result of this she came to me begging that I terminate the pregnancy at once. I refused to do this and urged her to go to term and be delivered by Cesarean section. I told her that the operation was a serious one, but that ninety-five per cent of the women operated upon recovered, provided the operation were done under the best of conditions, and that she could be quite certain of having a healthy, full-term baby.

After some days of deliberation the patient came to me bringing her husband with her. They declined to accept the risk of the operation, although understanding that any other operation at full term offered no hope of a living child. I then offered to induce labor at the eighth month, telling them that only one-half of the babies born in this way survived. This proposition was gratefully accepted and the thirty-sixth week of pregnancy was fixed as the time for the induction of labor. The patient remained in good health.

On February 14, 1902, she was etherized and a bougie inserted along the posterior wall of the uterus up to the fundus; a tampon in the vagina held the bougie in place. Labor pains began forty-three hours later, on February 16. Position of child, O. L. A. The membranes ruptured five hours after the beginning of labor, and the amniotic fluid escaped slowly. Although pains were severe, the os dilated slowly and was about the size of a silver half-dollar at the end of fifteen hours. The head could not be made to engage and remained free above the superior strait. Under ether the os was dilated readily and version performed easily; the child was delivered quickly and without any difficulty whatever. The child, a girl, was quite feeble and required some attention before it would cry well. It weighed 2,268 grammes (5 pounds) and was 45 centimetres (18 inches) in length. The finger nails did not reach the tips of fingers, there was an abundant growth of lanugo, and the skin of the face was wrinkled. The measurements of head were as follows: Biparietal, 8 centimetres (3¼ inches) ; suboccipito-bregmatic, 8 centimetres (3¼ inches) ; fronto-mental, 8 centimetres (3¼ inches) ; occipito-frontal, 10½ centimetres (4¼ inches) ; occipito-mental, 11½ centimetres (4½ inches). The circumferences were: Suboccipito-bregmatic, 29 centimetres (11½ inches) ; suboccipito-frontal, 29 centimetres (11½ inches) ; occipito-frontal, 33 centimetres (13 inches).

The child was wrapped in cotton, kept in an incubator, and disturbed as little as possible. For two days it was given five drops of cream in a teaspoonful of water every two hours. After the second day it was given two to three teaspoonfuls of its mother's milk every two hours. After the fifth day the baby failed gradually and, in spite of the best of care, died on the eighth day. Jaundice was marked from the beginning and did not clear up. There were four to six normal, yellow dejections daily after the fifth day. In view of the characteristics of the baby and an uncertainty as to the exact date of the mother's last menstruation, I think the age of the child was thirty-four rather than thirty-six weeks. Our inability to determine the exact age of the fetus *in utero* must always be borne in mind in esti-mating the chances of a successful result of induced labor.

The treatment of contracted pelvis, always one of the most interesting subjects in obstetrics, has been materially affected by the advance made in abdominal surgery, and the brilliant results of Cesarean section cannot be ignored. The mortality rate is not over five per cent when the operation is done under the best con-ditions, as is shown by a fairly large number of reported cases.

For many years the only treatment of. the cases of marked pelvic deformity which offered any hope for the child was the induction of labor. Many children were saved in this way, and the procedure was so much more successful than any operation at full term that it acquired a well-merited reputation. At the present time, however, the possible operations at full term are not limited to forceps, version, and embryotomy, but Cesa-rean section with its definite mortality rate must be considered.

The difficulty in properly contrasting the merits of the two operations, Cesarean section at term and induced labor at the eighth month, lies in the fact that we do not know the exact or even the approximate fetal mortality rate of induced labor. Recent statements upon this point are largely a matter of opinion and are not founded upon the results of reported cases. The successful cases are easily recalled, but many cases in which the

23

child did not survive have slipped from the memory.   The fetal mortality of induced labor is given by different men as 15, 30, and 40 per cent.   It is my belief that the true rate is at least 40 per cent.

By the kindness of Dr. Leonard Wheeler I am able to report eight cases of induced labor from the records of the maternity ward of the Worcester City Hospital:

CASE I.—Eighth month.   True conjugate, 3½ inches.   Baby survived.

CASE II.—Eighth month.   True conjugate, 3½ inches.   Baby survived.

CASE III.—Eighth month.   True conjugate, 3½ inches.   Baby still-born.

CASE IV.—Eighth month.   True conjugate, 3½ inches.   Baby died on third day.

CASE V.—Eighth month.   True conjugate, 3½ inches.   Baby survived.

CASE VI.—Eighth month.   True conjugate, 3½ inches.   Baby died on third day.

CASE VII.—Thirty-eighth week.   True conjugate, 3⅞ inches. Baby survived.

CASE VIII.—Eighth month.   True conjugate, 3¾ inches. Baby died on second day.

Adding my own case to these, we have a total of nine, with only four children surviving—a mortality rate of 55 per cent. Labor was induced in each case because diminished pelvic diameters made labor at term extremely dangerous for the child. Each woman was in good physical health at the time labor was induced.

It is to be hoped that more cases of labor induced at the thirty-sixth week may be reported, in order that the decision as to what is the best treatment of cases of contracted pelvis may be determined by fact rather than opinion.

3 ASHLAND STREET.

TRANSACTIONS OF THE AMERICAN GYNECOLOGICAL SOCIETY.[1]

PROCEEDINGS OF THE TWENTY-SEVENTH ANNUAL MEETING, HELD AT ATLANTIC CITY, N. J., 1902.

The next thing in order was the presidential address, by DR. SETH C. GORDON, of Portland, Me. Dr. Gordon selected for his subject

THE RELATION OF THE GYNECOLOGIST, OBSTETRICIAN, AND GENERAL SURGEON.

He said it was the custom of late years to say that gynecology had passed its usefulness and had become merged into general surgery, and that there no longer existed the necessity for attempting to prolong the life of this hopelessly doomed department of medicine. With this proposition he took issue, and maintained that until modern obstetrics approached more nearly to the ideal standard there would be a large field for the gynecologist proper. Scientific gynecology had its birth in America and was founded by Marion Sims. No gynecological surgery prior to his day had made any impression on surgical progress which had endured until the present time. That which the keen, brilliant genius of Sims made possible, the intelligent, patient, practical common-sense of Emmet made probable to every afflicted one of womankind. The field was wide, and from all parts of the country came the sufferers from childbed injuries, many of which were due to the faulty obstetric work of that day. Among the causes were long-delayed use of the forceps, careless and needless use of forceps, disregard of the accidents occurring, and a total lack of aseptic precautions during the progress of labor. From the first came vesico-vaginal fistula; while from the second came lacerations of the uterus and perineum, many of which could have been remedied had the accoucheur regarded them at all and treated them according to the best-known surgical principles. The great fault lay in entirely ignoring such accidents.

There were many faults yet to be overcome in the practice of obstetrics before the millennium would dawn for the gynecologist. While public institutions were doing good work in eliminating germ diseases and bringing the mortality almost to the vanishing point, much missionary work needed to be done among professional men in private practice.

The criticisms he offered were: 1. The too early use of the

[1] Concluded from p. 270, August JOURNAL.

forceps. When the pendulum began to swing from rarely using the forceps it went to the opposite extreme, using them far too often. A very large majority of cases would, if let alone, terminate naturally. 2. Cases of accidents occurring in labor were not properly repaired at the time.

The fashion of late seemed to be to prohibit antiseptic douches after labor. While it might be necessary in normal labors with no accidents, lacerations should be kept surgically clean, and this could be done only by frequent irrigation and germicides. Surgical cleanliness on the part of the accoucheur and patient, from the beginning of labor until convalescence, insured the safety of one and duty well performed on the part of the other.

As an additional safeguard against laceration of the perineum he believed the timely use of anesthetics was invaluable. It prevented the use on the part of the patient of the voluntary muscles, which did much to cause this accident. His preference as an anesthetic was the A. C. E. mixture, given only during pains. It acted promptly and did not excite the patient.

Postpartum hemorrhage was not due to the use of an anesthetic, but to the carelessness of the attendant. A steady, careful, persistent manipulation of the uterine tumor during the expulsion of the child and placenta, and continued until firm contraction was produced, insured safety in almost every case. His own experience fully justified him in making the assertion that a strict adherence to this rule would nearly always prevent postpartum hemorrhage.

The modern methods of Cesarean section had given such good results in diminishing mortality that the barbarism of craniotomy had practically ceased, and the morbidity which furnished such abundant gynecological material had correspondingly decreased. This great progress was practically due to anesthesia, asepsis, and improved technique, and for this credit should be given to gynecologists who had perfected operative details of abdominal section made possible by the discovery of anesthetics and cleanly surgery.

Laceration of the cervix, especially of long standing, was not always an indication for trachelorrhaphy, destruction or extreme atrophy of tissue of the cervix being a decided contraindication to the operation. Thousands of women suffered much more after trachelorrhaphy than before it. The cervical canal was closed too much, drainage prevented, and often infection developed in the uterus and tubes, and the last condition was much worse than the first. Emmet, he thought, never taught such gynecology as that. He did not even teach that all lacerations of the cervix required an operation. On the contrary, he believed that many of them did not require any surgical intervention simply because they were not producing any morbid symptoms. The tendency had been too much in the direction contrary to Emmet's teaching, with the result that gynecology had been brought largely into disrepute. Many of the symptoms attributed to laceration of the cervix had been found to be due to disease of the other pelvic organs.

The plastic operation of perineorrhaphy, so often done by the general practitioner, to say nothing of the general surgeon, was far too often apologetic, as compared with the work of Emmet, Thomas, Marcy, and others throughout the country.

The best work for malignant disease of the pelvic organs had been done by gynecologists, and to them, he said, we must look for further progress. Probably no man could show better results in the way of relief, and even cure, of cancer of the uterus than Dr. John Byrne, a former President of the Society. Whether hysterectomy in any stage of the disease was to be the ideal method was by no means well settled. The best did not give very satisfactory results from this operation, even when the most radical dissection had been done. He believed that a more careful examination and more close observation of women under the care of physicians would detect malignant disease in its earlier stages, at a period when hysterectomy would be the ideal operation.

Much yet remained to be done with plastic operations about the vagina, not only in relation to prolapsed uteri, but for vesicocele and diseases of the urethra, especially that of caruncle. Incisions into the posterior cul-de-sac for acute inflammatory conditions, whether attended with pus or not, deserved the attention of gynecologists.

Dr. Robert A. Murray, of New York, read a paper on

THE TREATMENT OF PLACENTA PREVIA—CESAREAN SECTION NOT
JUSTIFIABLE.

Dr. J. Whitridge Williams, of Baltimore, in opening the discussion, questioned the propriety of Cesarean section in many cases of placenta previa, and said this operation was done altogether too frequently. Recent statistics as to the great safety attending Cesarean section were liable to do almost as much harm as good. If the Society did not take a decided position in regard to Cesarean section in cases of placenta previa, he feared this operation might be practised as frequently and indiscriminately as oöphorectomy. There was a small field, in his opinion, for Cesarean section in placenta previa.

Dr. Edwin B. Cragin, of New York, said that the conditions which would justify Cesarean section in a case of placenta previa were so numerous that they were seldom all found present, and among them he mentioned a good condition of the child, good surroundings for the operation, and a cervix so rigid that there would be great difficulty in dilating it and doing version. Those three conditions were rarely met with in a case of placenta previa. As a fourth condition he mentioned central implantation of the placenta.

Dr. Philander A. Harris, of Paterson, N. J., said that when the statistics of Cesarean section in cases of placenta previa were analyzed as to the mortality to the mother and child, it would be found that the more rapid, prompt, and effective the delivery, the less the mortality and the better the general results. If the case could be seen when the first hemorrhage occurred, it would be a favorable time for Cesarean section. He would not, however, advise it. but would try to effect delivery by other methods.

Dr. CHARLES JEWETT, of Brooklyn. said the results under modern obstetric methods of treatment of cases of placenta previa were good: whereas the mortality from Cesarean section was much larger than had been claimed by its advocates.

Dr. EDWARD P. DAVIS, of Philadelphia, said Cesarean section in placenta previa must have a very limited application at present. Among the poorer classes of women with placenta previa the mortality among children must be great, with a considerable mortality among mothers. However, he was not willing to universally condemn Cesarean section in cases of placenta previa, for his personal experience with the operation had led him to look upon it as a successful operative measure under favorable circumstances.

Dr. A. PALMER DUDLEY, of New York, thought the general practitioner should be educated in regard to placenta previa. He should study his cases more carefully and make a diagnosis of placenta previa sufficiently early to refer them to specialists, thus saving the lives of many children and many mothers which otherwise would undoubtedly be sacrificed. There was no use in performing this operation after a profuse hemorrhage had occurred. The danger of Cesarean section, when properly and promptly performed, was almost *nil*.

Dr. EGBERT H. GRANDIN, of New York, said he would treat a case of placenta previa as radically as one of carcinoma or sarcoma of the uterus. He would go at it with hammer and tongs, just as soon as he was sure of his diagnosis, and, no matter what the period of gestation, he would empty the uterus. His experience had been fairly extensive, and his results from this hammer-and-tongs policy had been favorable as regards the mothers. He had never had a mother die in any case, although there might be considerable mortality as far as the child was concerned. But usually, he said, these children were nearly dead when the cases were first observed.

Dr. MURRAY, in closing the discussion, said his desire was to bring this subject before the Society at this time, and not to postpone it for another year, because in the discussion at the meeting of the American Association of Obstetricians and Gynecologists a very strong plea was made for the treatment of placenta previa by Cesarean section. Such treatment at the present time should be protested against, and he thought his paper and the discussion would show that with proper treatment such a grave operation could be avoided. Of course there was a very small minority of cases that could be treated by Cesarean section.

TWO CONDITIONS SIMULATING ECTOPIC GESTATION.

Dr. Edward P. Davis, of Philadelphia, Pa., read a paper on this subject.

Case I.—A multipara had pelvic pain at intervals with disordered menstruation for several months. Had been exposed to cold and wet during menstrual period. Her husband, a physician, had made intrauterine applications and had introduced a sound. After nine months of such' illness the patient developed a hematocele filling the cavity of the pelvis. Abdominal section was declined and vaginal section permitted. Considerable clotted blood was removed by vaginal incision, the cavity washed out and packed with iodoform gauze. This gauze was gradually removed in ten days after the operation. After the removal of the gauze the patient gradually developed symptoms of septic infection ending fatally. Abdominal section was declined and autopsy was not permitted. The examination of blood clot removed after section gave no evidence of ectopic gestation. This case resembles others recently reported by Kober[1] and also observed by others, in which pelvic hematocele has accompanied diseased conditions of the pelvic viscera other than tubal gestation.

Case II.—An emaciated, anemic woman aged 20 had previously had an abortion between three and four months. Bleeding was very profuse and was controlled with great difficulty. Several months after, she became pregnant and had attacks of intermittent pain with hemorrhage from the vagina and rapid, feeble pulse. Upon examination the pelvis was found filled with a soft, boggy tumor completely occupying the posterior cul-de-sac. The body of the womb could not be distinctly outlined, but was enlarged. The patient's condition indicated hemorrhage, and abdominal section was performed. A retroverted pregnant uterus was found, filling the pelvic cavity, the tubes and ovaries being normal. The womb was replaced, pregnancy proceeded for some time, and the patient left the hospital. She subsequently returned and aborted at six months. The uterus was found lined with clotted blood at the time of abortion. Ségond, Routier, and Varnier have recently reported to the Obstetrical Society of Paris similar cases. In obscure cases of hemorrhage in which a diagnosis is not evident, abdominal section is safer than continued uncertainty. Conditions simulating ectopic gestation usually require prompt interference and surgical treatment.

Dr. Egbert H. Grandin, of New York, said the diagnosis of ectopic gestation was not easy, because, in his experience, the symptoms usually laid down in text books did not exist in some cases. All the so-called classical symptoms were absent in some cases, yet on careful investigation one would always find a symptom which would leave him to believe that ectopic gestation

[1] Centralblatt für Gynecologie, No. 39, 1901.

probably existed, one which was not associated with any other intrapelvic lesion, except it be pyosalpinx or ovarian abscess— conditions which, from the position of the tumor, simulated ectopic gestation. This symptom was a colicky pain, the green-apple pain. Dr. Janvrin was the man who had taught him how to arrive at a diagnosis of ectopic gestation. This colicky pain was symptomatic of beginning rupture of the tube. While the rent did not occur in the tube, the tube was beginning to distend more than it was capable of doing, and a slight rupture occurred. This was the time to operate. If surgeons operated then all cases would be saved, provided they did not infect the woman. When the colicky pains recurred they were symptomatic of secondary rupture, and then waiting for further symptoms would possibly lose the patient. It was his custom now to make a posterior vaginal section for diagnosis. If primary rupture had occurred, or tubal abortion was apparent, and secondary rupture had taken place, one would get blood or clots low in the pelvis. The diagnosis once established, one should proceed at once to operate, provided he did not get either blood or clots. With the finger introduced he could palpate the mass and determine whether he had ectopic gestation or pyosalpinx to deal with. Credit for this symptom of colicky pain should be given to Dr. Janvrin.

DR. WILLIAM R. PRYOR, of New York, said there was one condition which the essayist did not mention, and that was acute hemorrhage of the ovary, which sometimes simulated every single symptom of ectopic gestation. There was more or less shock, high pulse, general depression of the vital forces, and the characteristic pain. He had had three such instances, and, being enthusiastic in regard to vaginal incision as a means of diagnosis, he had found blood and clots in these cases of acute hemorrhage of the ovary. He had taken them out by means of a vaginal incision, some of the ovaries being three and a half inches in diameter. This acute hemorrhage of the ovary had been recently written about. The condition occurred a little previous to menstruation, and apparently it was another explanation of what was described as ovarian hematoma or ovarian apoplexy. He had no doubt it was in the stroma of the ovary, and the capsule of the ovary would rupture, followed by an escape of blood into the peritoneal cavity. The pulse, in one of the cases he had seen, ran as high as 118, while the temperature was lowered. There was great pain, anxiety, pallid face, and symptoms indicating the presence of a mass on the side.

DR. FERNAND HENROTIN, of Chicago, said if there was any point in the paper to be criticised, it was to draw attention to one fact that was very striking, namely, it was absolutely necessary, when ectopic gestation was simulated, to carefully and completely analyze all points in a very deliberate manner. There was, no disease of the abdominal cavity in which the history of the case cut such a large figure. He could not emphasize too strongly the absolute importance of analyzing all the symptoms and of recognizing pregnancy by its usual signs, which was one of the things omitted so frequently in abdominal work in which pregnancy existed—as, for instance, the appearance of the breasts, the appearance of the vulva, the general characteristics indicative of pregnancy, etc. If there was one thing that had a tendency to mislead men in diagnosis, it was malposition of the uterus. He thought the essayist should have referred more to those cases in which extrauterine pregnancy was simulated but did not exist, and his mind naturally reverted to the many cases in which he had seen extrauterine pregnancy existing when he did not expect it. Several times he had been called upon to confirm a diagnosis of extrauterine pregnancy when there was apparently enlargement of one side of the uterus, but when it was simply retroverted and laterally inclined. Once intra-abdominal hemorrhage was diagnosed, the abdomen should be opened.

DR. WILLIS E. FORD, of Utica, N. Y., said that two cases had come under his observation recently which illustrated both phases of the question. The first case was put down as an operation for a fibroid with hemorrhage, in which the abdominal distension was considerable and the hemorrhage had been so profuse as to almost exsanguinate the patient. There was slight elevation of temperature. The physicians who had seen the woman judged that it was a case of fibroid from the history rather than from the physical signs. Physical examination by the family physician was not convincing. The speaker found what he thought was an ectopic gestation in the fourth or fifth month, with adhesion of the sac behind. He excised it, drained it, and got the fetus out all right. In cases of unruptured ectopic gestation he did not empty them, but excised, and drained off a small quantity of fluid, and in a few days it was gone.

Recently he had operated on another woman in a physician's office. She had been seized with pain a second time. She gave a history of pregnancy. She was a trained nurse originally, had borne two children, and supposed that she was pregnant again. The pain came on at about the seventh week of gestation, which was so severe that she fell and fainted and went into collapse in a water closet. The family physician thought the woman had a slight ruptured ectopic gestation. As soon as she was able to move about she was brought to the office of the family physician, and while there had another severe pain. The speaker was sent for at night, and on his arrival, after examination, thought the woman had a small ovarian tumor with twisted pedicle and hemorrhage. He operated and found a tumor as large as a double fist, which was easily lifted out of the abdomen. There were no adhesions or clots about it. A tuberculous mass surrounded the junction of the small and large intestines, in the midst of which was a ruptured appendix, also two or three ounces of pus. The adhesions to the intestines everywhere showed that it was a case of long standing. The adhesions were separated from the mass with difficulty, and in the midst of it was the ruptured appendix, which he tied off. The woman manifested all the symptoms which are generally attributed to ectopic gestation with rupture.

Dr. WALTER P. MANTON, of Detroit. Mich., had had two or three cases in which he had opened the abdomen for intraperitoneal hemorrhage after a diagnosis of ectopic gestation had been made, but ectopic gestation was not present. The most notable case he had had was published in the Transactions of the Southern Surgical and Gynecological Association in 1900. The patient had two distinct hemorrhages; she presented all the classical symptoms of ectopic gestation, even the colicky pains to which Dr. Grandin referred. The abdomen contained several quarts of blood clots, but there was no ectopic gestation. There was, however, a large ruptured vein at the lower portion of the broad ligament. Microscopic examination showed progressive fibroid degeneration of the ligament, this degeneration having begun below in the ligament, crept upward, and involved the upper portion of the ligament. Both tubes and ovaries were normal.

When called upon suddenly to see a case with intra-abdominal hemorrhage and obliged to operate immediately, one could not consider all the points in every case and make an accurate diagnosis. The diagnosis must be made from a scant history as to the previous condition of the patient.

Dr. JOSEPH E. JANVRIN, of New York, said that while he was probably the first man to recommend laparatomy for tubal pregnancy in its early stage, he did not claim any particular credit for it. He was driven to it by cases he had treated with galvanism. He found hemorrhage from the arteries in the peritoneal covering of the distended tube. The paper in which he recommended laparatomy in such cases was read before this Society in 1886 in Baltimore. In 1888 he reported additional cases. The principal points in diagnosis he alluded to at that time were similar to those that had been pointed out by Drs. Henrotin and Grandin, namely, symptoms of pregnancy plus colicky pains, plus tumor on either side, wherever it existed close to the uterus, evidently in the tube and ovary, strong pulsation in the tumor from its rapid growth, and distended arterial circulation.

CLINICAL REPORT UPON URETERAL SURGERY.

This was the title of a paper by Dr. CHARLES P. NOBLE, of Philadelphia.

CASE I. *Stone in the vesical portion of the left ureter; suprapubic cystotomy; incision of vesical wall and ureter; removal of stone; interrupted but good recovery.*—Family and personal history presented nothing of note. The bladder symptoms had persisted for nine years. From time to time she had been confined to bed. From November, 1891, to March, 1892, she was in

the Jefferson Hospital under the care of Dr. Parvin, who made a
fistula in the bladder, which was allowed to remain open for four
months and was then closed.   The symptoms were not at all improved.   The urine contained blood and pus.   Upon bimanual
examination a swelling could be felt in the region of the left
ureteral orifice.   The vagina was quite small from post-climac-
teric atrophy, and for this reason it was determined to open the
bladder by the suprapubic route.   As the stone was near the
ureteral orifice, the bladder wall and then the ureter were incised and the stone removed.   Drainage both by suprapubic
drainage tube and retention catheter was maintained.   The convalescence was interrupted by an attack of mania.   She made a
tedious convalescence, but when seen some months later was
entirely free from pain and bladder discomfort.

It is believed that this case is a type of many others in which a
stone in the vesical portion of the ureter has been mistaken for a
so-called encysted calculus of the bladder; or, in other words,
that many cases of supposed encysted calculus are really cases
of calculus in the ureter.

CASE II. *Ruptured tubal pregnancy; intraligamentous ovarian
cyst; hematocele partly subperitoneal; hysterectomy; removal of
lower half of ureter; ureter stitched in abdominal wound; subsequent nephrectomy; good permanent recovery.*—Abdominal section disclosed a ruptured tubal pregnancy and right intraligamentous ovarian cyst.   The patient's condition demanded a
rapid operation, which led to the removal of the ureter along
with the intraligamentous cyst.   The accident was discovered,
but the ureter was too short to implant into the bladder, even
had the patient not been in collapse.   It was therefore sutured
into the abdominal wall, and the kidney was removed by a lumbar incision at a later day.   The patient made a prompt recovery and has since enjoyed good health.

From the nature of the conditions present, the accident of removing the ureter in this case was probably inevitable.   Only
a careful, time-consuming operation would have prevented it, and
in the condition of the patient this would probably have led to a
fatal result.   In spite of later investigations concerning the implantation of the ureter into the bowel and the suggestion that
the ureter be implanted into the ureter of the opposite side, making a uretero-ureteral anastomosis, it was believed that under
similar conditions the plan adopted in this case was the best.
The ureter was so short that it would have been necessary to
select the cecum for implantation—a plan of procedure not warranted by the results of experimental studies.   The ureter was
too-short to implant into its fellow of the opposite side, even if
future experience should show that this operation gives good
results.

The writer's own experience with the permanent results of
nephrectomy when one kidney was sound, or even when it was
the seat of moderate degeneration from septic trouble, made him

believe that it was wiser to do a nephrectomy than to implant the ureter into the bowel. Such a procedure could properly be entertained when the remaining kidney was known to be diseased, or in the rare event of the patient having but one kidney.

CASE III. *Large multilocular bilateral ovarian cyst; double ovariotomy; injury of the right ureter; suture; death.*—The right cyst contained twenty-eight litres and the left four litres. The history was not definite, but it was probable that the tumors had been growing for six or eight years. In the course of the removal of the right cyst, which was partly intraligamentous, the right ureter was found to pass between two lobes of the tumor. Although the ureter was separated from the tumor with great care, its walls were so friable from edema that the lumen of the ureter was opened through perhaps one-third of the circumference of the duct. The rent was sutured and a vaginal subperitoneal drain was placed. The patient died about forty-eight hours after operation. There was no leakage of urine.

CASE IV. *Papillary cancerous tumor of the left ovary; occlusion of the ureter; atrophy of the kidney; division of ureter in removing tumor; recovery.*—The tumor formed a large mass filling the pelvis and lower abdomen. The cyst was peeled out of the left broad ligament, tied off, and removed. The left ureter was then found divided, but the patient was in such bad condition that it was deemed inadvisable to prolong the operation by the performance of ureteral anastomosis, and the end of the ureter was brought out of the abdominal incision, which was closed. No urine ever flowed from the kidney, showing that the kidney had undergone atrophy from the gradual pressure of the cancerous tumor upon the ureter. The patient made a good recovery from the operation, but her subsequent history was unknown.

The suturing of the ureter into the abdominal wall was not only justified by the result in this case, but was demanded by the condition of the patient.

CASE V. *Epithelioma of the cervix; combined hysterectomy; vesical and ureteral fistulæ; subsequent uretero-vesical anastomosis; recovery with vesical fistula.*—Examination showed an epithelioma advanced to the point at which it was doubtful whether or not a radical operation should be attempted. Vaginal hysterectomy was attempted. The vagina was extremely small and the cervical tissues so friable that volsella forceps would not hold. In attempting the separation of the bladder from the uterus an opening was made into the bladder. Owing to the lack of room in the vagina and the friable nature of the cervix, vaginal hysterectomy was abandoned and an abdominal hysterectomy was carried out. The bladder was sutured. The patient recovered from the operation and was discharged with a urinary fistula. When she was readmitted it was found that the fistula was ureteral in character. A uretero-vesical anastomosis was attempted. Etherization was very unsatisfactory, cyanosis and rigidity being present throughout the operation. It was soon evident that the operation had been attempted at too early a date, as there was extensive exudate in the pelvis, which greatly complicated the operation, making it much more difficult than ordinarily would be the case. In separating the bladder from the masses of exudate about it, an opening into the vagina had been made. The result of the operation was the cure of the ureteral fistula, but there resulted a small vesical fistula through which most of the urine still escaped. The patient had since refused operative treatment.

It was probable that the ureteral fistula in this case was caused by the thermo-cautery, although possibly due to the partial inclusion of the ureter in a ligature. The extensive exudate in the pelvis three months after the hysterectomy made the freeing of the ureter a matter of extreme difficulty, and would indicate that a secondary operation should not be attempted too soon after the formation of a ureteral fistula.

CASE VI. *Recurrent sarcoma of the uterus; hysterectomy; division of the left ureter; primary uretero-vesical anastomosis; perfect uretero-vesical union; death on the fifteenth day from chronic nephritis.*—Two years before coming under observation this patient was operated on in a neighboring city, the surgeon making a diagnosis of fibroid tumor. In a short time the tumor recurred, and the same surgeon operated a second time, making a diagnosis of recurrent fibroid. Seven months later a sloughing tumor was removed. The tumor filled the vagina and sprang from the posterior lip of the cervix. A diagnosis of sarcoma was made, which was confirmed by microscopical study of the tumor. Following the operation the patient was greatly prostrated and suffered from vomiting for ten days. During this time the urine contained hyaline and granular casts, and once epithelial casts. Two weeks later hysterectomy was performed by the combined method. It was evident that the left broad ligament was involved, and in the effort to keep beyond the area of infiltration the left ureter was divided. Primary uretero-vesical anastomosis was performed. A convenient point in the bladder was selected, the bladder was opened, the end of the ureter split, a transverse suture was passed through the anterior half of the ureteral end, and the two ends of the suture were passed through the bladder wall from within outward, so that when tied the ureter was fastened by a mattress suture to the vesical wall. Fine chromicized gut was used for this purpose. The bladder wall was then sutured with fine catgut and fine silk sutures, and a tension suture was passed fastening the bladder back to the peritoneum, so as to take tension off the ureteral sutures. The immediate operative recovery was entirely satisfactory. The anastomosis succeeded perfectly. The patient died, however, on the fifteenth day, of chronic nephritis. The technique of the uretero-vesical anastomosis was entirely satisfactory. The writer could see no possible improvement in the technique, unless it were to use two mattress sutures to fasten the ureter to the bladder wall, the one introduced through the anterior portion of the ureter as in this case, and the other through the posterior portion of the ureter, the free ends of each suture being passed from within outward through the bladder wall, the needle being introduced through the opening into the bladder. In spite of the fact that this patient died from chronic nephritis, she passed at least the average quantity of urine for some days after operation.

CASE VII. *Advanced epithelioma of the cervix; pregnancy advanced between fourth and fifth months; ovum dead; hemorrhages from the cavity of the uterus; vaginal hysterectomy; ligation of left ureter; death on the fourth day.*—It was evident that the left broad ligament was involved, and a radical operation would not have been done had it not been for the condition of pregnancy. A vaginal hysterectomy was not considered more dangerous than to empty the pregnant uterus through the sloughing cervical cancer. Owing to the involvement of the left broad ligament there was marked tendency to hemorrhage, and it was felt that some liberties were taken with the integrity of the left ureter. The amount of urine passed after operation did not indicate that the ureter had been tied, and there was no pain in the kidney involved. She died on the fourth day. Autopsy showed that the left ureter was occluded by one of the ligatures. The ureter and pelvis of the kidney were distended with urine. This was the only case in which it is known that a ureter had been tied in the experience of the writer, either in vaginal or abdominal hysterectomy.

CASE VIII. *Supposed calculus in left ureter; perforation of ureter and peritoneal cavity by ureteral catheter; celiotomy; no calculus found; ureter sutured; recovery.*—The personal and family history presented nothing of note. The history of the present attack was that she had had pain in the left side of the abdomen for over a year. The urine contained no blood nor albumin. An X-ray examination was made twice by Dr. Leonard, who reported a stone in the left ureter at or near the brim of the pelvis, and it was on this report that the patient was admitted for operation. The absence of blood in the urine was carefully noted, but the positive diagnosis by Dr. Leonard was accepted. A ureteral catheter was passed easily into the left ureter. This fact was also noted, but it was felt that the stone might be in a pocket in the ureter, which permitted the passage of the catheter. It was intended to pass a catheter into the ureter to serve as a guide in hunting for the ureter in doing an extraperitoneal operation. Some resistance was encountered in passing the catheter. A fair amount of pressure, which was not considered violence, was used, and the catheter seemed to pass readily. The peritoneal cavity was wounded accidentally, and the opportunity was taken to make an intraperitoneal examination in order to locate the stone. Instead of finding the stone,.

the ureteral catheter was found in the peritoneal cavity, showing that the ureter had been perforated. The ureter was carefully palpated, but no stone was found. The ureter was sutured with chromicized catgut. The ureter remained intact, there being no leakage through into the peritoneum or into the vagina. The original symptoms for which the operation was done still persisted. Should the writer encounter in the future a similar accident, he would perform uretero-vesical anastomosis in preference to suturing as in this case.

This case was reported to show two things: First, that perforation of the ureter was possible even when the catheter was passed by one having had considerable experience and when no apparent pressure was used. Second, that the report of an X-ray examination, even by an expert, was not absolutely reliable.

CASE IX. *Ureteral calculus, X-ray diagnosis; extraperitoneal operation; removal of stone; suturing of ureter; primary union; good recovery; stone situated two centimetres below brim of the pelvis.*—Personal and family history presented nothing of note. Two years ago the patient began having attacks of left renal colic with suppression of urine, which had recurred until the present time. At first the attacks came every two months and lasted two days, and recently they had come about every three months and lasted one day. Repeated examinations of the urine showed the constant presence of a moderate number of red blood cells. X-rays were taken three times by Dr. Leonard, who reported the presence of a stone in the left ureter at about the pelvic brim. An incision was made parallel with the course of the ureter, being partly above and partly below a line drawn from the umbilicus to the anterior superior spine of the ilium. The peritoneum was pushed off from the posterior wall of the abdomen until the iliac and abdominal vessels could be palpated. The ureter was not found upon the posterior wall of the pelvis, and was then sought in the fatty tissues behind the descending colon. The thickened ureter was found and traced into the pelvis. About two centimetres below the brim of the pelvis a stone was located. Having satisfied himself that the stone could not be displaced upward, the ureter was incised over the stone, which was removed. The incision into the ureter was then closed by interrupted fine chromicized catgut sutures, between each of which sutures a second suture of fine cumol catgut was placed. A small rubber tube was introduced and the abdominal wound closed with tier sutures. The patient made an uninterrupted recovery and was discharged on the twenty-sixth day.

This case contrasted strongly with the last in showing the importance of the X-ray in this department of surgery. In the last case an erroneous X-ray report was the cause of an unnecessary operation, and in this case it prevented the performance of an unnecessary operation. Without the X-ray a diagnosis of stone in the kidney would have been made, and the primary incision would have been a lumbar one to expose the kidney.

DR. FERNAND HENROTIN mentioned a case in which a well-known Chicago physician tied the ureter, in operating for the repair of a lacerated cervix, while going high up and pushing back the bladder.

DR. WILLIAM R. PRYOR stated that, as there were some moot points relative to the best methods of anastomosing the ureter, he desired to put on record the following case:

Mrs. H. F., aged 30, was admitted to the hospital March 24, 1902, and discharged April 29. Married eight years; had borne two children; oldest child 3 years old, youngest 7 months old. No miscarriages. First labor normal. Second labor difficult; in labor seventeen hours; no forceps used; had profuse hemorrhages after delivery. Suffered from severe pain in the abdomen, which radiated to the lumbar region and to the thighs; also constant hemorrhages during the past two months.

Past Personal History.—Negative until eight months ago; was at that time eight months pregnant and suffered from profuse leucorrhea. One month later the child was born. No bloody discharge during pregnancy. Labor was difficult. She had severe hemorrhage after delivery. Painful micturition for three weeks. In two weeks' time lochial discharge stopped, and patient did not notice any flow until two months ago, at which time she began to flow, and has been flowing ever since. Quantity slightly less than natural flow. No change in quality. No clots, except occasionally a small one, were passed at any time. Has had more or less pain in the pelvis since last delivery. Present illness began two months ago. Pain has increased gradually until two weeks ago, when it became unendurable. Pain in all pelvic organs, but most severe on the left side. The pain radiated to the lumbar region and down to the thighs. Severe pain on urination. The patient first menstruated at 14 years of age; regular; three days' duration. She suffered some pain up to the time of her first pregnancy. She has not ceased flowing during the past two months. Urinalysis: Specific gravity, 1029; urea, 1.5 per cent; pus, blood, and granular casts; albumin present. Specimen contaminated. Catheter specimen showed only pus.

Diagnosis: Squamous-cell epithelioma of the cervix and vagina, with involvement of parametrium and glands.

Upon the posterior vaginal wall, extending one and one-quarter inches below the cervical attachment to the vagina, was a corrugated nodule still covered with epithelium. The posterior lip of the cervix was livid, the difference in color between the posterior and anterior being very marked. Upon digital examination the posterior vaginal wall was found infiltrated, corresponding to the area of the corrugated nodule mentioned. Extending from this to the right side of the pelvis the parametrium was found thickened and the uterus immovably fixed.

Dr. Pryor opened the abdomen in the median line, the incision stopping one and one-half inches short of the umbilicus. He found glandular enlargements very distinct upon both sides at the bifurcations of the iliacs, and it was necessary to remove these glands before the iliacs could be exposed. Upon the right side the ureter was distended, so as to measure five-eighths of an inch in diameter, this hydroureter being evidently due to an obstruction of the ureter as it passed through the infiltrated broad ligament. He ligated the ovarian vessels, round ligaments, and internal iliacs, and then the obturators without very much difficulty. He found that the posterior cul-de-sac was so deep that the cancerous infiltration did not invade the rectum, but there was a clear portion of the vagina below the cancer. In attempting to separate the bladder from the uterus, he clearly demonstrated that it was impossible to release the ureter on the right side from the cancerous tissue. He therefore cut the ureter across one-quarter of an inch below the bifurcation of the right iliac and removed all the cancerous tissue in the right parametrium. The right ureter was again severed close to its insertion into the bladder and the stump ligated with kangaroo tendon. He found the uterus very friable, the entire cervical canal being infiltrated with cancer and tearing off under slight traction. He could not help soiling the field of operation by the cancer elements, much to his disappointment. However, he removed all the cancer, including the upper half of the vagina. He then dissected the bladder from the pubis, and made an incision just to the right of the median line transversely in that portion of the bladder covered by peritoneum. He passed two anchoring sutures of fine silk into the ureter at each side of its opening, and these same sutures again were passed through the mucous membrane of the bladder, this membrane being drawn out of the bladder by tenaculum one inch within the incision, so that when the sutures were tied the ureter was drawn well into the bladder. After this he approximated the peritoneum of the ureter to that of the bladder, and posteriorly the raw surface of the bladder to the raw surface of the ureter. He infused the patient with three quarts of saline solution, after closing the wound with through-and-through silver wire and introducing the self-retaining catheter. Time of operation, one hour and forty minutes.

May 15, 1902: Patient reported for examination. The vault of the vagina was found soft and elastic, but occupied by a few granulations due to the open treatment of the vaginal wound. Patient had gained in flesh, had no pain, and had to rise but twice during the night to relieve the bladder.

Dr. CHARLES JEWETT reported a case of Cesarean section and complete hysterectomy for cancer of the cervix, uretero-cystostomy, with recovery. The woman had been in labor for four days, in active labor for twenty-four hours. A cancerous growth involved the right and a portion of the anterior and posterior

24

aspects of the cervix.   The operation was performed in the night, with insufficient light.   The growth had extended somewhat further into the base of the right broad ligament than had been made out in the examination before delivery.   The ureter, which was enveloped in the growth and lifted with the uterus, was divided about one inch from the bladder.   An attempt was made to do a uretero-ureterostomy, but owing to the difficulty of manipulation, with poor light and deep down in the pelvic cavity, the attempt was abandoned.   The ureter was then implanted extraperitoneally in the base of the bladder higher up.   It was sutured with fine silk and covered with the anterior peritoneal flap.   The convalescence was entirely free from complications. The patient left the hospital at the end of four weeks, no leakage of urine having occurred.   The child was saved.

Dr. EDWARD REYNOLDS, of Boston, said that about two years ago Dr. E. C. Dudley reported a case in which the ureter was anastomosed into the bladder by the forcipressure method of Dudley.   When he saw and read Dudley's paper it impressed him as a very crude procedure.   He thought this was probably the reason why it had not gained ground.   Subsequent experience of his own, however, in which he adopted the method, prompted him to say that it was more expeditious, more secure in every way, and so much superior to the suture method that he thought it ought not to be overlooked in the discussion.   He reported a case in which he followed the Dudley method.

Dr. A. LAPTHORN SMITH reported a case of transplantation of the ureter by the Van Hook method, and his patient made a splendid recovery.

This paper was further discussed by DRS. REUBEN PETERSON, E. W. CUSHING, BACHE McE. EMMET, WILLIAM M. POLK, A. H. BUCKMASTER, J. WESLEY BOVÉE, B. B. BROWNE, who illustrated their remarks by the aid of blackboard diagrams, after which the discussion was closed by DR. NOBLE.

THE PRINCIPLES UNDERLYING THE REPAIR OF CYSTOCELE, AND AN OPERATION FOUNDED THEREON.

DR. EDWARD REYNOLDS, of Boston, Mass., read a paper with this title.   He said that there were two anatomical points which underlay success in the operation for cystocele, which were not original with him, but were worth reiterating.   The first point was, that to attain success we should ascertain and utilize the natural supports of the anterior wall instead of simply denuding and gathering together the overstretched portions; the second, that we should not only avoid using any part of the overstretched portion of the wall, but should actually excise and do away with it, both of which objects should be attained without the performance of an unnecessarily extensive or severe operation.   The anterior vaginal wall had naturally two fixed points of attachment.   The first, that of the lower end of the wall to the posterior surface of the pubes, was exceedingly firm and never yielded.

The second, the attachments of the upper end of the wall, was not so strong, but was sufficient for this purpose. In prolapse of the uterus all the attachments of the vault failed, but in prolapse complicated by cystocele we could not cure the cystocele without restoring the prolapse, and our experience of late years in the total extirpation of the uterus and upper portion of the vagina for cancer had taught us that the only attachment between the genital canal and the pelvic wall which was not readily separated with the finger was the insertion of the broad ligaments into the lateral edges of the uterus and the vault of the vagina. This only firm support of the vault was, then, the only upper point which could rationally be used in the restoration of the anterior wall. The utilization of the bases of the broad ligaments had, moreover, the very great incidental advantage that it not only relieved the uterus of the weight of the prolapsed anterior wall, but in itself tended to restore the prolapse by throwing the cervix backward. The first point in any operation should, then, be the attachment to each other of these two firm portions of the wall.

The second principle insisted upon was the excision of the weakened portion of the wall. The anterior wall in its natural condition was a short, firm fascial and muscular structure which extended from its origin at the firm bases of the broad ligaments to its still firmer pubic attachment, thus forming one of the strongest supports of the uterus and other pelvic organs.

In cystocele the condition found was that the central portion of the protrusion was covered by an overstretched, thinned, and weakened vaginal wall; thus the support of the uterus was weakened, while the base of the bladder had practically no support. The thin portion of the wall had lost its power of resistance to further stretching, and if we utilized for repair any part of this weakened portion of the wall we should have as a result a weak scar which was necessarily predisposed to further stretching.

Cystocele was in effect a hernia of the bladder through the muscular and fascial structures of the anterior wall of the vagina, and this second principle involved in dealing with it was essentially that which was already well established in the treatment of other hernias. It had been customary to treat cystocele by denuding the vaginal wall of its epithelium, invaginating the protrusion, and stitching the denuded surfaces together. No one would to-day think of treating any other hernia by denuding the protrusion of its surface epithelium, invaginating it, and sewing the surfaces together. We should not so treat the hernia of the bladder which we called cystocele. We were accustomed to treat other hernias by reducing them, and excising the sac until we laid bare strong, firmly attached fascial edges. We should so treat cystocele, if we could devise an operation which would enable us to do it without undue severity.

The essayist then described the operation, with the aid of numerous diagrams.

Dr. Isaac S. Stone, of Washington, D. C., read a paper entitled

ANTERIOR AND POSTERIOR COLPORRHAPHY BY A NEW METHOD.

Anterior Operation.—The vaginal wall is incised in the median line, and, after clamping the sides of this incision, the bladder is pushed away, upward and backward, until the entire base of the bladder is separated from the vaginal wall and from the anterior surface of the uterus, if desired. It is necessary to extend this separation as far out laterally as possible, for the whole pelvic roof shares in the prolapse. He proceeds now to lift the bladder with fingers or gauze packing, or with a sound inside the organ, as far upward as possible, to assure of the extent of liberation. The excessively long flaps which presented over the base of the bladder as a cystocele (the distended anterior vaginal wall) are now excised and the wound brought together edge to edge, taking care to entirely obliterate the cystocele and to leave the new anterior vaginal wall straight across. The method of applying the sutures is important, for the flaps are sutured near the centre of the wound to the anterior surface of the uterus with silkworm gut, silk, or chromicized catgut. This is done for the double purpose of holding the bladder high above the former attachment on the uterus, and to hold the uterus forward if it has been retroverted. The bladder is held away and the deep sutures passed through the uterine wall between the attachments of the round ligaments. The wound is then entirely closed with catgut sutures. It will be observed that the author has applied the Mackenrodt method of vaginal fixation to his operation, but it was primarily to hold the bladder higher upon the uterus rather than to cure the displacement. In very large cystoceles the vaginal wall is, of course, greatly lengthened, and one may shorten it by removing a V-shaped section from each side of the incision in front of the cervix. The longitudinal wound in the median line will then join one made transversely across the vagina in front of the cervix.

The Posterior Secondary Operation.—The injuries to the posterior vaginal wall and perineum differ greatly in their extent and in the direction of the tear. In short, the rent may be either longitudinal or transverse, and in any event needs to be fully exposed below the vaginal mucous membrane, which in the past has borne the brunt of surgical attack, while the fascia, the objective point, is hiding with the much-discussed and rarely seen levator ani muscle, and is only influenced by sundry excursions of needle and suture, which, after all, only hold a denuded or scarified mucous membrane together while union progresses. The crest of the rectocele is grasped with the left hand, making a transverse fold, which is divided with the scissors down to the rectum. Clamps are applied to the edges of the incision, and the rectum pushed away on both sides with a gauze sponge until it is quite free from all connection with the vaginal wall. The incision in the vaginal wall is extended above and below until sufficient narrowing of the vagina is secured to answer the purpose in view. The sutures are placed with greater facility when the rectum is separated freely on each side, and one need have no fear of not obtaining good union after the operation. After liberating the rectum and having clamped such hemorrhoidal vessels as give trouble, the wound is closed in the following manner: With tissue forceps (or tenacula, if preferred) the operator catches up two points, one on either side, which he wishes to unite in front of the rectum. These points are usually about one and one-half inches below the edge of each flap, but the size of the rectocele will necessitate a test in each case as directed, so that we may secure good approximation of the fascia over the rectum, and not. however, exert undue traction upon the sutures. The fascia is firmly and thoroughly united along the entire length of the wound. In some instances the speaker has used a double tier of sutures, which gives excellent support to the floor of the vagina and makes a firm obstruction to the exit of a procident uterus. After the buried sutures are placed, he excises the long flaps from each side and closes the vaginal incision with interrupted catgut down to, and rather below the former site, of the crest of the rectocele. Emmet's or Hegar's method may now be selected for the final stage of the operation, according to the predilections of the operator. The operation in some respects resembles that of Hegar, the chief difference being in the method of exposing the fascia.

Dr. REUBEN PETERSON, of Ann Arbor, Mich., read a paper entitled

A CONSIDERATION OF OVARIAN FIBROMATA, BASED ON A STUDY OF TWO RECENT CASES AND EIGHTY-TWO COLLECTED FROM THE LITERATURE.

In order to study the clinical features of ovarian fibroma, eighty-two cases of this disease were collected and tabulated by the writer. To these were added two recent cases occurring in his own practice. Only those cases pronounced fibromatous by careful microscopic examination or proved to be so by competent observers were selected. Borderland cases of ovarian cystic disease were excluded, as it was the purpose of the article to study solid ovarian fibromata presenting no or slight cystic degeneration.

The writer's first case was a woman of 64, who noticed a growth in the lower left abdomen five years previous to her entrance to the hospital. The growth had increased in size until it reached the border of the left ribs. There was little or no pain, in fact very little discomfort from the growth. Operation, December 24, 1901, disclosed a large tumor of the left ovary weighing seven and one-quarter pounds. The tumor was bilobed, the smaller lobe being edematous. The larger tumor showed points of calcification. Microscopic examination showed the tumor to be a fibroma. The patient made an uneventful recovery.

In the second case the patient was 61 years of age and entered the hospital for distension from ascitic fluid, of four years' standing. During this time she had been tapped sixty-five times. At the operation, April 25, 1902, was found an irregular, hard, fibromatous tumor of the left ovary which weighed three pounds. There were a few adhesions present, and the other ovary was the size of a hen's egg from a surface papilloma. Seven hundred cubic centimetres of clear ascitic fluid were removed at this time. The microscopic examination showed an ovarian fibroma of the left side. Except for an attack of gallstone colic, proved by the passage of four gallstones, the patient made an uneventful recovery.

The essayist then dwelt on the frequency, age, menstrual history, etc., in connection with fibroma of the ovary; also social state and fecundity.

The author thought that neither menorrhagia nor metrorrhagia was a very constant accompaniment of fibroma of the ovary. It was more apt to occur where both ovaries were affected by the disease. An ovarian fibroma might grow for many years before the tumor reached large proportions or gave rise to marked symptoms. In other cases the growth was more rapid, reaching considerable proportions and giving rise to noticeable symptoms in a comparatively short time, say a few months. Pain was present to a greater or less degree in nearly one-half the cases of ovarian fibromata. Freedom from pain meant, as a rule, the absence of adhesions of the growth to the surrounding organs. Pain was more frequently met with in tumors of moderate size. Dysuria was a symptom in about 15.6 per cent of the cases.

DR. MATTHEW D. MANN had seen six cases of fibroma of the ovary upon which he had operated, in each of which there was ascites. In the first there was so much ascites that he could hardly recognize the tumor. The tumor was situated deep in the pelvis; he could touch and feel something hard through his incision, and found, after getting the fluid out, there was a fibroid of the ovary. This was the first case he had operated upon.

DR. WILLIAM T. HOWARD, of Baltimore, had seen three cases of fibroma of the ovary, in each of which there was a large amount of ascitic fluid. All of his cases recovered. Sir Spencer Wells, he said, out of twelve hundred ovariotomies, saw but three cases of fibroma of the ovary. The late Dr. William Goodell saw three. Fibroma of the ovary was a rare condition.

DR. GEORGE J. ENGELMANN, of Boston, mentioned one case on account of the diagnostic difficulties. It differed from the cases that had been mentioned in that it closely resembled a uterine fibrocyst. There were no adhesions. It was not impacted, so that the uterus and tumor moved together. The solidity of the tumor and its movability with the uterus led to the diagnosis of a fibroid of the uterus. The uterus was elongated, very much enlarged, and there were menorrhagia and metrorrhagia. The case was operated upon in 1874. The pedicle was small. There was no ascites. He had seen two other cases of fibroma of the ovary in a clinic in Berlin, with no ascitic fluid in the abdominal cavity. In his case it was curious to note that one portion of the tumor was cystic and the other had undergone colloid degeneration.

DR. FERNAND HENROTIN had had the opportunity of operating on three cases of fibroma of the ovary. Two of them were small tumors, not larger than a medium-sized orange. The other one was large. In this case there was very little ascites. In the other two cases there was more or less ascites associated with the tumor, in one particularly, the whole abdominal cavity being completely filled. The tumor in this case could only be felt at times when in a certain locality. He had seen ascites occur in other forms of tumors in the abdomen, and it was a question whether ascites was not caused by the local irritation of the small tumor floating around and rubbing up against the peritoneum.

DR. J. WHITRIDGE WILLIAMS had likewise seen three cases of ovarian fibromata, not exceeding an orange in size. In two cases the tumor was completely calcified. He exhibited these two tumors before the Society some years ago. In the calcified case the tumor was not more than two inches in diameter, and the woman suffered from marked ascites. Since then he had seen a third tumor of the ovary which corroborated the conclusions of Dr. Peterson that they occur in early life. The patient was a young married woman, 24 years of age, and pregnant for the first time. She complained of some discomfort during pregnancy. He examined her carefully and made a diagnosis of ovarian tumor. He operated, found an ovarian fibroma, pregnancy went on to term, and the woman was delivered.

DR. BACHE McE. EMMET, of New York, recalled one case of multiple fibroids—he believed there were seven. These were movable. They were absolutely drowned in ascitic fluid. He could not recall having seen a case of a pure fibroma of the ovary. He mentioned a case of spindle-cell sarcoma of the ovary the size of an adult head. The patient was a woman of 60. There was no ascites.

DR. SETH C. GORDON, of Portland. Me., had had two cases of fibroid of the ovary, one about ten inches in diameter. It was a myofibroma. The other was three inches in diameter and was a pure fibroid of the ovary. There was no ascites in either case.

DR. A. LAPTHORN SMITH said that when he found ascites associated with an abdominal tumor he considered it strong presumptive evidence in favor of its being malignant. He mentioned one case of fibroma of the ovary in which there was no ascites; also another case in which he was called to see a woman who was gasping for breath. She was sitting in a chair. He drew off two pails of fluid with a small trocar, and found two tumors, one as large as an adult's head, the other as big as that of a child. On examination he found indications of malignant degeneration. He believed that where ascites was associated with these tumors the chances were that the tumor is either malignant or beginning to be so.

DR. ANDREW F. CURRIER mentioned a .case which occurred in the practice of Dr. Thomas twenty years ago at the Woman's Hospital. It was one of the first cases of fibroma of the ovary reported. The tumor was the size of a small orange. The woman was large, apparently in perfect health with the exception of the presence of a large quantity of ascitic fluid in the abdomen and an umbilical hernia. The tumor was movable. The diagnosis was made by Dr. Thomas before operation. The case seemed a favorable one for operation and recovery, but unfortunately the woman died.

DR. PETERSON, in closing the discussion, said many cases had been reported in the literature of so-called fibroma of the ovary which he had to ignore, for the simple reason that he had to take some standard, and this was a microscopical examination.

As to the cause and frequency of ascites, he mentioned that ascites occurred in five per cent of all the cases, thus confirming the conclusions of Dr. Henrotin. Large tumors of the ovary did not produce the greatest amount of ascites. The cause of the ascites had not yet been proved. Whether it is due to the irritation from the movements of the growth, or not, was mere speculation.

DR. PHILANDER A. HARRIS, of Paterson, N. J., followed with a paper on

THE CLOSURE OF SUPPURATING ABDOMINAL WOUNDS FOLLOWING LAPARATOMIES.

The author stated that when abscess formed in the abdominal incision the skin was reopened in the line of incision to the upper and lower limits of the mural abscess. The wound was then treated as an open one until the flow of pus became greatly reduced in quantity. All the granulations were then removed with a sharp curette until the muscle, fascia, fat, and other tissues were recognizable. The separated edges of the deep fascia were then drawn together by a series of silkworm-gut sutures, which interlocked each other at the apposition line of the fascia. Each one of these sutures was introduced through the skin about one inch away from the incision, and each one was brought out either just above or below the point of its introduction. If the first suture both entered and emerged from the right of the median line, the next one was introduced and emerged at a point to the left of the incision, and was so introduced as to interlock the first or preceding suture. The third suture was introduced and brought out from the same side as the first suture, and interlocked the second one. The fourth suture was introduced from the same side as the second suture and interlocked the third or preceding one. This singular suture had for its chief object the coaptation of the deep fascia, and, when properly introduced and tied, it was claimed that the fat and opposing edges of the skin fell in apposition, adhered and healed without additional sutures. Most of the few cases thus treated promptly healed and generally did so without suppuration. A not unimportant part of the technique of operation was the thorough and repeated washing with solution of bichloride of mercury, always followed by a normal salt solution irrigation. The stitches were all removed on the twelfth and fourteenth days.

Fifteen photographs illustrated much of Dr. Harris' work in this relation. A not uninteresting part of the photographic illustrations was the appearance of the wound after the sutures were introduced and tied, as they converted the area of the opened and large wound into an elongated mound at whose base on either side there appeared a row of knots, while at the summit of the mound the opposing edges of skin simply lay in apposition awaiting adhesion and healing.

Dr. Harris was of the opinion that the stronger solutions of carbolic acid or possibly other disinfectants might serve as good if not a better purpose than the solution of bichloride of mercury which he had employed for this work.

Dr. Clement Cleveland said that if the case was one of suppurative pelvic disease, the abdomen, the intestines, and the abdominal wound should be carefully protected with sterilized gauze pads. It was his habit always to put the patient in the Trendelenburg position, to draw the intestines as far back as he could toward the diaphragm, and to cover over a portion of the intestines with sterilized pads, having these pads wet with sterilized water or normal salt solution. He was also careful to cover the incision with sterilized gauze. In these cases he made a large incision, in order to have ample room to deal with all the structures in the pelvis.

In regard to closing the abdominal wound, in long operations he used the through-and-through suture to gain time, employing for this purpose silkworm gut almost exclusively. He passed every other suture through all the layers, and the alternate sutures through merely the fascia, bringing the fascial edges closely together; by that means they could be coaptated. This was first suggested by Dr. Wylie, and he had found it an excellent method in addition to every other suture through the fascial edges. He had never known a ventral hernia to follow this method.

As to closing wounds by layers, he believed that in many cases where he had had suppurating wounds it was due to the closure of the fascia in later years, and it was because he had employed either chromicized kangaroo tendon or chromicized gut. Chromicized gut often contained free chromin, which would certainly produce more or less irritation and sloughing. He had also found that some chromicized gut contained micro-organisms which were a fruitful source of suppuration. He had always been careful not to suture the fasciæ very closely together or to draw the edges very tightly together. If the fascial edges were drawn tightly together sloughing would occur.

Since the introduction of the rubber glove he believed that one very fertile source of infection had been eliminated.

He had never ventured to close by sutures an abdominal wound that was opened by suppuration. He watched such cases carefully, and, after pus had ceased discharging, he used some stimulating application, such as balsam of Peru, and drew the edges together very carefully with elastic straps. He could not recall a wound that had not perfectly closed after this method was resorted to, the line of incision being almost the same as though it were brought together by sutures.

Dr. J. M. Baldy wondered if it was not true that the decrease in the number of suppurative abdominal wounds, which was attributed to the use of rubber gloves, was not coincident with our better knowledge, the infliction of less traumatism to the fat, and the greater care taken now in handling wounds than formerly. He did not use rubber gloves very much, but he was extremely careful to cover the edges of the fat of a wound with gauze pads, so as to prevent bruising. He could not see why a man's hands could not be made clean enough for ordinary abdominal surgery without necessitating the use of the rubber glove.

He had never reoperated on a suppurating wound after an appendicitis operation. He left these wounds open. He had witnessed this: that as soon as the sinus had closed, after the drain was taken out and the appendical abscess had ceased discharging, if he had a large wound in the flank (and he left a large wound for the purpose of enabling him to see the sinus), almost as soon as the pus had ceased discharging from the abdominal wound one could begin to clean the fat and let it close. If the fat was kept clean and stripped it would close in two or three days a very long incision. He did not wish to be understood as saying that he had never seen any hernias follow open wounds for appendical abscess. However, he had seen only one or two.

So far as the closure of the abdominal wound was concerned, he believed one of the reasons why gynecologists used to have more stitch-hole abscesses and occasionally more suppuration than now was that dead spaces were left; but after beginning the use of tier sutures, sewing up the peritoneum first with catgut, and sewing the aponeurosis of the muscle with the same catgut, then using silkworm gut for the last tier of sutures, there were less stitch-hole abscesses and suppuration of wounds. His habit was to attach the last tier of sutures to the aponeurosis of the muscles, so as not to leave any dead spaces.

Dr. William E. Moseley, of Baltimore, stated that his method of closing the abdominal wound was different in some particulars from that of the essayist, and illustrated it by the aid of blackboard diagrams.

Dr. Fernand Henrotin said he varied the method of closure of the abdominal wound in accordance with the condition of the wound. In a large gaping wound, where there was a tendency to oozing, he put in a suture, going through all the structures, but not tying until the end, putting the layers in tiers, including both peritoneum and fascia, and afterward using horsehair sutures between the through-and-through supporting sutures. This prevented oozing, as also gaping of the wound. Where he had a wound that fell well together, that did not gape or bleed much, in the hospital with which he was connected they employed Brown's aluminum wire, using three wires, inserted as the essayist did his silkworm-gut suture, beginning half an inch below the wound, one passing underneath the muscle approximating the peritoneum, the next layer approximating the fascia, the next being subcuticular and bringing the skin thoroughly together as does any subdermal stitch. When the wound fell well together, all that was necessary was to bring the fascia together and then the other parts. The wire which pierced the skin was taken out at the end of two weeks.

Dr. Robert A. Murray called attention to the importance of avoiding traumatism to the edges of the wound during the operation.

Dr. Reuben Peterson spoke a word or two in defence of the rubber glove. He was a great believer in its use in surgery for the purpose of guarding against suppurating abdominal wounds. He knew from his own experience that the rubber glove was of inestimable value, and that ordinary wound suppuration was not more than one-half as frequent as formerly.

As to chromicized catgut, he did not think it had a place in the closure of the abdominal wound. He had gotten suppuration from it repeatedly when he was quite sure he and everything else were clean. Closure of the wound with catgut in different layers, then either a subcuticular stitch or an interrupted silkworm-gut suture, gave a good result.

Dr. Seth C. Gordon was very much afraid to close a suppurating wound in the way the essayist had described. It seemed to him unsafe. With reference to closing abdominal wounds, he used silkworm gut from within out, including the peritoneum, and always passed his needle from within out, never from without in. He then closed the fascia, including a portion of the muscle with it, with a small catgut running suture, and had never seen any trouble from it. He then tied his catgut sutures outside; he put in no intermediate sutures ordinarily, because if one took the forceps and pulled up the wrinkled portion to the median line where the suture wrinkled a little, he would straighten it out and intermediate sutures would not be needed. He left these sutures from two to three weeks, never less than two. He said that, according to Dr. J. Collins Warren, it requires at least three weeks to get absolute repair of tissue. Since he had followed that method of closing abdominal wounds he had seen no hernias, no stitch-hole abscesses, etc.

The paper of Dr. Harris was further discussed by Drs. Wil-

LIAM H. BAKER, EMORY MARVEL, MATTHEW D. MANN, J. WESLEY
BOVÉE, and A. LAPTHORN SMITH, and the debate was closed by
DR. HARRIS.

The following officers were elected for the ensuing year: *President*, Dr. Joseph E. Janvrin, of New York City; *Vice-Presidents*,
Dr. Edward W. Jenks, of Detroit, Mich., and Dr. A. Palmer
Dudley, of New York City; *Secretary*, Dr. J. Riddle Goffe, of
New York City; *Treasurer*, Dr. J. M. Baldy, of Philadelphia, Pa.
Washington, D. C., was selected as the place for holding the next
annual meeting, in connection with the Triennial Congress of
Physicians and Surgeons, May, 1903.

TRANSACTIONS OF THE
CHICAGO GYNECOLOGICAL SOCIETY.

Meeting of April 18, 1902.

The President, LESTER E. FRANKENTHAL, M.D., *in the Chair.*

CONSERVATIVE CESAREAN SECTION.

DR. JOSEPH B. DE LEE.—A primipara, aged 19, unmarried, had
been in labor from April 3 at 5 P.M., and the pains had continued at intervals of ten minutes during the night. The following morning, at 8 o'clock, the bag of waters ruptured, after
which the pains recurred at six-minute intervals. She vomited
several times during the day. Her pulse in the morning was
100, in the evening 94; temperature 98°. A diagnosis of face
presentation being made by the house physician, a careful examination was instituted at 8:30 on April 4. The following were
the findings: The woman was 4 feet 7 inches in height (137 centimetres); interspinal diameter, 22 centimetres; intercristal,
25 centimetres; bitrochanteric, 29 centimetres; Baudelocque,
18½ centimetres; diagonal conjugate, 10¼ centimetres; bi-
ischiatic, 6¼ centimetres; sacro-subpubic, 10 centimetres; circumference, 81 centimetres. True conjugate was estimated at 8¾
centimetres. On internal examination pelvis was found to be
very small, so that the inlet could be spanned with the two vaginal fingers. The sacrum had an infantile shape; there was a
distinct bowing-in of the inlet on both sides, at the site of the
ilio-pubic tubercle. The head was in a right occipito-posterior
position, with extreme flexion, so extreme that the small fontanelle was in the mid-line, and even, I think, a little to the left
of the middle line; the forehead could be felt abdominally high
up upon the left side. The baby was estimated to weigh 6½
pounds. Ossification of the head was very well marked. The
head was not engaged, but movable. Upon removing the fingers

from the vagina this little body came away upon the finger (exhibiting). It had a white color at the edge. What it was we did not know. A microscopical examination is to be made of it. I believe, however, it will turn out to be a cervical polyp which was flattened during pregnancy and was broken off by the frequent and strong labor pains.

Dr. Watkins was kind enough to see the case with me, and confirmed the diagnosis in all its points. There was a generally contracted pelvis; probably no rachitis. With a conjugata vera of $8\frac{3}{4}$ centimetres, and with marked lateral contraction, the baby was too large to come through unmutilated. That being the case, and since the woman was in good condition, an operation aiming to save the life of the child was to be selected, and the choice lay between Cesarean section and symphyseotomy. Owing to the fact that the bi-ischiatic diameter was $6\frac{1}{4}$ centimetres, the woman being a rather tightly built young person, it was decided to perform Cesarean section as the operation least likely to leave permanent damage. It was admitted, however, that the case was not as favorable as it might be, the patient being already three hours in labor. The operation was performed at midnight of that same day. A median anterior abdominal incision was made and the uterus was delivered through the small opening in the abdomen. We then determined that the placenta was on the anterior wall by the course of the round and broad ligaments. The median anterior incision was made, which went through the placenta, and there was considerable hemorrhage. The child was delivered as usual. It gasped while the head was still *in utero*—the first time such an occurrence has happened to me in the Cesarean sections I have done. Usually the child has been in a condition of apnea, but this child made a gasp while its head was *in utero*, and sucked some of the uterine contents into its bronchi. As I have said, there was considerable hemorrhage, which was with difficulty controlled. Massage, hot applications, and ergot hypodermatically were resorted to. Three layers of sutures were placed—a buried continuous catgut suture, then an interrupted catgut suture taking in the peritoneum and part of the muscle, then a superficial peritoneal running catgut suture, more or less a Lembert. The abdominal wall was closed in three layers. The patient was in good condition when she left the table. The baby was a girl. I have its cephalic measurements: Biparietal, $9\frac{1}{2}$ centimetres; bitemporal, 8 centimetres; occipito-frontal, 12 centimetres; suboccipito-bregmatic, $10\frac{1}{2}$ centimetres; occipito-mental, $13\frac{1}{2}$ centimetres. Circumferences of the head: suboccipito-bregmatic, $30\frac{1}{2}$ centimetres, and occipito-frontal, 34 centimetres. As was estimated, the child weighed $6\frac{3}{8}$ pounds; length of its body, 48 centimetres.

The woman immediately after labor felt very well, and was laughing when I left her; within a few hours thereafter the temperature and pulse arose, and the patient presented signs of serious illness. She was vomiting profusely; had a distended abdomen, with pains in the abdomen, and pulse varying from 140 to 150. Temperature rose to 102° several times the first three or four days. I have here the temperature chart, which shows that the case pursued an irregular course of fever, running from 99° to 101° in the evening. Pulse has remained below 100 for the last ten days, and the temperature now presents a normal curve. The sutures were removed on the eleventh day; primary union throughout. The child was alive at the time of discharge.

Dr. Thomas J. Watkins.—I had the privilege of controlling the hemorrhage in Dr. De Lee's case during the incision in the uterus and the delivery of the child and placenta, and also in a recent case operated by Dr. C. B. Reed, by manual compression of the broad ligaments. I was much surprised at the ease with which both of the broad ligaments could be grasped with one hand. In Dr. Reed's case some of the amniotic sac had apparently presented into the vagina, and was grasped by the hand which held the broad ligaments, so that for a brief time the condition simulated adhesions of the sac. In both cases the manual compression seemed to interfere with the contraction of the uterus, which is accounted for by the interruption of the arterial blood supply and the venous circulation. It would seem that this disturbance of the circulation would cause more loss of blood than would occur from incision of the uterus without any compression of the blood vessels. The elastic ligature that was formerly used would be more objectionable than manual compression.

Dr. Gustav Kolischer.—The indications for Cesarean section in this case were quite clearly pointed out by Dr. De Lee, and, considering the conditions given, I am sure symphyseotomy would not have given as favorable a result as the other operation. With reference to the technique, I will mention two points: One, the constriction of the lower uterine segment by means of an elastic cord, or the temporary compression of the broad ligaments in order to control hemorrhage. This has been abandoned for two reasons—first, because the child becomes easily asphyxiated by the interference with the blood supply; second, if we compress the ligaments energetically there will always be a paresis of the blood vessels following this compression. We observe the same in other surgical instances. I am sure the hemorrhage in the reported case was due to this compression. If we do not use any of those preventive measures, the hemorrhage stops quite soon of its own accord by the contraction of the walls of the blood vessels and by the retraction of the uterine muscle. So far as suturing is concerned. I would like to take exception to the use of running sutures. On account of retraction of the uterine muscle a part of the tissue which is caught in the loop of such a suture may slip, or if one part of the suture is closed too tightly the enclosed tissue may slough. On the other hand, if infection starts at one point we are sure it will run along the whole line of the stitches.

Dr. De Lee (closing the discussion).—The point Dr. Kolischer made regarding a running suture in Cesarean section is well taken. There are other accoucheurs who advance the same objection. The reason a running suture was taken in this case was on account of hemorrhage. An incision was made through the placental site; there were a number of bleeding sinuses which had to be closed, and I found that I could not close them fast enough with an interrupted suture, so I rapidly ran down the whole length of the uterine wall with a running suture, which controlled the hemorrhage so well that we could put in interrupted sutures, taking more time to insert them, so that this patient got the benefit of an interrupted suture. Where there is the least suspicion of sepsis in a Cesarean section, when it does not amount to more than a suspicion, it is wise to make as complete a closure of the uterine wall as possible and use three layers of sutures.

With reference to compressing the broad ligaments to arrest hemorrhage, I have learned my lesson regarding it in performing Cesarean section, and I shall dispense with it hereafter. In one case an assistant compressed the uterus, or rather the broad ligaments, so vigorously that he ran his thumb through the peritoneum into the connective-tissue spaces of the broad ligament, necessitating several sutures to close the rent.

I have been asked why I did not make a Fritsch incision in the uterus. I have done so and found that I had just as much hemorrhage as by making the other incision. The matter of making a Fritsch incision went through my mind at the time, as the placenta was on the anterior wall, but I saw no particular advantage in making the fundal incision. A transverse fundal incision would have gone along the edge of the placenta, and the difference in the size of the sinuses is not worth while considering.

With reference to delivering the uterus, in all cases of emergency Cesarean sections the uterus should be delivered and the peritoneal cavity protected from infection by cloths. You may open the uterus *in situ,* where it has not been infected before operation, as there is no danger of meconium and uterine secretions escaping into the peritoneal cavity.

A CASE OF ANENCEPHALUS.

Dr. Charles S. Bacon.—At the last meeting of the Society I showed a specimen of cranio-rachischisis. I have another one, this time a case of anencephalus, which was delivered a few hours ago, that I desire to show this evening. I present this case largely on account of the peculiar history of the patient, as having a possible bearing on the etiology. The patient, a primipara 30 years of age, is said to have had peritonitis when 14 years of age, since which time she has been well, except for some trouble with the stomach, of which very great belching is the prominent feature. She was married in August, 1900, and menstruated last on August 6, 1901, as much as usual. She had nausea on September

18, which continued until November 27, and was quite severe. The baby was born to-day, about four weeks before term. She felt fetal movements on January 2. At no time was I able to make out either the position of the child or any heart tones. About the first of March she had a great deal of disturbance, very much pain, and did not sleep for several days. Then suddenly she became much better and attributed her improvement to some salol powders which I had given her, but no fetal movements were noticed for the last month.

A peculiarity was the shape of the uterus; it was triangular, very much enlarged, and on each corner the enlargements were very marked. A suspicion of molar pregnancy occurred to me because of the inability to make out any fetal parts, although the hydramnion prevented an entirely satisfactory examination. For the last month she had had very marked uterine contractions; but labor may be said to have begun on Wednesday evening last, and continued until delivery at about 4 o'clock this afternoon— that is, about forty-six hours. There was nothing conspicuous about the labor. The impossibility of determining anything about the child beforehand was a marked feature of the case.

FIBROID TUMOR OF THE UTERUS.

DR. ALBERT GOLDSPOHN.—I have two rather interesting specimens which were recently removed. The first, the largest fibroid tumor of an ovary I have seen, was removed on March 31. The woman was 38 years of age, multipara, and well nourished. Bimanual examination led me to make a probable diagnosis of dermoid tumor of the ovary. The tumor lay anterior to the uterus, extending up not quite to the umbilicus, crowding the uterus to the right and backward, and being rather harder than we usually expect a glandular cystoma of the ovary to be. It proved to be a large fibroid, weighing one pound and ten ounces, which consumed the entire ovary. No vestige of ovary could be seen. The tumor was attached by a slender pedicle and removed with the greatest ease.

The case is interesting, I think, because genuine cases of fibroid tumors of the ovary constitute only about two or three per cent of all ovarian neoplasms.

BROAD-LIGAMENT FIBROID.

The other tumor is a broad-ligament fibroid. The case presented some clinical features such as I have never met with before, viz., prolonged suppression of urine by pressure against the neck of the bladder. It was evident that a fibroid existed somewhere in the uterus; but on examination of this woman, who was 50 years of age and who had had a child thirty years before, the condition within the vagina was very much as in a woman eight months advanced in pregnancy, with a very short, soft, stubby cervix presenting at the middle of the vaginal inlet, and the upper part of the cervix expanded. It appeared to me that I was dealing with a uterus with one or more fibroids posteriorly, and also a cystic ovarian tumor in front of it. In making an incision about four inches in length, there was beneath the entire length of the incision something that looked very much like some ovarian cysts, very much engorged with veins, and different from a cyst, however, in its consistence, in not being membranous, but thick-walled, of rather doughy, edematous structure. Examining for its attachments, it was evident that this mass was extraperitoneal, and it was soon demonstrated that it was the bladder; by simply squeezing upon it urine was extruded (several ounces), which could not be obtained by means of a catheter which was passed immediately before making the incision. This patient had had retention of urine some three months ago, and at that time required to be catheterized for a week or more; and recently, before coming to the hospital, she was troubled in the same way for nearly two weeks, and she came with a very pronounced cystitis of old standing which had infiltrated the bladder walls to that extent. The tumor was found to be this (exhibiting) lobulated fibroid, two pieces separated completely from each other, the tumor having developed entirely within the right broad ligament. The uterus is not enlarged, as it usually is with a fibroid of this size, because the fibroid lay entirely outside of its walls, and therefore this patient did not have the usual menorrhagia and metrorrhagia—a feature which cast some doubt upon the presence of a fibroid, in the diagnosis. In removing the tumor we first ligated the ovarian arteries which were accessible; the bladder was then detached from the tumor anteriorly. But with the tumor in the broad ligament the uterine arteries were wholly inaccessible. Therefore I simply incised the capsule of the tumor and enucleated that first. This allowed the whole mass in the region of the cervix to rise higher in the pelvis, and made it comparatively easy to ligate the uterine arteries and to do a supravaginal amputation. Both patients have had very smooth, normal recoveries, one of them being now about to go home.

DR. EMIL RIES.—Why was the uterus removed?

DR. GOLDSPOHN.—This was the case of a woman 50 years old.

DR. RIES.—I would like to ask Dr. Goldspohn whether he removes the uterus in every woman who is 50 years of age.

DR. GOLDSPOHN.—I would in such cases as this, because it is perfectly useless, and the operation is safer.

DR. FRANKENTHAL.—Do you not think that the uterine artery would have been accessible if you had started on the side on which the fibroid was not? Suppose it were right-sided, and you had operated on the left side of the broad ligament, ligating it off from that side, you would have struck the uterine artery on that side, which is frequently done.

DR. PALMER FINDLEY.—This ovary reminded me of a specimen which Dr. D. W. Graham removed at the Presbyterian Hospital. The specimen was fully as large as this tumor.

25

DR. GOLDSPOHN.—In answer to the question of Dr. Frankenthal, one side of the uterus was about as accessible as the other in the region of the uterine arteries, because the uterus itself was crowded against the left pelvic wall, and there was no advantage in trying to ligate the uterine artery before enucleating the tumor. Enucleation of the tumor was readily done and did not add to the danger of hemorrhage. After the tumor was enucleated the other parts became flaccid, so that they could be drawn upward, and a very material advantage was gained, such as Doyen obtains sometimes by his technique of drawing the cervix into the abdomen and upward through an incision in the cul-de-sac. The ligation of the uterine arteries is then much easier, and, what is more important, we can do it with perfect safety and not endanger the ureters. To tie the uterine arteries before the tumor was enucleated would have been practically an impossibility, and would have endangered the ureters in such a manner that I would then have chosen not to remove the uterus.

DR. S. L. WEBER reported

A CASE OF OBSTETRICS.

About three weeks ago I saw a case of obstetrics that presented some unusual features. I was called one evening to see a woman who, the messenger stated, was dying. It was a woman whom I had operated upon about two years before for appendicitis. When I arrived at the patient's house I found a woman with an enormously distended abdomen and in labor pains. Her pulse was about 160 and weak, her eyes deeply sunken, and the features pale and pinched; she was breathing with difficulty and rapidly. She was sitting on the edge of the bed, supported by her husband who was sitting beside her. The history I gathered was the following: She was pregnant, had been feeling as she had been during her former pregnancies (this was her sixth), and labor came on at about the expected time. Three and a half days ago she first felt labor pains. At first they were irregular, but in a few hours became of fair force and regularity. She called a midwife. Very soon after labor pains began she began to vomit, and ever since she had not been able to retain anything on the stomach; even a little water would be promptly expelled. As there was no progress in the case and the woman was becoming weak, they called in a physician the next morning. The physician examined her and said that there was nothing to do, that pains would soon increase in strength and the child be expelled. She went on like this all that second day of the labor, becoming weaker and weaker from exhaustion and lack of nourishment. The next morning, the third morning of the labor, another physician was called, who, after examining her, said that the labor was slow on account of "dropsy" of the abdomen that was present and complicating the pregnancy. He prescribed and told her that the labor would soon be completed. That same evening and the next morning—the morning of the day I saw her—

he called again and said that it was a bad case on account of the dropsy. I found the cervical os dilated about one-half of its full extent and a fetal head swimming near the inlet. I recognized the case at once as one of hydramnion, and, as the urgency was great, I ruptured the membranes boldly and let the amniotic fluid flow out freely. About six quarts came away at once into a basin held for the purpose, and a considerable quantity flowed out slowly later, keeping the bed saturated in spite of frequent changes. Her breathing improved at once, and the pulse within an hour was down to 120. Very soon afterward she was able to retain water, and in about one hour took and retained a cupful of half milk and half coffee. About six hours later I was called again, and found that the general condition of the woman was fair. She had taken tea with milk several times, had retained everything, had no temperature, and her labor pains had been growing in strength since I left. Upon examination I found the head well down in the pelvis, but it was a brow presentation. I tried every way to convert it into a face or an occiput presentation, but the head was large and firmly fixed in the pelvis and would not budge. After waiting about two hours and a half, and no progress made, I applied forceps, giving spinal anesthesia. With the use of considerable force the head was born, and then, taking off the forceps, I delivered, but with a great deal of trouble, the trunk. The child was very large and fat across the shoulders, which offered the resistance to the ready birth of the body. I omitted to state that it was a case of occiput to the right and posterior. The child was dead and the beginning of maceration showed that it had been dead for some time. The woman made a good recovery. There was no sign of Bright's disease.

There are two features of interest in this case: First, that the hydramnion gave the patient no serious discomfort until labor pains began. Before labor began, her abdominal walls being very lax, the great accumulation of fluid was accommodated and no pressure symptoms appeared. After labor pains began the contraction of the abdominal wall forced the fluid in the only direction it could—that is, upward—and then began the pressure symptoms, manifested by vomiting and labored breathing and heart action. This is a matter of hydrostatic principles. The second unusual feature was the causation of the brow presentation. Upon examination of the dead fetus—which, by the way, weighed twelve pounds—I found that its neck was so short and its chest so fat that it was impossible to flex or extend the head enough to make an occiput or face presentation.

Dr. Gustav Kolischer.—I would like to ask Dr. Weber what manipulations he used to change the presentation of the head.

Dr. Weber.—It was impossible to use any. The fetal head was wedged in so tightly that I could not push the occiput up nor the face down.

Dr. Kolischer.—I understood Dr. Weber to say that it was impossible by manipulation to change a brow presentation into either an occipital presentation or face presentation. I cannot imagine a reason which would induce an obstetrician to change any kind of presentation into a face presentation—one of the most difficult presentations to deliver a child we know of. I do not think any obstetrician could be induced to change a brow presentation into a face presentation—that is, change a less difficult presentation into a more difficult one.

The second point in this case is interesting, because it reminds us that, if we rupture the bag of waters, in particular if it is a hydramniotic bag, it is a paramount duty of the obstetrician to watch carefully, to do all he can to induce the appropriate part of the fetus—in this case the head—to enter the pelvis at once. It is a well-known fact that if we rupture the bag of waters the umbilical cord prolapses, etc., so it is the first duty of the obstetrician to induce the head to enter the pelvis in a favorable position. I do not think it is right to rupture the bag of waters and leave the patient for six or seven hours, then go back again and be surprised at a brow presentation. That is the most important point in this report.

Dr. JOSEPH B. DE LEE.—The points brought out by Dr. Kolischer are well taken in connection with this case. With reference to the causation of brow presentation, Dr. Weber will find reference to that in the last work of Ahlfeld; that is, short-necked, fat children are liable to be found in face and brow presentations. Second, the causation of the dyspnea and rapid heart in hydramnion; another explanation which is closer to the facts, and is a little more forcible to me, is that the hydramnion was getting worse toward the end of pregnancy, because the woman was in false labor two or three days before Dr. Weber saw her, which labor threw so much work upon the already overburdened heart that it had not sufficient strength to meet the demand. The hydrostatic explanation of the dyspnea does not appeal to me very much, because in analogous instances we do not find the uterus rises up and presses upon the heart and lungs.

Dr. RUDOLPH W. HOLMES.—In cases of hydramnion labor cannot advance until some, at least, of the liquor amnii is removed. Rupturing the membranes means more or less complete escape of the waters, which, without engagement of the presenting part, is unfavorable. Two courses are open: First, if the os admits two fingers the membranes may be ruptured, and, as the waters drain away, Hicks' version performed. By the time the version is consummated and the leg brought down sufficient liquor amnii will have escaped to allow proper uterine action; then the attendant is master of the situation. Second, if the os is closed the water may be allowed to escape slowly after rupture of the membranes by placing a rubber bag in the vagina and filling it; when the uterus is partially evacuated the fetus may be outlined, and then if the head presents it may be fixed by the method of Hofmeier. This latter method is open to criticism in that the fetus in cases of hydramnion tends to take abnormal positions, as it did in this case, although its position may be ascribed rather to the short neck than hydramnion. Generally it may be stated version offers better results in hydramnion when the head is floating than fixation of the head.

I cannot agree with Dr. Kolischer's statement that a brow presentation is more favorable than a face. I have always taught my classes to bring down the face, brow anterior, thus securing a mento-anterior position; for if the occiput is brought down an occipito-posterior is produced. This commonly is the cause of a brow or face presentation, and the same causes which originally resulted in the brow presentation would again operate. Here possibly a version would be better than manual correction and a secondary manual rotation of the occiput to the front. *Per contra*, if the brow is posterior, by bringing down the occiput we get a favorable occiput anterior. Brow presentations mean that the largest diameter of the fetal head must pass through the pelvis, which by no means is the case in face presentations. With a roomy pelvis and a head normally large it is an exceedingly slow and laborious task for the uterus to expel a fetus with the brow presenting, which is not the case in mento-anterior positions.

DR. WEBER (closing the discussion).—I reported this case very briefly, and on that account I did not bring out many of the points that have been touched upon. As to leaving the woman immediately after rupturing the membranes, I did not leave her until she was in fairly good condition and the head was presenting. I could not make out exactly whether it was a brow presentation at that time. There was no prolapse of the umbilical cord nor of the arm. I saw to this and other things before I left. As to the possibility of the baby being alive, I spent half an hour with the stethoscope, after relieving the woman of the hydramnion, trying to get fetal heart tones, but could not do so, so I felt sure that the baby was dead. The occiput was to the rear, in the third position.

DR. S. L. WEBER read a paper entitled

SPINAL ANESTHESIA.[1]

DR. GUSTAV KOLISCHER.—This paper is rather a surprise to me. I thought that spinal anesthesia had been sufficiently exploited by sensation and advertisement-craving surgeons. If we want to judge upon a method of anesthesia, we must first have clear ideas as to the demands which we put upon the method of anesthetizing a patient. First, we have to be sure that we are able to put a patient under general anesthesia with the same certainty as we can do so by administering chloroform or ether. Second, the new method should at least be no more dangerous than chloroform or ether narcosis. Third, the remote sequelæ of this new method should not be more serious than those of our usual methods. I would mention that, if we have to

[1] See original article, p. 297.

deal with very nervous patients, the administering of morphine or chloral before commencing with chloroform or ether is a very expedient means. It is to be admitted, I believe, even by the enthusiastic advocates of spinal anesthesia, that in a considerable number of patients they absolutely fail to produce any kind of anesthesia, so we never know whether we are going to succeed in putting a patient under anesthesia by spinal cocaine injection. As to the dangers, the rosy views of Dr. Weber can be easily dispelled by a little thought on this subject. Although his figures concerning the death rate are too low, we can even prove by his statistics how much more dangerous spinal anesthesia is than the use of chloroform or ether. He informs us that 11 deaths are reported in about 3,000 cases of spinal anesthesia, whereas the statistics of chloroform anesthesia show that 1 death occurs in from 6,000 to 12,000 cases, according to different statistics. Even the most unfavorable reports count only 1 death in 3,000 cases. That shows that spinal anesthesia is ten and twenty times more dangerous than chloroform narcosis. By a great many authors ether is considered less dangerous than chloroform. I think these figures speak for themselves. I furthermore want to mention that since Schleich's mixture was adopted, for instance at Schauta's clinic, no death was reported from narcosis inside of five years. Other operators report in the same way. Everybody who is familiar with the effects of cocaine on the human system knows how extremely dangerous the drug is. In Vienna, Paris, Berlin deaths have been reported immediately following the application of weak cocaine solutions in the bladder. In one case the patient died inside of a few minutes, although the bladder was washed out immediately and stimulants were used. We know of a famous physician in St. Petersburg who committed suicide after he had killed his mistress by a hypodermatic cocaine injection applied in order to produce local anesthesia. We know that a great many individuals manifest a decided idiosyncrasy against cocaine, and we have no possible way to recognize this idiosyncrasy before the fatal error has occurred. We have a great many effective methods of dealing with syncope and asphyxiation from chloroform or ether, but in cases of cocaine poisoning we can do nothing effective for the patient. As to the remote consequences of cocaine anesthesia, if we consider the reports of Dr. Weber, there were no bad after-effects in 150 cases. This statistic is rather unique. All other authors who report on spinal anesthesia admit that in quite a number of cases bad after-effects have been observed. As to the remote consequences, I know of two very serious cases right here in Chicago. One is a woman who is an absolute invalid now for almost two years since spinal anesthesia was administered to her. The other woman suffers since this method was tried on her, from an extremely severe hysteria. A prominent neurologist considers her incurable. I know of two cases of damage suits following spinal anesthesia, in which cases the physician had to settle with his victims, because a prominent medical man in town who is conversant with legal matters told him that he had no earthly chance to win his suits. The doctor has recommended spinal anesthesia in obstetrics and said that we can use it to great advantage in this kind of work. In most cases we do not care so much for the anesthesia, in obstetrical work, as for the relaxation of the abdominal muscles and of the uterus. The point that Dr. Weber made, that, on account of the contraction of the uterus which follows the use of cocaine, it is more difficult to pass the hand next to the fetus, does not count for much. The point is that the danger of rupturing the uterus is greater if it is in such a condition. If Dr. Weber informs us that Tuffier has never attributed any of the deaths he reported to the specific effect of cocaine, that only goes to show that Tuffier is not very particular about the method of painting his statistics. One of the originators of spinal anesthesia, Bier, stated in a recent publication that this method is by no means ready for general use, and he cautions most emphatically against its extensive adoption. Dr. Weber says that he uses it in cases where chloroform or ether is contraindicated. He enumerated so many different cases of surgical intervention that I can hardly see how in all these 150 cases there were contraindications to chloroform anesthesia.

In summing up I want to say: If we look over the statistics given upon spinal anesthesia, I cannot see how a physician could use this method if he does not want to take chances with his patients' lives in order to do and publish something new.

DR. EMIL RIES.—I believe Dr. Weber mentioned that, so far as he knew, no death from spinal anesthesia had been reported in America. I wish to say that Dr. Carl Andersen, of this city, reported such a death before the Mississippi Valley Medical Association at its meeting held in Asheville.

DR. CHARLES S. BACON.—Dr. Kolischer's criticism of the paper is too severe. His criticism is based on one or two statements for which we are obliged to accept the word of Dr. Kolischer, but which I think ought to be supported by references.

For example, the question as to the danger of chloroform and ether is not settled by the statement that 1 death occurs in 8,000 or in 20,000 cases. The statistics of both chloroform and ether deaths are notoriously difficult to get at. The figures given by Dr. Kolischer are too low. We are justified, with proper precautions, in continuing the investigation of anything, if it promises results, and so I think it is timely and wise that we have listened to such a report to-night.

An interesting and important question is that of the use of cocaine anesthesia in heart disease. Recent discussions on this subject seem to show that the danger from chloroform and ether is not particularly great in cases of simple valvular heart disease, but rather in cases of myocarditis. I should be glad to know what the prospect is for the use of cocaine anesthesia in such cases.

Furthermore, I was left in doubt a little as to the effect of subarachnoid anesthesia on shock. At first I got the impression that it was favorable to shock, but there were some things said which led me to believe that it was not favorable. That, of course, is an important question to be investigated.

DR. KOLISCHER.—I want to say, in reply to Dr. Bacon, that the figures mentioned by me were taken from the statistics of the Hyderabad Commission. Furthermore, I would ask Dr. Bacon what the proper precautions in the use of cocaine are.

DR. BACON.—I cannot answer that question; but I am not quite certain that Dr. Kolischer's statement in regard to the statistics of the Hyderabad Commission is correct.

DR. FRANK E. PIERCE.—I have never seen this method of anesthesia used, and consequently the impressions I have gained from it have come from reports of cases and statistics. I agree with Dr. Bacon that Dr. Kolischer is rather premature in making such a radical attack on this method. That this method of anesthesia, used as a substitute for general anesthesia, has a field in selected cases there can be no doubt.

There are a few points to be noted in connection with the paper which reports of other cases show, and those relate to the effect of the drug and substitutes for the drug. Tropacocaine is mentioned by him. A report of sixteen cases has been given to test this drug in comparison with cocaine, and it has been found that many of the depressing physiological effects of the cocaine are avoided.

As to the dose of the drug, I believe Dr. Weber stated that he had used three-tenths of a grain in his cases. In the majority of cases reported the dose is given as one-fifth of a grain, and the depressing effects which have followed in cases have been where excessive doses have been given, that is, above one-fifth of a grain.

Dr. Weber has mentioned the impracticability of resorting to this form of anesthesia in abdominal work. The percentage of cases where nausea and vomiting have occurred is shown in Tuffier's cases to be at least forty per cent; and while in Dr. Weber's cases nausea has disappeared a short time after the anesthetic has been given, in some of the cases reported by others the nausea went on to vomiting, and the vomiting had resulted badly for the patient during the operation, in that through the straining of vomiting the bowels were pushed down through the opening, etc. This method should not be selected unless other forms of anesthesia are contraindicated.

In relation to the zone of anesthesia, it may be interesting to mention a case which was reported to me by a physician who was present at the time of the operation. It shows the value of this form of anesthesia in selected cases and the area of anesthesia which is produced. This case was a woman, about 40 years of age, who first consulted the late Dr. Christian Fenger for a very large fibroid of the uterus which reached to the ensiform cartilage and caused a good deal of dyspnea. After a careful examination by him, Dr. Fenger referred the case to the Presbyterian Hospital for further examination. The patient was seen by Dr. Webster. Dr. Herrick examined the woman because she presented cardiac symptoms which were very distressing. It was the general opinion among all of them that no operation should be done, because the patient was unable to stand a general anesthetic. She was discharged from the hospital and came under the care of a physician who lives just outside of the city limits. He decided to try spinal anesthesia in her case. He had no hospital facilities or assistants; but in the kitchen of the house where she lived he injected cocaine solution into the subarachnoid space, the dose of which I am uncertain. Owing to the very large size of the tumor an incision had to be made as high up in the abdominal wall as possible, to the ensiform cartilage, from there down to the pubes. The tumor was removed through this incision, and a total hysterectomy was done. The operation lasted about two hours. The patient during the operation showed no signs of heart disturbance, and no pain, showing that the effect of the drug had reached a higher level than the umbilical line. The only pain the patient complained of was in placing the last three upper sutures in the abdominal wall. During the operation the patient was quiet; she had no nausea, no vomiting, so that these complications were avoided. She took some nourishment during the operation, namely, three glasses of milk and ate two or three pieces of bread, and her recovery was uneventful. She subsequently walked into the doctor's office in apparently perfect health.

This case illustrates in a striking manner how this method of anesthesia is of great value in selected cases. Unquestionably this woman would have died if she had taken a general anesthetic to be operated on, because of the bad condition of her heart.

Another point of interest is with reference to the physiological action of cocaine. Of 150 cases reported by Galvani, in Athens, in 12 there were involuntary movements of the bowels during the operation. This has been explained by some as being due to relaxation of the sphincter. Whether it is that or not I do not know, but in general the reports which have been given are to the effect that muscular tone is not lost. It would be interesting to know just what the cause of the bowel evacuation was in those cases.

DR. WEBER.—Dr. Kolischer is entirely too radical in his objection to this method of anesthesia. I distinctly stated in my paper that at present I would not use spinal anesthesia if chloroform or ether could be given. This method of anesthesia should be learned by all, so that in any case where ether or chloroform is contraindicated it can be used. Whenever general anesthesia is impossible or strongly contraindicated, this method comes in as a great aid. I do not wish to be understood as saying that general anesthesia was contraindicated in the 152 cases I have had in which I resorted to this method. In many of them I resorted to spinal anesthesia to familiarize myself with the method and to find out possibilities of it. There was only a small number of the 152 cases in which it was absolutely necessary to use spinal anesthesia; general anesthesia could as well have been given. I think it is the duty of every physician to familiarize himself with a method which may save life and enable him to do an operation which otherwise could not be performed. According to the statement of Dr. Kolischer, there were many cases in which no anesthesia could be induced. He does not speak from personal experience. In the literature of the subject a number of cases are reported where anesthesia could not be induced. Why? Simply because of lack of experience with the method. When one is thoroughly familiar with the technique of this method he can induce anesthesia in every case. In many cases failure to introduce the needle into the subarachnoid space and inject the cocaine solution while the cerebro-spinal fluid is escaping drop by drop is responsible for lack of success.

With reference to the mortality following this method of anesthesia, I wish to say that I have had no deaths and no alarming symptoms. I gave the number of deaths following this method in foreign countries, as found in medical literature. I do not claim infallibility for this method, and I am susceptible of change in my opinions with further experience. I think the method is valuable, and can be used in selected cases where ether or chloroform is contraindicated. Let us suppose that a physician in a small town is called to a patient with strangulated hernia which ought to be operated upon at once. He cannot get anybody to give anesthesia; what is he to do?

DR. KOLISCHER.—Use Schleich's method.

DR. WEBER.—I don't know about that. But one can resort to spinal anesthesia and proceed alone with the operation.

Stated Meeting, May 16, 1902.

The President, LESTER E. FRANKENTHAL, M.D., *in the Chair.*

A CASE OF MYXOSARCOMA.

DR. T. J. WATKINS.—I have a specimen to show of myxosarcoma. Pathological report by Dr. E. B. Hoag, Assistant Pathologist to St. Luke's Hospital:

The tumor mass removed weighed in the neighborhood of twenty pounds. Extensive degeneration and many large and small cysts were found. The uterus was much thickened and showed great increase in fibrous tissue. A large cyst containing perfectly clear serum was punctured and some of the fluid transferred to agar tubes. No growth was obtained. Sections were cut on the freezing microtome from various parts of the tissue removed. All of them showed about the same condition, namely, much myxomatous degeneration and the presence of round sarcomatous cells. A diagnosis of myxosarcoma was therefore made. There was also present quite an extensive small round-cell infiltration.

The history of this case is interesting, in that the increase in size of the tumor was very rapid during the last week. The tumor, extending from the bottom of the pelvis, filled the entire abdomen and involved the uterus and left ovary. It was so extremely friable that in removing it masses broke off, as you will see in examining the specimen, and the degeneration was so extensive that almost no bleeding occurred from the torn surface of the tumor. The degeneration was so far advanced that in about twenty of the first sections that were made only myxomatous tissue could be found, so that it was only after considerable investigation that sarcoma was diagnosed. The patient left the operating table in as good condition as when she was put upon it, the pulse practically the same; and the pulse remained of good character for about twelve hours, then it gradually began to get faster and softer. Patient died about thirty-six hours after the operation. It is difficult to know to what to attribute the death. The tumor was sterile, and, as great care was taken in the technique, I do not believe infectious material was introduced. There was practically no loss of blood, as all the surfaces were clamped before they were cut, and I feel certain that there was no hemorrhage after the operation. In the literature of this subject I find it stated that these degenerative tumors, which are sterile, do contain toxins; but I fail to find any experimentation along that line, and it would seem that death must have been due to an acute toxemia, the toxins having been liberated by the breaking-down of the tumor in its removal. In a few cases where large degenerative tumors have been removed the patients appear to have had an acute toxemia.

CARCINOMA.

DR. LESTER E. FRANKENTHAL.—I present this case on account of the unusual occurrence of malignant degeneration in a fibroid tumor of the uterus, Cullen reporting only two cases in his entire series. The patient, Mrs. A. D., 66 years of age, German, was admitted to the Michael Reese Hospital May 9, 1902. She had the menopause at 50 years of age. Five years after this, which was about ten years ago, the patient had profuse hemorrhages lasting for two or three months, but no more until about six weeks ago. Since then she has had profuse hemorrhages of "red" blood and large clots. No pain accompanied the hemorrhages. She has lost about twenty pounds in weight. She has been troubled with frequent micturition. She has had six children.

A physical examination was made May 10. Head and neck negative. Lungs: A few whistling râles anteriorly, otherwise negative. As to the heart, there is a slight accentuation of the second pulmonic sound, but no murmurs present. The sounds are somewhat distinct. Abdomen: Linea nigra to umbilicus, slight diastasis of recti. In the right inguinal region a hard tumor can be palpated, extending nearly to the umbilicus. Fingers are somewhat deformed, and a slight grating felt in phalangeal joints. Reflexes present. Patient is a well-developed individual, with abundant adipose tissue. She has some dyspnea. Skin soft and rather inelastic, showing a number of varices.

Examination of the genitalia discloses a perineal laceration, rectocele and cystocele. Vaginal walls very lax. Cervix points almost directly backward, is of normal size, and is harder than normal. The laceration is such that the os opens to the right, and to the left is felt a hard, irregular protrusion. Uterus is anteflexed, anteverted, and immovable, and about the size of a goose egg, very hard, and presents some irregularities of the surface. To the right of the uterus and intimately connected with it is a hard, smooth tumor about the size of an orange. This tumor is firmly fixed and gives no sensation of fluctuation. Large clots of blood were passed after she entered the hospital. During her stay in the hospital her temperature was not higher than 100° F.; the pulse ranged between 68 and 92, and the respirations between 20 and 28. Diagnosis: fibromyoma of uterus and probable malignant degeneration.

On admission to the hospital she was given strychnine sulphate, one-fortieth grain every six hours, and kept on a soft diet with quantities of fluids. On the fourth day she was prepared and taken to the operating room. The anesthetic used was chloroform, of which she received forty grammes in fifty minutes. After preparing both the vagina and the abdomen for operation. and after vaginal and abdominal palpation. a median incision was made, about four inches long, between the symphysis pubis and the umbilicus; the peritoneum was picked up and divided between tissue forceps, and the opening enlarged by digital traction. The intestines and omentum were pushed away from the tumor and retained by large gauze sponges. A slight intestinal adhesion on the left of the tumor was broken up, and a thin. grayish fluid oozed from the injured surface of the tumor. The tumor was examined and found to be densely adherent posteriorly and laterally; small nodules were found on the peritoneum. so that an operation was not deemed advisable. There was also lymphatic involvement. The wound was then closed with deep silkworm sutures and a few superficial stitches; a strip of gauze (iodoform) was left as drainage over the oozing patch on the tumor. The preparatory work took more than thirty minutes. which was criticised at the time. A dry dressing was applied; the patient was put to bed at 11:30 A.M. with a pulse of 72 and respirations of 28. About fifteen minutes later the pulse became weak, irregular, and at times imperceptible. The patient was dyspneic, cyanotic, and very restless. The extremities became cold, and cold perspiration broke out over the body. External heat was applied, one-thirtieth grain of strychnia was given hypodermatically, followed by nitroglycerin, one-hundredth grain, in a few moments, and the latter was repeated a few moments later. Inhalations of oxygen were given, but to the above measures there was no response, and the patient died at 12 M.

A postmortem examination was made. The incision was opened and slightly enlarged, and absolutely no hemorrhage was found. The uterus and tumor were removed with great difficulty because of the density of the adhesions posteriorly. The microscope showed that a portion of the tumor was a carcinoma.

EXTRAUTERINE PREGNANCY.

DR. FRANKLIN H. MARTIN.—Mrs. E., housewife, aged 23, American, married nine years, was referred to my service at the Post-Graduate Hospital by Dr. L. Price. Menstrual history: Puberty at 11 years, regular, no dysmenorrhea until the present condition began. Duration of menses, four days, and flow quite profuse. She was married at the age of 14; husband healthy; no children. One miscarriage five years ago, when she was confined to bed three months with chills and fever, since which time she has had general pelvic pain. Dysmenorrhea. Pain and tenderness in left inguinal region, at times so severe that patient is unable to be on her feet. Two years ago, while flowing, she had a sharp pain, when flow was very much increased, amounting to a hemorrhage. General pelvic pain and extreme tenderness, so much so that anesthesia was used for the purpose of making an examination. Nothing was done at these examinations. No curettement. The physician in attendance is reported to have said the mouth of the womb was closed. The pain and hemorrhage continuing, a second anesthetic was given, but nothing was done. This condition continued for about six weeks. Since then the patient has been an invalid.

Pelvic Examination.—External genitalia normal; no discharge. Cervix long and small, directed upward and forward, lying directly back of the symphysis; fundus posterior, so that the uterus lies in the same axis as the normal, but the poles reversed. A tumor, from one and a half to two inches in diameter, lies below the fundus and is the first object to be felt by the examining finger. Very slight pressure causes excessive pain. Examination under anesthetic. Tumor slightly movable; fundus adherent and cannot be replaced.

Operation.—Laparatomy. A median incision was made. Uterus was completely retroverted and adherent, as were the tumor, ovaries, and tubes. The adhesions were freed, when it was found the tumor was situated in the fimbriated extremity of the Fallopian tube, which was greatly enlarged and stretched over half of the tumor. The tube was ligated and the tumor removed. The uterus was brought up into its normal position and suspended on a strip of peritoneum. Abdominal incision was closed by three layers of sutures. The peritoneum and fascia were sutured with catgut, the skin by a subcutaneous silver-wire suture. The tumor contains the remains of a fetus, the skeleton being quite perfect.

Dr. Zeit's Report.—Prof. Zeit, of the Post-Graduate Laboratory, makes the following report: Diagnosis, lithokelyphopedion. Extrauterine pregnancy, tubo-abdominal. The fetus died while still small. The specimen consists of a sac, six by eight centimetres in diameter, the walls of which are formed of hard, calcified, fibrous tissue, to which the fimbriæ and tube are adherent. The fetus is adherent to the inside of this sac, a fairly well developed skeleton bathed in a mass of pigment, fat, and cholesterin. All the soft tissues are absorbed. The parts of the fetus which are adherent to the inside of the sac are calcified.

GALLSTONES.

DR. A. GOLDSPOHN.—I have something here that is not of frequent occurrence, and it may perhaps be an argument in favor of the removal of the gall bladder in gall-bladder operations. About six years ago I did a nephrorrhaphy and gall-bladder operation on the same patient, at the same sitting. A large tumor existed to the right of the navel, and I was not able to decide positively which one of these two it was. Therefore I cut for a floating kidney, and found that and anchored it, and then made an incision anteriorly and emptied over one hundred small gallstones. The fistula at that time closed in about five weeks. During that time several larger stones were spontaneously discharged. Patient made a nice and complete recovery. About a year ago, she says, she began to have pain again and consulted some other physician, who treated her evidently for recurrent gallstones, until the pains became unbearable, and she came back to me a few days ago, at which time I discovered this hard mass, which is evidently malignant, in the outer portion of the former sinus in the abdominal wall. It was partially movable. I think I could move it in all directions except inward, and the inward movement of it was impeded by its attachment to the rectus fascia. Yesterday I excised it, which, after an exploratory incision on one side, I found I could do quite completely, there being no perceptible involvement of the lymphatic glands. Quite a broad attachment to the omentum was ligated off, and the whole mass cut out in healthy tissues, a reasonable distance away from the induration. In connection with it I removed about two square inches of the adjacent thin border of liver, which I severed by means of the Paquelin cautery without difficulty as to hemorrhage. A piece comprising the greater portion of the almost obliterated gall bladder is shown on the specimen.

Dr. Rudolph W. Holmes presented

AN INSTRUMENT FOR THE MECHANICAL DILATATION OF THE OS AT OR NEAR TERM.

Manual dilatation of the parturient os by the method of Harris or Edgar is a tiresome procedure, by whose completion the hands are cramped, stiff, and tired, so the operator cannot do justice to himself or the patient in the subsequent operative work. Extensive lacerations of the cervix are prone to occur in the course of manual dilatations, as the obtunded sensibility of the hands prevents an exact estimate of the power used. In the hope of finding a substitute for manual dilatation I have devised the following set of instruments. As I have just to-day received the first number of the set from the instrument maker, I can speak of the instruments only from a theoretical standpoint.

I have devised a series of six cones made from hard rubber; their general outline is that of Hegar's dilators; if the instrument proves practicable it should be made entirely of metal. Each cone is split vertically down its length; in the proximal end of each lateral half is an opening into which the points of the ordinary Goodell-Ellinger dilator may be introduced. The length of each cone is 7.5 centimetres. The first five numbers have diameters of 2.5, 3.5, 4.5, 5.5, and 6.5 centimetres respectively. The usual Goodell dilator opens about four centimetres; when a cone is placed on the dilator, practically one centimetre of this spread is lost, giving three centimetres of effective dilatation. Therefore, when the cones are opened, practically ellipses are formed whose minor diameters are as above given, and whose major diameters are these plus 3 centimetres. For example: Number 1 has a sectional diameter of 2.5 centimetres; opened it will produce nearly an ellipse with the minor diameter of 2.5 and the major of 5.5 centimetres.

To produce complete dilatation the sixth cone has a vertical (major) diameter of 9.5 and a horizontal (minor) diameter of 6.5; opened, a circle with a diameter of 9.5 centimetres is formed.

Method of Use.—The os must be dilated by Hegar's dilators (preferably) or by Goodell's instrument until Number 1 may be admitted. The anterior lip of the cervix should be caught by a volsella, and the vagina opened by broad specula; this probably will be essential for the smaller numbers, and possibly unnecessary, if not impossible, for the larger numbers. The Goodell, armed with the cones, is introduced into the cervix, and dilatation is carried out as in the usual use of the Goodell instrument. As soon as full dilatation with the first number is secured the second is quickly substituted, and so on until complete dilatation is obtained. It will be a useful expedient to rotate the cones in the course of the dilatation with each number, so different areas of the cervix will be fully acted upon by the dilator.

The advantages of a mechanical dilator over a manual dilatation are material: there is no cramping of the hand, so the power

expended may be more exactly gauged; the operator is not
wearied before the crucial test of the delivery and the performance of the postpartum procedures; also, at least with the smaller
sizes, the eye may observe the effect of the instrument on the
cervix, that is, if there be a tendency to lacerate. Using the same
care as in the application of Hegar's dilators, there should be no
danger of prematurely rupturing the membranes. During contractions it would seem essential to remove, or at least to partially withdraw, the dilator. It would be most useful where the
presenting part was above the brim; possibly it might still be
used in appropriate cases when engagement had occurred.

The objections to the cones increase with the size of the instrument; probably the largest size, Number 6 (9.5 by 6.5 centimetres), will be found to be entirely inapplicable; possibly the
theoretical objections to this number will also obtain for Numbers
4 and 5. Generally the first half of the manual dilatation is the
most difficult and tiring, so even if the larger sizes are impracticable the smaller ones will be a useful adjunct in hastened deliveries. As I see them, the objections to the larger sizes would be:
(1) they would be unwieldy; (2) the cones would so com-

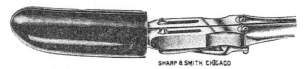

SHARP & SMITH CHICAGO

Uterine Dilator.

pletely fill the vagina that it would be difficult to ascertain the
effect of the instrument on the cervix, i.e., imminence of lacerations; the size has the advantage of preparing the vagina for
the delivery, which would be of advantage in primiparæ; (3) it
could not be used in prolapse of cord or extremity, as can the instrument of Bossi.

A Goodell dilator armed with the first number of the cones is
pictured above.

INSTRUMENT FOR INJECTION OF NORMAL SALT SOLUTION.

Dr. Joseph B. De Lee.—I have here an instrument which, I
think, possesses signal advantages over the instruments or
needles generally used for the injection of normal salt solution.
Without going fully into the disadvantages of the other needles,
I will mention the advantages of this, which are:

1. There is a handle with which to hold the needle in injecting
the solution. The ordinary needle has no handle, and the rubber
tube sometimes slips off during the process of forcing the needle
through the skin.

2. The needle consists of a single steel tube, which runs
through the handle, and there is no jog or offset, so that a piece

of cotton can be pushed through to rid the interior of any foreign matter.

3. It has small lateral openings, so that the fluid, instead of going through the point alone, has exits at the side, which is a distinct advantage—the fluid is more evenly disseminated.

4. The needle also has a guard, which is ventilated, to prevent rust, and to keep the point sharp.

DR. LESTER E. FRANKENTHAL.—I do not know how well acquainted the profession is with the Bossi instrument, but I did not know anything about it when it was published first—in 1897—until I read an article by Leopold in which he published eighteen cases, five or six of which were éclamptic and five or six were primiparæ. In some instances the os was so small that he had to dilate at first with a small dilator, like a Goodell dilator, in order to introduce the Bossi instrument, and in no instance did he have any tears. In every case he was able to dilate, the longest time being thirty-five minutes. I thought so well of the instrument—after reading his description of it and its use in these eighteen cases—that I was induced to get one. The advantage of it over the instrument exhibited by Dr. Holmes, to my mind, would be that the dilatation would go on better for the entire circumference of the os. Its branches, four in number, work like a Goodell. There is a central stalk, like the one in the Goodell, from which four branches bifurcate in pairs. There is another dilator which Dr. Holmes did not mention, and that is the Tarnier dilator. I have never used it.

OVARIAN CYST COMPLICATED WITH INFECTION BY THE PNEUMOCOCCUS AND STAPHYLOCOCCUS ALBUS.

DR. T. J. WATKINS.—The patient was sent to me with a pelvic tumor which extended from the pelvis above the umbilicus, and on examination before anesthesia it was diagnosed as a uterine fibroid. After the patient was anesthetized the body of the uterus could be made out separate from the tumor, but the uterus was considerably enlarged. On opening the abdomen quite a large ovarian cyst was found on the right side, which was firmly attached to the uterus and nearly covered over the fundus. The uterus was large and contained a fibroid. The tumor and uterus were both removed, and at the time of operation it seemed certain that the cyst was carcinomatous.

The pathological report by Dr. Robert Zeit, Pathologist to St. Luke's Hospital: Sections of the tumor were cut in celloidin. No indication of malignancy or tuberculosis was found, but there was an extensive purulent inflammation of polymorphonuclear leucocytes of all tissues, with much fibrinous exudate and necrosis. The appearance of the sections indicated either a staphylococcus or gonococcus infection. Some growth on agar tubes was obtained, which proved to be a pure culture of staphylococci. A direct smear on cover glasses made from the tissues under proper precautions showed a few diplococci (evi-

26

dently pneumococci). The infection was undoubtedly mainly due to the staphylococcus albus, but the pneumococcus may also have played a part.

This patient took the anesthetic badly. There was a profuse secretion of mucus, although she showed no signs of bronchitis before the operation. After the operation there was an acute laryngitis and bronchitis, and a suspicion of small patches of lobular pneumonia. She had a slight elevation of temperature, but this and the acceleration of the pulse were attributed to the bronchial affection. On the fourth day the dressings over the wound were completely saturated. On removing them it was found that the tissues which were included in the sutures in the lower angle of the wound had sloughed out, leaving quite a large opening. All sutures were removed from the skin, in order to give more perfect drainage, when it was found that the tissues of the peritoneum and fascia which were included in the sutures had entirely sloughed out. There were no adhesions, and the intestines presented freely in the wound. There was a copious exudation of serum, and macroscopically there was but little pus. A culture made from this fluid showed a pure staphylococcus infection. I may say that the peritoneum was closed by dry catgut, the fascia by chromicized catgut, and the skin by silkworm gut. Every one who had anything to do with the operation wore rubber gloves, and, from the precautions taken, I think there was very little chance of infection at the time of the operation, and that the infection existed previously in this tumor. Before the operation the patient was comparatively well, in that she was up and about, and all she complained of was the presence of this mass in the abdomen. Of course it is possible she had a general pneumococcus infection, but an examination of the profuse secretion from the bronchi failed to show the presence of any pneumococci. Two such examinations were made during the first two or three days after the operation, and were negative. So I believe it can be safely said that the suppuration that took place in this case was due to an infection which existed in the tumor prior to the operation. The patient died on the fifth or sixth day, about twenty-four hours after the escape of the infected serum through the abdominal incision.

A CASE OF BACILLUS COLI COMMUNIS INFECTION.

DR. JOSEPH B. DE LEE.—The woman had had several criminal abortions performed upon her, fourteen in all, at various times during her married life. In one of these criminal abortions, about six years ago, I treated her, when she was having a high temperature and a corresponding acceleration of the pulse. After cleaning out the uterus the symptoms subsided, but she carried away from the criminal abortion a bad endometritis, which was treated more or less successfully by local gynecologists. She has a retroversion. Eighteen months ago she was delivered of a living child after a rather hard labor, with some postpartum hemorrhage, adherent placenta, and with placental evidences of endometritis. She became pregnant again after this, and at three months had begun to vomit a good deal. I gave her three doses, five grains each, of oxalate of cerium; the emesis ceased. I flattered myself that it had cured her, but two weeks later she had a spontaneous miscarriage, with the expulsion of a macerated ovum. Her present illness: She again became pregnant, and when six weeks advanced in pregnancy went to a criminal-abortionist, who made four attempts to enter the uterus. She had a retroflexed and more or less adherent uterus, and the abortionist said it was difficult to enter it. Anyway, he produced considerable hemorrhage, and, as the woman was threatened with an abortion, I was called to see her. On my arrival I found she had a temperature of 101°. Her pulse was good. The temperature then declined to 100° and the bleeding subsided: she got up, went about her business, and had a normal temperature for a week, so I did not do anything. At the end of that time she began to flow profusely. Tamponade. The next morning the uterus was cleaned out by curetting, after slight instrumental dilatation, and subsequently she had a perfectly normal temperature for six and a half days. The temperature did not reach above 98.4° nor the pulse above 74 for six and a half days, and at the end of that time she got up and I was about to discontinue my visits. She had no lochia, but as she was apparently perfectly well I concluded that I had cleared out the uterus so thoroughly that there was no decidua left. Nor was there at any time during the whole course of the fever any real lochial discharge, that is, in the course of the four weeks' treatment. In the evening of the seventh day she was taken with a chill, when the temperature slowly rose to 104°, the pulse being correspondingly accelerated. Thinking that the uterus was full of decomposing lochia, I gave her a uterine douche. *Nothing* came away except fresh blood produced by the manipulations. The temperature declined to normal the next morning, and I could not explain the drop. The temperature rose again to 103.6°. I gave another douche and put a rubber drainage tube into the uterus with some difficulty, because the uterus was retroflexed and the cervix was higher than the fundus. Nothing came through the tube except a few drops of watery secretion. When the temperature went up again to 103° I gave another douche, and this time got a little clot, about the size of one-half of my small finger nail, and about as thick. The clot was darkish and slightly decomposed, and probably produced by the previous manipulations. The temperature took a slight drop. I again reintroduced the drainage tube, and nothing escaped except some few drops of secretion. The tube from the uterus was sent to Prof. Zeit for bacteriological report. Careful examination then showed that there was no inflammation, no tumor at the side of the uterus, no enlargement of the tubes, and the only finding was a rather tender uterus.

Temperature declined to normal, and remained so for about four days; then it rose again. I gave her another douche, thinking that something had accumulated in the uterus, but nothing came away. Again the temperature went down for a while, and then rose again. She now developed a small, movable, tender mass to the left of the uterus. I stopped giving the douches, and she continued to have a slight irregular temperature, until finally it came down to normal and remained so for eight or nine days. Here I will read the pathological report, prepared by Prof. Robert Zeit: "Direct smears showed great numbers of an irregularly staining bacillus, rounded ends, no spores, parallel arrangement, and cultures gave pure growth of bacillus coli communis. The examinations were by the whole class in bacteriology, and the results were the same in forty-five examinations."

There is no doubt that this was a case of bacillus coli communis infection.

Dr. A. Goldspohn read a paper entitled

WHAT ARE THE KNOWN FACTS ABOUT FOLLICULAR CYSTIC DEGENERATION OF THE OVARIES.[1]

Dr. Emil Ries.— I do not believe in Dr. Goldspohn's theories. What he has stated to-night is not his own work. If he had spent a little more time, zeal, and energy in making some examinations of his own we might have had something to discuss. The doctor has only given us what has been stated by others. In a number of fresh cystic ovaries which years ago were removed by a man who, I have reason to believe, does not remove cystic ovaries at present, I have had the pleasure of demonstrating normal ova in these so-called cystic follicles.

Now, there is no question about small cysts being developed from such follicles; but a slight pathological abnormality or a slight deviation does not warrant or necessitate surgical treatment. There are other organs which show similar deviations—as, for instance, the testicles in the male—and I have taken particular pains to examine a number of specimens of testicles and have been able to find numerous degenerations and cysts. Who operates on them? The tunica albuginea of the ovary is constructed very much like the tunica albuginea of the testicle. One may be thick and the other may be thick. In the ovary the tunica albuginea prevents the easy and rapid emptying of the follicles, to a certain extent. In the testicle, from the tunica albuginea processes of fibrous degeneration radiate into the substance of the testicle, and you can see in the testicle a great many abnormalities produced thereby. Who takes them out? Who punctures them? Who cuts them? Who cauterizes them with cautery or carbolic acid? There are other organs in which similar abnormalities take place very frequently. You will find such cysts in the kidney. You will find such retention cysts in the liver.

[1]See original article, p. 343.

What difference do they make? We find numerous cysts, of the size of these dilated or enlarged follicles of the ovary, in almost any inflammatory process of the peritoneum, around the tubes, the ovaries, among the intestines. Who cares for them? There is a difference between a deviation from the absolutely normal and a pathological condition. There is a difference between their pathological and clinical importance. Some physicians cannot see it. The symptoms produced by retention cysts and these follicles (let us assume that this is the correct theory) have never been demonstrated to be of great importance. Dr. Goldspohn says that the presence of such cysts alone would not induce him frequently to operate. If he finds them accompanying other pathological conditions which require surgical treatment, he goes for them. Well, if they need treatment in one case, why not in the other? He says he takes them out. He cuts through the thickened tunica albuginea. What does he leave behind? He leaves behind the thickened tunica albuginea. The next follicle develops. Does he operate again?. Why does he not take out the ovary? If it is the thickened tunica albuginea that prevents the escape of the ovum, that prevents the bursting of the follicle, why does he not take away the thickened tunica albuginea? Because he knows very well it would not do any good. Why not take out the ovary? Because he knows it is not necessary. Why does he take out a piece of the ovary? I do not know.

We come to the important point of cystic degeneration and its influence on the general health of the patient. If a woman complains about her general health, is nervous, worried, broken down, tired, and comes to a practitioner, in nine cases out of ten he looks at the cervix first, as if that were the seat of all evils that womankind is heir to. The more expert ones make a bimanual examination. Now, it is extremely rare that the experienced practitioner or specialist cannot find something wrong with the sexual tract that displeases his esthetic sense. Follicles of the ovary of large or small size are formed in such large numbers that if one wants to operate on these every time he finds them —well, the hospitals in Chicago will have to be increased tenfold. There will not be enough operators. Will the women be any healthier after these operations? Not a whit. The amount of tinkering that has been done on ovaries and cervices in this and other cities is something outrageous. If the gentlemen whose work is confined to the female sexual tract would take the trouble to examine the whole woman instead of the sexual tract alone, they might find as many enlarged cysts, but they might find more women who needed treatment for something else than their ovaries. It happens that women come to my office quite frequently with the statement that they need an operation on the cervix or an operation on cystic ovaries, and yet, after carefully examining them, I find that they have no local symptoms whatever, that they are neurasthenic or hysterical women, and that they need treatment at the hands of the neurologist. I may find a latent tuberculosis or a beginning psychosis, which is not at all rare, and these women are not a bit better off after an operation than they were before. My idea, therefore, is that these dilated or enlarged follicles are pathological conditions without any clinical dignity. They are not normal. But if you want to remove everything that is not normal, that is a slight deviation from the normal, there is not a person here to-night who does not require an operation at this moment. The fact that these women have such follicles does not necessarily mean they need to be treated. I do not deny that it is not a normal condition, but I do deny its importance. Many times women come to us with these enlarged follicles in the ovaries, and they have been told that their neurasthenia and similar nervous affections are the consequence of these cystic ovaries. To the men who believe in that I have nothing to say. My opinion is that these cases belong to the domain of neurology or general medicine, not to that of gynecology at all.

Dr. Gustav Kolischer.—I want to say, in connection with Dr. Goldspohn's paper, that every one who has seen a great many operations done, who has seen a great many postmortem examinations made, is familiar with these small cystic degenerations of the ovaries in individuals, but which were never complained of as producing any special disorder of the genital organs. We see women of all ages on the postmortem table who have had these degenerated cystic ovaries, which have had plenty of time to develop into tumors or into cysts, without proliferating into dangerous tumors.

I do not agree with Dr. Ries in his statement that one cannot discuss a paper in which there is no original work. Personally, I think a concise, complete report of a certain line of work is sometimes more worthy of consideration and discussion than original work which does not amount to much.

Dr. Ries said that there is too much operating done by gynecologists and other practitioners. He is certainly right.

Dr. Goldspohn (closing the discussion).—If any credible person says that two and two are not four, and claims that they are five, as illustrating what Dr. Ries has said in this instance, it behooves us first to make sure that two and two are four, and not five, before making further calculations.

It has been a question of real concern with me how far to go when we have an opportunity, without increasing surgical risk, or without hurting the patient, in destroying some of these follicles. I have followed, with a great deal of interest, the results of the various original workers in this line, to find out what they have to say, to guide me in my own practice. If the ovum does die early, as we see from most of these investigations, it is certainly not an innocent thing to allow a follicle or a cyst, that is assuming the size of a pigeon's egg or larger, to go on indefinitely simply because it is not of a proliferating character. I say that all of this work is practically incidental or auxiliary to other surgical indications. Rarely would this condition of the ovaries alone constitute a prime indication for operation, as I have distinctly stated. It is practically all auxiliary work. When the abdomen has been opened for other good reasons, from above or through the vagina, and the opportunity is afforded, how far is it our duty to go in destroying these cysts?

The remarks of Dr. Ries about operating on all these cases are out of order and impertinent. No one thinks that these follicles always cause symptoms. We all know they do not, and yet many of them do, as I have demonstrated to my own satisfaction dozens of times. He says it is not proved that they have any clinical significance; but if I have satisfied myself of one thing, I have of this, that by removing these follicles (and sometimes incidentally improving the position of the ovary) the patient has been freed from constant pain which she had theretofore, and this pain did not return. If one can do this in dozens of cases, namely, excite a given pain that is complained of, by careful bimanual palpation of an ovary in this condition, and do this repeatedly in each case, then merely exsect these follicle cysts and do nothing more on the ovary except possibly to improve its location a little, and then find that the various individually specified pains have quite uniformly subsided in all the cases, at once and permanently as a rule, I think we have ample data from which to draw the conclusion logically that many of these follicle cysts do cause pain, and then probably also other symptoms. Therefore, if an operation is done at all—which will usually be for other more important concomitant indications—it is our duty to attend to this lesser indication also in order to do complete work.

So far as the tinkering with cervices and the vagina is concerned, I agree with Dr. Ries most heartily. I called it "whittling on the cervix" years ago. Men stop in the vestibule and ascribe to superficial appearances there the symptoms that are due to lesions higher up in the generative organs or to disorders of other organs.

BRIEF OF CURRENT LITERATURE.

OBSTETRICS.

Blood Counts in the New-Born.—John Aitken *(Jour. Obst. and Gyn. of the Br. Emp.,* Apr.) has found that the red corpuscles in the blood of infants at birth are relatively more numerous than in adults. During the first forty-eight hours of life the number per cubic centimetre increases owing to the concentration of the blood. The child loses weight during this period. From the second day, as a rule, a gradual fall in number takes place. The child gains weight during this period. During the early days the blood shows variations in size and shape of the corpuscles and deficiency in rouleau formation. Nucleated red corpuscles are present at birth, normoblasts and megaloblasts. The hemo-globin is relatively high at birth and during the few succeeding days, usually over 100 per cent. The white corpuscles are two or three times as numerous at birth as in adults, increasing in number for the first two days. After the third day they decrease in number. Digestion leucocytosis is very marked, especially after the first feedings. The lymphocyte percentage usually exceeds that of the neutrophiles at birth. After the first feeding there is a relative and absolute increase in the neutrophiles. This gradually diminishes as the effects of digestion wear off. The percentage of eosinophiles is, as a rule, greater than the adult blood.

Treatment of Obstetrical Depressions of the Skull.—Villard and Pinatelle *(Ann. de Gyn. et d'Obst.,* Mar.) favor an open operation and elevation of the depressed cranial bones by a spatula in all cases of extensive or deep depression, even without symptoms. Their arguments are that without operation more than half the cases die, that the survivors are often mentally or physically degenerate, that the operation relieves cerebral compression and allows absorption of intracranial hemorrhages, and is not dangerous if properly done.

Metastasis of Chorionic Villi.—Introduction into the circulation of a kind of cell is followed by the formation of a corresponding antitoxin. The chorionic villi are surrounded by maternal blood, and separation of cells from their periphery must result in what may be called a syncytiolysin. To study this B. Scholten and J. Veit *(Cent. f. Gyn.,* No. 7) placed portions of placenta in the peritoneal cavities of rabbits, after removing the blood as far as possible and trying to introduce only cells from the periphery of the villi and connective tissue. Their results were: (1) Serum of rabbits, after introduction into the peritoneal cavity of .5-.10 gramme of human placenta, was no more hemolytic when added to human blood than that of normal rabbits. (2) Serum of pregnant women showed no hemolytic property toward blood of men and pregnant women, and only slight toward that of the non-pregnant. (3) Serum of rabbits treated with human placenta was innocuous to other rabbits. (4) Serum of two eclamptic women showed no hemolytic properties for blood of men, pregnant or non-pregnant women, and was not toxic when introduced in certain quantities into rabbits. (5) Urine of rabbits treated with human placenta or with that of rabbits showed albumin after twenty-four to forty-eight hours. (6) Pieces of human placenta placed when fresh in fresh serum from rabbits treated as above showed, after twenty-four hours, separation of the nuclei of the syncytium. The usual presence of albumin in the urine of rabbits treated as described above is held to suggest that the same is to be expected after wandering of villi. Certainly not all cases of albuminuria of pregnancy, however, are caused by this.

The Specific Gravity of the Maternal Blood, and its Relations to the Development and Sex of the Fetus.—Enrico Tridondani *(Ann. di Ost. e Gin.*, May, 1902) gives the results of his observations as follows: The specific gravity of the blood during pregnancy is always less than normal. It is lower in pluriparæ than in primiparæ, and diminishes with the progress of pregnancy. This diminution holds good both as to the blood as a whole and the serum without the corpuscles. It increases, as a rule, during labor. The specific gravity of the fetal is always higher than that of the maternal blood. With a lowered density of the maternal blood (1055 or less) there are more male than female fetuses (58:18). With increased density (1056 or more) the females predominate (50:28). The lower density corresponds to greater development of the fetus (3270:3150 grammes) than does the higher density. In the eclampsia of pregnancy the specific gravity is not above normal.

Urobilinuria as a Sign of Fetal Death.—Numerous observations by C. Merletti *(Cent. f. Gyn.*, No. 16) have shown that in at least the last quarter of pregnancy it is the rule to find an increased urobilinuria in apparently healthy women. The quantity of the pigment is two or three times as great as that excreted by non-pregnant healthy women. In five cases of intrauterine death of the fetus occurring between the fifth and seventh months, he found a marked urobilinuria which returned to the normal amount within five to ten days after delivery. In consequence of these observations Merletti calls attention to the existence of a physiological urobilinuria of pregnancy and to its marked increase in cases of fetal death *in utero*. He regards the latter as a reliable sign of death of the fetus.

Bacteriology of the Uterus and Vagina.—G. Drummond Robinson *(Jour. Obst. and Gyn. Br. Emp.*, June) finds that it is generally admitted that infection of the uterus, during or after labor, may take place from gonococci or from anaërobic saprophytic organisms which were present in the vagina before labor, but that, in spite of some observations to the contrary, the great weight of evidence is to show that forms of infection other than these are in the vast majority of cases due to the direct introduction from without of micro-organisms which are not previously in the vagina. He believes the researches emphasize the importance of asepsis in midwifery practice, and suggests that the douche, used as an antiseptic agent, is, as a rule, unnecessary, if not positively harmful.

Eclampsia.—H. O. Nicholson *(Jour. Obst. and Gyn. Br. Emp.*, July), in discussing the use of thyroid extract in eclampsia, states that deficiency or impaired activity of the thyroid secretion leads to a derangement of some part of the defensive mechanism. Toxic substances then gain entrance into the blood, and this coincides with the onset of the pre-eclamptic state. Diminution and ultimate arrest of the secretion of urine occurs, which allows absorption of the toxins, and this culminates in convulsions. By producing symptoms of thyroidism in an eclamptic patient the re-establishment of diuresis is secured. When the symptoms of thyroidism are produced the blood vessels are fully relaxed. Large hypodermatic injections of morphine or saline infusions produce similar effects. Diuresis does not occur as an immediate effect of the general enlargement of the arterial calibre, because the period at which relaxation of the renal vessels occurs is variable. Under thyroid treatment many of the unfavorable symptoms ameliorate before the functions of the kidneys are fully restored, and postpartum fits apparently do not occur. If this treatment be commenced early the prognosis as regards the mother should be very favorable. Thyroid extract may counteract the autointoxication by favoring metabolism in some unknown way. In view of a probable relationship between the thyroid-gland system and the conditions which lead to the formation and absorption of toxins in pregnancy, culminating in eclampsia, treatment by thyroid extract should be preferred to that of morphine or saline infusions. Thyroid extract would seem to act more powerfully and permanently on the circulation than these other agents, but a combination of morphine and thyroid extract is sometimes invaluable.

In the early stages of puerperal eclampsia W. E. Parke (Med. News, May 24) advises a diet with the minimum amount of nitrogenous matter. The bowels should be kept open and the skin active by hot baths every day, if necessary. The kidneys may be stimulated by Basham's mixture or calomel, squill, and digitalis. Nitroglycerin may be used to reduce the arterial tension. If the symptoms increase pregnancy should be terminated at once. For the treatment of the convulsions in full-blooded patients he advises venesection. Inhalations of chloroform can be used to avert the convulsive seizures. Veratrum viride has given good results in the author's practice. Normal saline solution infusions are valuable especially when blood-letting has been practised.

R. Abrahams (Med. News, May 24) has found that the abstraction of blood in eclampsia produces (1) an immediate favorable change in the woman's appearance; the cyanosis of the face; the rigidity of the muscles; the spasms and twitching which are often noticed even during the stage of deep coma. (2) The pulse loses its tension. (3) The coma yields. Transfusion (1) improves the pulse; (2) induces free sweating and free micturition; and (3) produces intense thirst in the awakened patient, which causes her to drink copiously, and this is very desirable.

Splanchnoptoses in Pregnancy.—Charles D. Aaron (Am. Jour. of Surgery and Gyn., July) finds that dispensing with the abdominal bandage after pregnancy predisposes to enteroptosis. Pregnancy favors and assists the cure of enteroptosis, hence patients suffering from it need not hesitate to be exposed to pregnancy. Its disagreeable symptoms seem to disappear while carrying the child. Keeping the patient in bed after delivery and

applying an effective band is very helpful in the cure of enteroptosis, while early getting-up after delivery and insufficient support to the abdomen predispose to the condition.

Cervicitis and Endocervicitis in Pregnancy.—L. M. Bossi
(*Archiv. Ital. di Gin.*, vol. iv., No. 5) holds that these conditions
are much more frequent during pregnancy than has been generally supposed. The cause may be found in abortions, premature
labors, abnormal pregnancies, and complications during labor
or the puerperal period. These causative factors are so often
ignored by both patients and midwives that it is of the utmost
importance to call attention to them. The gynecological examination of pregnant women under proper conditions, and made
when the symptoms point to the presence of some complications,
is harmless and allows of the treatment of lesions in time to avoid
serious results. The author has had success by the use of dis-
infectant vaginal douches, cauterization, and dusting with various powders. For the douches he advises a daily use of a litre
and a half of fluid, alternating a solution of 40 grammes borate of
soda in that amount of boiled water, with a half-gramme of corrosive sublimate in the same proportion. With improvement of
the condition the douches may be taken every two, three, four,
and five days and then stopped altogether. In order to avoid all
danger of causing uterine contractions, the douche must be taken
at low pressure, the bag being suspended not more than about three
feet above the pelvis of the patient, who should be in the gynecological position. The vaginal tip should not be inserted further
than half-way in the vagina. The water should be allowed to
flow slowly, by only partly opening the tube. The substances
used by the writer for cauterization are: carbolic acid in 50 per
cent of alcohol, and chloride of zinc in a 30 per cent solution, the
latter being used for the more severe cases. These should never
be applied during the menstrual molimen, but with that exception
may be performed once a week, vaginal douches being taken
daily in the intervals of treatment. After cauterization a tampon impregnated with a 1:3000 bichloride solution is applied to
the vagina, which is then dried with absorbent cotton and the
following mixture dusted over the surface:

℞ Salol,
  Iodol,
  Bismuth,
  Powdered starch,
  Powdered lycopodium...................... āā gramme i.

Emmet's operation may have to be resorted to in case of very
severe laceration.

The Anatomy of Tubal Pregnancy.—Andrea Majocchi (*Ann.
di Ost. e Gin.*, Dec., 1901) thus sums up the result of his researches: 1. In the gravid Fallopian tube we do not have the
formation of a true decidua, as in the uterus, but close to the
point of insertion of the ovum there is a slight decidual modification of the connective tissue of the mucosa and of the muscular

coat. 2. No true reflexa is found, there being merely an hypertrophied fold of mucous membrane, presenting the same modifications as occur in the mucosa itself. 3. The serotina of the tube is similar to that of the uterus, excepting for the fact that it is not sharply limited from the subjacent muscular tissue. 4. In the non-gravid portions of the tube the epithelium is normal, but in the vicinity of the ovum it undergoes numerous changes. 5. The author was unable to come to any conclusion in regard to the formation of the syncytium, but in all probability the maternal epithelium is not involved.

Tubal Gestation.—Francis Henry Champneys (Jour. Obst. and Gyn. Br. Emp., June) in a series of 75 cases finds that 34 cases recovered without operation, a proportion of 45.3 per cent. To these cases he adds 11 in which the cyst was evacuated by vaginal section, making 60 per cent of cases which recovered without abdominal section. As in all other departments of practice, in order to get the best results from operation the best course would be to operate on all cases; but this would include, according to the 75 cases referred to above, 65.3 per cent of unnecessary abdominal sections. If the patient is not fairly accessible, it may be safer, in any individual case, to do abdominal section than to watch the patient.

Primary Ovarian Gestation.—A. W. Mayo Robson (Jour. Obst. and Gyn. Br. Emp., July) reports a case of primary ovarian gestation upon which he operated successfully. The parts removed showed that the tube was not dilated. Two translucent cysts were attached to the fimbriated end. The fimbriæ could be distinctly seen. The ovary was seen to have ruptured into what appeared to be a small sac. The small ovum was found in a mass of clot taken from the top of the ovary. The tube was firmly adherent to the bottom of the pouch of Douglas, leaving the ovary free above. Robson suspects that the spermatozoa must have reached the ovary through the opposite tube.

Pregnancy after Removal of both Ovaries.—Alban Doran (Jour. Obst. and Gyn. Br. Emp., July) cites a case in which pregnancy occurred two years after the removal of the ovaries. The case had had one ovary and tube removed fourteen years previous to the time he operated for the removal of the ovary of the other side for a cystic growth. He supposed at the time that no ovarian tissue was left and that the tube was tied off with the pedicle of the growth.

Inversion of the Uterus.—J. Edson Kelsey (Amer. Med., July 26) reports a case of complete inversion of the uterus with prolapse immediately following labor. The delivery was instrumental. The placenta did not come away after a wait of fifteen minutes, so slight traction was made on the cord and the uterus came down with the placenta adherent. The uterus was replaced with difficulty. The cord measured thirteen inches.

Artificial Dilatation of the Cervix.—G. Leopold (Cent. f. Gyn., No. 19) reports the use of Bossi's four-branched dilator in five additional cases besides the twelve included in a previous paper. He finds that it gives, in twenty to thirty minutes, sufficient dilatation for forceps delivery or version without appreciable laceration of the cervix, and in nearly all cases starts uterine pains. The writer considers it particularly useful in eclampsia.

Deep Transverse Arrest of the Fetal Head.—Charles B. Reed *(Ann. Gyn. and Ped.,* July), in discussing this presentation, states that it is a relatively common complication of labor. The diagnosis is easily made from the position of the sagittal suture and the fontanelles. The normal termination of the case cannot be waited for in most instances, but forceps should be applied as soon as it is evident that rotation will not occur spontaneously. The blades should be applied in that pelvic diameter toward which the occiput lies. The occiput must be located before the blades are applied. Traction and rotation must be simultaneous.

Labor and Locomotor Ataxia.—Richard Cohn *(Cent. f. Gyn.,* No. 16) made the diagnosis, in May, 1894, of locomotor ataxia on account of the characteristic gait and loss of patellar reflexes of a 37-year-old multipara. In August, 1897, the woman was delivered of a child. Instead of dystocia on account of advanced age, the labor was so easy that the appearance of the head at the vulva was the first warning of its onset. The entire delivery was painless, the puerperium normal. The woman was not aware that she had given birth to a child until told on the next day.

Miscarriage and Difficult Labor after Ventrofixation.—H. Macnaughton-Jones *(Br. Gyn. Jour.,* May) reports a case of miscarriage at the fifth month one year after an operation for ventrofixation. The patient subsequently bore a full-term child, the labor being difficult. Shortly after this labor the patient was operated upon for a blood cyst of the ovary about the size of an orange. The uterus was found firmly connected to the abdominal wall by a band of fascia an inch in width. In only a limited class of cases and after a certain age is ventrofixation the operation of selection, ventrosuspension being the safer operation during the childbearing period.

Sepsis following Abortion or Labor.—W. O. Henry *(Med. News,* May 24) advises the early removal, with finger, sharp curette, and flushing, of all decidua, blood clots, and sloughing tissue which may be infected. He would dry all raw surfaces and freely apply to them 95 per cent carbolic acid, washing away the surplus with sterile water. Unless hemorrhage requires, no tubes or packing of any kind should be left in either vagina or uterus. A 2 per cent carbolic douche should be used twice a day. The bowels must be kept open freely. He gives quinine, three grains every four hours, followed by tincture of the chloride of iron, fifteen drops in water. Nourishing diet. If abscesses form in the wall of the uterus, that organ should be removed. If pus forms in the tubes they are drained through the vagina.

GYNECOLOGY AND ABDOMINAL SURGERY.

Tuberculosis of Cervix.—Arthur H. N. Lewers *(Jour. Obst. and Gyn. Br. Emp.,* June) reports a case of primary tuberculosis of the cervix occurring in a patient 36 years old. There were no signs of tuberculosis in any other part of the body. The case was operated upon for supposed cancer of the cervix, the correct diagnosis being made some time after operation by a pathologist.

E. Octavius Croft *(Jour. Obst. and Gyn. Br. Emp.,* June) cites a case of papillary tuberculosis of the cervix occurring in a patient 26 years old. Vaginal hysterectomy was performed. The disease was apparently local and showed well-marked miliary tubercles with giant cells.

Operative Treatment of Cancer of the Uterus.—W. T. Burrage *(Boston Med. and Surg. Jour.,* July 24) finds that absolute cure of cancer of the uterus by operation is rare. By the best methods of operation, only from 5 to 10 per cent of the cases are well five years later. The results of operation for cancer of the body of the uterus are much more favorable than those for cancer of the cervix. All cases of uterine cancer, except those advanced cases which develop vesico-vaginal or recto-vaginal fistula, should be operated upon, if not with the prospect of effecting absolute cure, at least to prolong life and relieve suffering. In early cases of cancer, where the disease has not gone outside the uterus and the patient is in good condition, the best operation is the abdominal operation. In advanced cases where the disease has gone outside the uterus and where the patient's condition is poor, vaginal hysterectomy, curetting, and cautery are to be chosen.

Edward Reynolds *(Bost. Med. and Surg. Jour.,* July 24) believes the abdominal method of operating easier, neater, more complete, and more satisfactory. It affords us the opportunity of making an exact diagnosis of the conditions. The danger of subsequent hemorrhage and infection is less: it is not likely to be followed by painful adhesions. The vaginal route should be the choice in enfeebled women, because it is attended with very little shock.

M. R. Richardson *(Bost. Med. and Surg. Jour.,* July 24) advises radical operations only in cases where the growth is limited to the uterus or cervix, though a cure may be attempted if a very limited area only of the vaginal membrane is involved. Thickened masses in the broad ligament, remote metastases, infiltration about the ureters, infiltrations of the vagina, the rectum, and the bladder, are all distinct contraindications to hysterectomy. Vaginal hysterectomy is preferable when the uterus is movable, when the disease is distinctly confined to the cervix and the vagina is capacious. When the uterus is fixed, the vagina small, and the fundus large, the abdominal route is preferable. In at least 90 per cent of cases a satisfactory diagnosis can be made that operation is not feasible.

John O. Polak *(N. Y. Med. Jour.,* July 19) states that an early diagnosis is possible. The earliest symptoms differ, depending upon whether the disease begins during menstrual life or after the menopause. During menstrual life one should compare bleeding with what has previously taken place in the same woman. Suspicion should be aroused by intermenstrual spotting and serous discharge. After the menopause any serous or sanguineous discharge is significant. Every woman over 30 who may exhibit any menstrual vagary or persistent leucorrhea should be examined. Radical operation should be limited to those cases in which the disease is confined to the uterine tissues.

Dysmenorrhea.—G. E. Herman *(Br. Med. Jour.,* May) finds that pregnancy is the natural cure for spasmodic dysmenorrhea, but the disease is often accompanied by sterility, which may be cured by dilatation of the cervix. The best drugs for the relief of uterine colic are antipyrin and phenacetin. In severe cases it may be necessary to use morphine or chloroform. In a few cases ten grains of guaiacum resin will remove the pain. The local treatment of spasmodic dysmenorrhea is to dilate the cervix. This is best done by bougies. In certain very severe cases it may be necessary to remove the ovaries.

Stone in the Female Bladder.—P. J. Freyer *(Br. Gyn. Jour.,* May) removed a stone by litholapaxy from the bladder of a young woman. The nucleus was a slate pencil about three inches long. The débris of the pencil and phosphates collected on it weighed 237 grains. Litholapaxy in females is eminently successful and the patient is able to be about in a few days; there is no incontinence of urine.

An Acquired Hernia of the Fallopian Tube.—A. T. Bristow *(Med. News,* July 12) reports a case of strangulated hernia of the Fallopian tube and ovary of the left side. The patient was operated upon with good results. Acquired herniæ of the ovary nearly all occur on the right side, probably because the right ovary is more nearly in the iliac fossa.

Hematemesis after Operation.—So far as his personal experience is concerned, Halliday Croom *(Br. Gyn. Jour.,* May) is disposed to think that most cases of hematemesis after abdominal operation are due to sepsis. Sepsis could produce congestion and small hemorrhages in the mucous membranes; and whether sepsis be the actual cause or not, the phenomenon was usually observed in cases which ultimately succumbed to sepsis in some form or other. It is, as a rule, a precursor of death.

Hematemesis after Hysterectomy.—H. Macnaughton-Jones *(Br. Gyn. Jour.,* May) reports a fatal case of coffee-ground vomiting and hematemesis following a hysterectomy for multiple myomata.

Operation for Cystocele.—M. Chiaventona (article in MS.) describes an operation which is the result of extensive studies on the cadaver and on animals, and which he has successfully performed on living human beings. The technique may briefly

be described as follows: 1. Laparatomy. 2. Incision and exposure of the utero-vesical peritoneum and exposure of the base
of the bladder as far as the interureteric ligament. 3. Suture
of the base of the bladder to the anterior wall of the uterus.
4. Suture of the incised peritoneum in such a way as to restore
the serous covering of the pelvic organs. 5. Fixation of the
uterus by hysteropexy, with shortening of the round ligaments
by the Ruggi Spinelli method, according to the degree of the
prolapse in the individual case. 6. Suture of the abdominal
wound.

Parovarian Cysts.—Giuseppe Coen *(Ann. di Ost. e Gin.,*
March, 1902) states that there are two kinds of cyst which
originate within the folds of the broad ligament—those which
develop in the pelvis and those which develop in the abdomen.
The diagnosis of the former, and more frequent, is often easy:
of the latter, difficult. The chief characteristics of these intraligamentous cysts are: the slight influence exerted on the patient's general condition, the easily perceived sense of fluctuation,
the regularity of the cyst walls, the fact that they are unilocular,
and the quality of the fluid contained within them. They are
most frequently met with during the period of sexual activity.
These cysts may further be classified as hyaline and papillary,
the first being the more frequent. Treatment of these cysts
should always be surgical, varying according to whether they
are pelvic or abdominal, and according to the adhesions formed.
Extirpation or enucleation is the operation of choice, marsupiali-
zation the one of necessity. A frequent complication of abdominal intraligamentous cysts is torsion of the pedicle. In this
case there are seldom adhesions with neighboring organs, the
inner cyst wall seldom shows any signs of impeded circulation
in its vessels, and the contained liquid is not altered in any way.
The diagnosis of the complication is easy, the treatment surgical.

The Practical Value of Umikoff's Reaction in Human Milk.
—As a result of his researches Alessandro Mariani *(Ann. di Ost.
e Gin.,* March, 1902) states that: 1. Umikoff's reaction, although
not absolutely constant, is very frequently found in human milk,
whether this be heated to 60° C., as the author recommends, or be
cold. 2. By treating the milk with a solution of ammonium a
purplish red coloration is obtained which varies in intensity, this
intensity having no relation, however, to the age of the milk.
3. By heating the milk to above 60°, or boiling it, a coffee-brown
color is obtained. 4. Neither the early appearance of the coloration, its character, nor its tenacity after cooling are data which
give any information in regard to the time of parturition in relation to the extraction of the milk for examination. 5. The
amount of fat does not in the least influence the coloration.
6. Mariani does not believe that this reaction can give any information as to the age of the milk.

Metastatic Carcinoma of the Ovary.—F. Schlagenhaufer
(Monats. f. Geb. u. Gyn., Bd. xv., Ergänzungsheft) finds that a

large proportion of bilateral, usually solid, malignant tumors are metastatic carcinomata. Cases of so-called combination of malignant ovarian tumors and tumors of the stomach, intestine, or other abdominal organs are metastatic. The chief primary growth, excluding breast, uterus, and vagina, is carcinoma of the stomach, intestine, or gall bladder.

Conservative Treatment of Interstitial and Submucous Fibroid.—The conclusions reached by D. A. Abuladse *(Monats. f. Geb. u. Gyn.,* Bd. xv., Ergänzungsheft) are that conservative treatment should be employed for interstitial and submucous fibroids. Conservative myomectomy has a lower mortality than hysteromyomotomy and also permits the uterus to exercise its normal functions. Before trying myomotomy an attempt should be made to enucleate the growth.

Myomata and Heart Disease.—L. Kessler *(Zeit. f. Geb. u. Gyn.,* Bd. xlvii., H. 1) records the removal by laparatomy from a woman 54 years of age of a fibromyoma of the uterus weighing about sixty pounds. Convalescence progressed well until the seventh day, when the patient died suddenly while sitting up in bed. The autopsy showed fibroid changes in the myocardium of the auricles and left ventricle. Kessler is inclined to attribute this cardiac lesion to circulatory obstruction by the tumor. If this effect of uterine fibroids is conceded, the practical deduction is that every myoma which may reasonably be supposed to exert such an influence should be removed.

Vaginal Morcellation of Uterine Fibroid during Pregnancy. —Reports of the performance of operations upon the genital organs without disturbance of an existing pregnancy are no longer rarities, but the following case is worthy of notice, as the traumatism was exerted within the uterine cavity. The woman was four weeks pregnant when there occurred a severe hemorrhage from the uterus which was not arrested by tampons in the vagina. L. Seeligman *(Cent. f. Gyn.,* No. 21) then removed a submucous fibroid by morcellation, and packed the uterine cavity with iodoform gauze which was removed on the sixth day. Convalescence was rapid and pregnancy went on to term in spite of the tamponade and operation, the ovum being implanted upon the anterior wall of the uterus while the fibroid was attached to the posterior.

Result of Presence of Cauterization Scabs in Peritoneal Cavity.—H. Franz *(Zeit. f. Geb. u. Gyn.,* Bd. xlvii., H. 1) has conducted a series of experiments upon guinea-pigs to determine the practical results of leaving charred tissue in the peritoneal cavity. By comparison of such an area in one set of animals with an area simply denuded of peritoneum in another, it was found that in the first series there was a tendency to the formation of adhesions, while in the second series this did not occur. Another series of experiments with reference to the occurrence of infection showed that this was favored by the presence of cauterized tissue.

27

DISEASES OF CHILDREN.

Acute Pyelitis in Infancy.—James Ritchie *(Scottish Med. and Surg. Jour.*, July, 1902) reports a case in a baby 7½ months old. He says that the condition may be suspected in any case which presents considerable and perhaps irregular variations of temperature with apparent integrity of other systems. The condition of the urine—acid, with pus and bacteria—will complete the diagnosis. Cystitis may be excluded by the absence of painful and frequent micturition. The amount of pus varies, as does the degree of tenderness. Treatment consists chiefly in rendering the urine neutral and so removing the condition necessary for the growth of the bacillus; maintaining a copious flow of urine, so as to render it as little irritating as possible to the inflamed tracts; and general hygienic care. In the case described, marked improvement followed the use of sodium salicylate, the symptoms becoming worse when it was stopped. The existence of constipation and anal fissure may require special treatment.

John Thomson (ibid.) concludes from his study of this disease that: 1. In infant girls, when debilitated by any cause, acute pyelitis may be set up by the immigration of the .bacillus coli from the bowel. 2. The presence of the disease is sufficient to occasion very high fever, extreme distress, and a copious deposit of pus and bacteria in acid urine. 3. Unlike any other disease except malaria, it frequently causes rigors, even in young babies. 4. The presence of anal excoriations has possibly an important etiological significance in these cases. 5. The prognosis (when the case is treated) is altogether favorable, although complete recovery is sometimes delayed for many weeks. 6. The only essential treatment consists in the thorough and long-continued neutralization of the acid in the urine by the administration of alkaline remedies.

Amaurotic Family Idiocy.—A. Hymanson *(N. Y. Med. Jour.,* July 12, 1902) reports the case of a child of 15 months affected with amaurotic family idiocy. His parents were healthy and not consanguineous, but the five children of the patient's great-uncle died of apparently the same disorder. The etiology of the disease is still obscure; it is common among the Hebrews, especially among the Russian-Polish Jews. Family predisposition is evident from the fact that 28 cases tabulated by B. Sachs occurred in fifteen families. There did not seem to be any history of syphilis, alcoholism, or nervous derangement in any of the cases. There was consanguinity in only four cases. The development of the affection was not prevented by change of feeding from the mother's breast to that of the wet-nurse or to artificial food. No prophylactic measures have been discovered, and treatment was of no avail. E. Frey, who has made an autopsy on a child a year and a half old, corroborates the statement of Hirsch that the degeneration occurring in this form of idiocy is not congenital, but post-natal. It is not due to a defect of development, and he and others have demonstrated that the form and structure, as well as the convolutions, of the brain were normally arranged. It seems that there is some inexplicable condition, probably of an infective nature. possibly derived from the mother's milk, according to Jacobi. which causes a progressive degeneration in the cortices of the hemispheres and affects the cells and fibres of the entire nervous system, although food has no influence on the disease. The chief features of the affection are: idiocy, weakness of all the muscles. terminating in paralysis, gradual loss of sight and characteristic changes in the macula lutea, marasmus, and death at the end of the second year.

Chorea Minor from Intestinal Intoxication.—Mario de Maldè (*Riforma Med.*, May 19, 1902) describes the case of a girl of 9 years affected with chorea, for which it was difficult to find a cause. There was no family history of nervous taint of any kind, and chorea from imitation, from previous disease or diathesis, or from fright or shock had to be excluded. The possibility of worms as a cause induced the author to suggest an examination of the feces. The child's mother then acknowledged that there was obstinate constipation, an evacuation occurring only once in ten or twelve days, and even then consisting of a few hardened and offensive scybalæ. Energetic intestinal disinfection was at once instituted by means of 50 centigrammes of calomel in two doses. This resulted in the expulsion of a few scybalæ which were almost petrified, black, and fetid. No ascarides lumbricoides or their ova were found. On the following day a single dose of 30 centigrammes was given, and was followed by a copious evacuation of hard, black, and offensive matters. A glass of fluid magnesia was given in the morning for about ten days, the discharges being at first diarrheal and then normal. To the author's surprise the symptoms of chorea disappeared one after the other, and in a few weeks there was a complete cure.

The Dietetic Causation and Treatment of the Gastro-intestinal Diseases of Infancy.—R. O. Beard (*Northwestern Lancet.* June 1, 1902) says that in calling attention to the question of the causation and to the possibilities of the prevention or the cure of these death-dealing disorders of infant life, it may be well to recognize certain facts upon which these disorders are conditioned: 1. Gastro-intestinal diseases are essentially prevalent in infancy; they decrease with every year of life; they neither occur nor do they kill to any notable degree those whose years lie between infancy and old age. 2. They are largely of seasonal occurrence; their ravages are felt during the summer and autumn months. 3. They are of bacterial or parasitic origin. 4. The intestinal tract is usually the arena of their invasion. The dietetic causation of the gastro-intestinal diseases being the primary one, their prevention and cure are only to be accomplished by dietetic means. There are but two principles which enter importantly into treatment. One of these is physiologic rest. The other is therapeutic cleansing. The former should be regarded as a means of prevention as well as a means of cure. It is to be attained in part by affording the digestive organs an easy task. Human milk is of course the ideal food of infancy. The author believes that the successful feeding of the infant by natural means depends upon a physiologic equation between the nursing mother and the individual nursing child, which begins, not at the moment of birth, but at the moment of conception. When the mother is unable to nurse the child, wet-nursing is not so good a substitute as modified cow's milk. Gelatin solutions and starchy gruels are sometimes of value in diluting this milk. Water is not good, as it is not the sum total of the milk which requires dilution, but the caseinogen. Sterilization is under the shadow of a doubt as a probable cause of infantile scurvy. Physiologic rest for the digestive organs is further to be attained by a careful graduation of the quantity of food supplied to the infant. The common practice is to fill up an ill-nourished and frequently-fed infant with as much food as it can carry, trusting to its readiness of overflow. This is to invite indigestion and to add to the tendency of "starvation upon a full stomach." It has been possible, by a careful study of the average capacity of the infant stomach, to construct the following table of gastric capacity at successive periods of infancy:

AGE.	QUANTITY.	
	c.c.	ozs.
One week	70	2¼
One month	95	3
Two months	120	3¾
Three months	150	4½
Four months	175	5½
Five months	225	7
Seven months	275	8½
Nine months	300	9½

Perhaps the most important element in the attainment of physiologic rest is time. The infant digestion is relatively slow. It has been the practice of the writer for the past eighteen years to feed infants at the breast, from birth on, not oftener than once in four hours, and to order an abstinence from food at night. In the supply of artificial foods or imitations of the human milk, still longer intervals, involving from three to five meals in the twenty-four hours, are demanded. This practice, with other observances of physiologic rest, has secured to over 800 infants so fed not only a practical immunity from gastro-intestinal disease, but a gain in weight (which is really the only true test of successful nutrition) above the average. In the treatment of acute forms of gastro-intestinal disease, physiologic rest has been successfully carried to the point of practical starvation for periods varying from one to seven days. In cholera infantum complete abstinence from food during the acute onset of the disease is invariably remedial. A material aid to physiologic rest is the therapeutic attainment of regular and thorough cleansing of the alimentary canal. By the use of large quantities of water given to the always thirsty infant, by the judicious employment of laxatives to clear away the débris of digestion in the small bowel, and by the systematic use of the colonic flush, a diminution of pain, of diarrhea, and of toxemia is always to be secured.

The Importance of Milk Analysis in Infant Feeding.—A. H. Wentworth *(Boston Med. and Surg. Jour.,* July 3, 1902) gives the following summary of the result of his researches: 1. The general statement that the upper one-fourth of one quart of cow's milk in which the cream has risen contains ten per cent of fat, represents the average of a large number of milks. There is too much variation in milks from different cows to enable one to figure modifications of milk on this basis with any degree of accuracy. 2. The results of the great variation in cow's milks would not be of so much consequence if the percentage of fat in the cream were always low. Too much fat in a modified milk is more likely to cause digestive disturbance than too little. 3. It is advisable, therefore, to have the percentage of fat determined in the cream at least once whenever an infant begins to use modified milk. It is also advisable to have the fat determination repeated at the times of year when the cattle's food is changed. 4. It is not advisable to modify milk with a cream in which the percentage of fat is too low—under ten per cent—because if one obtains a sufficient percentage of fat in the modification the percentage of proteids will be too high in many cases. 5. If the percentage of fat is too low in the upper eight ounces from one quart of "set milk," it is better to take fewer ounces off of the top, determine the percentage of fat in these ounces, and use such a number of ounces of cream as contains twelve per cent, or more, of fat. If more proteid is required it can be obtained by the addition of lower milk which is almost free from fat. 6. A safe rule would be to have at least one determination of fat made, no matter how many ounces are taken from the top of the "set" milk, and afterward to continue to take the same number of ounces off each time. 7. In order to make a modification of milk in which a high percentage of fat is combined with a low percentage of proteid, it is necessary to use a cream that contains a high percentage of fat. In general it is better to use a cream removed from the milk at home than to use cream bought for this purpose, because the latter is much more likely to be stale and to have undergone changes due to heat or to age. 8. Within certain limits, accurate percentage modifications of milk are not essential to the well-being of a majority of the babies that are fed on modified milk. Proof of this is afforded by the fact that so many infants do well when fed on modified milk, and yet it has been shown by the results of analysis that these modifications are rarely accurate. Unfortunately it is not always possible to tell beforehand to which class a given case belongs, and this is a sufficient reason, even if there were no others, for modifying the milk as accurately as possible. A complete analysis of the milk requires too much time and training to make it a practical procedure, except in special cases. The determination of the percentage of fat in the cream used for modification is easily made, requires but a few minutes to do, and enables modifications of milk to be made that are accurate enough for most cases, if in addition directions for modifying are carefully given and followed. 9. The *advantage* of modifications of milk furnished by establishments is that it is convenient. It relieves the family of all responsibility so far as the preparation of the infant's food is concerned. Three great objections to the use of commercial modifications of milk are: *(a)* inaccurate modifications, *(b)* stale milks, *(c)* expense. *(a)* The claim is made by those interested in the sale of commercial modifications of milk that the percentages of fat, sugar, and proteids are accurately determined in each modification. This claim of exactness forms the basis upon which such commercial modifications of milk largely depend for their success. Analyses submitted by the writer show how little dependence can be placed upon such statements. *(b)* People who reside beyond the limits of wagon delivery—and most people do so for several months each year—have to use on Sundays and part of Mondays milk that is delivered on Saturdays and of a necessity milked on Fridays. It is claimed that no deleterious changes take place in these milks if they are kept cold. A sufficient number of clinical observations have been made to show that such a claim is unwarranted. *(c)* The cost of modifications of milk made at home is less than twenty-five cents a day. Compare this with the cost of commercial modifications of milk, to which must be added in many cases the cost of transportation. 10. The technique of fat determination by the Babcock method is simple and easily acquired. The entire outfit, including a centrifugal machine, flasks, pipettes, and acid, can be purchased for nine dollars. The time required for a fat determination by this method is about fifteen minutes.

Intussusception in a Child; Operation; Recovery.—A. Primrose *(Canadian Pract. and Rev.,* Mar., 1902) reports the case of a child of 3½ years suffering from pain in the abdomen, an obstruction which the administration of purgatives was powerless to relieve. There was persistent vomiting, and from time to time she passed quantities of bloody mucus. On admission to the hospital her face was flushed, but she did not look very ill, save that she appeared to be in a condition of lethargy. The tongue was coated, temperature 100°, pulse 132, respirations 28 per minute. A distinct tumor could be felt on palpating the abdomen in the left lumbar region. Abdominal section revealed the intussusception, which was reduced. The following condition was noticed after reduction: extensive ecchymosis in the portion of the omentum which had followed the invaginated bowel into the intussuscipiens; the bowel above the tumor was quite collapsed; there had been absolutely no distension. A very much thickened piece of bowel formed the apex of the intussusceptum. The amount of thickening here was so remarkable that the author found it impossible to convince himself by manipulation that the lumen was pervious. It reminded one somewhat of the normal pylorus, but involved a much larger extent of the gut. To make sure that obstruction was not complete he had normal saline injected per rectum, and satisfied himself that fluid passed through the thickened portion. The little patient made an uneventful and uninterrupted recovery.

Measles.—An editorial comment *(Pediatrics,* Mar. 1, 1902) calls attention to the caution necessary in the treatment of measles in the tenements. Measles is regarded by many mothers who live in tenements as a very mild disease. They consider that warmth and exclusion of light are all that is required and that the services of a doctor are superfluous. The result is that the patient is often put in a dark inside room which is overheated and insufficiently ventilated. His resistance is so much the more lowered and he becomes specially liable to some secondary infection, most frequently broncho-pneumonia, diphtheria, or tuberculosis. A patient with broncho-pneumonia following measles who in addition contracts diphtheria is in a well-nigh hopeless condition. Yet this sequence does occur. The writer is cognizant of four intubations performed within the past two months for laryngeal diphtheria following measles. In each of the four cases the doctor who was called in when the symptoms of croup became marked attributed the condition to catarrhal laryngitis complicating measles, and did not administer antitoxin, or even make a culture, until the severity of the symptoms made operative intervention imperative. It should be kept in mind that symptoms of croup occurring during measles may not be due to catarrhal laryngitis, but to diphtheria. If the symptoms are at all severe a large dose of antitoxin will certainly be on the side of safety.

Marked Separation of the Pubic Bones.—J. E. Goldthwaite *(Boston Med. and Surg. Jour.,* July 10, 1902) reports a case illustrating an unusual condition. A boy 11 years of age had disease of the right hip joint, tubercular in character. At the time of the examination it was noticed that the pubic bones were markedly separated, there being seven and three-quarter centimetres between the spines of these bones. Both iliac bones had separated so that the anterior superior spines were the outermost portion of the iliac bones, instead of the middle of the crest as is normal. There was considerable motion owing to the looseness of the sacro-iliac articulation, but this did not prevent the child from walking freely, and had apparently caused no symptoms. The right pubic bone was more prominent than the other, and appeared on first inspection like a tumor projecting at what would ordinarily be the location of the external inguinal ring. The only thing to in any way account for the condition was that when 2½ years old the child was run over and was lame for a short time, but ultimately improved so that he was considered well until six months previous to the examination, when the trouble with the hip began.

Medical Examination of Criminals.—An item *(Northwestern Lancet,* June 1, 1902) states that the following is part of a resolution which was adopted at the last meeting of the Congress of Criminal Anthropology, recently held in the city of Amsterdam, Holland; it should be followed in the rules of procedure in all of our criminal courts: "1· Every child who has committed a crime should be examined by a competent physician before being summoned into court, and those discovered to be actual degenerates should be placed in pedagogic establishments organized for the purpose of training and improving them intellectually and morally. 2. The biologic record of the criminal should be appended to the court record in every criminal case. 3. Government should take effective steps to arrest the progress of alcoholism."

Otitis Media Purulenta Treated by the Dry Method.—F. W. Davis *(N. Y. Med. Jour.,* July 12, 1902) says that the natural resistance of the mucous membrane lining the tympanic cavity to micro-organisms is very great, and if drainage is effectually established recovery from disease is very rapid. Dryness is as fatal to most germs as strong chemical antiseptics, and in no way can the tympanic cavity be kept dry so effectually as by gauze drainage. After a thorough trial of dry cleansing and gauze drainage, the writer believes it to be more effectual than the use of watery injections, etc., in all cases, whether acute or chronic. It requires a little more skill than simple syringing and powder-blowing. The discharge should be thoroughly wiped away with the cotton carrier, exposing the drum, perforation, or the tympanic cavity if the drum is destroyed. In the latter case the cotton can be introduced into the middle ear and clean it of all secretion. A narrow strip of dry gauze should now be introduced through a speculum and the canal loosely packed to the meatus. This should be allowed to remain until soaked with the discharge, whether it takes one or twenty-four hours. It should then be removed, and a piece of dry cotton placed and left in the meatus until the next packing. The packing should usually be done twice daily in acute cases, once in chronic cases. No antiseptics or other medicaments are necessary. Plain sterile gauze is used. In chronic cases, where the discharge is offensive, a few instillations of boric acid in alcohol, before each packing, correct the fetor. The alcohol aids the treatment by its drying action, and the boric acid stimulates the membrane to healthy action. The draining away of the discharges accomplishes cures more rapidly than any other method, is agreeable to the patient, and keeps him under the direct care of the physician. The writer believes that there are few cases that will not yield to this treatment. He reports three out of a large number.

Primary Intestinal Tuberculosis.—M. Nicoll *(Arch. of Ped.,* May, 1902) reports the case of a child, 2 years and 3 months old, suffering from measles and ulcers about the eyes. Death took place very suddenly from broncho-pneumonia. At the autopsy an ulcer was found about two inches above the ileo-cecal valve, and corresponding to it, in the mesentery, a mass the size of a walnut composed of half a dozen or more cheesy lymph nodes. Many other of the mesenteric lymph nodes were enlarged, whitish or pinkish in color, with no evidence of tubercle. A very long and careful search was required to demonstrate the presence of tubercle bacilli in the sections. The point of interest in the case is the presence of a single primary lesion of tuberculous infection, without any evidence of tuberculosis elsewhere except in the lymph nodes of the immediate neighborhood. It cannot be doubted that death alone prevented the occurrence of a general miliary tuberculosis, and when one considers the general condition of the patient, and the well-known tendency of measles to light up a previously quiescent tuberculous process, it is rather remarkable that the tuberculous process had not made further progress. The case constitutes the sixth example of undoubted primary intestinal tuberculosis occurring at the New York Foundling Hospital among many autopsies performed by Drs. Northrup, Freeman, Bovaird, and the writer.

The Probable Injurious Effects of Caraway Seeds.—W. Bramwell *(Med. Times and Hosp. Gaz.*, June 7, 1902) says that one of his patients was suffering from ischio-rectal abscess, and, dreading anything in the shape of lancet or knife, had allowed it to discharge spontaneously. While pressing out the pus the writer caught sight of a little black speck which turned out to be a caraway seed. This was in a perfect state of preservation, and, in spite of the fact that it had been lying in pus, was not even softened or swollen from the absorption of moisture, but was as hard as ever and had many sharp points. The pointed extremities of many of these seeds are of needle-like sharpness, one of which projecting from a hardened mass of feces could easily become fixed in the mucous membrane, and when pointing downward be driven further into it by the downward passage of the feces during defecation, thus forming a suitable nidus for the commencement of abscess resulting in fistula. It is probable, too, from similar reasons, that these seeds may be the cause of some cases of peritonitis of obscure origin, and perhaps also of abscess and ulcer of the stomach, to say nothing of the irritation resulting in cancer. During the process of baking they soften and swell up, but as the loaf cools they contract and harden, changing color to black or dark brown. The increased hardness renders them doubly dangerous weapons in their passage through the stomach and intestines, especially the smaller varieties, which do not appear to soften while lying in the intestinal fluids.

Pulse Variations in Childhood.—G. A. Dotti *(Rivista Critica di Clin. Med.*, May 17, 1902) concludes from his studies: 1. That the normal and pathological pulse of children is more variable than that of adults. 2. Temporary changes are very frequent, and usually occur during convalescence from acute febrile diseases, even such light ones as mumps and chicken-pox. 3. Permanent arhythmia is much more rare. 4. Dicrotism is the most frequently occurring change, and its degree appears to be independent of the body temperature. It is present in all cases of typhoid, less characteristic and less frequently found in pulmonary affections, and more rarely still in diphtheria, scarlet fever, and meningitis. 5. The paradoxical pulse is distinctly felt in nearly all cases of stenotic diphtheritic laryngitis. It does not occur in catarrhal laryngitis, as a rule, but may be found in grave and diffuse pulmonary troubles. 6. Allorrhythmia is specially found in the convalescence from typhoid, allied to bradycardia. 7. False intermittence has no importance *per se,* but is probably a transition stage toward true intermittence. 8. As to the various diseases studied by the author, he has found that in *typhoid* the arhythmia appears from the fifteenth to the thirtieth day, disappearing from the thirty-fifth to the fiftieth. The earlier it comes the later it goes, and *vice versa.* In *pneumonia* the pulse is more similar to the typhoid pulse than in other pulmonary affections; in the latter there is irregularity rather than true intermittence. In *influenza* the arhythmia occurs early. In diphtheritic angina arhythmia is observed in less degree; in light cases there is tachycardia and a small pulse, in the grave cases bradycardia corresponding to severe lesions of the myocardium. In the convalescence from scarlatina the bradycardia is even more marked than in typhoid. The disappearance of the arhythmia coincides with the beginning of desquamation.

The School and its Effect upon the Health of Girls.—W. B. Drummond *(Scottish Med. and Surg. Jour.,* July, 1902) says that, considering how great a drain upon a girl's energy is the rapid development which takes place at puberty, the general line of treatment in schools should be such as to avoid undue dissipation of energy; to avoid all the known causes of that curious form of fatigue which has attained notoriety under the name of over-pressure. For many girls, rest during, or at least at the beginning of, each period, until the habit is thoroughly established, is a necessity if health is not to suffer. As Dr. Reynolds says: "The world has known for a great many generations that it could get more work out of itself in six days than in seven: it has come to know that employees must be given two weeks' vacation out of a year, and that the brain-worker can do very much more work in eleven than in twelve months out of the year. I believe, when we are a little bit more civilized, we shall know that, as a pure matter of economics, we can drive more work out of women in twenty-five days than we can in twenty-eight." If this is so, it rests with the school so to arrange its time table as to make this relaxation of work possible without embarrassment to the pupils. The following are a few general points which require consideration in the case of girls: *(a) Nutrition.* Periodical, but not too frequent, weighing and measurement of the children would give many a timely hint if all were not going well. *(b) Physical exercise.* This is of the greatest value and importance, but there must be kept in mind the danger of overexertion, strain, and fatigue at the time of puberty. For physical exercise, girls should be classed on a physical and not an intellectual basis. Even such an apparently trifling matter as the steepness of the school stairs, and the number of times the girls have to climb them in passing from class to class, deserves more attention than it receives. *(c) Suitable clothing,* both for ordinary wear and exercise. *(d) Abundance of interesting occupation* and a healthy mental environment, with plenty of rest between the periods of activity. *(e) Early hours* and *sufficient sleep.* Social and outside demands are often the disturbing factor here rather than the school. *(f) The school medical officer.* This applies, as a rule, to boarding schools. The author notices with pleasure that the school boards in England are tending more and more to appoint medical officers to act with and to advise the board as to conditions affecting health in the schools.

Spasmodic Wryneck Appearing in the Course of a Case of Exophthalmic Goitre.—Walter G. Stern *(Cleveland Med. Jour.,* April, 1902) reports the case of a girl of 14 years, suffering from exophthalmic goitre, who was troubled with torticollis. The case was at first diagnosed as one of Pott's disease of the cervical vertebræ, but the position of the chin, which, though deviated to the right, looked upward, should have sufficed to exclude that affection. Moreover, the pain was not constant nor localized, pressure upon the vertebræ was painless, there was no limitation of motion of atlas or axis, no swelling of the bodies of the vertebræ, no retropharyngeal abscess, nor did the child hesitate to jump from a chair without supporting her head with her hands. Under anesthesia the muscles relaxed completely and the neck was freely movable. From congenital torticollis the history, the symmetry of the head, and the absence of any permanent contractures, as shown under anesthesia, give the differential diagnosis. From scoliosis, or congenital elevation of the shoulders, the presence of the various contracted muscles speaks for wryneck. The youth of the patient is unusual, both for exophthalmic goitre and for spasmodic wryneck. Out of 32 cases of wryneck Walton reports only 2 under 20 years of age. Exophthalmic goitre has been reported by several French authors even as early as the second year. With the exclusion of the possibility of Pott's disease or congenital wryneck, all thoughts of laminectomy or tenotomy are dispelled. In this case the author would follow out the best course of treatment known for exophthalmic goitre. In other cases of spasmodic wryneck the best treatment is that advocated by Dr. Hamann in his splendid paper upon the treatment of spasmodic wryneck. The author wishes but to emphasize the fact that, when the operation of cutting the posterior nerve roots is performed, it be done on both sides, for if performed only upon one side the muscles of the other may take up the spasm, as one case under my care has well shown. Massage, electricity, and intermuscular injections of curare, hyoscine, belladonna, and like drugs produce few lasting effects, but may sometimes be tried with benefit.

Spinal Cocainization with Double Amputation on a Child.— William H. Brooke *(N. Y. Med. Jour.*, July 12, 1902) reports the case of a colored boy of 9 years, both of whose feet were frozen, with marked swelling of both legs and thighs. In a few days they were gangrenous. While waiting for a line of demarcation he had a septic temperature ranging between 99.2° and 106° F., with rapid, feeble pulse and marked delirium. Spinal analgesia was decided on, and thirty minims of a two per cent solution of cocaine were injected in the usual way. In three minutes there was complete anesthesia in the left leg; in five minutes it was complete in both. Both legs were amputated at the middle third, the stumps healing in nine days by first intention. One hour after the operation the temperature was 103.2° F., but it fell to 99.6° the next morning, and remained below 99.8° until complete recovery. Headache was mild and of short duration, with little nausea and no vomiting. The boy was fairly comfortable twenty-four hours after operation, which was remarkable, considering his poor condition before operation. The pulse remained full and regular, though a little rapid, during the operation and for two days after, when it became more slow.

Spindle-Cell Sarcoma of the Thorax in a Child.—Louis Fischer *(Arch. of Ped.*, May, 1902) reports the case of a boy of 8 years who had a number of tumors on the front of the thorax which felt quite hard on palpation. Operation was performed, but the child died shortly after. The tumor was found to be a spindle-cell sarcoma in a rather active state of growth, on account of the large number of mitoses present. Sarcomatous growths in children are quite rare. Manderli, in the Children's Hospital at Basle, Switzerland, reports ten patients in the past twenty years. The interesting points about the present case are: 1. That the heart was displaced, so that it was immediately behind the right nipple. ' 2. There was intense dyspnea, caused by the pressure of the tumor. 3. There were constant cyanosis and edema of the limbs, due to interference with the return circulation to the right side of the heart.

Strangulated Hernia in Nursing Infants.—E. Estor *(Rev. de Chir.*, June 10, 1902) reaches the following conclusions on the subject: 1. Strangulated hernia is rare in infancy, but not exceptional, as proved by his statistics involving 232 observations. 2. The rare occurrence of strangulation is explained by the slight resistance offered by the tissues composing the canal containing the visceral hernia. 3. Strangulation of appendicular and ceco-appendicular hernia is the most frequent in infancy. 4. The symptoms differ according to whether there is strangulated enterocele or hernial appendicitis.   5. The mortality from celotomy is a trifle less during the two first years of life than in adults.   6. Strangulation being less constricted than in adults, the time during which celotomy can be attempted is naturally prolonged beyond the same period in adults.   7. Hernial appendicitis is a more serious affection than strangulated enterocele. 8. The general condition of the child should have the greatest influence on prognosis.

Tetanus and Vaccination.—Joseph McFarland (*Medicine*, June, 1902), from an analytical study of 95 cases of this rare complication, reaches the following conclusions: 1. Tetanus is not a frequent complication of vaccination, a total of ninety-five cases having been collected.   2. The number of cases observed in 1901 was out of all proportion to what has been observed heretofore.   3. The cases are chiefly American and occur scattered throughout the eastern United States and Canada.   4. They have nothing to do with atmospheric, telluric, or seasonal conditions. 5. They occur in small numbers after the use of various viruses. 6. An overwhelming proportion occurs after the use of a particular virus.   7. The tetanus organism may be present in the virus in small numbers, being derived from manure and hay. 8. Occasionally, through carelessness or accident, the number of bacilli becomes greater than usual.   9. The future avoidance of the complication is to be sought for in greater care in the preparation of the vaccine virus.

Tuberculosis, The Infectiousness of the Nails of Children in Regard to.—Preisich and Schütz (*Berl. klin. Wochens.*, vol. xxxix., No. 20) examined the dirt scraped from under the nails of 66 children between the ages of 6 months and 2 years, and found tubercle bacilli present in 14, or 21.2 per cent.   Five of the infants had no tuberculous history.   In six there were cases of tuberculosis in the family, in two the infants themselves had the disease, and in one other the child was cared for by a family who had lost two children of tuberculosis, and one had cervical adenitis at the time of observation.   These examinations were made during the months of February, March, and April, a time when the children go out but little.   Animal experiments showed that other pathogenic germs besides tubercle bacilli were present, and this fact explains the frequent occurrence of cervical adenitis in young children.   The observations further demonstrate the infectious nature of the dust of living rooms.

Urine, The Study of, in Young Children.—J. Madison Taylor (*Internat. Med. Ann.*, May, 1902) says that it is becoming well understood that urinalyses reveal significant clinical facts far beyond the mere evidences of disease of the kidneys.   The trouble of bedside urinalyses is not great, but unless one becomes habituated to making them it seems a grave burden.   In conditions of infectious disease this should be invariably done, or a standing order be left for specimens to be sent to the laboratory at regular intervals for a number of days.   As to the difficulties of obtaining a specimen, these seem greater than they really are. A piece of absorbent cotton surrounded by a bit of oil silk, rubber dam, or waxed paper, and laid over the genital organs and under the buttocks, will usually suffice for the youngest infant. For older infants, a month or more, the habit can readily be established of passing water at fairly regular intervals in a vessel on which they are placed. The total quantity passed in twenty-four hours should be ascertained; the time when the specimen is passed in relation to food and drink; the color described; the reaction and specific gravity stated. The tests used for albumin should be specified; if present, the percentage; so of tests for sugar. Tests for indican, acetone, and bile are of importance. The urea should be estimated in percentages. The sediment should be described. Then any special tests for the particular specimen may receive attention. Finally, a clear statement should follow of the microscopic findings after centrifugation.

Floyd M. Crandall (ibid.) says that the character of the urine in infancy must be fully understood, lest erroneous conclusions be drawn. After the third day the specific gravity is very low, ranging on the fourth or fifth day from 1003 to 1007. During the first six months it is rarely over 1010; before the beginning of the fourth year it is not often found above 1014; after ten years it may be found as high as 1020, but it is more commonly about 1015 until the fifteenth year. After the first days of life, when the urine is apt to be scanty and high-colored, it is commonly pale or colorless. The amount of urine is comparatively large in young children, because their food is largely liquid and because of the active metabolism of infancy. The reaction is commonly faintly acid, but may be neutral or even faintly alkaline without being abnormal. The ratio of uric acid to urea steadily decreases after infancy, but is larger throughout childhood. The brickdust deposit of new-born infants and young children consists of crystals of uric acid. The urine is usually sharply acid, of comparatively high specific gravity, and sometimes very irritating. It is best relieved by giving freely of water, especially alkaline water. The lithuria of older children requires thorough examination to determine the underlying cause—indigestion should especially be sought for and corrected. Albumin during the first week of life has little significance; after that its occurrence has usually the same significance as in later life. The chief exception to the rule is the so-called cyclic or functional albuminuria which is occasionally seen in children between 5 and 15 years. Hyaline and sometimes granular casts may be found in the urine of perfectly healthy infants during the first week— sugar during the first three or four weeks. During the second or third month its appearance is usually accompanied by symptoms of impaired digestion. In these cases the sugar may sometimes be detected by Fehling's test when it cannot be found by the fermentation test. The diagnosis of functional glycosuria should not be made too quickly, for diabetes may occur very early in life. Blood in the urine of children is probably always pathologic. In addition to the causes which may account for its appearance in later life are melena, purpura, scurvy, and new growths of the kidney. Pus in the urine of young children may have its source in any portion of the urinary tract, but is most frequently derived from the pelvis of the kidney. Acute pyelitis and pyonephrosis are not uncommon in infants. Chronic pyuria is commonly due to a calculus or to tuberculosis of the kidney. The author frequently makes use of the lactometer accompanying Holt's milk-testing apparatus, in examining the urine of infants. It requires but little more than a tablespoonful of fluid, and is as accurate as one requiring several ounces.

Vaccination.—William L. Welch and Jay F. Schamberg (*Therapeutic Gazette,* June 15, 1902), referring to their experiences at the Municipal Hospital of Philadelphia during the recent epidemic, give a table showing the comparative mortality rates in the vaccinated and the unvaccinated; it also gives the mortality percentage in individuals with good, fair, and poor vaccination scars, respectively:

	Admitted.	Died.	Per Cent.
Vaccinated in infancy (good mark)	268	7	2.61
" " " (fair mark)........ ..	83	10	12.04
" " " (poor mark)..........	98	14	14.28
Vaccinated cases	449	31	6.90
Unvaccinated cases	465	131	28.17
Vaccinated after infection	63	12	19.04
Total.......................	977	174	17.80

This table shows that the danger from smallpox in vaccinated persons can be measured to a considerable degree by the character of the vaccination scars. It is seen that those showing good scars were better protected than those showing fair scars, and that the latter were better protected than those showing poor scars. It should be stated, perhaps, that we have classed as "good scars" all those distinctly excavated, having a well-defined margin reticulated or foveolated, and altogether presenting the appearance of having been stamped into the skin with a sharply-cut die. Under the head of fair scars are classed all those presenting the same general characteristics, though much less distinctly marked. Under the head of "poor scars" are classed all those which are said to have resulted from vaccination, but which very often were so indistinct or uncharacteristic as to make it difficult and sometimes even impossible to recognize them as vaccination scars. The author calls particular attention to the great difference in the death rate between the vaccinated and the unvaccinated patients. Those who were vaccinated in infancy and showed good scars gave the remarkably low death rate of 2.61 per cent, as against the high death rate of 28.17 per cent in the unvaccinated. There is no doubt that all those who showed either good or fair scars were successfully vaccinated in infancy. If we consider them together, therefore, the death rate is 4.84 per cent. In making a comparison between the vaccinated and the unvaccinated cases, it is scarcely fair to include as vaccinated all the cases showing poor scars, as very many of them doubtless were never successfully vaccinated at all. The table further shows that sixty-three patients had been vaccinated after exposure to the smallpox infection, therefore during the period of incubation of the disease.

The following table shows the cases vaccinated after exposure, divided according to the period which elapsed between the vaccination and the appearance of the smallpox eruption:

Vaccinated seven days or less before eruption.			Vaccinated more than seven days before eruption.		
Cases.	Died.	Per cent.	Cases.	Died.	Per cent.
14	5	35.71	49	7	14 28

When vaccination is performed soon after the exposure to smallpox, absolute protection is not infrequently conferred; but when it is delayed a few days the protection may be only partial, and when delayed too long there is usually none at all. The table shows that the patients who had been vaccinated seven days or less than seven days before the appearance of the eruption of smallpox gave a death rate of 35.71 per cent, while those who had been vaccinated for a longer period than seven days before the outbreak of the efflorescence gave a death rate of only 14.28 per cent.

Vermiform Appendix of a Child as Found after Death.— John D. Malcolm (*The Lancet,* July 5, 1902) reports the case of a little girl of 6 years who died after two days' illness, unattended by any physician. Dr. Rendall was sent for after her death, and was told that while at school she was suddenly seized with violent pain in the abdomen, vomiting, and diarrhea. The next day she was better off and on, but died suddenly on the succeeding day. The body was opened by order of the coroner. The small intestine and mesentery were found to be glued together by inflammatory adhesions so as to shut off the pelvic cavity. The appendix was in a gangrenous state beneath the adherent coils. and close to the peritoneum covering the sacrum. Liquid feces had exuded and had filled the pelvic cavity. On incising the appendix a concretion was exposed, and was found to be formed about a pin, the point of the pin being directed toward the tip of the appendix. The case is interesting, as it shows that the most serious mischief connected with the vermiform appendix may excite no real anxiety in the minds of a patient's friends.

THE AMERICAN

JOURNAL OF OBSTETRICS

AND

DISEASES OF WOMEN AND CHILDREN.

| Vol. XLVI. | OCTOBER, 1902. | No. 4. |

ORIGINAL COMMUNICATIONS.

REPORT OF TWO ' CASES OF GASTRECTOMY:
WITH REMARKS.[1]

BY

ALBERT VANDER VEER, M.D.,

Albany, N. Y.

At one of the meetings of the Medical Society of the County of Albany, I think during the winter of 1885, in presenting a number of pathological specimens, I exhibited a stomach that I had removed post mortem, a case of carcinoma, and in my remarks I said to the gentlemen present that this organ could have been removed with probable success. In all my abdominal work from that time on I did not meet with another case that offered any encouragement in doing this operation until the following:

Case I.—Mrs. B. S., Albany, N. Y., æt. 42, married, housewife by occupation. Entered the Albany Hospital February 12, 1900.

Present Illness.—More than one year ago noticed that when taking solid food she would vomit five or ten minutes afterward. Liquids did not distress her, nor did she have any pain. During the past year she has not been able to take solid food of any

---

[1] Read at the meeting of the American Association of Obstetricians and Gynecologists, Washington. D. C.. September 16, 17, and 18, 1902.

kind. Once in a great while would vomit, even if strictly on a liquid diet, never any great amount. Has lived mostly on milk. Has lost considerable in weight. For about two months has noticed a bunch in left side, which has gradually increased in size. On physical examination this can easily be made out, just above the umbilicus, and a little to the left of the median line— a tumor, lobulated and size of her fist, with slight tenderness on palpation.

Past History.—Married at 21 years of age; has had six children, four living; no miscarriages; menstruation always regular.

Family History.—Patient has four brothers and four sisters alive and well. No history of malignancy or tuberculosis. She remained in the hospital until operation, vomiting more or less continuously. Diagnosis made of carcinoma of the stomach, probably involving omentum and transverse colon. The case was thoroughly explained to the husband and patient, and their consent readily granted to an exploratory incision, with the understanding that if the diseased mass could be successfully removed we would go on with the operation. The patient, while in the hospital, had been given one grain of calomel, in divided doses, followed by two A. S. and B. pills, and apparently producing a good movement of the bowels. The intestinal tract was thoroughly emptied by means of rectal enemata. Pulse previous to the operation did not go above 100 at any one time. Respiration was slightly increased and temperature normal. She had slept very well, although somewhat restless the night previous to the operation.

Operation February 20, 1900. Gastrectomy. Median incision between ensiform cartilage and umbilicus. Upon opening the abdomen a hard mass occupying the greater curvature and cardiac end of the stomach was found. There were a few adhesions, but the neighboring glands were not infiltrated. The omentum was ligated in sections, and stomach loosened from all of its attachments. The duodenum and pyloric end of the stomach grasped with forceps and section made well below the tumor, the stomach being gradually worked out of its bed up to the cardiac end. Cardiac end of the esophagus grasped and stomach removed. Duodenum joined to end of the esophagus by means of a medium-sized Murphy button. In the entire operation very little blood was lost. There was considerable tension observed at the time, the disease extending so close to the diaphragm, and the esophagus was loosened by lateral incisions. The abdominal wound closed by silkworm-gut sutures and standard dressings applied. Anesthetic fairly well taken, operation lasting one and one-half hours.

Patient returned from the operating room with a cold, uncomfortable perspiration over the surface of the body, which was relieved by brisk rubbing and wrapping up in flannel blankets. Pulse 126. She complained of a good deal of difficulty in breathing; could not take a full inspiration, at times gasping for breath, and had a great desire to sit up. Mouth very dry. Hot bottles applied to extremities.

February 20, 3 p.m.: Pulse 114. 4 p.m.: Pulse 108. Mouth occasionally cleansed with hot water; patient apparently reacting very well, much warmer, and a better pulse of good volume. 5 p.m.: Was turned on her side and a pillow firmly applied to back: complained of pain through abdomen. 6 p.m.: Pulse 116; rectal enema well retained. 6.30 p.m.: Pulse 126: one-sixth grain of morphia given hypodermatically. 7 p.m.: Pain much less severe; patient said she felt better. 8 p.m.: Pulse 124, temperature 98.8°, respiration 30. 9 p.m.: One-thirtieth grain of strychnia continued every three hours, rectal stimulating enemata every four hours, hypodermatically; has slept a few minutes and feels quite comfortable. 9:30 p.m.: Sleeping. 10:10 p.m.: Rectal enema well retained; pulse 128. 10:45 p.m.: Pulse 118, good volume; very quiet; not sleeping. 11 p.m.: Voided four ounces of urine; position changed more to side. 11:30 p.m.: Complained of sharp pain in right side of abdomen; position changed, by great desire of patient, and she was made much more comfortable.

February 21, midnight: Temperature 100°, pulse 124, respiration 26; perspiring very freely; hot-water bottles continued to feet. 12:30 a.m.: Sleeping; pulse good. 1 a.m.: Slept fifteen minutes: belching up a little gas; no nourishment allowed, but mouth rinsed frequently. 1:10 a.m.: After sleeping ten minutes, awoke with a start, giving herself quite a severe movement of the body; pulse soon after became weaker and rapid, about 140. 1:20 a.m.: Hypodermatic injection of brandy, repeated in a few minutes: legs and arms rubbed with warm alcohol: skin cold and unpleasant to the touch. 1:45 a.m.: Dressings changed and wound found to be in good condition. From this time on the patient grew more restless, pulse much weaker, respiration increased to 36, very labored, gasping and sighing for breath, and she died at 3:30 A.M.

Upon opening the site of the incision it was discovered that the attachment between the duodenum and esophagus had given way; that the upper segment of the Murphy button had loosened in its attachment to the esophagus, allowing what little fluid contents were present to escape into the peritoneal cavity.

I cannot conceive of a more embarrassing position than in doing an operation of this kind, as it becomes very difficult to make attachments to the under surface of the diaphragm only.

CASE II.—Transferred from the medical side by Drs. Ward and Neuman. Mr. H. M., æt. 55 years; native of Canada; blacksmith by occupation; residence, Turner's Falls, Mass. Entered Albany Hospital January 1, 1902. Diagnosis, sarcoma of the stomach. Operation, gastrectomy. Result, recovery.

Family History.—Mother died, æt. 70, of heavy cold; father, æt. 63, of pneumonia: one sister and two brothers living and well. One brother died, æt. 28, of inflammation of bowels; one brother, æt. 35, from disease contracted from a horse, possibly actinomycosis.

Previous History.—Patient had ordinary diseases of childhood; pleurisy in 1873. Has had occasional attacks of vomiting since 1877; hernia in 1883, for which patient has since worn a truss. He has used tobacco for forty years—chews it and smokes a pipe. Has used alcohol for about twenty years in the form of beer and whiskey. Is a hearty eater. No further history of specific trouble. Bowels always regular.

Present Illness.—Began in October, 1900. Pain in epigastrium, independent of food, and especially marked between 4 and 5 o'clock P.M., with vomiting any time during the day, which generally relieved pain. Quite diffuse burning sensation after vomiting. Considerable eructation of gas occurred. Appetite very poor since onset of disease. Vomitus had a sour, bitter, disagreeable taste. Bowels constipated; no bladder symptoms. Chilly sensation occasionally at night. No cough or shortness of breath. No night sweats. Has lost about 44 pounds in flesh since beginning of trouble, and much strength. Has been spitting some blood since having pleurisy, more especially since present trouble came on. Vision and hearing impaired; general sensations normal.

Physical examination, January 1, 1902: Patient 5 feet 10 inches; weight, 148 pounds; well developed; lies on right side;

expression cheerful; skin and mucous membranes rather pale; face slightly flushed; tongue slightly fissured; pupils medium-sized, equal and react to light and accommodation; pulse 80, regular and full; arteries atheromatous. *Thorax*—Normal in shape, symmetric, clavicles somewhat prominent, costal angle wide, expansion fairly good; palpation and percussion negative. Auscultation : Breathing harsh at apices, with prolonged expiration. *Heart*—Dulness begins above at upper border of fourth rib, limited externally by nipple line and internally by left sternal border. First sound at apex extremely loud, and second aortic sound exaggerated. *Abdomen*—Oval, symmetric, respiratory movements transmitted; percussion note tympanitic; tenderness in epigastrium; muscular resistance all over upper half of abdomen ; reflexes normal.

The case was explained to the patient, and the operation of gastro-intestinal anastomosis suggested, believing that this was all that could be done. The patient readily consented, being desirous of obtaining relief, even temporary, if possible.

Operation January 4, 1902, at 11 o'clock A.M. Ether and A. C. E. administered. Median incision four inches in length. Entire stomach (which was quite movable), with the exception of about two inches at the cardiac extremity, found involved, as were also the surrounding glands. It seemed possible to do a gastrectomy, which I proceeded with.

Mesentery tied off with fine silk. Stomach clamps applied, and, after thoroughly walling off the surrounding parts with tampons, the stomach was excised at about two inches anteriorly and three inches posteriorly from the cardiac end and just below pylorus. The posterior and all involved glands thoroughly removed. Excised ends brought together and sutured with silk sutures, and all raw edges invaginated by peritoneum. Abdominal wound closed with interrupted silkworm-gut sutures, and one vaginal iodoform gauze left in for drainage. Iodoform gauze and standard dressing. Operation lasted one and one-half hours. Anesthetic (ether) well taken.

After operation, patient at times restless and weak, highest temperature 102°, pulse 126, but he responded well to stimulating enemata, and went on to uneventful, complete recovery, the only complication being some delirium for a short time after the tenth day, and a stitch-hole abscess. The after-treatment of this patient consisted in giving nothing by the mouth for forty-eight hours, and several saline injections. He was allowed to rinse out his mouth with hot water occasionally. Stimulating rectal enemata given every four hours, patient retaining same very nicely. His thirst was quite distressing for a time. At the end of forty-eight hours the dressings were removed and found somewhat stained from the drainage from peritoneal cavity. Part of the iodoform-gauze drainage was removed, the balance at the end of the fifth day. Aside from this, no unusual treatment was called for.

Pathological report was as follows: Anatomical diagnosis, carcinoma of stomach in region of pylorus. Microscopical diagnosis, round-celled sarcoma of stomach, with metastases to neighboring lymph glands.

Patient returned home on the twenty-fourth day, and the following is from Dr. Houle, his attending physician:

February 3, 1902: "Mr. M. arrived home January 30, and, although a little fatigued, yet he bore the journey remarkably well. I dressed abdominal wound on the evening of his arrival and found it in very good condition. His appetite is very good indeed, and he would eat more if I dared let him. Have seen him every day since, and his pulse and temperature have been normal at each visit. He is in good spirits and feels confident that many more will be sent *ad patres* before him. His mental condition was somewhat disturbed Thursday and Friday A.M., but to-day it is much better. Will advise you from time to time about his progress."

April 12, 1902: "I told you Mr. M. had a stitch abscess. This healed, another formed near it, and yesterday I located a buried suture, situated in centre of abdominal incision, just to right of median line. There has been more or less oozing of seropurulent matter from this location, and is annoying my patient; otherwise he is the picture of health and weighs 165 pounds. I did not care to remove suture without getting your opinion in the matter." Answer sent to remove suture at once.

Patient exhibited at meeting of American Surgical Association, Albany, N. Y., June 4, 1902, and presented the following history: Appetite excellent; bowels in good condition; wound thoroughly healed; is able to eat any kind of food, and in increased quantity. Mr. M. has gained over 30 pounds in weight.

On September 13, 1902, a letter received from his physician states that on August 1 Mr. M. purchased a blacksmith shop, is able to work at the anvil, and is apparently in full health.

Remarks.—The rarity of this operation impresses itself upon one who is doing much abdominal surgery. Very few cases present in which the operation of gastrectomy can be performed. Partial resections are not infrequent, gastro-intestinal anastomosis by no means uncommon and a very satisfactory operation.

My first case presented the most serious complications in regard to the disease, extending up to and implicating the diaphragm, and were I to operate in another similar case I would certainly close the duodenum, bring up a fold of the jejunum and attach it to the under surface of the diaphragm, including the esophagus, and not attempt the use of the Murphy button, thus relieving the parts from any strain. Undoubtedly it was this traction that caused her the severe pain in the back and the difficulty in breathing, the parts dragging upon the diaphragm, ultimately separating it from its attachment to the friable portion of the esophagus.

It is a question whether the sudden start from her sleep did not have some bearing upon the action of the diaphragm, causing loosening before adhesions had taken place.

The second case is very remarkable, regarding the complete recovery the patient has made, and in the great amount of comfort attained, not only in his ability to attend to work again, but in his pleasure in the variety of diet he is able to assimilate. His increased nutrition illustrates the fact that the stomach can be removed and the remaining portion of the intestinal tract perform the necessary functions.

28 EAGLE STREET.

NORMAL INVOLUTION OF THE APPENDIX AS A MATTER OF SURGICAL INTEREST.[1]

BY

ROBERT T. MORRIS, M.D.,
New York.

SENN and Ribbert first called attention to the fact that the vermiform appendix normally undergoes an involution process which is marked by a gradual disappearance of the mucous coat, with obliteration of the lumen of the appendix. These cases have received attention in anatomical literature rather

[1] Read by title at the meeting of the American Association of Obstetricians and Gynecologists, Washington, D. C., September 16, 1902.

than in the literature of surgery; but I wish to show their importance in the field of the surgeon and to state the reasons why we ought to have collective data upon a class of common cases that go the rounds of the medical profession, seeking relief that has not been given very often, because the nature of the cases was not clearly defined in medical literature.

At various times in the past patients were sent to my office for examination because they complained of a sense of discomfort in the appendix region, but with no history of acute attacks. As these patients gave no history of acute infective attacks of the appendix, and as nothing abnormal was discovered on palpation, I dismissed the patients as not presenting surgical cases, and believed that their symptoms of intestinal indigestion and of general malaise were due to some of the common causes that required analysis by the physician.

I remember well one gentleman who was certain that his appendix was at fault, and who had been advised against operation by several authorities, but who was so insistent upon having the appendix removed that he offered a very large fee if any one would do the work for him. He was dismissed with the advice to take a trip around the world and to engage in enterprises which would have a tendency to take him away from the habits of a valetudinarian. And yet, as I now look back upon the case, he gave a good description of symptoms that may be classified distinctly as belonging to normal involution of the appendix. The patient was undoubtedly an "appendix invalid," but he died of pneumonia some years before I had begun to classify observations for an understanding of this subject.

The first case of normal involution of the appendix that engaged my attention because of its symptoms was in 1895, in a surgeon whose work in appendicitis is well known, and who was convinced that something was wrong with his own appendix, although he had suffered no acute attacks of inflammation of that organ. During the previous four years he had been conscious of an area of discomfort localized in the appendix region, with occasional neuralgia of the ileo-inguinal and ileo-hypogastric nerves. There was no actual pain, and there were at first periods of complete relief; but these became shorter and shorter, until finally the discomfort was so persistent and accompanied by so much intestinal indigestion that he sought relief. His appendix was readily palpable, and, to my touch at that time, seemed to be perfectly normal. There was no local tenderness on pressure. but the abdominal walls were unnaturally resistant. I advised against operation, and expressed the opinion that the symptoms were caused by intestinal fermentation and that the condition called for medical treatment. After some months of careful medical treatment the patient reported that he had received much benefit and that he was better in every way, but there was more or less of the local appendix discomfort at various times during the day, and this increased whenever medical treatment was relaxed, so that the patient preferred to have the appendix placed ''where he could look at it.'' The appendix was about three inches long and presented no external evidence of infection changes. On longitudinal section it was observed that nearly all of the distal half of the appendix had undergone a normal involution process, with obliteration of the lumen and replacement of the lymphoid and mucous layers by connective tissue. The part that showed involution change had a slightly lesser diameter than the part that still possessed a lumen.

I still had doubts about the appendix having been any very important factor in the production of symptoms, but asked Dr. H. T. Brooks to make a report upon microscopical findings. He reported that in the involution area of the appendix the outer peritoneal covering was normal. The two muscular coats were undergoing a degeneration process. The lymphoid and mucous layers had entirely disappeared, and were replaced by connective tissue. The smaller blood vessels were becoming obliterated, but the nerve filaments persisted, and these were surrounded by groups of new cells in such abundance that there was presumptive evidence of the presence of inflammation of the nerve filaments.

The line of reasoning then included the deduction that the solid replacement tissue was practically scar tissue, and that this scar tissue of the appendix was acting precisely as it does in the scar of an amputated leg when it contracts and irritates nerve filaments that are engaged in the scar tissue. The primary effect of the irritation of nerve filaments by contracting connective tissue in the appendix was presumably the production of a sense of discomfort in the appendix region. A secondary result was probably a sympathetic irritation of Auerbach's and Meissner's plexuses of the walls of the colon and ileum, with resulting loss of function to an extent which allowed intestinal fermentation to take place. A third result would naturally be the chain of phenomena which are commonly associated with the absorption of saprophyte toxins from the bowel.

In this first case of mine, which was typical, and in a patient whose observations were particularly valuable because of his understanding of the whole subject, the treatment by removal of the appendix was completely curative. He has been relieved from all discomfort in the appendix region and from the intestinal fermentation, and is to-day in robust health.

The specimens from similar cases which are here presented illustrate the condition resulting from normal involution of the appendix. In this first specimen the longitudinal section shows almost the entire appendix involved, with very little lumen remaining, and at the cecal end. Involution change begins usually at the distal extremity of the appendix and proceeds toward the cecum regularly; but in some cases, as illustrated in this second specimen, it apparently occurs irregularly, with the production of stricture bands and a narrowing of the lumen of the appendix at one or more points. I am under the impression that the narrowing of the lumen with consequent mucous inclusion, upon which Abbe lays so much stress, is due to such irregular normal involution as this specimen shows. It has been my belief that appendices undergoing normal involution changes were not apt to be the seat of acute infective processes; but if irregular involution with mucous inclusion occurs, it would be fair to assume that the conditions are favorable for acute infective attacks proceeding from decomposition of incarcerated mucus.

The microscopical specimens here presented are from cross-sections of appendices undergoing the regular form of normal involution, and they show the condition described by Dr. Brooks in the first specimen which he examined.

The symptoms accompanying normal involution of the appendix belong particularly to middle life, although they sometimes become marked as early as the twentieth year. They persist over a series of years, and probably disappear in later life when the appendix has become transformed into a string of looser connective tissue.

In making a differential diagnosis we find, in regular normal involution cases, an appendix which feels harder than normal on palpation. The abdominal muscles are unnaturally resistant, protecting the irritated appendix very much as they do an infected one, but not to such a marked degree. There is a sense of discomfort amounting almost, if not quite, to pain in the appendix region; and while this may be absent for hours or for days at a time, it is persistent in its recurrence. Intestinal fermentation is a characteristic accompaniment of involution irritation of the appendix, and there may be an associated neuralgia of the ileo-inguinal and ileo-hypogastric nerves.   There is little or no tenderness on pressure upon the involuting appendix.

In tuberculosis of the appendix we have the same symptoms as in regular normal involution, but there is a marked degree of tenderness on pressure, and the tuberculosis is distinctly progressive in its infection area, with eventual wide involvement of the peritoneum or mucosa of the bowel.

In cases of benign mucous inclusion or of appendix irritation due to torsion or angulation, we have the same symptoms as in regular normal involution, but the attacks are much more acute; they are apt to be associated with nausea or vomiting; and there are longer periods of complete relief.

In cases of hysteria with simulation of the symptoms of appendicitis, we have the collateral neurotic history for guidance.

The treatment for the disturbance caused by regular normal involution of the appendix is treatment for the symptoms only, unless the disturbance is sufficient in degree to call for removal of the appendix.   I have a number of these patients under observation, and they have been given to understand that the question of operation is one of comfort rather than one of necessity.   The majority of the patients prefer palliative medical treatment, but some of them choose operation.   On account of my exhibition of normal involution cases before the class at college, they are sometimes spoken of as "Morris appendices"; but I wish to have them called "scar appendices" instead, for the reason that the former nomenclature has been taken to mean that I favor the removal of normal appendices, and has resulted in unwarranted criticism.   I have never, in speaking or in writing, advocated the removal of normal appendices, and I fear that even this article may lead to the removal of some normal appendices at the hands of colleagues who are not quite as careful as I try to be in making a selection of cases.   The matter should be left entirely to the patient in cases of disturbance from regular normal involution of the appendix, and our attitude is very different from the one that we are to assume when we are responsible for the outcome of a case of true infective appendicitis that has been entrusted to our care.

58 WEST FIFTY-SIXTH STREET.

NORMAL SALINE SOLUTIONS BEFORE, DURING, AND AFTER ABDOMINAL OPERATIONS.[1]

BY

WILLIAM H. HUMISTON, M.D.,

Associate Professor of Gynecology in the Medical Department of Western
Reserve University; Gynecologist-in-Chief, St. Vincent's Hospital;
Consulting Gynecologist to the City Hospital, etc.,
Cleveland. O.

IN 1895[2] I first published my method of allaying thirst following celiotomy, and again in 1898, in the same periodical, I gave the results of the observation of twenty-four cases in which this method had been used upon the excretion of the kidneys. I showing an average of 31½ ounces of urine and 90 per cent of the normal quantity of total solids passed during the first twenty-four hours succeeding celiotomy.

This satisfactory condition was obtained only in those cases in which a sufficient time for preparation could be had prior to operation, and left those usually more grave and disastrous emergency cases without this material aid; and usually at that time recourse to intravenous transfusion or subcutaneous injection was postponed until complications with heart or kidneys had already arisen.

It was not until June of 1897, in a case to be hereinafter detailed. that I used the peritoneal cavity as the inlet to large quantities of salt solution. During the remainder of the year I used in a cautious way this procedure in a few seemingly hopelessly desperate cases, with such satisfactory results that I soon adopted it as a routine.

The technique is simple. After partially closing the wound I pour into the cavity through a glass funnel not less than two quarts of normal saline solution at a temperature of 112° F., and quickly tie the few remaining sutures previously introduced. Within a few minutes the anesthetizer notes a marked change in the character of the pulse, its rate diminishing, lowering ten-

[1]Read by title at the meeting of the American Association of Obstetricians and Gynecologists, Washington, D. C., September 16 and 17, 1902.

[2]AMERICAN JOURNAL OF OBSTETRICS.

sion and increasing fulness. The color of the face more nearly approaches the normal, and usually the patients have little or no thirst for the first eighteen hours, have less pain, and require no enemata of any kind, and are thus kept absolutely at rest and free from the annoyance of *too much nursing.*

In vaginal celiotomies where this method cannot be employed I begin to have the saline administered subcutaneously; the trocar entering at the junction of the anterior axillary border at a line on a level with the upper border of the right breast, the trocar being plunged downward, backward, and inward, so that the fluid finds the loose tissue in the axilla and backward underneath the scapula rather than under the breast. In this position, with a very little massage, three or four quarts can readily be injected with four feet of pressure. In emergency work outside of hospitals, where assistance is limited and sterile salt solution is not to be had, I have used a hastily-prepared non-sterile salt solution during an operation by allowing the sigmoid and colon to be slowly filled with the fluid. This is easily accomplished when the patient is in the Trendelenburg posture and the peritoneal cavity opened to permit of the ready guidance of the tube above the pelvic brim. Large quantities may be used in this way without hindrance in the field of operation, and the rapidity of absorption can only be appreciated by actual observation.

Another use of the salt solution which I have made of late has certain theoretic, and proven practical, grounds for its adoption. For a number of years I have not flushed the cavity nor used a drain. I do, however, occasionally employ the Mikuliez tampon to control general oozing; and in this latter class I have found that the filling of the peritoneal cavity after the tampon has been placed tends toward the dissolution of clots and the carrying off of effete material within the pelvis through the capillarity of the tampon.

I have never had a bad result which could be attributed to this use of the saline. There are no certain indications to its use, but, on the other hand, I am certain that many a case of sepsis, of septic nephritis, and of low cardiac vitality has been saved.

CASE I.—June 18, 1897. Mrs. P., aged 50 years, had a tremendously large ovarian cyst, which had become adherent to almost all the structures within the abdominal cavity, excepting the spleen and the left kidney and the anterior abdominal wall, the latter escaping through the intervention of the omentum.

The cyst was a large multilocular óne, containing the products of suppuration familiarly known as "peasoup." After the contents had been carefully and slowly withdrawn and the cyst wall freed and removed, the patient suddenly collapsed. During the flushing of the peritoneal cavity the patient recovered slightly. and it gave me the thought to leave some of the fluid to replace the weight which I had removed. Four quarts were used. She was placed in bed in an almost moribund condition, but in a very few minutes the radial pulse was again to be felt. Within an hour the rate could be readily made at 160, and it gradually dropped to 90 within the first twenty-four hours, and the patient made a rapid and uninterrupted recovery.

CASE II.—Mrs. L. J., aged 34 years, had been married sixteen years and had given birth to two children, the youngest being 8 years old. She had two miscarriages prior to the birth of the last child. Her early menstrual history shows no divergence from the normal. In later years she has been troubled with dysmenorrhea and pain in the ovarian region, but her general condition has been excellent. The last menstrual period began on January 18, 1901, and continued throughout the usual length of time, without any deviation from the course of previous epochs. There was no appearance of the menses either in February or March, but a week after the expected period of the latter month the patient "took something." For ten days there was a bloody discharge, but on March 28 the patient had a severe pain in the left groin and was faint and nauseated. At this time a probable diagnosis of gallstones was made, but a second physician decided that a pregnant uterus was misplaced to the left and an abortion was threatened. On April 4 a second and more severe attack occurred, followed by collapse. The patient was then kept in bed till May 12. Two distinct attacks occurred during this period of forced quiet. Pain, nausea, and vomiting with tympanites were the chief symptoms. During one of these attacks one-half grain of morphine was administered before relief came. The bedside record shows with each attack a rise in pulse rate from 80 to 100 and 120, followed in about twelve hours with a rise of temperature from the normal to 100° or 100½°, with rapid declination of pulse rate and temperature to the normal. The nurse was discharged on May 12 and the patient rapidly improved in general condition. The bloody discharge from the vagina, which had occurred almost continually through the month of April, had ceased.

During the first week of July she came from her home to Cleveland to recuperate. On July 9, at 10 A.M., the fifth distinct attack of pain occurred. At this time the patient sank into collapse. The history and clinical picture made the diagnosis of extrauterine pregnancy with internal hemorrhage positive. Dr. F. S. Clark, who first saw the case, called me to operate. I found the patient in an extremely low condition, with sighing respiration, blanched skin, cold extremities, and small, feeble pulse whose rate was scarcely distinguishable at 170 to 188, temperature 95°. The operation was quickly arranged for at her sister's home. Under anesthesia the diagnosis was confirmed, the body of the uterus being easily distinguished from the large tumor mass, and in the latter fetal parts could be felt to the left and posterior to the uterus. Such, in brief, was the typical course of this case; and now I desire to call your attention to the value and necessity of certain operative procedures.

As soon as partial anesthesia was induced the introduction of salt solution beneath the breast was begun, and when the patient was taken from the table two quarts had been given and most of it had already been absorbed. The placenta was found attached to the posterior surface of the broad ligament and to several coils of small intestine in the cul-de-sac. The posterior wall of the gestation sac was coherent to the colon and small intestines. In the abdominal cavity there were clots, in various stages of organization, representing the different periods of previous ruptures. Ligatures were immediately placed on the ovarian artery, and a clamp applied over the tube and broad ligament along the left side of the uterus. With the checking of the main blood supply the fetus and the various blood clots were removed from the pelvis and the placenta was carefully detached. The posterior wall of the gestation sac was carefully handled with a view to leaving it as a shield for the general abdominal cavity. No attempt was made to clean the general peritoneal cavity, but as much salt solution as the space would contain was poured into it and left when the stitches were tied. The posterior wall of the gestation sac was sewed to the upper portion of the wound in the abdominal wall, and the cavity of the gestation sac was packed with gauze to control the general oozing.

The patient's condition when first placed upon the table was very precarious, but with the absorption of the salt solution beneath the breast and the use of strychnine sulphate, one-fifth grain. the pulse gradually grew stronger and fuller, and at 4 P.M. was 140 in rate. One-half pint of salt solution was given per rectum every hour. one-thirtieth of strychnine every two hours. and four minims of fluid extract of digitalis each four hours hypodermatically. At 7 P.M. the pulse again began to waver, and again a subcutaneous injection of two quarts of salt solution was given, and at midnight the pulse was 160 and rapidly growing stronger and slower. Twenty-four hours after operation it was 128 and never again went above this point. The stomach was irrigated thirty hours after the operation. and undigested food, with a large amount of raspberry seeds, was removed. The nausea ceased and nothing further complicated convalescence.

The rapidity with which this patient responded to the use of submammary injections of salt solution when the conditions seemed most hopeless. and the ease with which the general peritoneum cared for the blood and clots that were left in the cavity, are the two important facts to be deduced. To one other point must I call your attention : however hazardous seems the attempt, my own conviction is that all of the placenta should be removed in every case. The danger of intoxication or general sepsis from this (usually sloughing) mass is avoided and the convalescence shortened. And. lastly, I have seen many accidents happen because of the early removal of the gauze packing. My own practice is to wait until Nature has made a firm wall about it and the granulation tissue which early permeates the gauze has sickened of its work and died.

CASE III.—Mrs. A. G.. aged 23 years. came into the hospital with a tentative diagnosis of old ruptured tubal pregnancy with general pelvic peritonitis. She was much reduced in weight and color, having suffered for six months with intermittent abdominal pains. with more or less severe internal hemorrhages. The history rather pointed to intrauterine gestation, with miscarriage followed by a septic peritonitis. At the operation the latter proved to be the correct conclusion. The pelvis was completely filled with enlarged, thickened inflammatory tubes and exudate. The usual landmarks were obliterated and the pelvis was cleared with great difficulty. The rectum was accidentally torn, and it was found necessary to resect about three inches of it, making an end-to-end anastomosis. The patient was given two quarts of saline into the axilla during the operation, with good results, noted in the condition of the pulse. A Mikulicz tampon was placed in the pelvis to control oozing and to protect the rectum at the junction of anastomosis, and two quarts of saline were placed within the abdominal cavity. The greater portion of this was drained through the Mikulicz, the gauze dressing being changed frequently. The patient passed through the first twenty-four hours in fair condition. The pulse, weakening twelve hours after operation, was readily helped by a quart of saline given subcutaneously. From this time the patient steadily improved toward convalescence without an untoward symptom.

The three cases detailed are sufficient to show the range of applicability of this invaluable agent. I have used it in those extreme cases of prolonged pelvic suppuration where the vitality was so low as to preclude the possible hope of recovery; beginning its introduction subcutaneously, after partial anesthesia, and continuing it throughout the operation with the effect to *prevent shock* or seemingly loss of strength, as in many instances the patient left the operating table with a better pulse than at any time noted for days before.

I have given you but the clinical experiences that I have enjoyed in the use of normal saline solution. The theories and speculations in regard to its actions and results must be determined by the laboratory workers. That it has a wide range of applicability I believe all will agree.

536 ROSE BUILDING.

THE MANAGEMENT OF CASES OF EMERGENCY ARISING FROM RUPTURE IN ECTOPIC PREGNANCY.[1]

BY

AUGUSTUS P. CLARKE, A.M., M.D..
Cambridge, Mass.

THE subject here presented must always be of deep concern both to the physician in the city provided with every means for reasonable care of patients, and to practitioners residing in places at considerable distance from the greater medical centres. The occurrences of the more seemingly desperate cases coming

[1]Read at the meeting of the American Association of Obstetricians and Gynecologists, Washington, D. C., September 16, 17, and 18, 1902.

29

to the treatment of any one obstetrician do not appear, upon the whole, to have been very numerous, for many physicians who have had quite an extended experience have scarcely met with a case. This may sometimes be due to the fact that cases of extrauterine or ectopic pregnancy having been early diagnosticated may have been brought under appropriate treatment before the more dangerous symptoms had supervened. The occurrence of cases of alarming nature to treat will now and then take place, and this may at times happen when the practitioner, even if he should be a most skilful operator, feels the least prepared to meet such an emergency.

Operators have also recognized the difficulty that may sometimes be met with in the differentiation of the various forms of ectopic pregnancy, if not as to their always being certain as to the existence of such a kind of pregnancy, and so measures may be delayed as to the safe management of such a case. Some forms of pelvic hematocele are no doubt due to the presence of ectopic gestation. I can enumerate quite a few of such cases that were evidently the result of this cause. In cases of hematocele there is often more or less shock attended with considerable free hemorrhage and a marked exsanguine appearance of the patient. Cases of this character, so far as I have been able to observe, have occurred in the very beginning of the pregnancy. I shall never forget my experience in a case seen some few years since with the late Dr. Nelson, of Boston. We had seen the patient three weeks previously and had concluded that the case was one of tubal gestation. Rectal indagation, as well as bimanual examination, revealed that there was a circumscribed mass in the right iliac fossa; the patient had passed over a menstrual period. Other phases also pointed toward pregnancy. Early in the morning, on being called to the patient, I found her in a state of much collapse; the pulse was weak and the heart's action was greatly depressed. The sudden enlargement in and about the mass in the pelvis afforded almost unmistakable evidence of rupture of the fetal sac, and of hemorrhage. An abdominal incision, made in the median line, showed at once that the condition of the patient was due to hemorrhage from rupture near the fimbriated extremity of the Fallopian tube. The mass was brought forward and secured by aseptic animal sutures and then incised. The abdominal cavity was thoroughly irrigated with warm water. The incision was closed without resort to further drainage. The patient made an uninterrupted recovery. The fetus was of the size of one of about forty-five days' duration.

In another case to which I was afterward called the patient had sustained sudden shock from an apparent loss of blood: a small mass just above the left iliac fossa could be made out. An abdominal incision disclosed the presence of quite a considerable clot about the distal extremity of the Fallopian tube, but no fetus could be found. Though the hemorrhage had ceased for the time being, the point of a small artery from which the blood had escaped was made safe by ligature; the cavity in and about the site of the hemorrhage was cleansed and drainage by the insertion of iodoform gauze was established. The incision was then practically closed; recovery took place without any serious mishap, all drainage having been dispensed with on the fourth day.

In considering the condition of this last case I have sometimes felt that the patient would have, by means of more palliative treatment, recovered without having been submitted to an abdominal section. In the first case the chances without the patient's yielding to operative measures would have been against her recovery, because the abdominal section showed that considerable hemorrhage was still going on and that the patient's strength was gradually being diminished; besides, there were dangers incident to infection and to the presence of the foreign mass.

In the consideration of the question of the proper management of any case of rupture in ectopic pregnancy, it should not be overlooked that patients meeting with such mishaps do not infrequently, by the aid of the more general measures of treatment, recover. This is evidenced by the cases coming from time to time, long after reaction has taken place, to the surgeon for operative interference. The history of such cases often shows that the patients had suffered from severe shock from hemorrhage, but must have, of course, recovered.

On referring again to my own notes made in regard to unusual sequences of pregnancy, I find that, in three cases of undoubted rupture occurring in the early stage of ectopic gestation, two of the patients recovered without having to submit to radical operative measures; in the third case, however, the ending was fatal, the patient's family declining to have an operation undertaken. In this last case the surroundings of the patient and her own condition at the time being so unfavorable, it appeared extremely doubtful whether an abdominal incision would have been of any particular benefit. There was a well-defined mass to be felt extending from the right toward the left iliac fossa.

Another class of cases to be mentioned is that in which patients have recovered from the immediate effects of rupture and have subsequently presented unmistakable evidence of having suffered from the mishap. The number showing the various phases of having been the subject of such a condition has not been a few. These I merely mention as tending to show that rupture and other accidents may take place and yet be recovered from. Dr. John C. Irish, of Lowell, reported some time since to the Gynecological Society of Boston two cases of extrauterine fetation in which sudden rupture had occurred, in both cases the surroundings and the condition of the patients being so unfavorable it was deemed that operative interference would be in such cases an unwise measure of proceeding. In one of the cases the patient had missed one menstrual period; in the other case the extrauterine pregnancy had advanced two months. In both cases active palliative treatment was resorted to. The use of opiates, stimulants, and restoratives was followed by such a degree of reaction that abdominal section was considered unnecessary. Dr. Irish, in carrying out the treatment in these two cases, seems to have been strengthened by the fact of his experience in operating for final relief in twelve cases of extrauterine pregnancy, in which it had been manifest that at some time previously hemorrhage from rupture had taken place and had been accompanied with more or less collapse. The practice of waiting, therefore, in some extreme cases, he felt could not always be considered as inadvisable. If all patients. it may be remarked, who may sustain hemorrhage and shock or great exhaustion resulting from the incidents of ectopic pregnancy, would, without submitting to surgical interference. perish, the duty of the surgeon, when called on in such an emergency, would undoubtedly be always most plain.

In estimating the amount of danger the rupture of the sac or the sudden occurrence of shock may entail, much will have to be taken into consideration as regards the quantity of blood that may have been lost and the probable degree of hemorrhage that is still going on. The loss of only a little blood will sometimes produce apparently as much collapse of the patient as that of a larger quantity. In the lighter grades of hemorrhage the shock is not likely to be so continuous or so profound as it is in cases in which a larger volume has escaped. In the former grade the employment of stimulants is of more avail. Salt solutions can be used with great advantage.

Dr. A. L. Norris, of Cambridge, has reported a case of rupture that terminated fatally. He had waited with the hope that the patient would rally. At the autopsy a large amount of blood was found in the pelvic cavity. In another case of tubal pregnancy occurring in a woman aged 21 years, he did not wait long after the occurrence of the rupture, but had the patient taken to a hospital, where an operation proved successful. The incident of the rupture was accompanied with considerable degree of shock, though the loss of blood was not large.

Dr. George W. Jones, of Cambridge, reported to the Society a case of ectopic pregnancy in which great collapse followed rupture of the tube and hemorrhage took place. The case was seen in consultation. He thought, as it was evening when he was called. it would be best to wait until some reaction had taken place. Though the patient next morning had rallied somewhat. Dr. Jones felt that it was wisest to resort to abdominal section: he then could feel quite distinctly a large mass of exudation low down in the right of the abdominal cavity; it had become very evident that hemorrhage to some extent was still going on. The patient, however, declined to submit to operative measures. A little later, while he was still with the patient, there suddenly took place another collapse, in which the patient within a short time expired. Had Dr. Jones been permitted to operate as soon as he became satisfied that the hemorrhage was not being arrested. he would undoubtedly have had a fair chance of saving the life of the patient.

In a recent discussion of this subject Dr. Henry O. Marcy mentioned a case of rupture in which the shock was so great that the patient died within an hour after its occurrence. He spoke of another case in which the shock and hemorrhage were quite considerable. but the patient recovered nevertheless without resort to operation.

Judging from my own experience. and also from that of my confrères in whose ability, judgment, and sagacity I have high regard. I am satisfied that no hard-and-fast rule alike should be established for the management for all cases of shock or collapse from rupture occurring in ectopic gestation. In some cases. even when the shock is quite profound, the amount of hemorrhage may not be great; and even if it should be. it may not continue long. In such cases much can be successfully effected, as before remarked, by the way of stimulants, opiates, and by the employment of salt solutions. The constitution and condition of the patient should be considered. Perfect quietude should be enjoined. In some cases, no doubt, an attempt to remove the patient to a hospital or place of better situation or convenience may sometimes prove to be an unwise measure of proceeding. The first case mentioned by Dr. Marcy shows how small would have been the chances of accomplishing anything by the way of removal to a better situation or by the aid of operative interference. The case mentioned by Dr. Jones brings out another phase in the consideration, such as the "patient's objecting to operation"; the occurring of another collapse soon after the patient's expression of denial shows that complete mental as well as bodily rest is a most essential factor of treatment. The operative interference in the second case reported by Dr. Norris, as referred to, seems to have been particularly urged because of the adverse results obtained through milder measures in the first case. In that case it appears that the loss of blood had been considerable. The question naturally arises whether the patient could have really borne the fatigue incident to removal to hospital or the additional shock more or less attendant on a radical surgical measure. Such an ordeal to submit a patient to often brings to the mind of the experienced operator many misgivings. To operate in some cases of this character is not always an easy task, and the results are sometimes far from being satisfactory.

Dr. A. H. Tuttle, of Cambridge, in speaking of this subject, said that he had operated a number of times; in some cases the operation became a most desperate measure. He also says that in almost any case something can in the way of relief be accomplished to arouse the flagging powers of the patient. In some cases it is true that the mass. occurring as the result of hemorrhage, may gradually enlarge and the hemorrhage, continning, may lead to rapid death. In many cases, nevertheless, the choice of waiting may prove better than that of resorting to immediate operation. It is the quantity of blood lost, and not the character of the shock and other symptoms, that should always be considered in determining what would be the degree of danger to be encountered in a case. These remarks of Dr. Tuttle bear the impress of being the outcome of wisdom born of experience. The results of my first case reported seem to have been obtained by a wise method of proceeding; and though the outcome of the second case was fortunate, it would have undoubtedly been better, had the surroundings been less favorable for operative measures, to have waited and trusted more to stimulants and other palliatives for overcoming the shock and other grave symptoms. The features presented in the two cases as reported by Dr. Irish are most interesting, and the results obtained by the treatment are highly instructive. His experience in operating in the later stages in twelve different cases of extrauterine pregnancy, in which there had been shock and other serious symptoms, and from which the patients had rallied and lived on, served to have impressed him with the fact that much could be accomplished under unfavorable conditions by waiting and endeavoring to bring about reaction, as he did, as reported, most effectually.

I am not unaware that in the discussion of the subject of rupture or great shock some consideration, it may be urged, should be had in regard to the variety of the ectopic pregnancy. We know that the interstitial form is the most uncommon kind likely to be met with. Perhaps it may be said that in cases of accidents of rupture the hemorrhage occurring may be more easily controlled by operation in the tubal form. When rupture or shock occurs in abdominal pregnancy the implantation of the ovum to the peritoneum may be more difficult to remove. It should not be forgotten, however, that when the surgeon is not called until the occurrence of shock or rupture a differential diagnosis is often far from being easy to make. Especially is it so when it becomes essential to disturb the patient as little as possible in order to prevent further shock and hemorrhage. The object of immediate treatment, of whatever character it may be deemed most expedient to carry out, is to lessen suffering and to save life if possible. The subsequent management is always to be a matter for later consideration. If it becomes reasonably manifest that serious hemorrhage is still going on and that it is not likely to cease, an abdominal section, if the circumstances are such that it can be done with any probable chances of obtaining success, should of course be resorted to at the earliest moment after other measures appear unavailing. If, however, in a time of such an extreme alarm, an operation can be safely dispensed with until conditions more favoring, it would undoubtedly be a far better course to pursue, for it becomes in such cases, as it is in all other abdominal surgery where the work is in danger of being hastily or inconsiderately performed, most unfortunate for a surgeon to open the abdomen and then to discover that he has erred in his diagnosis; this is not only true in the case of a woman who may be a leader or most influential in society, but also in the case of one who may be in the more humble walks in life.

SO-CALLED NEURASTHENIA AND HYSTERIA IN THEIR RELATIONS TO ABDOMINAL SECTION.

A CLINICAL STUDY.

BY

J. STEWART NAIRNE, F.R.C.S.,
Senior Surgeon. Glasgow Samaritan Hospital for Women.

It is evident that this subject must be approached from two very different points of view—viz., the psychological and the physiological—if it is to have justice done to it. It is not my purpose to proceed from the former point just now, as it is quite enough, for all that I have in view, to deal with the conditions that are apparently directly concerned with ordinary physiological and pathological exhibitions.

Some years ago I had the pleasure of reading a paper at Edinburgh to the Psychological Section of this Association on a subject which had the very abstruse title of "The Psychology of Muscle." In it I dealt especially with what might properly be called the automatic phenomena of muscular movements in relation to their significance as psychological expressions.

I then stated as probable correct deductions from psychological phenomena many physical conditions that I am now prepared to uphold with practical clinical and physiological observations to support me.

To bring the matter to a point, I do not believe that any psychological phenomena can occur without a corresponding physiological condition, to which the relationship is absolutely direct as effect and cause.

Thus I dealt then with the value that was to be attached to muscular action as indicative of a corresponding psychological condition, without which psychological condition no similar muscular phenomena could exist.

To my mind then the argument on *a priori* grounds was unassailable; and to my mind now, after many years of observation and practice, the position is absolutely correct.

I do not venture to give any distinct definition of either hysteria or neurasthenia. It is not necessary to add to the confusion that already exists in the use of these words. It would be better if they were abolished, if they cannot be used without having a universally accepted clear definition attached to them.

For my present purpose this is of no importance, as I use the term "so-called" in order to clearly state that they are used here to indicate only a "set of anomalous nervous symptoms for which no organic lesion is apparently responsible." I say "apparently responsible," because I believe it is quite impossible for any vital phenomena, whether normal or abnormal, to occur without specific affection of the organs involved in their demonstration. Whether this specific affection is amenable to any kind of treatment is another question. The general opinion that in so-called hysterical and neurasthenic affections no organic lesion is to be detected is one that needs much consideration and modification. So I feel I am on safe and neutral ground when I use the terms hysteria and neurasthenia to indicate conditions of mind and body and exhibitions of vital phenomena for which no apparently organic condition is openly responsible.

The majority will agree with me that, as one goes on in life in the gynecological groove, it becomes more and more painfully apparent that the female sex suffers much in some kind of unstable physical equilibrium, and that organic diseases manifest themselves in pronounced psychological conditions which are of such a nature as can be traced only with the greatest difficulty back to their probably organic source.

In many cases, of course, the skilled diagnostician can easily fix the cause, while the unskilful man must grope in the dark, wonder how such and such a diagnosis can be made, and doubt, with a very sincere doubt, if it is ever made at all and not a haphazard guess. He naturally asks the question, "How do you know?" and as naturally the answer is, "I do not know how I know, but I know." So the gifted player on the violin to the untuneful amateur. No amount of training, teaching, exposition, labor, to the latter could bring the perfection and delicacy that naturally belong to the former.

The description of the circumstances that have accompanied the cases under my own personal observation compels me to ask whether it is not necessary now to reconsider many of the popular. views of these so-called nervous affections, and to ask whether our ordinary methods of diagnosis are quite sufficient for them, and further to mark down as two special points for consideration:

1. The non-possibility of neurotic condition without organic lesion or disturbance of physiological phenomena.

2. The possibility of direct nerve stimulation leading to neurotic conditions without apparent or appreciable organic affection.

Almost without exception, abdominal section has shown gross lesion of some abdominal organ.   In some cases there was kidney or ureter disease.   Some showed subperitoneal pelvic disease, suppuration, or tumors of various kinds.   Cystic disease of ovaries, broad ligaments, tubes was of almost constant appearance.   Simple inflammatory conditions, flexions, versions, dislocations of all kinds and of every organ, were frequent.   But the most marked pathological condition of all was what I may term "rigid uterus."   It occurred without exception in all cases where neurosis had been a prominent clinical symptom.   It was a great surprise to me in my earlier cases to note this strange condition.   And many times I missed it; in fact, did not recognize it at all until a pronounced case occurred when the uterus stood up rigidly, almost perpendicularly, and forced itself on my notice.   Once seen, it is readily found afterward.   The condition naturally varies in many degrees.   It is not necessarily, but frequently, associated with fibroid degeneration of the corpus uteri.   There may be a condition of fixity of the body downward and backward, either with or without flexion; and this fixity varies in degree also.

So far as I am aware, this is an undescribed condition and can readily be accounted for by some lesion in the cord in the region controlling the nervous supply to the uterus.   If this be so, it is easy to see how cures can be accounted for from the application of electricity internally or externally, from the application of counter-irritation, blistering, etc., to the spine, and from the cold douche and baths. It also explains the failure of what, for want of a better name, may be called moral-suasion methods.   I should like to know what good could be expected from encouragement, or seclusion, or Weir Mitchell's treatment, or anything of that kind, if it were a fact that there did exist an actual lesion somewhere and that we had to some extent means of diagnosing it.

Taking for granted that what I say is correct about this spasm of the uterus, what else could account for it other than the condition of its nerve supply? It explains the failures in relieving neurotic diseases by abdominal section and removal of the appendages. The failures follow quite as naturally as the cures. Should the ultimate disease be central, and should the cutting-off of its nerve supply to the organ not be sufficient to alter it beneficially, then the case must be regarded as a failure. Similarly with all other nerve diseases, e.g., neuralgia, tic. If one can only go far enough back in section of the nerve the disease can be cured. Pains and aches and physical discomforts are not necessarily the only resultants from uterine disease. In a very finely balanced human being pain is a factor that has seriously to be reckoned with. Pain is not always only a physical condition—the psychological element comes in and complements all our being. Pain can not only make us nervous, hysterical, neurasthenic, but can drive us mad.

I would not say that the inflammatory conditions of the appendages that one so frequently finds in an abdominal section are of themselves sufficient to produce the troubles we are considering. I would say that frequently they are of no consequence whatever, that they are merely subsidiary, sometimes only concomitants of the obscure disease that is behind. Similarly I, and, I am sure, most of you who have removed ovaries, have come to place but very little value on the cystic disease that is almost universally present. No doubt it is a satisfaction, a kind of quasi-proof that an operation has not been done unjustifiably when we can puncture those cysts and show the disease. But in themselves they argue nothing. In many cases they are of no importance whatever.

The argument is not from one condition. It must be from all the conditions together.

There must be, in such serious cases (for neurasthenia and hysteria are serious enough to threaten both life and reason), a consensus of, at the very least, probabilities. One symptom must be added to another; and when they are all added together, and we find not only some degree of error in position, condition, and feeling, but can also diagnose a rigid uterus, then I think we have fairly made good our claim to a probable diagnosis.

In order, however, to put my work as clearly before you as I think I have it before myself, I give you the following table as a summary of results:

1. Abdominal section: no disease found, patient informed; nothing removed; patient apparently cured.

2. Abdominal section: tubercular condition; nothing removed; patient apparently cured.

3. Abdominal section: fibroid condition (uterus, ovaries, or other organ); nothing removed; patient apparently cured.

4. Abdominal section: no disease found; nothing removed; patient not informed; patient apparently cured.

5. Abdominal section: no disease found; patient and friends informed; patient apparently not benefited.

6. Patient under anesthetic: no section done; patient apparently cured.

7. Abdominal section: appendages removed; patient apparently cured.

8. Abdominal section: uterus removed; patient apparently cured.

9. Abdominal section: appendages removed; patient sent to asylum.

10. Abdominal section: uterus removed; patient sent to asylum.

11. Abdominal section: tubercular condition; nothing removed; patient not cured.

Suggestions and Conclusions.—I would not be understood as advocating abdominal section in all cases of neurasthenia and hysteria. This would be too dreadful to contemplate. It is the other way about. Some cases of, neurasthenia and hysteria demand for their successful treatment abdominal section. And it is because, in the course of the major operations which I have performed, I think I have discovered a valuable sign indicative of the kind of case to which the operation is applicable, that I have bracketed "neurasthenia, hysteria, and abdominal section" together. It is not necessary to perform a section to diagnose this condition; it only requires greater practice in examination, greater patience in observation, greater discrimination in the valuation of the general signs and symptoms. It does not follow, even if one is convinced that the conditions are all there, that an abdominal section will be followed by a cure; and therefore it becomes doubly necessary that everything medical that is possible should have been done before resort is had to major operation.

Some time ago our very excellent member, Dr. Rabagliati, published a book on "Ovarian Neuralgia," which I heartily recommend to you and which will well repay a careful perusal. Many of these nervous, hysteric, and neurotic women have been treated by us too lightly, indifferently, callously sometimes. To tell the truth, we have good reason to be afraid to deal at all with some of them. When they are not regarded as nuisances they are often considered pests. And without doubt the nature of their trouble tends to render them somewhat irresponsible for their actions. When we come, however, to realize absolutely and clearly that many of these obscure complaints have a real, substantial foundation in some physical condition, although the physical signs may not be sufficiently gross for us to put our fingers on, then our efforts to relieve receive an impetus that they could not have had before; seeing, we now know that it is only our knowledge that is at fault, and that it is a reasonable thing to suppose that we may, by perseverance in observation and increased skill in management, enlarge that knowledge sufficiently to enable us to discover a remedy or remedies. No man can labor diligently in treating diseases unless he has a decided conviction that it is at least possible for him to provide remedies.

In bringing this paper before you I have done everything I could to eliminate sources of error. I have gone carefully over the records of the last 500 cases admitted into St. Margaret's Home—a private hospital for women—and the cases I have described have been especially selected as types of the conditions here considered. They are naturally of a better class than the ordinary hospital patient, and therefore, I think, better suited for any kind of demonstration of diseases which are certainly more prevalent in that class. Still I am sure that were I to enter on the same investigation among my public hospital patients I would arrive at a similar result. Among the poorer classes, so-called hysterical women meet, after a short time, with very little sympathy. They have no means to pay for attendance; ordinary hospitals fight shy of them; special hospitals are frequently so guarded by regulations to prevent either the staff or the directors from getting into trouble that they are excluded; and I have often thought that herein is one of the fruitful causes that drive so many poor women to drink.

ILLUSTRATIVE CASES SELECTED FROM THE RECORDS OF ST.
MARGARET'S HOME.

33. Miss A., Busby, aged 18; admitted February 7, dismissed March 12, 1890.

Condition.—Distension of abdomen: ovarian and tubal disease (?); hemorrhage; neurasthenia.

Treatment.—Dilatation of anus; cautery to cervix uteri.

This is probably the earliest case in which I made deliberately a diagnosis of neurasthenia and a trial of minor surgical means to meet the condition. She was a very young girl, of an amiable disposition, and I look back on her case with the most vivid recollection. Her old father and mother came with her—decent country people, who had never had any personal experience of neurasthenias or hysterias or anything of that sort. They said she was always ailing; pains here and there and everywhere: could do nothing—was always willing to do anything, but failed: pains in her back and side; great distension of the abdomen: rollings and rumblings of flatulence; a restless sleeper, a bad eater, with constipation, sometimes of nearly a week's duration. She had been under treatment for a considerable time with tonics and purgatives, till finally it was considered a case of nerves and both she and her parents were disheartened. Nothing seemed to do her any good. If she felt well for a little while she was bright, cheerful, and always working about. But these intervals were inconstant and short. The family were all willing and anxious to have anything done that might make her better. I cannot say that I was very hopeful of results from any treatment. for I was undoubtedly considerably in the dark, as there was nothing very definite organically to go upon. There was certainly the distension of the abdomen, but that was clearly only a symptom of some other disease; there was also the dysmenorrheal pain, but that was not particularly excessive: and the diagnosis of ovarian and tubal disease was made from the symptom as a tentative or possible condition. She was a virgin, and an examination under chloroform in that condition is deceptive unless there is gross organic disease of the appendages.

In any case she was an exemplary patient while in the Home, had few attacks of pain, and made few complaints. Of course she was resting all the time, which was very much in her favor. When she was dismissed on March 12 she was much better, and I, as well as her parents, had good hope that the improvement would continue.   It did so for a few months. Then she became worse than ever, and more than ever all those about her, with the steadfast exception of her father and mother, declared that she was putting it on and could help it if she liked.

Perhaps I, too, had a kind of half-idea that there was an element of voluntary deception in the matter, but I did not say so. I am saying so now because I am so sure now that I was absolutely wrong, that the apparently voluntary part of it was the involuntary automatic connection between her physiological and psychological condition, and that there was no more a separate voluntary action on her part than there is on the part of the governor on an engine when the safety valve is pressed open by excess of steam.

She was readmitted on May 12, 1891, and dismissed on the 23d of the same month.   She was under observation only during that period, and, although her record of residence was again favorable, I made up my mind to advise a major operation if she again relapsed.   I said that I believed that there was a deep-seated organic disease at the bottom of all her symptoms; that, as she was now suffering from distinct ovarian pains and abdominal tenderness, the most effectual method of dealing with them would be by means of an abdominal section, and then acting according to whatever internal conditions might be found.

She was then dismissed.   It was not long till she was worse than ever, and she was readmitted on November 15, 1891, for the purpose of major operation, which was performed.   I was very anxious not to sterilize the patient, if it could be avoided, and examined both ovaries and tubes carefully.   Both sides were affected.   The ovaries were cystic and the tubes were inflamed and thickened; the fimbriæ were edematous.   It was difficult to choose between them, if one set only was to be removed.   I then discovered that the appendix vermiformis was enlarged, apparently under an acute attack of appendicitis, but was quite loose.   That decided me.   I removed the appendix, and the ovary and the tube on that side, and punctured all the cysts I could find in the left ovary.   She made a very easy recovery and was better.   She went home and at first everything seemed to be going on well.   Menstruation had continued at first without pains, and if she had then passed totally from my sight I would have been hugging the delusion that she had been cured.

As it was, I learned subsequently that she had relapsed, at first slowly, then more rapidly, till she became as bad as, or worse than, ever, and ultimately died, after no long interval, under the care of the doctor at home.

Having pondered much over this case, I am sure that I did too little, and that it is quite possible that had I done more the ultimate issue would have been different. And what I argue from is this: The uterus itself partook of the general congestion, but it had also the special rigidity to which I have referred so frequently; and while an ordinary metritis may naturally be considered to subside under a simple blood-letting process, this kind of condition, dependent, as I think it is, on immediate or remote nerve irritation, can only be dealt with in a manner that radically deals with the nerves. Hence I think I ought certainly to have removed both uterine appendages completely, not sparing the cornua of the uterus.

198. Miss B., Glasgow, aged 31; admitted May 14, dismissed June 5, 1894. This girl, unmarried and a virgin, kept house for her father and brother. An invalid a long time, still had to work, as there was no other person in the house to help. She had been under medical treatment for several years, but became gradually worse. She complained of pain in both sides, mostly in the left, and the back far down over the sacrum. She suffered very much from dysmenorrhea for one day.

Examination by vagina and rectum revealed a thickened and hard uterus retroposed, without any flexion; firm pressure on it caused the usual pains.

In this case I had no hesitation in doing the complete operation, and the result was immediately beneficial. It has remained so. She does all her work, is never ill, and takes an active interest in all the affairs of life. She called on me last June; was never better in all her life. She has no nervous symptoms, does not cry or get morbid. She is happy.

218. Miss C., Ayrshire, aged 29; admitted January 8, dismissed January 18, 1895 (went to sister's house). Had not been very happy at home for a long time, domestic arrangements with stepfather not making things any better. Found she was not able to work, however much she tried. Had backache and headache and spineache, and anomalies of sight and hearing. She was regarded as pretty much of a nuisance at home and

"invited to make her own way in the world." All this she felt very much and was becoming gradually and absolutely quite unstrung; could not settle her mind to any kind of work and was developing a most alarming state of hysteria.

Examination revealed a small, hard tumor of the uterus, which discovery fortified my proposal to do a major operation.

Abdominal section was performed and I found it fairly easy to shell out two subperitoneal uterine fibroids. Under ordinary circumstances I might have been induced to do no more. But I am sure every operating surgeon has had many cases where the presence of uterine fibroids had not the slightest apparent effect on the health or spirits of the patient. In fact, she did not know they were there. I have at the present moment dozens of cases going about and coming to no harm. But in this case I had a special condition to consider, and, more than all, I had a spasm and fixity of the uterus before me which I could not attribute to the presence of these fibroids. Therefore I determined to take no risks, and removed the appendages on both sides as completely as I could.

I feel satisfied with what I did. She did not make an easy recovery—her record runs over weeks and weeks; but when she did get well she was fit for duty. She was a well-educated girl and is now in a position where ability and hard work are both necessary, and she is practically never off duty.

231. Mrs. D., India, aged 33; admitted March 27, dismissed April 17. 1895. This patient was married four years; had no children; well educated, far-travelled. She had never felt well since her marriage, although neither she nor her husband attributed her ill health to her marriage. She was strongly marked with smallpox, but notwithstanding had a considerable share of good looks, of which she was not unaware; and perhaps there may have been an idea in some minds that part of her trouble consisted in realizing she might have been still better-looking if she had not been marked with the smallpox. Be this as it may, she was of variable temperament—now up, now down; happy and miserable and morbid by turns. Indefinite pains troubled her—pains that she could by no means locate; and other physical pains and aches troubled her definitely enough in the usual sites of loins, flanks, back, spine, and head. She suffered from dysmenorrhea, and the menstrual flow was clotted, dark, and tarry, with sometimes an odor.

Her husband was an educated gentleman who dabbled in

30

hypnotism, braidism, and spiritualism. Both he and she told me
that he had frequently put her into the mesmeric sleep, and
especially when she was very ill he had sent her off into this
sleep and given her rest when nothing else did her any good.
They were both anxious that something radical should be done,
if there was a prospect of definitely and permanently curing her.

I examined her; found the pelvic conditions sufficient to justify
me in saying that I believed a laparatomy, with liberty to remove
the appendages if I thought it necessary, would probably result
in a permanent cure. Both parties said they had had such an
idea in their minds and were prepared to abide by my decision.
The gentleman suggested that, instead of the ordinary anesthetic,
he should put his wife into the mesmeric sleep. I consented with
alacrity; but I am sorry to add that the lady was never put to
sleep. His power had gone, and, try again and again as he
might, nothing came of it. The lady remained wide awake.
Nevertheless the operation was still determined on, and we over-
came the difficulty with the usual anesthetic.

At the operation I found the left ovary grossly affected with
cystic disease, and the right not visibly so. The uterus was rigid,
but not very markedly. Under these circumstances I gave her
the benefit of the doubt and removed only the left appendages.
She made an easy recovery and was well when she left the Home.
So long as she remained in Scotland she was well, but when,
in the course of a few months, she had to leave for India my
repentance began. It was, I am sure, misjudged mercy—a
fallacious conservatism; for she slowly relapsed into her former
condition, and I heard from her last year as desirous to return
and have a complete removal of the other appendage. I believe
she is right, and I believe also that, granting she recovers from
the operation, she will be quite rid of all her troubles thereafter.
I do not reckon this case as a success, but as one that has many
plain lessons on its face.

300. Miss E., Greenock, aged 27; unmarried; admitted February 6, dismissed February 26, 1897. Had been under treatment
for a long time with no benefit. Was generally considered a
nervous subject, quite hysterical. Complained of strange pains
in her side, her body generally, her bowels and stomach; felt
generally ill, and especially at menstrual periods had strange
stomachic and abdominal disturbances. Was rendered quite
unfit for housework; day after day she could hardly be induced
to exert herself in the slightest degree. I examined her and

satisfied myself that without doubt there was distinctly marked disease of the appendages. Her parents were extremely anxious that something should be done for her, as so far everything had failed. I did the operation and found distinctly marked signs of ovarian and tubal disease, but not such as I would recognize as sufficient to account for all the symptoms. In addition I found a rigid and hard uterus. I made the operation complete. From that day to this there has been perfect health. She has returned to her work and has no complaint. I saw her at the end of last year, and after the lapse of such a time I would regard the cure as permanent.

301. Miss F., Glasgow, aged 34; admitted January 10. dismissed February 4, 1897. Unmarried; works in a mill; lives at home with her mother, whom she keeps. Has been complaining for years, and has had much advice from many physicians; feels as if she would go mad. Suffers from dysmenorrhea and many nervous pains everywhere. Appetite bad, bowels constipated. When she feels well, is very happy and takes an interest in church affairs and Sunday-school; when she feels ill, is full of despair. Vaginal examination confirmed my preconceived notion that it was a suitable case for abdominal section. The complete operation was done. From that day to this she has remained well.

342. Mrs. G., Kilmarnock, aged 33; admitted November 29, dismissed December 13, 1897; readmitted February 15, dismissed April 2, 1898. This patient was under observation for a long time before she finally had abdominal section performed. I considered it a typical case and was very much disappointed with the result. She had, however, been ill for years—as, indeed, most of these cases are—and there were other complications which may have assisted in delaying the benefit. For one thing, she had persistent cystitis, from which she obtained no relief at all till I did a cystotomy (vaginal) and left the wound open.

She was a very voluminous correspondent and the following letter very fairly represents her condition:

April 22, 1898.

DEAR SIR:—I would have written sooner, as promised, but waited to feel if the pain would not get less with the change home. I am sorry it has not. I am constantly passing urine which is thick and bad-colored and never more than half a cupful at a time. When passing, and after, the pain is very severe; indeed, it is quite as distressing as the day after the operation. Nor is the pain in my left side better either. I am rather afraid it has started the old trouble again. At least it feels the same. I am nearly constantly in bed, only getting up for half an hour at a time. Might I venture to hope you will write me, if but to cheer me up, for I am sadly disappointed the operation was not successful.

353. Mrs. H., Paisley, aged 27; March 3, 1898; married six years; children, three, one alive. the other two premature. Never well since last child was born. two years ago. Complains of swelling on right side which goes away after diarrhea: nervous, irritable, unable to work; has seen many doctors, and got a pessary, for which she paid five pounds, from a travelling woman doctor from America, whose escape from justice was generally due to the celerity of her movements. She was much the worse for this treatment.

Considered to be a case of ovarian disease with appendicitis.

Both a median and a lateral incision were necessary. The appendix vermiformis was removed. The uterus, which was adherent to the floor of the pelvis and retroverted, was liberated. Neither tube nor ovary was removed. The abdomen was flushed out. She made a fair recovery. All the bowel symptoms were relieved, but not the general nerve condition. Again I believe it was a mistake not to have removed completely both uterine appendages.

403. Mrs. K., India, aged 40; admitted May 27, dismissed July 28, 1899. Chief complaint, pain; this begins at sacrum on left side, comes around to left iliac region and extends down thigh; and similarly on right side. Also during first and second days of period pain is severe all round.

In 1891 the patient was treated for ulceration of the womb. and since then she has complained more or less. Last March (1898) she was seized with dull aching pain in the pelvis, which continued and is present now. She has been treated in India medically for many years. She has had five children. Labors were tedious, but she was never given chloroform. On vaginal examination there is found fibroid degeneration of the cervix; the uterus is acutely retroflexed, movable, and firm. Sound passes three and three-quarter inches. There is a fibroid on the posterior wall. When the uterus is replaced it falls back at once. There is a ruptured perineum.

The uterine appendages were removed completely, running well into the cornua: the fibroid was not interfered with; the perineum was repaired. She made a tedious recovery. but the ultimate result has been all that could be desired. She is herself again, fit for work, happy and full of energy—no more talk of the burden and misery of life.

409. Miss L., Dumfries, virgin, aged 26; admitted July 18, 1899. Has suffered since March, 1897, with pain over uterus and left ovary.

Menstruation regular until last two times, when it became very scanty and lasted two days. Used to be ill about a fortnight. Menstruation began when she was about 11 years of age; the flow occurred probably three times and then disappeared till her eighteenth year. Dysmenorrhea had always been bad and she had to go to bed. Bowels were constipated and bladder more troublesome than formerly. Said she did not feel nervous at all. In appearance was fresh, fair, bright, vivacious when well, but with a hurried, anxious, and quick look of a purely neurasthenic type.

Rectal and vaginal examinations: Ovaries and tubes distinctly in spasm; the uterus is distinctly enlarged and in rigid spasm. Operation July 20, dismissed August 19.

The relief was immediate and permanent. In November her only complaint was the discomfort of wearing an abdominal belt.

425. Mrs. M., Berwick, aged 45; admitted October 16, dismissed November 16, 1899. Whatever shadow of a doubt I had had with regard to the diagnosis of neurasthenia and hysteria in association with the uterine condition was dissipated by my study and treatment of this case.

Mrs. M. had been under treatment for a long time by a most intelligent and well-educated practitioner. She herself was a woman of outstanding simplicity of character, full of sense as well as sensibility. None of us were in any special hurry to anticipate trouble, and so long as we could keep her going on reasonably we did not consider it was wise to perform or even suggest an operation. By and by, however, the condition became unbearable and her distress increased every day. She suffered constantly from pains and aches, fears by day and terrors by night, only now and again snatching an easy hour of peace of mind and body when her pains ceased. At last an operation was suggested, and on June 29, 1899, she writes: "You don't know how an operation haunts me and consequently unnerves me. For the last two days I have had constantly that horrid dull pain in my left side—not the bowel, you know. My headache is gone. I am sleeping well at night and don't feel so tired through the day because I am taking more rest.'' The operation was done and the conditions were found exactly as I had anticipated. The ovaries and tubes were distinctly inflamed and cystic, but not more so than one might reasonably expect in a long-standing case of pelvic disease, and certainly not beyond what one would expect to yield to ordinary medical treatment. But the uterus itself, enlarged with fibroid degeneration, stood erect in the pelvis and was the prominent sign immediately on opening the abdomen.

She was upset and hysterical for several days after the operation, but soon settled down. Her recovery was uninterrupted and has remained permanent. From being a wasted and anxious creature she wrote on March 11, 1900: ''I am getting fine and well, rosy, plump cheeks. I weigh nearly nine stones. You would not recognize me as the fretful lady you had in St. Margaret's Home.''

426. Mrs. N., Glasgow, aged 32; married eight years; one child; admitted November 2, abdominal section November 4, dismissed November 25, 1899. This patient's medical record under my own observation in consultations with her ordinary medical attendant began in 1896. It was a continuous history of ill health. Day in and day out she was never well. She was not of a complaining disposition; rather inclined to be cheerful and happy whenever her pains and aches would let her. As is usually the case in such troubles, the localizing of the pains is always, or nearly always, a difficulty, so that when friends, instead of getting a categorically plain answer to the question as to where the pain is, only get a general and indefinite statement, as here, there, and everywhere, no wonder a certain degree of scepticism is aroused. Medical resources, and perhaps patience, were exhausted and ultimately I advised removal of one or both appendages. I did this as the result of repeated and careful vaginal examinations. I became convinced that there was undue rigidity of the uterus, and that, although the ovaries and tubes were not apparently grossly diseased, there was a deep-seated nerve condition that would probably yield only to section.

At the operation the uterus was visibly and tangibly enlarged and hard, but the left ovary was so distinctly cystic and the tube of the same side so thickened and contorted, while those of the right side were almost normal, that I determined to save the latter. I did so. This is usually a mistake, I must repeat again, and the ultimate result of the case serves to emphasize my opinion. She is vastly better, has been very much better from the time of the operation; but she became pregnant and was delivered of a rather puny child which survived only a few months. She recovered from her confinement quite well and remains well now, but I think it was a mistake to let her have all the risks of childbearing after such a plain demonstration of her uterine condition.

445. Mrs. O., Middlesborough, aged 36; married sixteen years; three children. Menstruation regular, but with great pain; dark, tarry, sticky discharge. Pains left side, back, legs, ankles. Very nervous, and getting worse month by month. Admitted August 1, operation August 3, dismissed August 27, 1900.

Both ovaries were removed and the tubes also, cutting as deeply into the uterus as possible.

Her history was as the others in ordinary, and at the operation the pelvic condition was completely confirmatory of the foregoing descriptions. She ultimately did well and is now in good condition. I insert the following letter, received at an early date from her husband, which contains several extremely important observations:

MIDDLESBOROUGH, October 24, 1900.

DEAR SIR:—I am sorry that I have to inform you that my wife is not getting on as well as she would like since she came home; the reason why, she cannot understand, because she has given herself every attention and complete rest. She complains very much of a pain in her back, and menstruation has come as usual. This last two days it has been alarming, in fact the worst she has ever been, and cannot stir out of bed. I got so afraid that I was for calling in a doctor; but she thought it best to hear what you said first, if it was necessary to do so. Now, doctor, will you kindly tell me if that should be, because she was given to understand that she would not be troubled with menstruation again. She also has an irritable pain on the left of the wound. Will you kindly write by return and let us know what to do, as she is very bad.

446. Mrs. P., Stranraer, aged 30; married eleven years; four children. Menstruation too frequent. Pain on left side very severe. Doctors said she had rheumatism very badly. Suffers from palpitation of the heart, but no organic disease discoverable.

Vaginal examination: Metritis, ovaritis, salpingitis; uterus, ovaries, and tubes all easily palpated, enlarged, and tender. Fibroid and rigid condition of uterus.

Breathless. anxious, nervous, hysterical.

Operation, removal of both tubes and ovaries as completely as possible, August 10, dismissed September 11, 1900.

I was almost afraid to attempt this case. I had more than one hundred letters, telegrams, and communications about it from first to last, and the best way would be to let some of them speak for themselves. It was a typical combined neurasthenic and hysterical case clinically, and I had to box the compass twenty times as to the disease in nomenclature. diagnosis, treatment, and result. I could not improve on the patient's own description of her case before operation.

STRANRAER, Monday Evening.

DEAR DR. NAIRNE:—My husband informed me on his return from Glasgow that you intended writing me, and indeed I shall be delighted to hear from you when you can spare time.

Meantime I should like you to know my symptoms, and perhaps, dear Mr. Nairne, you will explain them a little to me. To begin with, I am suffering a deal of pain, sometimes in my body and then in my limbs. When in my body it is of quite a different character to the limbs. It is a burning, tingling pain, very disagreeable, but not nearly so acute as in the hips, leg, or ankles. Would you kindly say if it is muscular rheumatism or neuralgia, and is it due to weakness or have I caught cold? Then I have very heavy sweats and also shivers. I have not been out for some time, as even when the weather is good I find it so difficult to keep myself warm, and my limbs seem so weak and so sore that they will scarcely carry me.

Dr. M. proposed to give me sweating powders to try and carry the pain away, but as yet I have not made up my mind, as I do not feel quite sure of that being correct. I am so weak already, and if these pains arise from bodily weakness there is nothing to be gained by sweating me any more than can be helped. My head is fearful sometimes. but I could stand that if I could only feel myself getting free of the bodily pain. Would you please let me know what I should do? If there is nothing but rest for these pains, I am quite agreeable to lie: but I would feel relieved if I only knew what was best to do. I have been taking salicylate of soda powders, not very many as yet. but I do not feel benefited. I feel sorry for troubling you. but trust you will excuse me. as I am very lonely here without a mother or sister or any one to speak to. and it is dull ailing day after day like this. I pray for patience and feel sure it will be granted me, but still I would like to know what is best so that I might do it. Awaiting your kind reply, I wish so much I was nearer you. so that I might consult you when I feel so ill. It is so awkward here.

One cannot help saying, "Poor creature!" and wondering how much of this description is pictorial and how much real. Then comes a letter on the following September 15. four days after returning home:

DEAR DR. NAIRNE:—I have delayed writing you each day since my return, in the hope that I would feel better.   I have kept my bed to-day until just now, 5 o'clock, and feel a little better from the long rest.   I have had a deal of pain from left and right side where ovaries were removed, also a severe pain all up left side as far as shoulder blade.   There is also a deal of yellowish discharge from passage.   Indeed, dear Dr. Nairne, I never, never expected such bad effects, else I would never have faced operation.   I had poor health before, but nothing compared with this. I am mentally and physically wretched and I am at a loss what to do with myself.

The only other letter I take the liberty of transcribing is a fortnight after the last:

October 29. 1900.

DEAR DR. NAIRNE:—I trust you will not think me troublesome, but your last letter and advice proved helpful to me, so that I cannot resist the temptation to ask still further.   I have been keeping a little better since then, but, O dear! far from feeling happy about my condition.   I am resting nearly all day, and still with the slightest exertion the burning pain in the left side is very bad.   Now tell me, dear Dr. Nairne, should I confine myself entirely to bed, or is that sort of pain to be expected?   I would not get so worried about it if I knew it was just what should be and would pass away.   I have used the douche and sanitas. and the discharge is much improved.   I think it was caused by the pessary being misplaced.   Indeed, I did not know it was in; perhaps you forgot to tell me.   Dr. M. has taken it out, and I miss it very much, but you, too, may think it better to do without it.   I am trying to wear my corsets. but the skin irritation worries me very much.   I wear them very loosely at present.   Will I ever, dear Dr. Nairne, be able to wear them firmly?   Now do not laugh. please, at me being worried about the wearing of my corsets.   You know I am not an old woman yet and would still like to look smart.   By the bye. doctor, would you approve of me taking tepid salt water baths?   I was thinking they might help to strengthen me a little.

These three communications throw more light on a case of this kind than a whole volume of impersonal observations.   Here is practical experience, sad, controlling, and deeply disappointing.   Had the case ended here one would have been driven to different conclusions.   One might have been that the diagnosis was wrong and that it was a case of actual central (cerebral) disease; an absolute want of mental balance which an operation of this kind might only aggravate.   On the other hand, the cases where mental balance has been restored by complete oöphorectomy, although not numerous, are sufficient to show that the diagnosis might have been correct in spite of the apparent untoward result. About one thing there is no question, that the balance was very waveringly hung between sanity and insanity. Both follow. In this case, fortunately, I can wind up with a comforting report. After the lapse of another year, at Christmas, things have put on a new aspect and mind and body are declared both well. Thus in our practice, medical and surgical, we have to deal with an unstable system, a mental balance, that automatically is being continually readjusted. If we succeed, especially in those apparently violent although often necessary surgical methods, we get praised frequently far beyond our deserts; and if we fail, broad indeed require our shoulders to be to endure the weight of recrimination that is so unjustly, needlessly, and, as a rule, thoughtlessly thrown on us.

I do not think any one will imagine that the practice of surgery, especially in this branch, is an unadulterated joy. Disappointments meet one on every hand, and it is only the faith that one has in the honesty and single-hearted purpose of his endeavors to do good that can enable him to endure the burden. I have put down plainly, as far as possible, the patients' own words and descriptions of their troubles, very frequently distressingly pictorial and not always flattering, but, taking them all in all, satisfactory and encouraging, and indicating pretty certainly that, with a few discomforts and dangers, a large measure of success may be predicted and gained in this direction.

AN OPERATION FOR STRICTURE OF THE RECTUM IN WOMEN.

PRELIMINARY REPORT OF A CASE.[1]

BY

THOMAS J. WATKINS, M.D.,

Professor of Clinical Gynecology, Northwestern University Medical School, etc., Chicago.

(With seven Illustrations.)

As the operation was devised after failure to give relief in a case of stricture of the rectum by the use of the procedures which are usually recommended, I will first report the case.

[1] Read before the Chicago Gynecological Society, June 25, 1902.

Mrs. B., aged 33 years. Consulted me in February, 1899, for rectal symptoms which on examination proved to be due to a stricture of the rectum. She gave a history of syphilis, and when first seen she was suffering from alopecia, and examination revealed some enlarged lymphatic glands. The stricture was an annular one of the lower part of the rectum. The calibre of the rectum at that point was about that of a No. 22 sound (American scale). She was sent to Provident Hospital, and a few days later I attempted a resection of the strictured portion through an incision in the posterior vaginal wall according to a plan presented to this Society some years ago by Dr. L. L. MacArthur.

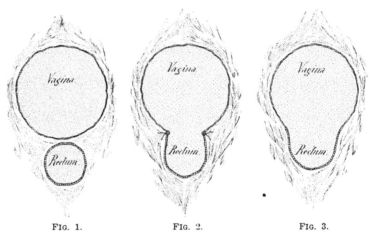

FIG. 1.   FIG. 2.   FIG. 3.

FIG. 1.—Transverse section of Vagina and rectum through the stricture. (Diagrammatic.)

FIG. 2.—Recto-Vaginal septum divided and mucosa of rectum sutured to Vaginal mucosa on either side. The two are made into one canal.

FIG. 3.—Result of first step of the operation.

This was abandoned on account of the absence of normal mucosa below the stricture. The recto-vaginal septum was then incised in the median line through the entire perineal body, the strictured portion of the rectum was excised, and the end of the bowel was sutured to the skin and perineal wound. This left a condition similar to a complete laceration of the perineum. She was given mercury and iodide of potash, and one month later an operation for complete laceration of the perineum was performed and the result seemed ideal, except that the calibre of the bowel at the uppermost angle of the wound was somewhat less than normal. She was entirely relieved of the rectal symptoms. and was instructed to- continue the use of anti-syphilitic treatment and to report at regular intervals.   She neglected to continue the treatment. and when. in February, 1902. three years later, she consulted me, examination revealed a stricture which extended from the anus to a point nearly opposite the cervix uteri and through which I could pass an index finger with difficulty.   She had a profuse discharge of pus and mucus.

The conditions contraindicated an attempt to use divulsion, resection. or excision, and I believe the operation saved her from a colotomy which otherwise would soon have become necessary.

The operation consisted in:

1. Division of the recto-vaginal septum along the median line through the perineum and to a point above the stricture.

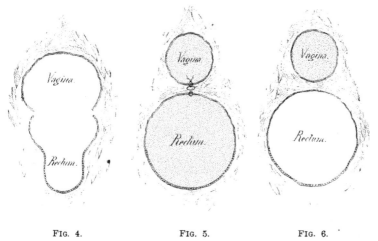

FIG. 4.   FIG. 5.   FIG. 6.

FIG. 4.—Vagina inCised on either side to form new reCto-Vaginal septum.
FIG. 5.—Sutures inserted and tied.   New septum is formed.   The dotted portion shows the relatiVe amount of original rectal mucosa
FIG. 6 —Completed operation.

through the perineum and to a point above the stricture.   This included nearly the entire vaginal wall (Figs. 1 and 2) and made the rectum and vagina one canal, as would result from a complete laceration of the perineum extending nearly throughout the entire length of the vagina.

2. Suture of the rectal to the vaginal mucosa on either side with fine catgut. (Fig. 2).   This completed the first step of the operation.   The second part of the operation is not performed until the healing becomes firm and the suppurating surface of

the rectum recovers. In this case the interval was four months. On exposure of the rectal canal the strictured portion showed the mucosa much contracted and the site of a large amount of granulating surface and cicatricial tissue. The dotted portion in the figures shows approximately the relative amounts of rectal and vaginal mucous membrane.

Second portion of operation (formation of a new septum).

3. Section of the vagina on both sides (Fig. 4). Formation by blunt dissection of two flaps on either side. The place of this incision depends upon the amount of vaginal and of mucous membrane present. The two posterior flaps were turned into the rectum to form the anterior portion of the rectum. and the

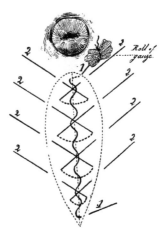

FIG. 7.—1, longitudinal suture closing "posterior flaps"; 2, figure-of-eight sutures closing "anterior flaps" and subVaginal tissue.

two anterior flaps were united to form the posterior wall of the vagina.

4. Suture of the vaginal flaps (Fig. 5).

The posterior flaps were united by a continuous silkworm-gut suture. It was inserted to the side of the wound near the cervix; to its end was tied a roll of gauze (Fig. 7, g) and passed through the edges of the two posterior flaps and brought out through the skin lateral to the anus. This was drawn taut and tied to a superficial suture near its point of exit and thus completely closed the rectal wound. This suture is similar to one which M. L. Harris described for the closing of the peritoneum in abdominal wounds. The wound that remained was similar in contour to an extensive Hegar perineal denudation. The suture illustrated for closure of the anterior vaginal flaps and the subvaginal tissue was a figure-of-eight one (Fig. 7). That for the perineal body and the sphincter ani was the same as is used in operations for complete laceration of the perineum.

It would seem difficult, after turning a large amount of vaginal mucous membrane into the rectum, to restore the sphincter ani. This is not, however, difficult, as the lower end of the two flaps mentioned are in close proximity to the ends of the sphincter muscle. Fig. 1 shows approximately the relative size of the vagina and the rectum at the site of stricture before treatment, and Fig. 6 shows approximately their relative size at the close of the operation.

The principle of the operation is simple, as the first step consists in division of the recto-vaginal septum, and the second step in making a new septum.

The change, if any, that will take place in the vaginal mucous membrane that is turned into the rectum remains to be determined; but the probabilities are that no pathological change of any importance will take place, as in complete laceration of the perineum and in cases of recto-vaginal fistula the feces do not irritate the vaginal mucous membrane. Observation in this case will be interesting, as three-fourths of the rectal wall now consists of vaginal mucous membrane.

The result in this case cannot now be estimated, as the operation was completed only one week ago. There will probably be very little danger of stricture forming in the vaginal mucous membrane that is turned into the rectum, if the syphilis is cured.

The convalescence has been much the same as is usual after operation for complete laceration of the perineum.

I have not had the opportunity to make an extensive perusal of the literature, but from a moderate investigation I am unable to find this principle of operation mentioned for stricture of the rectum. It makes little difference, however, whether the operation is new or not, if it proves of service in the treatment of some cases of stricture of the lower part of the rectum.

1800 MICHIGAN AVENUE.

PLASTIC SURGERY OF THE FEMALE URETHRA,

WITH REPORT OF A UNIQUE CASE.[1]

BY

HENRY P. NEWMAN, A.M., M.D.,

Professor of Gynecology and Clinical Gynecology, College of Physicians and
Surgeons, Chicago. Medical Department of the University of Illinois, and
Professor of Gynecology, Chicago Policlinic.
Chicago.

(With two illustrations.)

THE restoration of the female bladder, when extensively torn and its floor practically destroyed by the original injury and subsequent unsuccessful surgery, is in itself difficult enough, sometimes impossible, but where a new urethra must also be constructed and means of controlling the flow of urine must be devised the problem is indeed perplexing. Many methods of reconstructing this membranous canal with its mucous lining have been tried, some of them with marked success; but the literature of the subject shows that the same method can rarely be applied twice, since each of these accidents happens in its own way and calls for a new and specially devised operation. In presenting this report I had hoped to give final results in a very interesting case now under treatment at the Marion Sims Hospital, but its progress, while satisfactory, has been tedious and I am obliged to give only such data as I have secured up to the present.

The patient, Mrs. S. W., referred to me by Dr. Inks, of Nappanee, Ind., is 39 years of age and has been married three years. She is only four feet eight inches in height, undeveloped, with a generally contracted pelvis, and an ankylosed hip resulting from a severe attack of Pott's disease in early childhood. Two years ago she gave birth to a full-term stillborn child. The delivery was accomplished without instruments, but was a forcible extraction through a narrow pelvis with a distended bladder. The resulting rupture involved extensive tear of the bladder floor and complete obliteration of the urethral tract, which was laid open along its entire length. By subsequent re-

[1]Read before the Chicago Gynecological Society, June 25, 1902.

traction of the torn surfaces even the landmarks of the previous urethral channel were lost. Six weeks afterward, while the patient was 'still in bed from the results of her severe delivery, an attempt was made to repair the injury. This was repeated in April and September of the following year. The first two operations were done in a private dwelling, the last in a small country hospital. These were conscientious attempts and were done probably as well as limited facilities and experience would permit. The results, however. were most discouraging. When the patient came to me last December she had a veritable

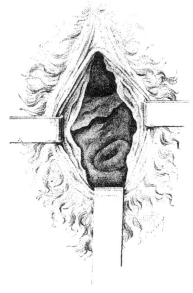

Fig. 1.

exstrophy of the bladder. The organ was everted through the large rent in the floor and the reddened and inflamed bladder walls were thickened and covered with mucus. The vulva and thighs were excoriated, and she had a large inflamed surface over the lower sacral region, in the centre of which was an ulcer the size of a half-dollar. The left hip was ankylosed, the pelvis narrowed. and the rami of the pubes, practically denuded of all but a thin covering of scar tissue, formed a very acute angle. No trace of a urethra could be made out in any of the surrounding tissues. The small, hyperinvoluted uterus was deformed by tears and resulting scars, the cervix drawn forward and downward by the large cicatrix in the small vagina, as will be seen by the accompanying illustration (Fig. 1). I operated in January last, attempting to constrict the large opening in the gaping bladder wall as a step toward subsequent closure. Flaps were taken from the vulva on either side, and, after splitting the bladder and vaginal wall, a considerable closure was accomplished by means of silver-wire sutures, a drain or retention catheter being inserted in an opening behind the line of sutures and the patient kept in the exaggerated dorsal position until the wound healed. It was desired to prevent in this way the urine from accumulating and soiling the sutures. The second operation was done in February, when still further closure was accomplished by a similar suturing of flaps. this time with silkworm gut. My further aim in both

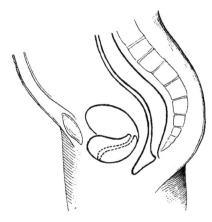

FIG. 2.

instances was to construct a urethral channel from the soft parts about the vestibule and from the labial mucous membrane. The results obtained left much to be desired; but the patient, feeling herself greatly improved over her former condition, left the hospital during my absence in the South and has but just consented to return for completion of the work. The operation which I have just performed, and which was along the same lines, bade fair to be successful in closing the entire bladder and obtaining a urethral canal, and its partial failure is due to an accident. An attendant unfamiliar with the case, in replacing a drainage catheter, pushed it through the newly-formed urethra instead of into the artificial opening provided for the purpose. As it is. the patient can hold her urine for a consider-

31

able time when in the recumbent position, and I believe some mechanical appliance can be provided which will prevent involuntary evacuation and leakage. Since the work I have already done has proved so successful, I shall abandon the intention I had when this report was projected.

In another case presenting all the formidable features of this one, I should be disposed to do the operation I have devised, and which I will briefly outline, rather than to expose the patient to the annoyance and distress—amounting. in a tubercular subject, to danger to life—incident to prolonged confinement and repeated operating.

Operation.—After the usual aseptic and antiseptic preparation, the patient is placed in the lithotomy position, the uterus drawn down with volsella forceps, and a semilunar incision made through the mucous membrane of the vaginal vault behind the cervix. This procedure and the opening of Douglas' cul-de-sac are the classical first steps in vaginal hysterectomy. The tubes and ovaries are now ligated with catgut and severed with as much of the broad ligament as is necessary to allow of the uterus being turned downward through the posterior vaginal opening and sufficiently inverted to close the gap in the floor of the bladder (see Fig. 2). The mucous and serous surfaces coming in contact with each other and intended for approximation are denuded and stitched together by interrupted silkworm-gut sutures.

An opening is now made through the wall of the uterus into the uterine cavity at a point corresponding to the location of the external meatus, and a retention catheter is inserted up through the dilated cervical canal into the bladder. The parts are approximated with sufficient firmness to prevent leakage from the now fully reconstructed bladder. The vagina is loosely packed with iodoform gauze and the patient put to bed. Permanent drainage is established by means of the catheter and extension tubing leading into a receptacle containing a 1:2000 bichloride solution.

The newly-formed bladder is washed out with a saturated solution of boric acid every eight hours and the external parts bathed with the bichloride solution. followed with sterile water, and dusted with aristol or some antiseptic powder.

This operation should not be confounded with the simple drawing down of the uterus without inversion for plastic work, nor with Freund's procedure in cases of vesical and rectal fistulæ. In this latter, only the body of the uterus is used, the cervix above being curled on itself and walled off by cicatricial tissue.

When we consider the horrible state the patient is in. the danger of infection extending to ureters and kidneys, the depressing mental effect, the impairment of general health, the danger to life, some radical procedure for relief seems imperative. Again the usual methods will not suffice. Entire closure, whether or not it includes the vagina as in urinary fistulæ, makes no provision for voluntary urination. A suprapubic opening, as used in the male, would be inapplicable. The gradual drawing downward of the uterus until it can be used for plastic closure of the bladder opening could not be done in this case, owing to the adhesions and fixation. Rolling up of vaginal tissue to form a urethra. after the unique method of MacArthur, and subsequently using the device of Kolischer, so ingeniously perfected by Fletcher. for controlling the flow of urine, was not possible because scarcely any anterior vaginal wall tissue was available. The transplantation of the trigone into the rectum was contraindicated by the insufficiency of the rectal sphincter. Indeed, all known methods seemed impracticable. The method proposed has in its favor these points: The entire operation for closing the bladder and furnishing a urinary tract can be done at one sitting with a strong probability of its successful issue. The saving of time and suffering to the patient is a great consideration.

The possible sources of failure might be: Insufficient collateral circulation in the uterus separated from its posterior attachments; the use of serous instead of mucous membrane for the bladder floor might be more or less objectionable, though this has already been reported as successfully done; the uncertainty of inducing sphincter-like control of the circular fibres of the cervix uteri. In spite of these difficulties I believe it is possible to use as an agent in forming another urethra the hyperinvoluted, deformed uterus, which has now no functional value proportionate to the service it may thus be made to perform.

100 STATE STREET.

SOME RECENT SURGERY FOR BILIARY OBSTRUCTION.[1]

BY

I. S. STONE, M.D.,
Washington. D. C.

THE study of biliary obstruction is of ever-increasing interest to the abdominal surgeon. The experience that he has gained will prove equally interesting and profitable to the physician, for the diagnosis of these diseases has been wonderfully facilitated since we have dared to attack surgically the various forms of obstruction.

Experience in pelvic surgery has enabled us to deal with many of the difficult cases of biliary obstruction with the greatest satisfaction, especially those having had acute infectious mischief with the resulting adhesions between peritoneal surfaces.

Operations upon the common duct are generally difficult owing to the location of the parts deep down in the abdomen; on the contrary, the gall bladder, which furnishes by far the greater number of pathological conditions, is easy of access.

It is a beautiful and satisfactory operation to cut down upon a distended gall bladder, to locate and remove a stone, or to aspirate the pus or bile-colored mucus. to suture the bladder to the wound, place a drainage tube, close the wound. and see your patient promptly recover. But all cases of biliary obstruction are not so "beautiful," nor are the difficulties encountered fully understood when one looks upon the small and comparatively insignificant objects often removed. The stones do not represent the difficulties one must encounter if he operates upon many patients with cholelithiasis. It is not my intention to dwell upon this portion of the 'subject, but rather to outline some of the indications for operative treatment. in order that we may become as familiar with gall-stone surgery as with other abdominal work.

Frequency.—Gall stones do not always give rise to pain or obstruction. They may be found by chance when the abdomen has been opened for other reasons. It is estimated that perhaps 5 per cent of gall-stone subjects feel the presence of calculi. while

[1]Read before the Washington Obstetrical and Gynecological Society, May 16, 1902.

95 per cent are totally unaware of their possession, although they may have some vague distress, such as eructations from the stomach or possibly some "dragging" in the right side. If one may rely upon medical literature as a guide, it would appear that operations upon the bile ducts are more frequent in England and in Europe than in America. For instance, Kehr, in his book published in 1900, reports over five hundred operations. He is located in Halberstadt, a small German town, although he has the whole of Europe for a field, and even has patients from the United States of America. His work and that of others in Europe is being closely followed, and their experience is only a little greater than that of some American surgeons. In a recent visit to a Western city the writer saw about twenty patients, in one hospital, in various stages of convalescence from operations upon the liver and gall ducts. A recent journal has a report of "328 operations upon the gall bladder and bile passages" by William Mayo, of Rochester, Minn.[1]

When we remember that gall-stone operations were exceptional before their popularization by Lawson Tait, we cannot fail to note how rapidly and universally they have come into professional favor. In some hospitals we have visited we saw nearly as many patients under treatment for diseases of the liver and its ducts, including gall-stone obstruction, as for appendicitis.

Symptoms.—The cardinal indications of biliary obstruction, jaundice and pain, with bile in the urine and its absence in the stools, are well understood as associated in nearly all cases of biliary obstruction. But there are many cases of gall-bladder and cystic-duct obstruction or inflammation which rarely cause jaundice. and there are often calculi present and possibly doing mischief without great pain.

Diagnosis.—It is now possible to reach, without great delay, a fairly accurate diagnosis in cases of biliary obstruction, thus affording patients greater security and safety from the various distressing complications. All surgeons and physicians know the dangers incident to operation during cholemia, and I need not mention how desirable it is to avoid delay on this account. In the examination of the gall bladder we need to have developed a perfect sense of touch and a refinement of the art of palpation. The cases of empyema, or indeed any case of moderately distended gall bladder, are easily made out. But we find the greatest diffi-

[1]Chicago Medical Recorder, April 15, 1902.

culty in correctly estimating its size, location, and condition
when contracted. These cases of contracted gall bladder are as
productive of unpleasant and dangerous symptoms as they are
difficult of palpation. While we may easily reach a conclusion
as to the cause of the symptoms when there is jaundice, it is possible to have many serious results of stones in the gall bladder
and cystic duct which rarely cause jaundice. In my own experience the most difficult of all have been these neglected or delayed
cases. An early resort to operation will enable the surgeon to
remove the stones before perforation occurs; therefore let us see
what may be done to throw light upon this part of our subject.

First we must learn that many of the symptoms heretofore
known as gastric, hepatic, or catarrhal may not have their origin
in these organs, but in the gall bladder or ducts. A perusal of
hundreds of cases in Kehr's book and elsewhere will show us that
anorexia, nausea, and vomiting were frequent, and indeed almost
constant, symptoms when the patient had gall stones or inflammation of the biliary passages. These symptoms, with a degree of
enlargement, or even tenderness or pain, on pressure under the
liver, furnish strong presumptive evidence that a cause for these
may be found in the biliary passages. Perhaps we would accomplish the same result by suspecting these ducts when we find no
solution for the symptoms after due examination of the stomach
and other viscera. By far the greater number of these cases
occur in women, and many more occur in persons of middle age
or in elderly people than in young persons. The diagnosis between cancer of the liver or gall ducts and obstruction from
stones is difficult in patients over 50 years of age. But we find
the two frequently associated, and unfortunately, in many instances, we find the evidence of cancer so unmistakable as to
negative any surgical treatment. The association of gall stones
with malignant disease is well known, and we fully agree that
malignancy favors cholelithiasis, and are almost ready to say
that the opposite proposition is also correct, namely, that the
development of cancer is favored by the presence of gall stones.

In making a diagnosis of biliary obstruction we must remember
that other causes exist besides stones in the ducts and cancer.
We have occasionally disease of the pancreas or its ducts which
may exactly simulate the symptoms above mentioned. A stone
in the pancreatic duct may press upon the common duct, or a
pancreatic stone may enter the common duct through an anomalous connection. (The pancreatic duct varies greatly in its

course, distribution, and its exit into the duodenum.) But the most important and probably the most frequently observed disease of the pancreas is chronic inflammation resulting in induration and hypertrophy. I have seen at least one instance of this form of obstruction, and cases are reported by Mayo Robson, England (who has seen several), McKenzie (Montreal), Fenger, Riedel, Kehr, and others. Before operation it is almost impossible to decide between this form of obstruction and malignancy and gall stones in the common duct. Still, I am convinced that diagnosis will be greatly facilitated when aided by the experience of the surgeon who operates after studying the symptoms. The diagnosis of suppurative diseases of the liver and bile passages is always difficult. Acute infectious cholangitis simulates liver infection and abscess. The presence of gall stones may add to the severity of the attack. but we do not find gall-stone colic in these cases. The high temperature, quick pulse, and chills will suggest operation in any event; but we should be very careful about the prognosis, as we have already diagnosed a condition demanding operative treatment if the patient's condition is such as to suggest a reasonably safe operation.

In empyema the fever is not very high, while in liver infection or abscess it is always much elevated. In cholangitis we may have a temperature to 104°, but generally without repetition of the first chill. We always look upon repeated chills as an indication of abscess of the liver and not simply due to inflammation of the bile ducts. Pain is almost invariably present. It is, as a rule, severest at the seat of the obstruction, but nearly always radiates or extends elsewhere. We know of few instances where this is so often observed as it is in the conditions now under discussion. The "gouty man" with a "bad liver," who may. or may not have gall stones, will say his pain extends to his shoulder or subscapular region. The severest gall-stone colic is rarely localized. It always means a pressure from behind, a distension of the gall bladder and hepatic and cystic ducts, if the common duct is the seat of obstruction. But it also means a dilatation of the duct, a scraping or maceration of the lining of the duct itself. The pain of cancerous obstruction, or that due to obstruction from pancreatic disease, is different from the regulation gall-stone colic. In two recent cases, very similar in many respects, this remark is fully exemplified. These forms of obstruction cause pain at intervals of three or four days. It is inconceivable that so many gall stones pass through the ducts, or that many cases of "ball valve" stone actually occur. A persistent pain in the region of the gall bladder or ducts demands explanation and relief. The pain in a case of obstruction due to chronic hypertrophic pancreatitis is chiefly in the epigastrium and extends upward in the median line. A diagnosis by exclusion is always possible, which should with sufficient accuracy enable us to decide to operate in time to prevent serious complications.

Nearly all patients have nausea and vomiting, but there are some very ill patients without either. One case formerly reported by the writer had vomiting of such persistence that the operation was done with this symptom as the chief guide. She had, however, tenderness upon deep pressure upon the gall bladder. Four small stones were removed and the patient was promptly cured and has remained well ever since. In reading Kehr's book one is struck with the large number of cases having symptoms referable to the stomach. In many of his cases he practised "stomach washing" after operation.

Loss in weight is almost invariably observed; the apparent exceptions are those in which the obstruction is in the cystic duct, which does not greatly interfere with the passage of bile into the intestine.

Obstruction of the cystic duct occasionally produces jaundice when the stone is a large one and presses upon the common duct. Obstruction is due: 1. To twisting, kinking, or inflammation of the cystic duct or tumefaction of its mucous lining, or to impacted calculi. 2. To obstructed hepatic duct. 3. To obstructed common duct, which may be due: (a) to calculi, (b) to cholangitis, (c) to diseased pancreas or carcinoma of ducts or organs adjoining.

Authors mention pancreatic calculi as responsible for obstruction of common duct, but we have no positive data as to frequency.

The question arises, What is catarrhal jaundice? What is its pathology? How many cases of purely catarrhal jaundice does the surgeon see which he believes due to duodenitis or gastroduodenal catarrh? We confess to a feeling of doubt regarding these questions, and think future experience will show very few such cases without cholelithiasis or other physical obstruction. Just as the number of severe intestinal colics diminish before the ever-growing science of physical examination aided by surgical exploration, we will find the cases of catarrhal jaundice disappear. As the number of renal and liver calculi increase, or, rather, as we learn how to find them, so will our cases of intestinal colic and perhaps some other of our vague gastro-intestinal disorders disappear.

When Lawson Tait first popularized cholelithotomy, it was thought a very serious matter to attack gall stones even in the gall bladder. But in the twelve or fourteen years since that time scores of surgeons have operated for biliary obstruction. With the writer as with many others, the work had come to be as much a necessity as any other surgery. It has been developed gradually, and increasing experience has shown good results in a comprehension of hitherto difficult work or obscure conditions.

Some of the Aims of Gall-stone Surgery.—Besides cystotomy for empyema or other distension of the bladder, we find a growing inclination to remove the gall bladder entirely—"cystectomy." In any contracted gall bladder it may be necessary to do this if unable to suture the bladder to the wound, or if the bladder be the seat of incurable disease and consequently demand removal. Besides the incision into and removal of the bladder, we have the following: Incision of either cystic, hepatic, or common duct for the extraction of calculi, or for purposes of drainage, etc., also anastomosis between the gall bladder or cystic or common duct and intestine or stomach.

Thus far we have found no necessity for anastomosis of cystic or common duct with intestine or stomach, but have been contented to remove stones, to drain the gall bladder and ducts, and to perform anastomosis between gall bladder and intestine. There may be in rare instances some need of anastomosis of the common duct with the intestine, as in certain cases of obstruction in the pancreas. Such occlusion of the duct would generally result in a dilatation, which would facilitate the operation.

RECENT CASES NOT REPORTED ELSEWHERE.

Mrs. A., white, aged 40. Operation in Columbia Hospital November 2, 1898. Had a dermoid cyst of ovary, which had become detached from its pedicle (migrating ovarian cyst). Her tumor was attached to the large omentum and parietes in the region of the umbilicus. Her symptoms of pain under the liver and those due to the condition of her stomach were all set down as due to the presence of the tumor, which weighed several pounds and greatly distended the abdomen. After removal of the tumor, the gall bladder was found about the size and shape of a hen's egg, filled with many stones which were impacted. The removal of the gall bladder was imperative. "Cystectomy." Recovery.

Stones in cystic duct; perforation; hemorrhage from stomach.
—Mrs. McP. (Dr. Moran). Operation March 7, 1896. Patient
had severe pain and inflammation with tumor in region of liver
and transverse colon. Hemorrhage from stomach of severe
character. A tumor found under the liver, at first thought due
to malignancy. The transverse colon was found firmly adherent
under the liver, entirely obscuring the gall bladder. Separation
of bowel caused free bleeding. Finally, when the gall bladder
was reached, presence of stones helped to clear up doubts as to
cause of her symptoms. It was discovered that the stones had
perforated the cystic duct, and, aided by adhesions of bowel to
liver and duct, they escaped into the intestine, making a natural
cholecystenterostomy. Drainage. Wound closed as usual, silkworm and catgut. Recovery.

*Stones in gall bladder; perforation; peritonitis; operation
June 1, 1898; recovery.*—Mrs. C., aged 28. Patient had been
treated in my private hospital about one year before for salpingitis. Pain, fever, and other symptoms of empyema finally
resulted in peritonitis, from which she barely recovered, causing
her to leave her distant home in Virginia to try an operative
cure. The stones were impacted in the remnant of a collapsed
gall bladder and were removed along with the greater part of
the viscus. Adhesions separated, and drainage by gauze and
tube instituted. Patient has continued in excellent health until
the present time.

*Stones in gall bladder and cystic duct; tumor due to distended
gall bladder; patient in bad health; has lost flesh, is anemic, and
has pain; operation June 2, 1898.*—Mrs. H. (care of Dr. D. O.
Leech), aged 44. Had never been very healthy; was thin, pale,
and nervous. History of long suffering, due to pain in region
of gall bladder. Had gastric symptoms, anorexia, occasional
vomiting, poor appetite. Had never been jaundiced, nor had
she had distinct gall-stone colic. Heart normal. Kidneys and
other abdominal organs not apparently diseased. She had a
slight elevation of temperature. Many large gall stones were
removed from the bladder, but one, at least, was left in the cystic
duct. The gall bladder was sutured to the wound and drained
with rubber tube. She made a symptomatic recovery, with a
fistula remaining which refused to close. This I attribute to a
stone in cystic duct, as the discharge is not colored with bile.

*Stones in the gall bladder and appendicitis, both of which
cause symptoms demanding operation.*—Mrs. C., of Virginia,
white, aged 38. (Care of Dr. Ransom, West Virginia.) Operation November 24, 1898; private hospital. A thin, delicate
woman with nervous temperament; had symptoms clearly indicating presence of gall stones for some months before pain
developed in the region of her appendix. The two diseases were
in no way associated. Her urine was thought bile-stained prior
to her visit to Washington. It was now free from bile. She
experienced severe pain on pressure over the enlarged gall blad-

der. She was not distinctly jaundiced, although I thought her complexion influenced by her septic condition. She had fever, and doubtless cholangitis had caused the acute symptoms referable to the gall bladder. Operation was quite easy, no complications. Drainage and wound closure as usual. Recovery uneventful from both operations, which were done at same sitting.

Stones in gall bladder; pigmentation of skin; easy operation, no complications; patient attacked by pneumonia on evening of second day; fatal result in nine days.—Mrs. F., white. Operation at private hospital October 27, 1899. The patient had been ill several months before the writer first saw her in consultation. She was somewhat emaciated, was anemic, and skin decidedly dark from pigmentation. She had in addition some evidence of bile-poisoning. She had a tumor in the region of the gall bladder, and her right kidney was somewhat prolapsed. No other evidence of kidney disease. There was distress and dull aching in her side, but no history of gall stone or renal colic. Feeling absolutely sure of the diagnosis, operation was advised. Ether anesthesia. Many stones found in gall bladder, which were removed and suspension practised. No stones were found in other ducts, and I was at a loss to explain the discoloration of the skin. Writing now, with nearly three years' additional experience, it is possible that improved methods would enable one to discover the hidden factor in a similar case.

The patient had no trouble from her gall-stone operation, but succumbed to an attack of pneumonia, due, in my opinion, to the administration of ether, and also in part to her lowered vitality from causes above mentioned.

Stones in cystic duct.—Mrs. W., aged 47. (Care of Dr. Dillenback.) Mother of several children. In usual good health until three months prior to operation at Sibley Hospital, May 28, 1900. Pain in gall bladder and region of bile ducts; no jaundice. Tumor distinctly outlined. Gall stones removed from gall bladder, and at least one from cystic duct. Suspension and drainage; cure.

Stones in gall bladder, cystic and common ducts; operation December 11, 1901; recovery.—Mrs. J., white, aged 30. Weight in health, 160 pounds; now reduced to 110 pounds. Had been sick several months with jaundice, but *unaccompanied by pain.* No stones found in stools. Intense icterus, and persistent nausea and vomiting. Gall bladder not distended. Diagnosis, obstruction of common duct by gall stones. The gall bladder was firmly contracted around a large stone, with a small amount of pus present. Another stone was firmly impacted in the cystic duct, which was badly lacerated and almost obliterated by the manipulations necessary for its removal. Two other stones, equal in size to those above mentioned, were found in the common duct. No effort was made to effect complete closure of the duct. A few catgut sutures were applied to hold the edges of the duct nearly together. Two drainage tubes were placed with

gauze packing under the liver to aid in protecting the peritoneal
cavity from bile, which poured out freely after removing the
stones from the common duct.   The patient was greatly shocked
by the prolonged operation, but made a complete recovery.

*Jaundice with pain simulating gall-stone colic, due to either
pancreatic hypertrophy or cancer; operation January 11, 1902,
at private hospital; symptomatic recovery.* – Mrs. H.. white. aged
60.   Was sent to me by Dr. H. T. Harding.   She had suffered
from symptoms of gall-stone colic and had been jaundiced for
more than two years.   Between the attacks she would improve,
but never entirely recovered.   Finally, for some weeks prior to
my visit, she had attacks of pain every three or four days, and
increasing jaundice with emaciation, which caused her to consent to the operation which her physician advised.   She had the
characteristic and classical symptoms of bile-poisoning, but not
so severely as to be called "cholemia."   Still she appeared so
ill as to give us much anxiety to avoid a protracted operation.

Incision in usual location outside right rectus.   The evidence
of long-standing disease of the gall bladder and ducts was quite
well marked.   The omentum and peritoneal surfaces were fairly
healthy, except for discoloration from bile-staining.   The liver
was not enlarged, but had a mottled appearance; was either carcinomatous or cirrhotic.   Pancreas was not examined as carefully as it should have been, owing to condition of patient.
Stomach and intestines healthy in appearance.   The gall bladder
was enormously enlarged and nearly empty of bile.   Her attacks
of pain were due to distension of gall bladder with bile.   The
dilated bladder would disgorge a quantity of bile every three
or four days and then would come cessation of pain.   We performed cholecystenterostomy without a button or mechanical
device, using rapid suture method.   The patient had considerable discomfort for the first two weeks from "gastric irritability."   She had no desire for food and would occasionally vomit.
Strychnia acted most happily upon this patient and appeared to
give prompt relief when administered for a weak pulse and
general depression.   The patient was able to leave the hospital
in four weeks, and made a splendid recovery.   The jaundice
rapidly disappeared, her appetite returned, she gained in weight
until she is apparently as well now as for many years.   We are
yet anxious to know if her liver may prove to be the seat of
cancer.[1]

*Five-year history of chills, followed by spitting of blood
during two years past, which is not due to malaria; diagnosis
of gall stones in contracted bladder; operation May 10, 1902, at
Columbia Hospital.* —Patient sent by Dr. H. M. Clarkson, of Virginia.   Mrs. C., aged 60.   Mother of several children.   Had
good health until five years since.   A residence in a malarial
locality caused her to seek treatment for supposed malarial
poisoning.   All of these efforts to cure her chills ended in absolute failure.   She had a good healthy appearance. is bright and

[1]Patient perfectly well October 1. 1902.

cheerful, and did not look as if her illness had influenced her general health. The chills occurred at intervals of four to seven days. The slight hemorrhage began soon after the subsidence of the chill and lasted about twenty-four hours. It was evidently not from the lungs or nasal or pharyngeal surfaces, therefore it may have come from the stomach. Its color showed that it had not long remained in the stomach, as it was bright in color. She had a movable right kidney, which descended to crest of ilium. As this patient gave no history of severe pain, we were surprised to find so much evidence of former mischief about the liver. The peritoneal surfaces of the superior and right side of the organ were adherent over a large area to the corresponding surfaces under the diaphragm and ribs. It was possible to separate these over the upper right lobe, but not on the extreme surface, as the danger of hemorrhage caused us to desist without completing the liberation. There were also adhesions under the gall bladder and liver, all of which were well organized and firm. The gall bladder was rather smaller than normal, was not thickened, and did not present evidence of past or present disease.

A medium-sized double dumbbell-shaped stone was removed from the gall bladder. It was quite black in color from the dark bile which filled the bladder. Careful search failed to reveal further disease, and we were obliged to content ourselves with suspension and drainage in the usual way. The patient had no vomiting, chills, or other symptoms to cause anxiety during her stay, and made a perfect recovery.[1]

Empyema of gall bladder; obstruction of cystic duct; large tumor reaching to appendical region; thought by family physician to be "appendicitis."—Mrs. A., white, aged 40. Residence, Virginia. Mother of several children. Had been in good health until three weeks before consultation with family physician, Dr. C., in February, 1898. Attack of continued pain in abdomen, a little to right of umbilicus, with great amount of tenderness which prevented a careful examination by the physician in charge. She had no jaundice, stools normal in appearance, urine not colored by presence of bile. She had vomited and had been kept under the influence of morphia for several days, which to some extent masked the symptoms. A hasty examination revealed an oblong or heart-shaped tumor, which was thought either a hydronephrosis or distended gall bladder, and operation advised as soon as patient could be sent to the hospital. When the patient was admitted her pulse was 120, temperature 103°.

Operation February 19, 1898. Incision outside right rectus, extending four or five inches below ribs, revealed the tumor, to which were united the adherent omentum and coils of intestine usually seen in such cases. A stone was easily detected in the cystic duct in this case. Before the fluid was evacuated by aspiration, gauze pads were placed carefully around the gall

[1]Patient had return of symptoms, then greatly improved.

bladder to protect the viscera. Then followed incision of the bladder and removal of the stone by forceps, aided by external pressure of the fingers on the cystic duct. The stone was oval in shape, weighed forty-five grains, had a rough exterior like a mulberry, and was evidently the only one present, being without facets, and the patient presenting only symptoms of cystic-duct obstruction. The gall bladder was sutured in the wound, a rubber drain tube inserted, and the wound closed by silkworm-gut sutures. The patient made an uneventful and permanent recovery.

Cholangitis.—Miss M., white, aged 26. (Care of Dr. Moran.) A clerk by occupation. Patient is a large woman, weighing 160 or 170 pounds. Previously healthy and had been ill for several weeks with acute jaundice before seen in consultation by the writer. The patient was deeply jaundiced, being of a deep yellowish-green color and quite saturated with bile. All of the characteristic symptoms were present—putty-colored stools, urine, skin, and conjunctiva deeply colored. The patient had pain in the region of the liver and in the epigastrium. She had no characteristic attack of gall-stone colic, although we were positively sure of partial, if not complete, obstruction of the common gall duct.

As the patient had resisted the usual treatment, operation was advised, and she was sent to Georgetown University Hospital. Operation February 15, 1901. Incision in usual place, just outside right rectus, extending downward five inches from the angle of ribs. The peritoneum, viscera, and especially the liver were all decidedly colored with bile. The appearance of the viscera in this case made an impression never to be forgotten. I had never seen such evidence of saturation with bile in any previous instance. The gall bladder was small and contracted so much that its upper extremity barely reached the margin of the liver. Evidence of acute inflammation in the gall bladder and ducts was abundantly shown in the recent adhesions forming around the ducts under the liver. As we had suspected stone in the common duct, a careful search was made along the course of the duct, but with negative result, much to our regret, for we both feared we might have overlooked the cause of the trouble. Finally deciding the cause of obstruction to be "cholangitis." a rubber tube was placed in the gall bladder and gauze packed around it and brought out of the wound. with the intention of preventing the escape of bile into the foramen of Winslow or into the larger cavity of the peritoneum. It must be remembered that we had here a patient with fever, temperature to 104°. pulse 120 to 130, with rigors and evidence of dangerous infection. It was, therefore, with grave reluctance that we were obliged to rely upon our rather limited experience in gall-stone surgery to aid in the diagnosis of this patient's condition; to exclude obstruction of the common or hepatic duct by gall stones, as well as to affirm that no inflammation or abscess of the liver existed; and, finally, to trust to drainage of the gall bladder and cystic duct for the relief of the patient.

I am fully convinced that my colleague (Dr. Moran) also shared with me some apprehension, although, in his kindly way, he spared my feelings by carefully avoiding criticism during the anxious days immediately following the operation. One source of anxiety was our inability to suture the gall bladder to the wound or even to the peritoneum. Knowing the intensely infectious nature of the contents of the gall bladder, it was with no little misgiving that we must rely upon gauze packing for protection against peritoneal infection. We dared not attempt cystectomy, because we would add greater dangers without the possibility of disposal of the entire area of disease. The patient gradually recovered from the operation and then rapidly from her cholemia. Large quantities of bile poured out of the wound, and, strangely enough, the stools ere long showed the presence of bile. The gauze was gradually withdrawn from the wound, all of it being removed in less than a week after operation. The drain tube remained a week after this, and was removed because the bile flowed freely around it. The patient remained in the hospital for six weeks and went to her home with a fistula, which finally closed. The patient is reported in good health at the present time, having regained her health and her normal weight.

Stones in common duct.—A patient was admitted into the hospital having sustained a blow over the lower border of the liver in region of gall bladder, which was followed by severe pain. No jaundice. Diagnosis of incarcerated stone in cystic duct.

Mrs. G., white, aged 45, a rather thin and somewhat anemic woman, was admitted into Columbia Hospital February 20, 1902, with the following history: She had no previous illness which seemed to have the least bearing upon the present attack, and appeared to be in good health and attending to the ordinary duties of housekeeping, including the care of a family which required pretty active exercise on her part, as she was in rather straitened financial circumstances. When examined by the writer no tumor could be found in the liver or region of the gall bladder. She had no history to give with the least relation to the present condition. She had a fall upon her right side four days before admission, since which time the pain had required anodynes. Her temperature had not been much elevated, and her pulse, while quick, was not indicative of any inflammatory condition or infection. Pressure over the gall bladder caused pain, and we consented to operate with nothing to guide us but the one symptom of pain and the patient's account of how she had been injured.

Operation February 22, 1902. The patient was placed on the table with shoulders well elevated. Incision in usual location. Careful examination of the gall bladder revealed no calculi. Further search, however, rewarded us by disclosing stones of small size in different locations, one of which was in the common duct. As the patient had not had jaundice, we were not surprised to find stones which did not entirely obstruct the flow of bile. These were, therefore, of small size and merely served to rather more than fill the ducts. It would be interesting to know if stones really cause entire obstruction, or if patients would not become cholemic with far greater rapidity if the ducts were actually closed. In this case, as in all of the operations upon the biliary passages, some interesting facts developed which at the time added interest, if not anxiety, while they also served to add to our stock of experience with possible advantage in future operations.

When the incision was made in the common duct, in order to remove the stone or stones with little delay and some effort of pressure upon the duct above the stone, it was caught with forceps and, although fractured, was removed. At once the wound and region about field of operation was covered with what appeared to be venous blood.

To all who know how near the duct lies to the portal vein must come the appreciation of what one suffers when confronted with the possibility of such an accident as wounding this important vessel. I was unable to think of any other important vein but this, and was at a loss for a moment to know what course to pursue. By pressure we could control the flow momentarily, but the blood would gush out again when an attempt was made to ascertain the source of the hemorrhage. Finally it was possible to encircle the duct and supposed vein together, when by careful examination it was found that the flow of blood was due to injury of the gall bladder and cystic duct while sounding and trying to remove the stone from the latter. I was cautious, however, and threw a catgut suture loop around the duct and vein, which was kept in position until absorbed. The severed gall ducts were only slightly closed by small catgut sutures and a rubber drainage tube placed, without gauze, down to opening in common duct. The gall bladder was sutured to the wound and a small rubber catheter inserted. The discharge of bile was abundant from the larger tube, and all the bile appeared to flow from the lower opening. The patient gave us some anxiety for two weeks or more. She did not improve as rapidly as such patients usually do. At first I was fearful lest the drainage was defective, yet I was unable to observe any symptom due to this cause. The patient is still nervous, but is free from pain and is doing, in almost every respect, perfectly well.[1]

[1] I find, by reference to notes made immediately after the operation, that I had torn a vein while removing a phlebolith. The presence of phleboliths in one or more superficial veins of the peritoneum over the hepatico-duodenal ligament gave rise to the impression that the hemorrhage came from a vein from which I had removed a stone. 'boliths, owing to their obliteration, and I also found the flow out of But there was no hemorrhage from the veins containing phleboliths, owing to their obliteration, and I also found the flow out of the duct had ceased before closing the abdomen; moreover, the abundant flow of bile proved the opening of the duct.

Pancreatic obstruction.—A patient had jaundice for several weeks with pain simulating gall-stone colic. Diagnosis of stones in choledochus. Operation. No stones, but a hard and greatly enlarged pancreas found, the only definite lesion. Drainage. Recovery.

Mrs. C., white, aged 47; married, one child 18 years old. A lady of fine, healthy appearance. Had had both breasts removed for suspected cancer, the last operation in 1900. No other history with least bearing upon the present illness. Mrs. C. had jaundice beginning eleven weeks before admission to Columbia Hospital on January 11, 1902. With the jaundice arose attacks of pain, requiring morphia for relief. The attacks were three or four days between, and she had the characteristic symptoms usually attending jaundice, such as nausea, anorexia, loss of flesh, with bile in urine and white alvine discharges. The pain was not near the gall bladder, but nearly in the median line just above the umbilicus in the epigastric region. No tumor could be detected in or about the liver, and a diagnosis of gall stones. in the choledochus was unhesitatingly made.

Operation January 13, 1902. The patient was placed on the table with shoulders elevated and incision made in usual place. Careful search failed to explain the cause of the prolonged jaundice and severe pain. At least, no stone was found. The pancreas was large, hard, and thought to be carcinomatous. A gloomy prognosis was made, and after placing the usual drainage tube in the gall bladder it was sutured in the upper angle of the wound. Silkworm-gut closure and the usual dressing applied. Abundant discharge of bile followed, then relief and cure of the symptoms. The patient recovered completely.[1]

1449 Rhode Island avenue.

SECONDARY PUERPERAL HEMORRHAGE.

BY

L. W. ATLEE, M.D.,
Philadelphia.

"Though much less frequent than primary hemorrhage, yet in some instances it proves as grave in its results; death may be as certain and as sudden in the one case as in the other" (Theophilus Parvin, M.D., Gyn. Trans., 1880.)

Mrs. D., a strong, healthy woman 26 years of age, was delivered on June 7, 1902. The labor was natural and easy (it was her second child). The child is a healthy male. The patient states, the placenta not appearing immediately, the attending

[1] Patient is still perfectly well October 1, 1902.

32

physician pulled it away by traction on the cord. Nothing unusual was noticed about her condition until June 11 following, when she began to lose considerable quantities of blood, both clotted and liquid, at varying intervals. This continued until June 16, when she was first seen by me. Upon inquiry I was told three physicians had seen her during this time, but nothing had been done to stop the flow; the last one had said "there was nothing in the womb." Some time before my arrival the nurse had taken it upon herself to buy some fluid extract of ergot and to administer a teaspoonful. The prognosis given by the last medical consultant had been so hopeless that the woman's death was momentarily looked for. Her condition was certainly perilous enough, but I could find nothing but what could be produced by the great loss of blood. The skin and visible mucosæ were blanched, the surface of the body was bedewed with cold sweat, and hunger and some nausea were present; the pulse was small, from an empty vessel, and 160 a minute.

Upon placing the hand on the hypogastrium the fundus of the uterus was found to reach nearly to the umbilicus, and was soft and distended; grasping and kneading it caused clotted and fluid blood to gush profusely from the vagina. A tablespoonful of brandy was given the woman, her head lowered and the hips brought to the edge of the bed, when a vaginal examination showed the os dilated sufficiently to admit two fingers easily. The fundus being controlled by the abdominal hand, the uterus was emptied of clots. The placental remains were attached to the right lower segment and were easily detached by gentle scraping with the finger, but to accomplish this it was necessary to introduce the whole hand into the vagina. The uterus after this contracted well, and the patient's condition was apparently none the worse generally. A teaspoonful of Squibb's fluid extract of ergot was now given, a number of tightly rolled napkins were applied around and over the fundus, and a smoothly applied binder put on. Rigid instructions were given as to keeping the patient horizontal. A weak mixture of brandy and water was to be administered, teaspoonfuls at a time. This was to be followed later by easily assimilated foods, such as beef juice, soft-boiled eggs. milk and broths. A prescription for two-grain ergotin pills was left, these to be given one every four hours.

The patient lived far out in the suburbs and was not seen again until the 21st instant, although some instructions had been given by telephone concerning a more liberal diet and the administration of a laxative. Since June 16 there had been no chill, no abdominal tenderness or pain develop. The lochia had a slightly stale odor, due, no doubt, to a mild endometritis, and not to be wondered at considering the history and the primitive precautions against sepsis. The pulse was 128, tongue clean, appetite normal, uterine involution was progressing, and there was no uterine tenderness. Hot vaginal douches were ordered three times a day, and a tonic of iron, quinine, and strychnine citrate in sherry wine was given before meals. Before leaving, the woman was advised not to leave her bed for at least ten days, but she got up and spent the whole day of the 25th about the house. The same night a phlebitis of the left femoral vein developed, the leg being much swollen and very painful over the course of the vein. By complete rest and appropriate treatment this had entirely passed away by July 3, when she was allowed to commence her household duties, wearing a well-applied rubber bandage from the foot to the groin. Since this date her health has been perfect, but the milk was dried up, most unfortunately for the child.

From the small amount of space allotted to the subject of secondary puerperal bleeding of a serious character in our text books on obstetrics, it must be regarded as of rare occurrence; but the history of the case related shows the seriousness of such conditions and should impress the obstetrician with the importance of losses of blood at these times. We are convinced the above case would have terminated fatally had it been left to Nature or a continuance of the "folded hands" policy. We confine our attention to those hemorrhages which cannot be properly classed as postpartum, and not due to inversion of the uterus or lesions of the genital tract. Parvin *(op. cit.)* divides the causes of these hemorrhages into:

1. Alteration of the blood—albuminuria, purpura, malaria.

2. Psychic causes.

3. Direct causes belonging immediately to the uterus may be included under two general classes—those which prevent uterine retraction and those which produce uterine congestion. Secondary uterine inertia, uterine fibroids, and possibly uterine adhesions may be included in the first.

We are inclined to believe that the hemorrhage caused by a uterine fibroid would manifest itself more as a primary than as a secondary bleeding, and that serious loss of blood of this latter nature will most frequently be due to the presence in the uterus of clots, placental remains, or that unusual but possible cause, a placenta succenturiata.

The sudden assuming of the erect or even a sitting posture has brought on serious hemorrhage in cases where the uterine contraction was poorly developed, the sudden filling of the unguarded uterine vessels causing the washing away of the clots closing the sinuses. Lusk[1] mentions a case of serious flooding in the second week, due to "the uterus being crowded back and downward to the pelvic floor by the compress, which had been too tightly bandaged upon the abdomen by the indiscreet zeal of the nurse."

Bleeding is seen. in cases where the uterine involution has been retarded owing to mild septic endometritis, when the patient begins to walk about and remain erect for any length of time; but that the loss of blood ever approaches the seriousness of the hemorrhages we wish to call attention to is improbable.

Parvin (op. cit.) regards the presence of clots in the uterus as a not infrequent cause of these bleedings, and quotes from McClintock: "A coagulum of any size is not apt to be found in the womb beyond the first few hours after delivery, as a very moderate degree of uterine contraction would be sufficient to expel it or to prevent its formation. Should it occur, however— and experience abundantly proves that it may—there will be a constant risk of hemorrhage so long as the clot remains in utero." That this is not an infrequent cause of secondary puerperal hemorrhage is shown by the statistics of Contamin: six out of fifty-six were attributed to it. The older obstetricians, such as Mauriceau, Dionis, Astruc, Smellie, and Baudelocque. recognized the danger of this cause. Madame Lachapelle had a fatal case of hemorrhage from retained coagula, the patient dying on the eighth day.

The following history of a case of the form of hemorrhage we are discussing is of great interest. It was reported to Dr. Parvin (op. cit.) by Dr. Allison Maxwell. "Mrs. B., aged 26, primipara, was confined August 7, 1880. The patient was a strong, healthy woman of German extraction. No family history of importance. except that a year ago a sister came very near dying of puerperal fever. The labor pains began about 12 o'clock. noon. and twelve hours after a healthy male child was born. The position was L. O. A. and the labor was natural.

[1] Science and Art of Midwifery, p. 592.

After the umbilical cord was severed the placenta was found in the vagina and was removed without much difficulty. I examined carefully and found the placenta intact, but was not so positive about the membranes, as they were somewhat ragged; but I did not consider it necessary to introduce my finger into the uterus, as there was but little hemorrhage and the uterus could be felt, a hardened ball the size of a child's head, through the abdominal walls. Everything went on naturally, except there was no lochial discharge save a slight colorless fluid. A firm coagulum could be felt obstructing the os uteri, but could not be reached and broken up by the finger. The uterus for the first five days did not appear to diminish any in size. On the afternoon of the fifth day an offensive sanguineous discharge began to flow, and some small clots were expelled during the night, showing that the coagulum which had occupied the womb for five days was disintegrating. Up to this time a vaginal injection of carbolized water had been used night and morning. The morning of the sixth day the patient nursed her baby, looked cheerful, and was apparently doing well; pulse 80, temperature 99½°. The lochia still continuing very offensive, I used the double catheter and washed out the uterus with a weak solution of carbolic acid and water; and just as I concluded the injection the uterus contracted firmly and ejected the water out of its cavity on to the floor. Almost immediately the patient had a chill lasting a half hour; but the uterus during this time remained firmly contracted, and there was no sign of internal or external hemorrhage. At this time I left the house, and two or three hours afterward hemorrhage must have begun, for when I was summoned at 3 P. M. the bedding was saturated with blood, the uterus completely relapsed so that no uterine globe could be felt, and the patient, pulseless and *in articulo mortis*, died within ten minutes. Immediately after the delivery of the placenta she was given a half-drachm of Wyeth's fluid extract of ergot, and the dose was twice repeated the next day. On the day of the fatal hemorrhage, soon after the chill, fearing hemorrhage, I gave her one drachm of the fluid extract of ergot.''

Fibrinous and placental polypi have been the cause of serious and even fatal hemorrhage in the puerperal condition. Parvin (*op. cit.*) mentions a case of Bailly's where a fibrous polypus appeared at the mouth of the uterus eighteen days after labor, and though it was removed the patient died. Death was attributed to the presence of more polypi in the interior of the uterus.

Among the unusual causes may be mentioned the presence of a rapidly growing ovarian cyst crowding the uterus upward. In the same class such causes as coprostasis, distension of the bladder, coughing, aneurism of uterine artery, and thrombus of the cervix are referred to by Parvin (*op. cit.*). The treatment of secondary puerperal hemorrhage must be directed to the removal of its cause; its prevention is part of the art of midwifery. Our attention should be directed primarily to the uterus, particularly its interior, which should be explored by the finger, as no instrument can take its place for this purpose. Not finding cause here, the other pelvic organs should receive our attention, particularly the condition of the bladder and rectum. If we can find no cause in the pelvis, the blood condition should be looked into as to purpura or albuminuria, as suggested by Parvin, as also the valvular condition of the heart itself. No matter what the cause of the hemorrhage, the after-treatment must be directed to maintaining the uterus firmly contracted, and this is best accomplished by the use of a reliable preparation of ergot. In conjunction with this the value of compression of the uterus through the abdominal walls by compresses and a smoothly applied binder will be evident. Stockings or small socks filled with sand or salt, or a partly filled water bag, will answer. Should these measures fail to bring about the desired result, it may be necessary to resort to packing the uterine cavity with some aseptic gauze. When reduced to the last extremity intrauterine injections of very hot water may be given, or, as suggested by Barnes, a 1:3 solution of the liquor ferri perchloridi may be used.

758 SOUTH FIFTEENTH STREET.

THE TIME OF THE OCCURRENCE OF OVULATION AS DEDUCED FROM SOME CLINICAL OBSERVATIONS.

BY

JENNIE G. DRENNAN, M.D.,
St. Thomas, Ontario, Canada.

OUR knowledge of the physiology of the female organs of generation is very much of an empirical nature, and a wide field for research is therefore open to the present and future physiologists.

One almost fears to enter into it, as her ignorance is so great and her knowledge so scant; but a few small observations may pave the way for others.. As yet the exact date of ovulation—whether it occurs once a month or oftener, or whether it occurs at the same time as menstruation or prior to it—has not been ascertained. I shall state the following cases and then draw my conclusions. The first is that of a healthy young woman, while the other two are those of women with diseased pelvic organs.

CASE I.—Æt. 30; single and healthy; of a nervous temperament; bright, active, energetic, intellectual, full of ambition; but not with the least neurotic tendency; not given to thinking of herself save in a healthy, reasoning manner, to know herself as we would all know others; given to self-analysis. All thoughts of the ordinary pains and aches, which so many women cherish as their own individual property, she will not tolerate. She is one of those few people who always say they are well, and for this reason I feel that in her case there are no imaginary symptoms. Her menstrual periods are always painless—only at rare times a feeling of lassitude and headache—and last for five days and are moderate in amount. During the intermenstrual period, about twelve days after the preceding menstruation, there have been symptoms which have led me to think that it is at this time that ovulation occurs. On May 2, 1902, she menstruated. Preceding this for some days there was soreness, fulness, and hardness of the right mammary gland, which continued until the onset of the menstrual period, when it began to decline and gradually disappeared. No other discomfort accompanied this menstruation. The next menstrual period occurred on June 1, and during this intermenstrual period there were no mammary symptoms, but instead a discharge of clear mucus from the uterus. This commenced about the twelfth day after the cessation of the preceding menstruation and continued until the following menstruation. The next menstrual period was on June 30, and during the intermenstrual period preceding it the same discharge occurred and no mammary symptoms. Then the next period, and last so far, was on July 29, and during this intermenstrual there was no discharge, but soreness, fulness, and hardness of the left mammary gland; and this symptom occurred on the twelfth day after the cessation of the preceding menstrual period, and disappeared with menstruation. A sense of slight heaviness was noticed in the left inguinal region on walking.

    April 4: Menstruation.
    April 20 (about): Pain in right breast (ovulation?)
    May   2: Menstruation.
    May   18: Leucorrheal discharge (ovulation?)
    June   1: Menstruation.
    June 15: Leucorrheal discharge (ovulation?)
    June 30: Menstruation.
    July 16: Pain in left breast (ovulation?)
    July 29: Menstruation.

CASE II.—Æt. 37; had suffered for thirteen years from pelvic disease following puerperal infection, and when I saw her was a physical wreck. She had never consented to a thorough examination. She was now menstruating fairly regularly, but with pain, and during the intermenstrual period there was a profuse muco-purulent discharge, which she described as the bursting of great ulcers. There was at all times some discharge, but this profuse amount was noted at about the middle of the intermenstrual period. She had an old chronic endometritis and a chronic interstitial ovaritis and salpingitis of the right side. She suffered much from sacral pain radiating down the right thigh and even extending to the right heel—she had been treated for sciatica —and over the right inguinal region. This pain was most marked during the profuse discharge. She passed out of my care while I was endeavoring to build her up for an operation, owing to over-anxious relatives. I was unable to obtain any history of specific infection, but as, during the administration of calomel to relieve a congested portal system, the discharge ceased for two months, and the fact that she improved on potassium iodide in large doses, becoming less anemic, I have my suspicions.

CASE III.—The patient was of a nervous temperament well controlled. During an acute attack of pelvic inflammation I made some observations. Eight years prior to this she had had an illness—"symptoms of typhoid" (?)—but which from the history I should say was an acute attack of pelvic inflammation. When about 18 years of age, at the commencement of her menstrual life, she had another illness, diagnosed as "inflammation," but which, I also fancy, was an ovaritis. The second illness was shortly after her marriage, but I know for a certainty that there was no chance of its being specific. By her first illness a disabling of the right ovary had resulted, and on the assumption of the married state an old ovaritis was relighted. From the second illness she experienced a certain amount of discomfort in the right inguinal region, pain on coition, and there was a leucorrheal discharge, but menstruation was painless, although irregular. Sometimes during the menstrual period she experienced headache and a slight elevation of temperature, especially during the spring and fall months, and these attacks had been diagnosed as malaria. At an operation later on the ovaries were found to contain pus, which accounted for the "malaria." She had never been pregnant. This last attack came on about September 22, 1901. She complained of pain in the back and thighs and lower abdominal region, accompanied by a profuse watery discharge—she had noticed a similar one at the commencement of the illness eight years previous—and thought that she had taken cold and continued to go about the house. On the 27th she menstruated, but this ceased on the 28th, and, as she was suffering severe pain, she sent for me, when I diagnosed an acute ovaritis which developed into a pelvic inflammation.

TABLE, CASE III.

Sept. 22, 1901:	Pain and watery discharge.
Sept. 27, "	Menstruation commenced.
Sept. 28, "	Menstruation ceased; ovaritis diagnosed.
Oct. 17, "	Pain increased. Ovulation (?)
Oct. 25, "	More discharge.
Nov. 7, "	Menstruation occurred, preceded by a distinct rise of temperature on the left side on vaginal examination and soreness.
Nov. 17, "	Pain on right side (ovulation?)
Dec. 6, "	Menstruation.
Dec. 26, "	Bloody discharge for one day.
Jan. 4, 1902:	Menstruation.
Jan. 14, "	Another attack of ovaritis, after which there was the removal of the ovaries and tubes.

In the first case the attack evidently began during the physiological congestion incident upon ovulation, and although the rest of the history is irregular, still one can see that exacerbations were due to it.

It is an admitted fact that there is a physiological pelvic congestion incident on ovulation, evidenced by discomfort at such times, but this is generally conceded to occur at the menstrual period. In cases of chronic pelvic disease we find an exacerbation of symptoms at certain times, with nothing else to explain them. The majority of healthy women in this age of civilization —for none are as healthy as they ought to be—experience a sense of general lassitude, irritability of temper, and sense of weight in the pelvis, which is relieved by the menstrual flow.

Distant organs, as the brain, at times show signs of congestion. Attention has, as a rule, been drawn to the condition solely at the menstrual period, save in those few observed· cases of intermenstrual pain; but I think there are symptoms which point— symptoms so slight in themselves as to often escape notice,. which indicate that ovulation occurs in the intermenstrual period about the twelfth day after the cessation of the last menstruation, and therefore about twelve days before the succeeding one. In my first case, that of a healthy young woman, there were one month the mammary symptoms and in another the uterine, showing signs of a congestion. Now, I have concluded that ovulation occurs at this intermenstrual twelfth day or thereabouts, and if the person is in *perfect* health no signs of the congestion may show themselves. Elastic ovaries will accommodate themselves to an increase of blood; but supposing in their delicate structures there is some impediment to this compensatory accommodation, then other organs concerned in the generative cycle will have to relieve this congestion and the brunt will fall on them, viz., the mammary glands and uterus; and if they in their turn are not physiologically perfect they will show evidences of congestion, evidenced by mammary soreness or uterine leucorrhea—there are many cases of vicarious functions in the body: kidneys relieved by skin, epistaxis during menstruation, etc. There is a physiological generative cycle during pregnancy and its preceding ovulation and succeeding lactation. First the ovarian congestion incident on ovulation; then the uterine congestion resulting in formation of the decidual membrane and the placenta; and on the termination of the pregnancy the uterus is depleted by the moderate hemorrhage, the lochial discharge and the determination of a greater supply of blood to the mammary glands, evidenced at first by the colostrum, which is composed mainly of the watery elements of the blood and a few more fully developed milk globules; on lactation being fully established the increased amount of blood is necessary for the formation of the mammary secretion—milk; then on the cessation of lactation the ovarian function is again resumed. Herein lies a perfect physiological cycle on a large scale, of which ovulation followed by menstruation is the same cycle on a small scale. Here the ovulation congestion is the same probably in both instances; there is at the same time a compensatory congestion in the mammary glands and uterus which in the perfectly (?) healthy will give no evidence of itself, but the least little cause may lead to a faint discomfort or sign of congestion. This congestion in the unimpregnated is relieved after an interval by menstruation, which is a means of depletion to the disappointed pregnancy. Now, in this person whom I call perfectly healthy there may have been some factor to cause at these times an interference with the compensatory congestion. I do not exactly like the term compensatory, but rather cyclic congestion; for although an ovary were unable to accommodate the increased amount of blood incident on ovulation, and the uterus and mammary glands relieve it, still if this cycle is only a prototype of the larger cycle of pregnancy there would be also congestion of these organs at the same time, unnoticed if in a healthy condition.

Unimpregnated Cycle.

Ovulation—Ovarian congestion; mammary congestion not often evidenced and uterine congestion depleted by menstrual flow.
Ovulation again.

Impregnated Cycle.

Ovulation—Ovarian congestion.
Pregnancy—Uterine congestion.
Lactation—Mammary congestion.

In the intermenstrual period in which mammary symptoms were complained of there was no leucorrheal discharge, so evidently the brunt of the congestion fell on the mammary gland; only one was affected and this leads to an inquiry: Does ovulation occur alternately?—Aristotle's idea that one ovary, the right, produces males and the left females. The fact that the mammary symptoms preceding the menstruation of May 2 occurred in the right breast, and those preceding that of July 29 in the left mammary gland, almost points to an alternate function of the ovaries: preceding May 2, right ovary; preceding June 1, left ovary (?); preceding June 30, right ovary (?); preceding July 29, left ovary.

There may be more truth than fiction in the old idea. That determination of sex rests on the temperament of the parents—a father more passionate than the mother producing a female child, and a mother more passionate producing a male—seems altogether too haphazard a method for Nature. In animals producing more than one offspring at the same time, has any one observed, as in the cat, for example, whether the different sexes are in different sides of the uterus? Some women during the intermenstrual period claim that they can feel the ovum pass from them, and at one time I gave this credence; but now I believe that it is only a mucous discharge from the uterus, caused by a compensatory or cyclic congestion of that organ at the time of ovulation, whereby ovarian congestion is relieved. The cases of intermenstrual pain of a colicky nature I believe are due to an engorged state of the tubes or uterus, which, on account of some pathological condition of their muscular structure, leads to painful contraction. Some of these cases are relieved by dilatation of the os, which would relieve an existing stricture preventing a free uterine circulation; and others are relieved by removal of the ovaries, which would put an end to the congestion dependent on ovulation. Slight symptoms, such as occurred in the first case, could be caused by any slight variation in methods of living or thinking, and by atmospheric changes. One's attention has of late been directed more toward the effect of mind on matter, of the psychological causes of disease; and at such a time as ovulation, when most likely the sexual appetite is more easily aroused, anything, no matter how chaste and pure the person—and I know that this one is so—may have the effect of disturbing the normal painless cycle. In reading Mr. Havelock Ellis' "Psychology of Sex," one cannot but see how interwoven in the being of all is the sexual element and how it must affect the organism in multiple ways. No law is recognized in the sexual life of the married of to-day, and how can such beget children not intoxicated with sexuality? What is sown is reaped! The need of the public to-day is not gynecologists who cure disease, but those who will prevent disease, and this can alone be accomplished by studying the physiology of the sexual apparatus and the sexual psychology of the individual. Arch. Reid says "teetotalers are born, not made." and so are sexual teetotalers born, not made.

My conclusion is that ovulation occurs in the middle of the intermenstrual period. The Levitical law, which was probably obtained in part from Egyptian learning—and this was far advanced—forbade coition during the week following menstruation, but allowed it during the rest of the time up to the commencement of the menses: and this points to ovulation recurring after the first week after the cessation of the menses, for thus during the forbidden time there would be no ovum to be impregnated.

HYDRORRHEA GRAVIDARUM.

BY

W. SINCLAIR BOWEN, M.D.,
Washington, D. C.

A SUDDEN discharge of watery fluid from the vagina during pregnancy naturally suggests the commencement of labor, and it is of practical importance to determine in a given case the source of the flow. The fluid may not have come from the amniotic sac, but from some portion of the decidua owing to a "deciduitis." Since hydrorrhea gravidarum is the resultant of one form of deciduitis, it might be well just here to outline briefly the other varieties of that disease.

Deciduitis is an endometritis modified by the changes in the uterine mucosa peculiar to pregnancy. The disease may be acute or chronic. The acute form may be due to trauma, sepsis, or certain infectious diseases, and it occurs in three forms, namely: (1) the infectious or exanthematous, (2) the hemorrhagic, and (3) the purulent. The infectious or exanthematous occurs with the development of the exanthematous diseases during pregnancy. The mucous membrane of the body of the uterus participates in the eruption and becomes intensely inflamed, causing abortion with high maternal mortality. The hemorrhagic variety is rare; it may accompany the acute infectious diseases, and is characterized by profuse hemorrhage. The purulent form is more common and often rapidly fatal following attempts at criminal abortion or other traumatism. The treatment of acute deciduitis consists in the management of the complications as they arise, the control of hemorrhage, and the application of aseptic principles.

Chronic deciduitis is a much more common complication of pregnancy and is the predisposing cause of a majority of early abortions.

Causation.—We may have a pre-existing endometritis becoming more inflamed in pregnancy, due to an increased vascularity

¹Read before the Washington Obstetrical and Gynecological Society, March 21, 1902.

of the tissues involved. Syphilis and other diseases have a causal relation. There are four varieties of chronic deciduitis, differing in clinical history, severity, and in the constituent element of tissue affected: (1) the diffuse hyperplastic, (2) the polypoid, (3) the cystic, and (4) the chronic catarrhal. The hyperplastic variety consists in an inflammatory hypertrophy of the decidua vera, with hemorrhage into its structure, producing a firm sarcous mass which is thrown off during the abortion, presenting what is known as the fleshy mole of pregnancy; or, if the hyperplastic growth occurs later in pregnancy and the fetus goes on to further development, adherent placenta is likely to occur, requiring considerable force to separate it from the uterine wall. The polypoid variety is characterized by the same hyperplastic inflammatory change, but occurring at different points over the decidua vera instead of over a broader surface, resulting in hemorrhage at these points into the decidua and the formation of polypoid masses and abortions. The cystic variety results from an inflammatory closure of the ducts leading from the utricular glands, with consequent accumulations of fluid forming retention cysts. The fourth and last form, the chronic catarrhal, occurs later in pregnancy, as a rule, usually after the sixth month, and pursues a more gradual course than the other three varieties. It consists of an excessive secretion of the utricular glands with some amount of hyperplastic inflammation of the decidua. It is more common in multiparæ. Adhesions form between amniotic sac and decidua vera, preventing the escape of the glandular secretion, which accumulates in quantities sufficient to break the adhesions, and it then makes its way with a sudden gush, constituting hydrorrhea gravidarum, or false waters, closely resembling the escape of amniotic fluid when the membranes are ruptured.

There is an uncertainty as to the exact etiology and pathology of hydrorrhea gravidarum. Braun believed it to be due to a pre-existing endometritis. Hegar considered it to be a hypertrophic growth of the utricular glands. Scanzoni, Tini, and Chozan attribute it to the conditions of the blood, to a transudation of serum from the watery blood of pregnancy or an extravasation from the hyperæmic uterine mucosa. The exact source of the fluid is as uncertain as is its pathology, and it is more than likely that all the constituent elements of the decidua contribute to the formation of the fluid. The discharge may take place suddenly without any warning, or there may be some discomfort due to slight uterine contractions. It is difficult at times to distinguish such discharges from the liquor amnii by any chemical test. The fluid is clear, thin, or pale yellow, containing albumin. It may be discharged while the patient is in any position, whether in bed or walking around. Usually the discharge occurs before the end of pregnancy and without any premonitory signs of labor. The flow occurs several or more times. The os is closed. Ballottement may be found. The fluid contains much albumin. In rupture of the amniotic sac, the occurrence is usually at the end of pregnancy and immediately precedes delivery. Labor pains have usually been going on for some minutes or hours. The discharge occurs but once. The os is open. There is no ballottement. The liquor amnii contains only a trace of albumin, but an abundance of urea.

In connection with the above remarks I will report a case which occurred recently: Mrs. B., 30 years old, a well-developed and healthy woman, has one child 10 years old. Her second pregnancy began about a year ago and progressed normally until about the middle of the sixth month, when suddenly, while asleep in bed, a large gush of fluid occurred from the vagina, watery in character and of sufficient amount to wet the bedclothing and nightgown. I was sent for at once, and supposed labor would come on, but found the patient in no pain and ballottement could be easily detected. I concluded that the source of the fluid was other than that of the amniotic sac. The os was closed and no uterine contractions felt. I administered a sedative and encouraged the patient to go to sleep. She rested well and remained in bed several days until another large gush of fluid occurred, and, becoming very nervous in bed, I allowed her to sit up. One week later a third discharge took place, and so it occurred from time to time, until about the end of the eighth month a large discharge was followed by uterine contractions which developed into true labor. The amniotic sac protruded through the external os and was ruptured. Delivery was easy and quickly accomplished, and the fetus was well formed, with the exception of the right leg, which was entirely absent, presenting the appearance of a knee-joint amputation. Without any traction on the umbilical cord the placenta was easily delivered, but entirely devoid of membranes, as though the amniotic sac had been carefully cut away from the circumference of the placenta. I continued to apply Credé's method of expression, hoping to see the membranes come away, but without success. I placed the patient across the bed and with a speculum and good light carefully inspected the external os. I could plainly see the edges of the sac. but on applying a small pair of forceps it would tear away in pieces, and after introducing my fingers it was evident that the amniotic sac was closely adherent to the uterine wall as far as the fingers could reach. I made no further efforts at its removal, trusting to natural processes. The lochial discharge was more or less offensive, and some elevation of temperature occurred, ranging between 100° and 102°. These symptoms were controlled by daily intrauterine irrigation with hot normal salt solution. Each napkin worn and each douche was carefully inspected, and I was surprised to find so little evidence of actual membrane removed, only a few particles and threads at times. The patient has since menstruated regularly and is in good health.

Since writing the above I have been fortunate in securing a reprint of a paper read before this Society more than seventeen years ago by Dr. Thomas C. Smith, entitled "The Watery Discharges of Pregnant and Puerperal Women—Hydrorrhea Gravidarum et Puerperarum." In this paper the etiology of hydrorrhea gravidarum has been most fully dwelt upon, and a number of most interesting cases have been described in detail.

1228 SIXTEENTH STREET, N. W.

THE DEGENERATION OF GYNECOLOGY.[1]

BY

W. P. CARR, M.D.,
Washington, D. C.

SURGERY has been called the opprobrium of medicine; and if we may consider surgery and medicine as separate entities, this dictum in a sense is certainly true, for medicine only invokes the aid of surgery when it has acknowledged its own defeat. In the same sense, if we may separate the two, we must consider pelvic surgery the opprobrium of gynecology; for it is, or should be, only when gynecology fails that pelvic surgery is invoked.

[1] Read before the Washington Obstetrical and Gynecological Society, April 19. 1902.

If surgery is the opprobrium of medicine, it is equally true that amputation is the opprobrium of surgery, and that pelvic surgery, with its numerous amputations and "ectomies," is the opprobrium of opprobriums. Therefore the gynecologist who becomes a pelvic surgeon degenerates as a gynecologist. He acknowledges his inability to cure without resort to the opprobrium of opprobriums. All of us who were in practice fifteen years ago remember the days of so-called "tinkering" at the uterus and pelvic organs, when women came week after week, and month after month, for bi-weekly or tri-weekly treatments at the offices of gynecologists; and we recognize the change in the methods now in vogue, whereby such patients are promptly curetted, relieved of their appendages, or otherwise rapidly and radically cured—or buried. And though the pendulum has swung back to some extent from the operative furor of a few years ago, when we first learned to remove ovaries with comparative safety, and though there is now no wholesale removal of healthy organs, still the field of gynecology is nearly covered to-day by the pelvic surgeon, and non-operative gynecology has degenerated into a shadow of its former self. Is this degeneracy the atrophy of a useless art, or is it the result of neglect for more brilliant and showy methods?

Many complex questions arise in this connection, some of which I shall present for your consideration and discussion. For the sake of convenience I shall restrict the term gynecology so as to exclude all operations except plastic and minor work done through the vagina, and all major operations, whether done by the vaginal or abdominal routes, will be included under the head of pelvic surgery.

There can be no question that the perfection of pelvic surgery is a blessing to many suffering women; but it has been, and is now being, invoked in some cases where it is not needed and where it may prove a curse. We have learned many important truths from the rich store of experience in the past decade, but have we read aright and fully all its lessons? We have learned not to remove healthy ovaries, but have we learned that many diseased ovaries and tubes do not need removal? Experience has plainly shown us this fact. It has shown us that there are many varieties of diseased adnexa, some of which, even though very grave, require neither removal nor patching up. Surgery has shown us what havoc pus can create in the pelvis; but Nature has also shown her marvellous powers of reconstruction. When

33

first the surgeon became familiar with the gross organic lesions of parametritis as viewed through an abdominal incision, no wonder he thought them beyond the reach of anything but the amputating knife. But larger experience has shown him that Nature, properly assisted, may do what the knife cannot—heal without destruction. He has learned, by forced experience in cases that refused operation and in cases that were too ill for radical operation, that Nature may perform the apparently impossible task of completely restoring some of the worst pelvic inflammations, even where pus had formed.

I shall never forget a case I saw with Dr. Atkinson about six years ago. This young woman had a severe metritis and parametritis following a criminal abortion. The uterus was large, boggy, and fixed, the vaginal vault was everywhere hard and thick, and the whole abdomen tympanitic. She had had a high septic fever for six weeks, and, while we had no doubt that there was a large quantity of pus in her pelvis. we agreed that her general condition was so bad that no operation could be done. I fully expected her to die within twenty-four hours. But she recovered without any form of operation and without the discharge of any pus either through the vagina or intestine, and her recovery was complete. I examined her carefully two years later and could detect absolutely no sign of disease or abnormality. I have seen many similar cases. but none quite so striking.

There was much to condemn in the old tinkering gynecology, but there was much also that was good that is worth preserving and improving; and when our eyes are less dazzled by the brilliancy of operative measures, and we turn to account the new light gained from operative treatment, we will get better results than in the past, when pathology was dark and the benefits of rest, drainage, heat, and many other valuable therapeutic measures unappreciated. The lesson we now have to learn is this: what cases may be cured without operation, or with minor operation, and what cases must go to the pelvic surgeon. The principal gynecological diseases may be roughly divided into a few classes as follows: tumors, congenital malformations, dislocations of pelvic organs, lacerations, and inflammations acute and chronic. We all agree that tumors and lacerations require appropriate surgical treatment. The other classes I shall briefly consider.

Acute inflammations, unless I have read very badly the lesson of the past ten years, should be taken from pelvic surgery and restored to gynecology. On November 6, 1896, I read a paper before this Society on the "Treatment of Acute Salpingitis," in which I endeavored to show that thorough and systematic treatment of this condition in its earlier stages would usually bring about resolution and recovery; that even when pus formed it should be evacuated per vaginam; and that in this way we could almost invariably, by safe palliative measures, tide the patient over the acute stage, and perform a radical operation later, if necessary, with comparatively little danger. Further experience has confirmed and extended these views, and I now believe that the radical operation will seldom be found necessary if proper treatment is continued, and that equally good results may be obtained in nearly all acute parametritic inflammations. There are several points in the treatment that I would emphasize:

1. *Rest.*—The importance of absolute rest in bed can hardly be overestimated. As long as there is hope of resolution, the patient should not be allowed to get up to evacuate the bowels and bladder, nor be propped up in bed, but should be made as comfortable and kept as cheerful as possible, so as to conduce to mental as well as physical rest.

2. *Nursing.*—A good trained nurse is invaluable in these cases. She can enforce rest, cheer and entertain the patient, keep her clean and comfortable, and in many ways increase her chances for recovery, besides carrying out the treatment ordered.

3. *Food and General Medicine.*—I think far too little importance has been attached to this part of the treatment. With increasing knowledge of Nature's methods of dealing with invading bacteria, we recognize more and more the importance of the part played by the leucocytes and blood serum. We look to these agents to perform the actual work of repelling the invaders and bringing about resolution. But no laborer can perform his best work upon a short ration, and it is a matter of first importance to supply the blood cells with the best possible ration in the form of rich serum. As our only ways of enriching the blood serum are by increasing digestion and checking waste. it becomes apparent that digestants and digestive stimulants, such as hydrochloric acid, pepsin, strychnia, and alcohol. may play no small part in the final result. The food should be of the most nourishing and easily digestible kind, and the quantity limited only by the ability to digest. Proteid food. beef, eggs, milk, etc.,

should be the chief reliance; but great care and judgment are necessary in regulating the quantity and frequency in individual cases.

It is also necessary to prevent the blood from becoming charged with excretory poisons, as far as possible, by keeping the bowels open and the skin clean. The bowels should be moved freely at least every other day by salts, calomel, or enema. It is of great value in the beginning to keep the bowels a little loose with re-peated small doses of salts. Opiates should not be given unless, during the formation of an abscess, the pain is so great as to demand them, and then only until the abscess can be located and opened. Such abscesses can usually be opened quite easily under eucaine anesthesia. As a rule, pain is controlled by rest and local treatment.

Complicating diseases should be looked for, and appropriately treated if found—particularly syphilis, malaria, and grippe. I believe that many acute inflammations of the ear, pleuræ, ab-domen, and pelvic organs may be traced to grippe as an exciting cause, and that such inflammations frequently go on to pus for-mation. The salicylates, particularly salicylate of cinchonidia, do much good in such cases.

4. *Local Treatment.*—Thorough uterine drainage should be at once established and maintained. I do not consider gauze drainage effective, and prefer the Outerbridge drainage tubes for this purpose. These tubes can usually be inserted without diffi-culty or pain if the cervix can be got in proper position. Where there is difficulty, eucaine anesthesia may be used to advantage. Many uteri that seem to have large cervical canals do not drain well, and a proper-sized Outerbridge tube, made preferably of silver wire, will make drainage efficient. Curage and intra-uterine douching may be advisable where there is abundant or offensive discharge, and these measures are necessary when the uterus contains placental tissue, clots, or other débris. Local anesthesia will usually be sufficient for this purpose. Vaginal douches, hot as can be borne, continued for fifteen or twenty minutes, are very effective in relieving pain and promoting resolution, and if one-half per cent of carbolic acid be added they are more effective. These douches may be followed by tampons of glycerin and iodine and adrenal extract. Adrenal extract is the most powerful vasomotor and heart stimulant known, and is readily absorbed by mucous membranes. It is doing much for the ophthalmologist, and is, I believe, from my

limited experience with it, destined to be of great help to the gynecologist. Local applications to the lower abdomen are also useful. Hot turpentine stupes aid considerably in relieving pain, and may be followed by painting with iodine.

I believe that everything should be done that may be of benefit, however small, and that these various measures are not usually practised in a careful and systematic manner. Some physicians use one part of the treatment, others another; but it is only by combining all that the best results are to be obtained. This systematic treatment will result in a cure in the great majority of cases, and will reduce the inflammation in the remainder to a chronic stage.

I have taken much time with these details, because I wished to bring to mind the many useful means we have at command. I might speak for hours on the proper and improper ways of using these various means, for as much depends upon the minute details of technique as upon the remedy used; and I believe that gynecologists, in degenerating into pelvic surgeons. have forgotten these details to a great extent in learning the equally important details of surgical technique.

I will speak more briefly of chronic parametritis, but I must insist that surgery is not the only hope for chronic salpingitis, ovaritis, metritis, endometritis, and other conditions included in this term. I have had many such cases sent me for operation that I have cured without operation, and I would urge surgeons to give gynecology a fair trial in all cases, not really urgent. before operating. The cause may often be discovered and removed. and Nature will do the rest. Flexions and stenosis will be found a very common cause and one usually removable.

Two striking articles have recently appeared, one by E. Kehrer[1] and one by A. Müller,[2] in which a new light is thrown upon parametritis posterior. Both these papers are compiled from careful examinations of large numbers of cases, and show that most cases of posterior parametritis, not gonorrheal, are of intestinal origin; that they begin in catarrhal conditions and ulcerations in the lower bowel; and that removal of the uterine appendages is useless as a treatment. We have long known that constipation and other gastro-intestinal diseases are closely associated with uterine complaints, and in my early days I found it impossible to cure some uterine catarrhs that were

[1]Centralblatt für Gynäkologie, 1901, No. 52.
[2]Ibid., 1902, No. 52.

associated with gastro-intestinal catarrh; but it has apparently remained for these gentlemen to put a proper interpretation upon these facts.

Curetting does these cases no good, and removal of tubes and ovaries sometimes only aggravates their condition. I have seen some of these women cured, or at least greatly improved, by the stomach specialist. But there are cases of chronic salpingitis and parametritis that are curable only by pelvic surgery; and when other means fail after careful trial, I think they should by all means have the proper operation. I only ask that it be not done without due consideration and after failure of other treatment.

Some cases of congenital malformation or lack of development from their very nature are remediable only by plastic operation; and others, such as chlorosis and infantile uteri, are as plainly medical cases. But the most common cases are flexions, and these are best treated by gradual dilatation and the wearing of drainage tubes.

Such dislocations as procidentia or prolapse of the uterus or bladder frequently require operation for their cure, but I believe that anteversions and retroversions can usually be remedied by curing the endometritis that usually accompanies them, and by the use of tampons and the gradual breaking or stretching of adhesions with the finger.

1418 L STREET, N. W.

CORRESPONDENCE.

DR. ROSS' CASES OF ECTOPIC PREGNANCY.

TO THE EDITOR OF THE AMERICAN JOURNAL OF OBSTETRICS, ETC.

SIR:—As an addition to my paper I would like to insert the following:

Note 1. "On June 2, 1902, I operated on another case of extrauterine pregnancy. There were no symptoms of pregnancy present. Patient was suddenly taken with pain and prostration, and I operated on her successfully within four hours. removing a large quantity of blood from the peritoneal cavity."

Note 2. "I have also met with another case of pregnancy occurring twice in the same patient, making my fourth case.

"Four years ago the patient was operated on by Dr. Temple, of our city, for extrauterine pregnancy with rupture. She recovered. I saw her on July 1, 1902, with Dr. A. D. Watson, of Toronto. She had missed a monthly sickness and had gone two weeks over her time. Complained of pain such as she had four years before when she was ill with extrauterine pregnancy. Breasts looked suspicious of pregnancy. No enlargement of uterus to be made out. Had nausea. She felt satisfied that she was pregnant. On examination under chloroform, I made out a club-ended tube on the right side. On July 3, at the operation, a very early, unruptured extrauterine pregnancy was found occupying the tube near its abdominal opening."

Yours truly,

JAMES F. W. ROSS.

481 SHERBORNE STREET TORONTO.

TRANSACTIONS OF THE
CHICAGO GYNECOLOGICAL SOCIETY.

Stated Meeting, June 25, 1902.

The President, LESTER E. FRANKENTHAL, M.D., *in the Chair.*

TUBAL ABORTION.

DR. HENRY BANGA exhibited a specimen from a patient 30 years old, a multipara, who on May 28 missed her regular menstrual flow. She experienced instead vague pains in the lower region of the abdomen, especially on the left side. Eight days after the expected time a scant bloody discharge began. Four days later he was called on account of pains growing worse and being of a labor-like, bearing-down character. There was no fever, pulse 80, slight bloody discharge with a few shreds, the uterus in median line, apparently somewhat enlarged, soft; in the left broad ligament a certain fulness and pronounced tenderness. The patient did not think that she was pregnant and had not done anything to bring on the flow. During the next few days the bloody discharge continued, and the pain at times could be controlled only by a morphine suppository. On the sixth day of observation a very tender swelling was first noticed in Douglas' pouch, extending down from the mass in the region of the left broad ligament. At the same time the uterus was pushed forward, upward, and to the right. During the following three days the tumor gradually increased until it reached the size of an orange, displacing the uterus still more in the direction described. Meanwhile he had become fully convinced that the case was one of extrauterine pregnancy which was undergoing rupture. This diagnosis was based on the following symptoms: (1) Missing of the menstrual period, slight flow setting in eight days later and lasting two weeks; (2) pain off and on in the left side, low down in the pelvis, beginning before the flow started and continuing ever since; (3) bimanual examination showing a certain fulness and tenderness in the left side, in which the patient had never before had any pain; (4) the sudden development, within a few days, of a large-sized tumor in Douglas' cul-de-sac, apparently extending downward from the mass in the region of the left broad ligament; (5) slight change in the complexion, the lips having become somewhat paler; (6) absence of fever.

In view of the steady continuance of the hemorrhage, as demonstrated by the gradual growth of the blood tumor in Douglas' cul-de-sac; in view, also, of the severe paroxysms of tearing, labor-like pains, which began to wear out the patient and caused her to beg for immediate relief, laparatomy was performed at the Policlinic. The left tube was removed and a large hematocele of the size of two fists was evacuated. Sixty hours after the operation she had a normal temperature and looked in every respect as though she were on the road to a rapid recovery. The specimen was an instructive illustration of what is called an abdominal abortion. It showed the wide-open, gaping fimbriated end of the tube, through which the ovum was ready to pass to be expelled into the abdominal cavity. The real ovum had, of course, been destroyed long ago. This lump contained what was left of its histological structure embedded in coagula formed by the original hemorrhages which led to the detachment of the ovum and to its destruction.

DR. T. J. WATKINS.—Many cases of so-called tubal pregnancy are cases of tubal abortion, and tubal abortion is frequently mistaken for inflammatory disease of the appendages. This probably accounts for many of the so-called cures of pyosalpinx without operation, as most cases of tubal abortion will recover without operation.

DR. LESTER E. FRANKENTHAL.—The history of the patient is exceedingly instructive, for it shows that the chief point in the differential diagnosis between tubal abortion and tubal rupture is the slowness of the onset. The symptoms of shock are less pronounced in tubal abortion than in tubal rupture. We know that the causation of the symptoms of shock following rupture is twofold. First there are symptoms produced by a loss of blood, and, secondly, those produced by the presence of a foreign body in the peritoneal cavity. In this patient the hemorrhage was slow, and the formation of the hematocele was likewise slow, consequently the chief symptom was that of pain and not shock.

Dr. Charles S. Bacon reported

TWO CASES OF INVERSION OF THE UTERUS.

This extremely serious complication of labor was fortunately very rare, as is seen from the oft-quoted statement that in the Carl Braun Clinic in Vienna no cases occurred in 250,000 confinements. The cases reported were interesting as illustrating two different etiological factors: one, efforts at expression of the placenta, and the other an unknown factor. In one case the best method of reduction was also demonstrated.

The first case happened in the speaker's practice about twelve years ago. The patient was a multipara who had had a rather free postpartum hemorrhage in a previous labor. After a short normal labor, in which only a very little chloroform was given at the end of the second stage, considerable blood appeared shortly after the expulsion of the child, before the birth of the placenta. The uterus did not contract very well, although abdominal massage was kept up, and, as the hemorrhage continued, Credé expression was resorted to. During the act the hemorrhage suddenly became greater, the patient complained of severe pain, and the uterus disappeared from the abdomen. The right hand was immediately introduced into the vagina and discovered the body of the uterus inverted into the lower uterine segment. In other words, the inversion had reached what is usually called the second degree. The placenta was quickly detached and the uterus easily reinverted. The hemorrhage was quite severe for a moment, but was quickly controlled by a hot intrauterine douche. This case illustrated the danger of early expression, and especially expression in the absence of uterine contraction.

The second case of inversion occurred a few months ago in the practice of a colleague who had had an unusually thorough obstetrical and surgical training. The patient was 32 years old and had had two induced abortions. The pregnancy had been normal. The labor was rather short, lasting about ten hours. There was no obstetrical interference whatever. After the birth of the child the physician massaged the abdomen slightly, but made no attempt to express the placenta, which came away completely and spontaneously in from ten to fifteen minutes. There was no hemorrhage following the expulsion of the placenta. Before the delivery of the placenta one drachm of fluid extract of ergot was given. After the delivery of the placenta the uterus was felt firmly contracted. The physician waited forty to forty-five minutes longer to care for the mother and supervise the care of the child. At the end of this period, everything seeming to be in good condition, the physician was about to take his departure when suddenly the patient complained of severe pains and a large quantity of blood poured forth from the vagina. A hand on the abdomen disclosed the absence of the uterus, and the other hand in the vagina showed the presence of the inverted uterus. The speaker was at once sent for, and in the meantime the attending physician attempted to reinvert the uterus by pressure on the fundus, but in vain. A hot douche then controlled the hemorrhage to a great extent.

Reaching the house about half an hour after the occurrence of the inversion, the patient was found in a condition of extreme shock, with a scarcely perceptible wrist pulse, and suffering great pain. The vaginal examination showed a complete inversion of the uterus, which was quite well contracted and not bleeding very much. Having pressed on the fundus and been convinced that restitution by that method would be very difficult or impossible, the hand was then carried behind and to the left side of the uterus up to the junction of the cervix and the vagina, and pressure was made upward. The cervix and lower uterine segment yielded easily and was followed by more and more of the uterus, until in a short time, perhaps one minute, the whole uterus had been reinverted. The patient was at once much relieved of her pain, but the hemorrhage became somewhat more severe. The uterus did not contract well in spite of a hot douche. On account of the desperate condition of the patient, the douche was stopped in order to give a hypodermatic injection of salt solution, the uterus tamponed with gauze, and about one quart of salt solution then injected into the thigh. The absorption was, however, very slight, the pulse did not react, and the patient died about half an hour after the speaker's arrival, or one hour and three-quarters after the end of labor. This case was of interest on account of its bearing on the question of spontaneous inversion of the uterus after expulsion of the placenta. Its relation, however, contained no clue to help in solving the question. Although there was at first contraction of the uterus, and at no time before the occurrence of the inversion any hemorrhage of importance, it was not impossible that at the time of the inversion the uterus was in a state of complete relaxation. According to the best teaching on the subject, such a state of relaxation is highly probable. It was the opinion of the attending physician and the speaker that shock was quite as important a factor in causing death as was the hemorrhage. It was possible that an intravenous injection would have been of greater value than the subcutaneous injection.

DR. RUDOLPH W. HOLMES.—Three years ago I presented to the Chicago Medical Society a paper on the etiology and mechanism of inversion of the uterus; the mechanism was considered from the point of view of anatomical relations as obtained by the study of frozen sections, and from the unique opportunity of studying the mechanism with inversion in progress in my case. My conclusions were directly in consonance with the teachings of Matthews Duncan. He taught that there were two kinds of inversion, the active and the passive; each of these two classes could be spontaneous or artificial. Active inversion is where either spontaneous (abdominal pressure) or artificial causes start the inversion, and uterine contraction continues the process in a manner somewhat analogous to intussusception; the passive inversion is carried on to completion by the primal causes without the aid of uterine action. The passive type is undoubtedly the most frequent form. In times past it was held that all inversions of the uterus were due to faulty technique of the attendant in the third stage. I found that, so far as figures would show, only twenty-five per cent were directly traceable to this cause. Traction on the cord was the most frequent fault in the technique of the delivery of the placenta; Credé's method with a lax uterus was the next in frequency. Because it has been so generally taught that inversion was always an artificial condition, few had the temerity to report their cases. I know about half a dozen men in this city who have had one or more cases of inversion. I am convinced that time will show that artificial causes are less operative than spontaneous ones. In a large proportion of women post partum there is a depression of the placental site, and this is more marked when the site is fundal, or especially over one of the ora Fallopii. An exaggeration of this depression will produce the first step, or introcession; the second step is that of intussusception; the third, that of inversion, or, where the fundus appears between the thighs, inversion with prolapse.

It is not sufficiently impressed upon students that the part that comes out last should be returned first. It is generally taught that the fundus should be pushed back first. This is wrong. Push back the lower uterine segment first, and then the upper segment, and in so doing direct the pressure to one side of the promontory, for a projecting promontory may be the only obstacle to a return. After reinversion is accomplished there should be no temporizing, but the uterus should be tamponed at once. It is interesting to know that the uterus may exceptionally return spontaneously, even after a protracted period. A London obstetrician tried to return a chronically inverted uterus before his class and failed; the next day he was to perform amputation, but when the case was presented to the class it was discovered that reinversion occurred during the night. Baudelocque also reported a case where the uterus reinverted itself after a lapse of eight years.

Dr. HENRY P. NEWMAN read a paper on

PLASTIC SURGERY OF THE FEMALE URETHRA, WITH REPORT OF A UNIQUE CASE.[1]

Dr. JOHN FLETCHER, of Winnetka.—You probably all remember my case for which these pessaries were made. The bladder at first was very small and urine ran constantly, but after treatment it held four ounces of urine. The woman was very uncomfortable when she came to me. Dr. Kolischer had a pessary which we tried to use, but the vagina was so small

[1]See original article, p. 479.

because of an attack of diphtheria that it could not be inserted. She came here from Boston and infected her vagina with a sponge that lay on the wash bowl. I tried to devise something that would help her, and this pessary is the result. She has worn it now two years and with great success. The pessary itself is quite stationary, but the bulb moves around with every movement of the patient. No soreness of tissues results, and there is no leakage at all until the bladder fills. This releases the spring slightly and there is some dribbling of urine. If she urinates often enough there is no leakage at all. She can urinate voluntarily, and without any more effort than if there were no trouble.

Dr. Jacob Frank.—I would like to know whether there was any loss of tissue.

Dr. Fletcher.—Yes, a great deal. Dudley operated for stone in the bladder, and she also had one kidney and one ureter removed. Consequently the bladder was considerably smaller than normal.

Dr. Charles S. Bacon.—I should like to ask whether the patient can remove and replace the pessary herself.

Dr. Fletcher.—No, she cannot. She has two pessaries, and one is removed once in three months. She lives in Boston now, and her physician removes it, inserts the other, cleanses the old one thoroughly and keeps it in a sterile solution until it is ready to be inserted again.

Dr. Palmer Findley reported

A CASE OF CARCINOMA CERVICIS IN A WOMAN NINETY-THREE YEARS OF AGE.

He was indebted to Mrs. Dr. Charles Becktol for the privilege of seeing the case.

Mrs. B., born in Pennsylvania in 1809, was at the age of 93 in remarkably good physical condition, save for the following complaint: During the last six months she had from time to time noticed a discharge of blood from the vagina, which she thought to be a return of the menstrual flow. The hemorrhage was associated with no pain, no intermenstrual discharge, and she suffered no discomfort whatever. At first the flow lasted for four or five days and was not unlike her previous menses. It recurred at intervals of from three to five weeks.

The patient began menstruating at 14 years of age. Her menstrual periods were regular in time and the quantity was normal. Her only illness was typhoid fever at 42 years of age. She was married at 19 and had given birth to eight children, all of whom lived until adult life. One died at the age of 48 from cancer of the uterus. Her mother probably died of a cancer located in the pelvis. She reached the menopause at 45 years of age. During the following forty-eight years and until six months ago there had been no sign of hemorrhage or a discharge at any time from the genital tract.

Examination showed a cauliflower growth, the size of a hen's egg, friable and bleeding, located on the anterior lip of the cervix. The vagina was as roomy as is that of a woman in the period of sexual maturity. The mucous membrane was dry and smooth. The vaginal portion of the cervix was perhaps one-quarter of an inch in length. No uterine body could be felt by rectal examination, and no sign of uterus, tubes, ovaries, or tumor mass could be found in the pelvis. This was the first examination of the patient that had ever been made in her ninety-three years of life, and now that she was in her dotage it was difficult to proceed with a thorough examination. A diagnosis of a cauliflower cancer of the vaginal portion of the cervix was based wholly upon the bimanual examination, in which was found the characteristic tumor upon the cervix with friability and bleeding on handling. So far as the writer could determine, this was the oldest reported case. He found in literature one case of cancer of the cervix occurring at 79 years of age. Dr. Effa Davis had told him of a case in her practice 82 years of age.

Dr. F. A. Stahl read a paper, illustrated with the stereopticon, entitled

INTERPRETATION OF THE HISTOLOGY OF THE VILLI FROM EARLY INTRA- AND EXTRAUTERINE SPECIMENS.[1]

Dr. Henry T. Byford read a paper on

LAPARATOMY FOR PUERPERAL INFECTIONS.

Dr. A. Goldspohn.—I understood the doctor to say that his first two cases did not present tumefactions of any size in the immediate vicinity of the uterus, in the places where we find them so very commonly in the puerperal state when infection occurs. If I am correct in supposing that perhaps even the uteri were somewhat movable, then the foci of infection could be assumed to be high up and multiple and not accessible by way of the vagina. Those two cases I would regard as properly treated by abdominal section, as he did. But in the third case there was tumefaction low down at the principal focus of infection. There will, of course, be tenderness of the appendages, even in connection with a parametritic abscess or common cellulitis. Those cases are not properly approached from above. The third case, as I understood him to describe it, I would open by a thorough transverse posterior colpotomy, preferably with the Paquelin cautery, making a sufficiently large opening. Then the finger should be introduced upward or sideways as required, breaking down all septa and converting the abscess cavities into one distinct cavity, then packing this and leaving the packing for a week, aiming to secure a solid wall around it, so that the cavity will not collapse when the drain is removed, and the opening in the vagina will remain widely open and can be repacked after the first packing is removed, if desirable, and large enough to irrigate as long as may seem desirable. The failure of these

[1]To appear in a succeeding number of the Journal.

vaginal-drainage operations comes very much from not establishing a large enough opening from the vagina into the abscess cavity, and also from insufficient exploration with the fingers at the time of the operation and incomplete breaking-down of septa. When this opening is thoroughly established we get very good results in the majority of these cases, especially if they present tumefactions in the connective tissue of the broad ligament.

In regard to the route of infection in the puerperium, I must contend that in the majority of cases it is not the route that infection travels in non-puerperal or ordinary gynecological cases, in those of gonorrheal origin, for instance, where the infection will practically always be through the entire depth of the uterus, out through the entire length of the tube, and will cause a pelvic peritonitis, the beginning of which is at the abdominal opening of the tube. Therefore we find in operating for retroversions, etc., later on, that adhesions at this point are exceedingly frequent, while real adhesions of the uterus itself are more rare, because if any pelvic peritonitis occurs it occurs near the tube opening first. That is the main type of infection in non-puerperal cases. But in the puerperal uterus we have an entirely different structure and process. The uterus having been recently distended, its wall is soft, thinned, and areolar: the lymphatics are wide open; the veins even are permeable, and infection readily passes directly through the reticular cervical wall, so that there is primarily a pelvic cellulitis rather than a pelvic peritonitis as in other cases. Puerperal infection frequently results in large tumefactions behind or at the side of the uterus, easily distinguished by vaginal or bimanual palpation. Sometimes the uterus is raised by the exudate and brought forward, and it is always held immovably by it. In these cases the route of infection is direct by way of the vagina and cervical walls. Inflamed but not distended tubes and ovaries, as in Dr. Byford's third case, are also present; but this inflammation will usually subside after removal of the principal foci of infection below from below. It is not good practice to enter the abdomen from above in these cases, because we are uncertain how much to remove, for everything looks inflamed and we are tempted to remove things unnecessarily. Such infection of these parts will subside and a good many menstruating women will be saved, while some of them will also retain the ability to conceive.

DR. CHARLES S. BACON.—Dr. Byford's description of how he kept the patient alive for operation is interesting. The use of alcohol hypodermatically and by rectal injection is undoubtedly of great value in cases that cannot be fed in any other way. Alcohol is a better energy-producer than the carbohydrates. It would also be of great value in all these cases that are not operated on. I believe that the medical treatment of inoperable cases of puerperal infection is of great importance. Too much attention is given to local and not enough to general supporting treatment. The subject of the operation in puerperal fever is largely a question of diagnosis. It is difficult to know when there are collections of pus present that ought to be evacuated. The conclusion of Dr. Byford cannot be accepted: that, after curettement and washing out, the continuance of the temperature is a safe diagnostic point. Many cases of general infection finally yield to proper medical treatment, and the great danger of operation in these cases must be considered.

DR. T. J. WATKINS.—I am entirely opposed to the use of alcohol in septicemia, as it increases the work of the already overtaxed kidneys and interferes very much with the administration of nourishment. I will cite briefly a case of severe septicemia following miscarriage without any local manifestations of infection. Two or three weeks after the infection occurred a consultant was called; the patient, at his suggestion, was put upon alcohol and rapidly became worse. The tongue became furred, the urine diminished in amount, and it was difficult for her to take nourishment. She also became restless and somewhat delirious. This continued for four or five days, when the alcohol was stopped and the patient rapidly improved. Another consultant was later called and alcohol was given and stopped with the same results. In septicemia I prefer to force nourishment. When stimulants are needed I depend upon strychnia, camphor, or some ammonia preparation. It is extremely difficult in cases of puerperal infection to determine whether to operate or not. In deciding this question it is most important to observe the progress of the case. We should never operate without first thoroughly exploring the uterus and cleansing the uterine cavity, if indicated, after which it should be let entirely alone. If the case afterward tends to get worse, an exploratory section is then indicated.

When in doubt whether to employ the vaginal or abdominal route, I always make a vaginal, posterior cervical incision for exploration, and then complete the operation by vaginal or abdominal section, as indicated. Cases of infection low down in the pelvis should be treated by very thorough incision and drainage. Cases of puerperal infection are excellent for drainage, as in these cases the inflammatory exudate usually tends to entirely disappear by absorption.

DR. LESTER E. FRANKENTHAL.—I would like to ask Dr. Byford whether any bacteriological examinations were made of the first two and the last case. Postpartum abscess formations not due to the gonococcus are nearly always found in the ovary and never in the tube. I do not wish to be understood as saying that the gonococcus is never found in ovarian abscesses, but that whenever an abscess is found in the adnexa after abortion or labor, which abscess was not present before pregnancy, and this abscess be not caused by the gonococcus, it then is nearly always in the ovary and not in the tube, the route of infection being through the lymphatics and blood vessels of the ovarian ligament.

DR. BYFORD (closing the discussion).—I did not have a bac-

teriological examination made, because I did not have the time
to attend to it.

Dr. Bacon's stricture is, I think. based upon a misconception
of my meaning, as I meant to say, if the symptoms continued,
and not the temperature only.

With regard to the third case. mentioned by Dr. Goldspohn,
he spoke more of cases immediately after labor. My case was
one of abscess of the ovary, the trouble originating probably
five years before, although she had been having an acute
inflammatory attack for eleven weeks. The ovary was not in
the cul-de-sac of Douglas, but on the posterior surface of the
broad ligament. The temperature indicated pus, and I do not
see why the doctor would wish to drain per vaginam when there
was practically no danger in operating radically from above
and curing the patient immediately. The patient got well without any trouble, except a little rise in temperature when the
vaginal opening was allowed to close.

I did not refer to cases with laceration of the cervix. absorption
of septic material, and extension in the broad ligament. I
mentioned only cases of pus in the ovary, which I said very
seldom came from infection through the uterine walls. The
ovary is very resistant to infection. and in nearly all cases there
is some evidence of infection in the tube, and even in cases of
old abscess of the ovary the tube is apt to acquire a normal
appearance.

Dr. Thomas J. Watkins read a paper entitled

AN OPERATION FOR STRICTURE OF THE RECTUM IN WOMEN.[1]

Dr. Jacob Frank.—I wish to verify the statement that the
rectum can easily be shelled out by making a posterior vaginal
incision. I have performed some of these operations, and I
cannot understand why the doctor cut entirely through the
perineum, except that the entire perineum was involved and
the sphincter as well. If the rectum was not diseased I do
not think it was necessary to cut through the perineal body.
I have shelled out a cancer of the lower part of the
rectum in almost the same way, dissecting it entirely, leaving
it attached to the anus, however, and after getting out the
entire mass I cut out the diseased portion, pulling the upper
end of the bowel down to the anus, and sutured it there. In the
female it is a simple operation. The bleeding is slight, the bowel
can be enucleated en masse, and the sphincter can be saved.

Dr. Emil Ries.—The operation described is unique as far as
I know. Where the entire rectum down to the anus is diseased
it is probably as good as anything that could be devised. I
operated six years ago on a case. which I afterward presented
here, of extensive stricture of the rectum, where only the mucous
membrane of the anus was left intact. The stricture extended
as high up as could be felt through the vagina, and a second

[1]See original article. p. 474.

stricture was found in the sigmoid, so that I had to bring down the sigmoid above the second stricture, so that fecal matter did not pass through the diseased rectum, but through the healthy bowel, which I pulled down into the anus. I saw the patient again about a month ago, and I am glad to avail myself of this opportunity to report the case, because cases are rare where the results have been observed for more than weeks or months after operation. The woman, when operated upon, was extremely emaciated and weighed about eighty pounds. She now weighs one hundred and eighty. She has daily bowel movements without any medicine, and the switched-off portion of the rectum and sigmoid now shows none of the discharge which was present during the first year after operation. That operation has one advantage over the one described by Dr. Watkins, inasmuch as it can be done in one sitting. If we follow Dr. Watkins' plan we have to leave the rectum open for an indefinite length of time until the mucous membrane has healed, if it ever does. During that time the woman has a fecal fistula, or practically the same thing, as she has no control of her bowels. Of course, where the entire mucous membrane is diseased and where there is no possibility of getting healthy mucous membrane, the operation I described would be more difficult, and that of Dr. Watkins would have to be considered.

DR. J. RAWSON PENNINGTON.—Dr. Frank and Dr. Ries both claim to have pulled the colon down and fixed it at the anus. This, in view of its attachments, seems to me to be impossible, as the colon is quite firmly fixed at the splenic flexure and at the external border of the psoas muscle, where it terminates. Of course it is possible to shell out the internal tunics of the bowel from the external, which, doubtless, is what these gentlemen did.

DR. JACOB FRANK.—This same question was debated when Dr. Ries presented his case a few years ago. I do not know whether Dr. Pennington has ever tried it, but I think he can get out the entire bowel through that incision by tying and cutting. I had my doubts about it at one time, but they were soon dispelled by a personal trial myself. Once the bowel commenees to run, it is one of the easiest things you can imagine to do. The rectum is the most difficult part, and after it is loosened the sigmoid and colon readily follow.

DR. EMIL RIES.—It is certain that the descending colon may have a mesentery, and it is not at all rare to find this mesentery of some size and extending high up. Rotter, of Berlin, says that it is possible to bring down not only the sigmoid but also the descending colon, and where a chronic dilatation exists, due to stricture, the colon pulls out peritoneum and makes a mesentery of it. There is no doubt that the colon may have a mesentery, but even where it is not present it is very easy to pull down the bowel, if one is careful and pulls slowly. It has been done.

DR. WATKINS (closing the discussion).—In reply to Dr. Frank's remarks, the first part of my paper distinctly says that

34

I attempted to resect the rectum, but had to abandon it because of the absence of normal mucosa below the stricture.

DR. JOSEPH B. DE LEE exhibited a specimen of

PLACENTA MEMBRANACEA.

The woman from whom I procured this specimen had a difficult confinement lasting three days, nine years ago, which resulted in spontaneous delivery of a dead child. Eight years ago she had a prolapsed cord, with anterior parietal bone presentation, and while we were getting permission to operate the child died. It was necessary to perform a craniotomy. She has a contracted pelvis of the rachitic variety, with a conjugata vera of between seven and eight centimetres. Subsequently she had an operation performed, version and extraction, for shoulder presentation, which resulted in a stillbirth. She tried another obstetrician in the fourth confinement. I understand that she was placed in the Walcher position over night, and in the morning the forceps was applied, resulting likewise in a dead baby. Finally she came under my care again a few weeks ago and was very anxious to have a living child. I immediately proposed a Cesarean section, having in mind my previous experience and that of the other obstetricians, but she refused this or any other operation which would endanger her life. She finally consented to a premature delivery. This noon, at 12 o'clock, I put a colpeurynter into the uterus, with twelve ounces of water, and the pains came on in twenty minutes. I removed the colpeurynter in two hours and the pains continued strong. At 8:40 the bag of waters ruptured, and on examination I found that the position had changed from the cephalic to the breech. The cord had prolapsed and it was almost pulseless. The feet and one arm had come down with the cord. I immediately put the woman on the table and made an extraction; the indication for rapid extraction being the almost absent pulsation of the cord. The child was deeply asphyxiated, but was resuscitated by means of a tracheal catheter. It cried vigorously. Hot baths were also given, and it was soon breathing pretty well and had a fair color. Immediately after delivery the woman began to bleed, so that it was necessary to remove the placenta. It was a large, membranaceous placenta, covering almost the whole extent of the membranes. In putting my hand into the uterus for the purpose of removing the placenta on account of hemorrhage, the hand went into the uterine wall and, as I first thought, through it into the peritoneal cavity. I found that the placenta fitted into the uterine wall in folds—dovetailed, as it were— and in trying to get it out my finger passed into these folds and, as I thought, into the wall of the uterus. That is the condition which I have found in several other cases, but never as prominently developed as in this. It illustrates very forcibly the danger of manual removal of even the normal placenta and the possibility of perforation of the uterus.

I do not know much about this condition pathologically. That endometritis will cause adhesion of the placenta is well known. If I had tried to remove the placenta in the ordinary way, I would certainly have gone through the uterus. I contented myself with merely scraping the surface with the finger, removing small shreds of the placenta at a time. The placenta was in the left upper corner of the uterus and tightly adherent. I have met this condition in placenta previa, where the placenta was grown fast into the uterus, and where it was impossible to distinguish between placental and uterine tissue. The child weighed four pounds and seven ounces, and it was very difficult to extract even so small a baby. It required the extreme Walcher position, strong pressure from the outside, and Smellie-Veit extraction.

DR. FRANK A. STAHL.—An important feature of this interesting case might be mentioned here. About a year ago I was sent for from a neighboring town to attend this patient. She was down with a serious general, systemic toxemia from a septic sapremia following an incomplete abortion in the third month. How it was produced I do not know. Perfect restoration followed a simple digital removal of the foul-smelling adherent particles, removed under chloroform. Dr. De Lee's report shows that conception must have followed shortly after this curettage. That this placenta membranacea should have produced such grave changes in the walls of the uterus as suggested by his report is unusual. In fact, as I heard him speak of his curettage, I thought it was due to the fact that many particles of this placenta remained adherent to the walls. The appearance of the placenta would suggest such a condition. Though late, it is still refreshing to hear Dr. De Lee laud the versionist over the craniotomist. In this particular case, after his craniotomy she was some weeks in convalescing; after my version she walked into my office on the tenth day, reporting herself able to resume her household duties. That this placenta should take on such an abnormal development is quite natural after the septic endometritis following the sepsis of the abortion.

TRANSACTIONS OF THE
NEW YORK OBSTETRICAL SOCIETY.

Stated Meeting, May 13, 1902.

The President, MALCOLM MCLEAN, M.D., *in the Chair.*

DR. HERMAN J. BOLDT presented the following:

MYOMECTOMY FOR INTERSTITIAL FIBROID.

The patient, S. O., æt. 38 years, had been troubled with menorrhagia since last July. In addition there was a constant bearing down in the pelvis, so that she could not attend to her duties of a maid without much discomfort. Examination showed an interstitial fibroid in the posterior wall. The abdominal route was chosen, because in such instances conservative surgery can be carried out easier and more successfully than by the vaginal route. Submucous neoplasms and the growths on the lower segment of the uterus, especially when not very large, may be removed per vaginam equally well, thus avoiding an abdominal scar. Convalescence in this instance is progressing normally.

PUERPERAL OVARIAN ABSCESS; ABDOMINAL SECTION; RECOVERY.

Mrs. R., æt. 32, had been delivered of her third child four weeks ago. Beginning on the third day after delivery she began to complain of pain in the right iliac fossa. The pain increased in severity for about one week and then remained steady without further exacerbations or remissions. The temperature remained between 101° and 102.5° F., pulse varied from 100 to 110. There was no other sensitiveness of the abdomen except in the right hypogastrium. Bimanual examination showed the uterus to be somewhat enlarged and relaxed in consistence. To the right there was a semi-fluctuating tumor about the size of a goose egg. It was seemingly not adherent to the pelvic floor. The diagnosis of ovarian abscess was made and confirmed on the following day by operation. While the adhesions were not very firm, they were extensive, but it was possible to remove the pyovarium without rupture. Convalescence smooth.

OVARIAN HEMATOMA; REMOVAL BY VAGINAL SECTION.

The ovary was so much increased in size (to that of a large hen's egg) that it was thought to be a small cystoma. The cause for intervention was constant pain in the left ovarian region, which increased in severity at every menstrual epoch for the past four months. It was removed by posterior vaginal section, that appearing to be the most desirable point for incision.

CHRONIC OVARITIS; VAGINAL OÖPHORECTOMY.

The patient, J. G., had been a sufferer from severe ovarian pain for a number of years. The pain was intensified so much during the menstrual flow that she was compelled to remain in bed for a week to ten days about that time. All remedies which had been used had failed to give any appreciable relief. It was decided to remove the ovaries. The glands showed the characteristic changes of chronic ovarian inflammation. Three months have elapsed since the operation, and the patient has enjoyed better health than since the beginning of her illness.

FIBROMYOMATOUS UTERUS; ABDOMINAL HYSTERECTOMY.

The fibromyomatous uterus was removed from a patient who had passed the menopause and about three months ago began to bleed irregularly. With the bleeding it was thought that the abdominal tumor also increased in size. From that time on it began to give discomfort from its weight. It extended a little above the umbilicus. As an additional source of discomfort there was present an umbilical hernia. The panhysterectomy proved unusually difficult because on a very long cervix (supravaginal hypertrophy).

SUPPURATING FIBROMYOMA WITH LARGE GAS CYST IN THE ANTERIOR WALL OF THE UTERUS; VAGINAL HYSTERECTOMY; RECOVERY.

The opportunity to operate upon the patient was tendered me through the courtesy of Dr. Abram Brothers, in whose service she was in Beth Israel Hospital. I beg to express my appreciation here for the privilege. The woman had been previously operated upon for a large ovarian abscess, and because of rupture during operation the operator had placed a Mikulicz drain in the pelvis. Although the patient did nicely for a couple of weeks, the temperature then began to rise again and the abdominal fistula resulting from the previous operation persisted. Bimanual examination revealed what was diagnosed to be a right pyosalpinx and a fibromyomatous uterus. A radical vaginal operation was decided upon. Because of the local conditions present a paravaginal section was made to enable me to get more room to work. On making a hemisection of the anterior uterine wall into the fibroid a considerable quantity of foul pus escaped from the tumor, showing that the suppurating fibroid was probably the cause of the fever. After washing out the pus, the section was carried higher up on the anterior wall, when suddenly a large volume of gas escaped with a hissing noise, distinctly audible to those near by. The first thought was that I had cut into a distended intestine. Such was not the case; it turned out to be a gas cavity, undoubtedly due to an invasion of bacillus aerogenes capsulatus. The clamp method was used. A rectovaginal fistula developed subsequently; it was of small size and low down. It healed spontaneously.

MULTILOCULAR SEROUS CYSTOMA OF THE OVARY OF THE PAPILLARY FORM, PROBABLY DUE TO REMNANTS OF THE WOLFFIAN BODY.

The tumor was in the left lower abdomen, extending but slightly beyond the median line toward the right, so that it was thought to be a tumor of the ovary. The uterus was pushed toward the right side and in position was anterior. The operation was done by my house surgeon, Dr. Vincent. On opening the abdomen it was found that the tumor was intimately adherent to the intestines and peritoneum of the pelvis on the left side. During enucleation, however, its origin was shown to be from the right side, the tumor twisting behind the uterus over to the left. The adhesions were universal, so that it proved a very tedious enucleation. Because of the oozing from the adhesions the doctor drained the pelvis per vaginam. The woman did not rally from the shock of operation.

Accompanying is the report from Dr. Bandler, who kindly examined the specimen:

The Pathologist's Report.—The cyst sent me by Dr. Boldt is of the size of a large cocoanut and is composed of (1) a larger, thin-walled portion containing fluid and (2) a smaller, fairly hard portion. Over the outer surface of the cyst is the abdominal or fimbriated end of the tube, while the abdominal end is apparently enclosed by a ligature.

On opening the cyst the large portion is found to contain a dark, thin fluid, not blood-stained. The inner surface shows several papillary excrescences and is otherwise smooth. Scrapings did not show positive evidence of ciliated epithelium.

The smaller, hard portion, on opening, is composed of two parts: *(a)* a smaller cyst like the larger one, and, like it, containing papillary excrescences; and *(b)* a thick-walled cyst containing a thick pseudo-mucinous secretion.

Diagnosis: Multilocular serous cystoma of the ovary of the papillary form.

Etiology: Probably due to rests of the Wolffian body.

DR. EGBERT H. GRANDIN.—In reference to the specimen of supposed large hydrosalpinx presented by Dr. Boldt, I would say that I believe it is quite likely that it is such. Only six weeks ago I operated upon a woman under the assumption that I had to deal with a large myoma posterior to the uterus, and, after enucleation, it proved to be a thick-walled hydrosalpinx.

LARGE FIBROID TUMOR SHOWING IN ONE PART SARCOMATOUS DEGEN-
ERATION, AND WITH A PECULIAR APRON-LIKE GROWTH
OVER ITS ANTERIOR SURFACE.

DR. HIRAM N. VINEBERG.—This tumor was removed from A. L., a spinster 50 years of age. The patient could not give a very clear history of herself. All the information I could obtain was that she had had a growth in the abdomen for years, but that it gave her no trouble until about a year ago, since when it has been growing rapidly. During the same period she has suffered with profuse uterine hemorrhages, and for the past five or six months she has practically been an invalid. Her left lower extremity began to swell about a year ago; now it is treble the size of the opposite one.

The patient is extremely emaciated, being nothing but skin and bones, and all the visible mucous membranes are blanched. The abdomen is uniformly distended by a semi-elastic growth which reaches from the symphysis to near the umbilicus. There is no evidence of fluid in the flanks. The superficial veins of the abdominal wall are very much enlarged. The vagina is small and atrophic, and on vaginal examination the pelvis is found pretty well filled with the abdominal tumor. The cervix passes into the tumor.

The diagnosis was made of a fibrocyst of the uterus, or a fibroid which was undergoing malignant degeneration. The patient was in a very feeble condition, having been bed-ridden for the past couple of weeks.

She entered St. Mark's Hospital and was operated upon by me March 31, 1902. On opening the abdomen a peculiar bluish-red mass presented itself. On enlarging the incision it was found that the mass covered the greater part of the anterior surface of the tumor. It was very vascular and was extensively adherent to the abdominal parietes. At first I thought it might be the altered omentum, but the omentum was found moved upward and normal in appearance and very much atrophied. It was then thought it might be a thin-walled ovarian cyst which had ruptured, but on removal of the tumor the two atrophied ovaries were found attached to the tumor.

It was a question whether it would be safer to make the attempt at removal of the tumor, in view of the great vascularity of the outgrowth and its extensive adhesions to the parietes, but I decided in its favor. I separated a portion of the outgrowth from the abdominal wall on the left side; then, by ligating in succession the left ovarian, the left uterine, the right ovarian, the right uterine arteries, I succeeded in ablating the tumor together with the cervix and adhesions, thus far with little or no loss of blood. The tumor was now free, excepting its attachments through the outgrowth to the abdominal parietes. I was now enabled to separate these with scarcely any loss of blood. It was remarkable how well the patient withstood the operation. But such was her lowered vitality that, in spite of there being no complications and in spite of everything in connection with the operation having progressed satisfactorily, she died on the ninth day, simply from progressive asthenia and emaciation.

At the postmortem inspection of the interior of the abdomen there was no trace of any pathologic change. The main tumor and the outgrowth has been kindly examined for me by Dr. F. S. Mandlebaum, the Pathologist at Mt. Sinai Hospital. One section of the tumor showed at one point a sarcomatous degeneration; the remainder was of a fibroid character. The outgrowth was found to be of an inflammatory nature.

SPECIMEN OF FATTY DEGENERATION OF AN OVARIAN CYST.

Dr. Brooks H. Wells.—The patient, Mrs. A. D., aged 65, had borne six children. She had had no miscarriages. Menopause occurred at 45. She had complained for a number of years of dull aching pain in the hips and thighs, and the abdomen had been enlarged. For two years she had noticed spotting of blood from the vagina. For several months there had been severe and increasing pain in the lower abdomen, rapidly increasing anemia and loss of flesh and strength. There was complete anorexia, insomnia, and marked constipation. Her physician, Dr. A. I. Miller, of Brattleboro, had strongly advised operation two years ago. The physical examination showed extreme emaciation. Heart, lungs, and kidneys were normal. The abdomen was dis-

tended by what was apparently a multilocular ovarian cyst reaching to half-way between the umbilicus and the ensiform.
Vaginal exploration revealed a firm, smooth, fibroid-like, rounded
mass filling the true pelvis and pushing the uterus sharply backward and to the left. A diagnosis was made of multilocular
ovarian cyst, or fibrocyst of the uterus with probable malignancy.
The patient came into my service at the Polyclinic, and on February 3 an abdominal section was made. Very dense adhesions
were found everywhere, especially between the cyst and the
omentum and intestines. With much difficulty these adhesions
were separated on the left side, and by evacuating the larger
portion of the cyst it became possible to reach and tie off the attachments of the tumor to the uterus. The mass was then separated by the finger from its inferior attachments and moved out
on to the abdomen, when it became possible to deal with the adhesions to the intestines. In spite of care and leaving portions
of the outer wall of the cyst in places, several areas of intestine
were denuded and had to have peritoneum sewed over them with
fine catgut. The abdomen was closed and the patient put to bed.
She received a high enema of a quart of hot normal salt solution
every four hours. She rallied well from the operation, made
an uneventful but very slow convalescence, and has now gained
greatly in color, weight, and strength. The tumor when removed was of a yellow-pink color and its cavity was filled with
yellowish-gray masses and old blood clots. A microscopical examination by Dr. Jeffries, of the Polyclinic Laboratory, showed
the tumor walls and its blood vessels to be in a condition of extreme fatty degeneration. The grayish masses were coagulated
fibrin. The increasing anemia and weakness of the patient were
caused by repeated hemorrhage from the degenerated blood vessels into the cavity of the cyst. There was nowhere any sign of
malignancy.

EDEMATOUS FIBROID.

DR. BROOKS H. WELLS.—Mrs. V. D., a widow of 38, came to me
March 19 complaining of a rapid increase in the size of the abdomen which she had noticed for five months. Menstruation
had been more free than usual during the same time and she
had suffered with backache and pain over the pelvic region. I
had examined her four years before and found the pelvic organs
normal. She now had a uniform ovoid enlargement of the
uterus similar in shape and size to a seven and a half months
pregnancy. This enlargement was soft and semi-fluctuant, but
the cervix was hard. A diagnosis of rapidly growing soft
myoma of the uterus was made, and, a few days later, the tumor
was removed by abdominal hysterectomy. Convalescence was
rapid and uneventful. The main interest of the case is in the
tumor. Microscopically it is an ordinary fibroma. When removed from the patient the vessels were all held in the grip of
clamps, and, in freeing these, so large an amount of blood escaped

that the tumor shrank visibly. On making a longitudinal median section it is seen that the uterine muscle is so filled with venous sinuses as to appear like an angioma. The fibroid itself was soft and spongy and several ounces of clear watery fluid drained from it in a short time.

GLANDULAR POLYP.

DR. BROOKS H. WELLS.—I have also to show a glandular polyp, the size of a hen's egg, removed from the uterus of a single woman of 42 years. Her menstruation was normal until two years ago. Since that time it has increased in quantity and for four months has been profuse. She has also had a watery discharge from the vagina for four months and is very anemic. Examination showed the polyp protruding from the uterus. The bladder having been separated and pushed back, the anterior lip of the cervix was divided in the median line for an inch and a quarter, so that the attachments of the polyp to the uterine fundus could be reached and severed. The cervix was then closed by interrupted catgut sutures and the cavity of the uterus packed with gauze. Convalescence has been uneventful.

DR. HERMAN J. BOLDT.—The specimen of myofibroma I saw in its fresh state, and it was full of vessels which were so tortuous that it simulated an angiomatous condition. Such a specimen I think is rare.

ECTOPIC GESTATION.

DR. EGBERT H. GRANDIN.—I wish to present a specimen of ectopic gestation with the right tube being in the process of aborting and the left tube being distended with a large clot. I exsected this tube, leaving the ovary. As is customary with many cases of ectopic gestation which I have seen and the histories of which I have recorded, there were no symptoms present which suggested the condition beyond slight irregularity in menstruation followed by irregular spotting. There was no pain and the uterus was small and empty.

A second specimen which I expected to present is being examined by the pathologist. It consisted of the left ectopic tube removed from a patient from whom, two months previous, I had removed the right tube for the same affection. In this case as well, the diagnosis had been in great doubt until a posterior vaginal section established it by giving exit to the blood which had been extruded into the peritoneal cavity. I again wish to lay stress on the value of the posterior section in diagnosis, and to call attention to the fact that nowadays only those cases of ectopic are fatal where the surgeon is undecided instead of being bold enough to make a diagnosis by posterior vaginal section.

DR. SIMON MARX.—The remarks made by Dr. Grandin as to the value of the vaginal section appeal to me very strongly, especially in view of the fact that within the last few weeks I have had three cases under my care which bring out the value of his suggestion. I do not believe that the diagnosis is always as difficult as Dr. Grandin states, provided we have such complication in mind and are looking for it. If we think of such a condition existing and there are present certain symptoms which warrant it, we at once make a vaginal section—*i.e.*, hemorrhage and pain, especially when these coexist with what is supposed to be a normal pregnancy. If bleeding occurs in a supposedly pregnant woman I think it should place us on guard, and if suspicious we should make a vaginal section for exploratory purposes. I do think that there is some risk run in such a procedure; but such risks seem to be warrantable in the face of the good that may result from the relief of worry and the value of having a correct diagnosis of the cause of bleeding.

I have in mind three cases, one of whom died from the shilly-shallying and procrastinating. She was treated by a neurologist for splanchnic paralysis; if this be the new name given for a rupture of an ectopic sac, it was correct, for upon opening the abdomen it was found to be filled with blood. This patient died.

In another case there was no tumor and very few symptoms were present, but I made a presumptive diagnosis from the dripping which took place for three weeks. Examination under chloroform anesthesia revealed nothing; curetting the uterus and examining the scrapings revealed nothing. I then made a vaginal section and found I had to deal with an unruptured tubal gestation. This was tied off, the wound sewn up, and the patient was out of bed on the tenth day.

The third case was a young woman who presented the typical history of an extrauterine pregnancy. She had a tumor to one side of the uterus and she discharged a decidual cast which was carefully examined by myself and a pathologist; I pronounced it a decidual cast, and the pathologist agreed and further said it contained no chorionic villi, which tended to verify my diagnosis. A brief history of the case is as follows:

She was a young woman who had given birth to two children. When she had gone six days over time she began to bleed. This kept up for three weeks continuously. She had severe paroxysmal pain which her family physician attributed to a peculiar neurosis. Upon examination a tumor was found to the right of the uterus, the size of a small bologna sausage; the uterus was not much congested. While preparing to operate she passed a complete decidual cast; in spite of this I was advised by the consultants to wait—why, I did not know. Within one week severe pain occurred, rupture took place, and the entire abdomen filled with blood.

I simply want to state that I agree with what Dr. Grandin has said, and wish to emphasize the fact that in atypical cases, with hemorrhage, we should think of ectopic gestation. If we have any presumptive evidence of its existence, I think we are justified in assuring ourselves of the correctness of diagnosis by making a vaginal section. I have seen this year fifteen or

eighteen cases. Why? Because I look for them, and if I have
the least suspicion that an ectopic exists I make a vaginal section.
So far I have not killed a woman by such an incision, nor have
I ever been sorry that I made it, for I almost always have found
something pathological to account for the symptoms.

Dr. Dougal Bissell read a paper on

IMPLANTATION OF THE URETER INTO THE BLADDER.[1]

Dr. Florian Krug.—I have here a reprint from the *American
Gynecological and Obstetrical Journal* for November, 1894, being
a "Report of a Successful Case of Implantation of the Severed
Ureter into the Bladder," done by me in the spring of 1894.
The patient, 30 years of age, had large multiple fibroids, intraligamentous, and had been treated by all sorts of electricity.
Her condition was complicated by the presence of many abscesses all over the peritoneal cavity, not only of the ovaries and
tubes, but also between the intestines; in other words, it was one
of the worst cases one could possibly meet with in performing
hysterectomy. Dr. Baldy had invited me to operate upon this
case in Philadelphia. With Dr. Baldy's assistance and in the
presence of Dr. Henrotin and Dr. Etheridge, of Chicago, hysterectomy was performed, and during the course of the operation
I severed the left ureter. It was an excusable mistake, for the
ureter had an anomalous course, running in front of the tumor
near the parietes. The ureter was severed at a point where one
would never look for it. After completing the enucleation of the
tumor and the ablation of the uterus, the stumps were turned
into the vagina and the peritoneal flaps closed. One of the gentlemen present suggested that the kidney be removed on that
side. However, being familiar with Dr. Penrose's case, I proceeded to engraft the ureter into the bladder. Dr. Penrose's case
was the only one I knew of in America in which the severed
ureter had been implanted into the bladder; I also knew of a
case in which an end-to-end anastomosis had been performed by
Kelly. From the reprint referred to I read:

"The distal end of the cut ureter having been tied off, an incision of about an inch and a half was made into the bladder near
the vertex. A fine needle, threaded with finest catgut, was now
passed into the bladder from without at a point about half an
inch below the incision. The needle was then passed out through
the incision, then through the ureter from without within, again
through the incision into the bladder, coming out at a point near
the original insertion. A second suture was passed in the same
way, taking hold of the other side of the ureter. The proximal
end of the ureter was now split between the two sutures, and
each of the two sutures loosely tied so as to suspend the ureter in
the bladder. The incision in the bladder was then closed up by
four tiers of running and interrupted sutures, the first two tiers

[1] Will appear in a succeeding number of the JOURNAL.

including the mucous and muscular layer of the bladder, while
the next two brought the peritoneal investment together. In
applying these sutures I had in view not to constrict the ureter
by too much pressure, and at the same time to close the incision
tightly enough to prevent leakage. The abdominal wound was
now closed and a self-retaining catheter inserted into the bladder.
The latter was removed on the fourth day after operation. The
patient was catheterized regularly during the next few days, and
attended to that herself for another week. The bowels moved
on the third day.'' Entire convalescence smooth. Cystoscopical
examination proved the patency of the implanted ureter. As
far as I know, she was cystoscoped by Dr. Kelly some years after
the operation and the ureter was found still patent.

I want to say that, if the same accident should occur to me
again, I should proceed to anchor the ureter in the same way and
not depend upon pulling the ureter down by means of forceps.
In order to prevent leakage we should introduce several tiers of
sutures tightly around the ureter, and be careful not to have
them too tight, producing a stenosis. The doctor included part of
the ureter in his sutures, stitching it to the bladder wall; I think
they might easily tear out. I believe the use of guy ropes in suspending the ureter into the bladder wall, as it was done in my
case, would be the preferable operation.

DR. BACHE McE. EMMET.—Dr. Bissell is to be given much
credit for his method of implantation of the ureter into the
bladder. By his technique he opens up the peritoneum, obtains a clear field for work, provides good drainage per vaginam, and has no fear of accidents following. Of course in
inserting his stitches he must guard against the possibility of
leakage in the peritoneum. When he places his patient in the
Trendelenburg position and works underneath the peritoneum,
this is certainly a step in the right direction and promises the
best results. The same principle, working outside of the peritoneum, has always been a leading feature in ureteral work. Dr.
Bissell will doubtless recall the case of Mr. Arbuthnot Lane, who
discovered a calculus in the ureter by an incision through the
abdominal wall. He closed this and sought the stone later and
removed it by an incision in the lumbar region, working outside
of the peritoneum. Similar work was done by Mr. Twynam, removing a stone from the ureter by raising the peritoneum in the
iliac fossa. To my mind it matters little what particular kind of
stitch one uses, nor how it is placed, provided one makes a tight
job and does not constrict the ureter. Whatever operation is
done in ureteral anastomosis—in the lateral position. in the
oblique, side-to-side, end-to-end or end-in-end, or in implantation
—it must be kept in mind that the stitches should be covered
over with peritoneum, in order that rapid healing may occur, and
in many of these cases no drainage is necessary. But, of course,
where there has been much dissecting, as in this case, with the
breaking down of cellular tissue and capillaries, drainage is very

essential, to guard against a pelvic abscess rather than leakage of urine, and that by the vagina is well conceived.

I wish to congratulate Dr. Bissell for opening up a new field of work and for the marked advance he has made in our resources.

DR. HERMAN J. BOLDT.—I wish to congratulate Dr. Bissell upon his paper. The method I have adopted in my first instance of uretero-vesical anastomosis I considered at that time applicable to most cases. I have seen two instances since where it was absolutely impossible to get a catheter into the ureter through the vaginal opening, although in one instance I was able to find the opening but unable to introduce the catheter. Later, on abdominal section, I found that the passage was false and the cut end of the ureter high up. The reason why I adopted such a method in the instance quoted by Dr. Bissell was because it was my first experience and it seemed most feasible.

I beg to report another case which has also not yet been placed on record. The operation was a resection of a septic uterus with the broad ligaments; there were multiple abscesses of the broad ligaments and uterus which necessitated radical operation. The ureter was severed, but it was not discovered until the abdomen had been closed. The patient recovered from the primary operation and two months afterward she was operated on again. Dr. Charles Jewett, of Brooklyn, was present. It was impossible to insert the catheter per vaginam, and so the ureter was found by tracing it down from the pelvic brim. The bladder was opened with a one-inch incision near its base and the ureter was implanted there, the peritoneum closed, and so the work was done practically extraperitoneally. It seems to me it is immaterial how a ureter is implanted into the bladder so long as the bladder opening surrounding the ureter is not made so tight as to cause a constriction.. In two instances I have had it made no difference. The main feature is not to make the sutures in the bladder, which surrounds the ureter, too tight. Also, they should be applied extraperitoneally and so close the incision about the ureter extraperitoneally.

The work of Dr. Krug I think is extremely commendable, and we should be pleased to know that it was one of our New York men who performed the operation in that way. Dr. Bissell's operation offers a certain number of advantages, especially in the way of finding the ureter by opening the broad ligament.

I have had two cases of implantation of the ureter into the vagina; one case failed entirely; the second case died. I did it just prior to my leaving for Europe and unfortunately could not learn any particulars on my return.

DR. CLEMENT CLEVELAND.—The operation described by Dr. Bissell is certainly a very interesting one, and I was impressed with the ingenious way he performed it and also his dexterity. It was particularly interesting to see with what ease it could be done with the patient in the Trendelenburg position. The point made of transplanting the ureters into the bladder extraperitoneally, entirely shutting off the abdominal cavity, is an important one.

DR. HIRAM N. VINEBERG.—The deposit of phosphates may have been due to the presence of the raw surface in the interior of the bladder.　I have now a case under observation in which the gentleman under whose care she was sewed the cervix into the bladder in order to cure a vesico-vaginal fistula. She menstruates through the bladder, and every now and then there occurs a thick deposit of phosphates upon the eroded cervix.　From time to time I remove the deposit of phosphates through a large-sized Kelly cystoscope, and she then has relief until the next menstruation.

DR. EMMET.—In those experimental cases in which end-to-end anastomosis has been attempted, done upon a catheter, there being no raw surface except at the edges, yet the catheter has been found so encrusted with phosphates that its removal caused the operation to fail utterly, which shows that the urine itself is at fault.

DR. DOUGAL BISSELL.—The method of finding the ureter and the point of *selection* on bladder wall for anchoring the ureter are the features of my paper I wish to lay emphasis upon.　As stated by Dr. Emmet, all methods of anchoring the ureter seem to meet with success; but I believe that the orifice can best be kept open by the procedure adopted by Krug and Baldy or that suggested in the paper.

———

TRANSACTIONS OF THE WASHINGTON OBSTETRICAL AND GYNECOLOGICAL SOCIETY.

———

Meeting of May 2, 1902.

The President, G. WYTHE COOK, M.D., *in the Chair.*

DR. J. WESLEY BOVÉE presented a specimen of

FIBROMATA OF BOTH OVARIES

he had removed that morning, and, as it was the first of the kind he had seen in the peritoneal cavity, he was willing to accept the statements of other surgeons that it was an extremely rare condition.

The patient was 40 years of age and first married at the age of 16 years.　About one year after marriage she noticed a severe sore on the vulva and in the groin.　Concluding this was a venereal disease contracted from her husband, she refused to live with him longer.　A few years ago she was again married, living with this husband until her admission into Columbia Hospital, when her husband left for Porto Rico with another woman.　She had never been pregnant.　She had suffered considerable pain during the past few years, and believing. from her own sensations and the opinion of the physician, that she was near the end of a pregnancy, she had made elaborate preparations for her accouchement. This coming to naught, she had called another physician, who diagnosed a uterine fibroid and sent her to the hospital for operation. She had a very large abdomen, which was in part due to the very thick abdominal wall and to gaseous distension, as well as to the presence of the new growth. Notwithstanding this statement of hers regarding the sore and the presence of a scar on the vulva, such as is usually seen after the healing of a chancre, he was led to think the lesion was not syphilitic. Upon examination the cervix was found to be hard and the body of about normal size. The appendages were not easily distinguishable because of exquisite tenderness and the physical conditions above mentioned. But at about the brim of the pelvis on the left side could be felt a fixed, hard, solid tumor that was flattened anteriorly and seemed disconnected with the uterus and appendages. Believing this to be retroperitoneal, it was thought to be a migratory uterine fibroid dissecting upward.

The operation, made through the abdominal wall, nearly six inches in thickness, revealed the growth to be an ovary that had undergone fibroid degeneration. It was flattened on the anterior and posterior surfaces, having a thickness in this direction averaging two inches, and its marginal circumference was nearly circular and about sixteen inches. It was nodular, had an unusually well-developed ligament, and was intimately adherent to the posterior peritoneum and omentum. The opposite ovary, considerably enlarged and adherent. was also undergoing the same change apparently. The tubes were both adherent to the ovaries and contained a muco-sanguinolent fluid. They had several nodules from previous inflammation—probably gonorrhea—early in married life. These fibroids evidently developed as a result of inflammatory disease of the appendages, the same as is occasionally noticed in the uterus under similar conditions.

DR. BOVÉE also presented a specimen of ruptured

TUBAL PREGNANCY

removed from a woman, 37 years of age, who gave absolutely no history of pregnancy. Her menses occurred at intervals varying from twenty-one to forty days, but she had not missed any period during the past year. A mass bulging the thin abdominal wall in the hypogastric region, that was sensitive and painful, together with her pulse of high rate and small volume, led him to operate under the impression that she was suffering with tubercular disease of the appendages. Upon opening the abdomen, April 30, he came in contact with a ruptured tubal pregnancy in which the living fetus was developed to about three and a half or four months and the placenta was attached to the right broad ligament and the intestines. In the sac was much fluid and coagulated blood. The clots were also found in the peritoneal cavity above the sac wall, and there were four distinct crops of them. The tube was found ruptured for an inch and a half at the outer end. This was the second living fetus he had delivered, although he had operated in periods of from two weeks to nine years. May 2 tubercle bacilli were secured from her sputum, and during the third night after operation, while coughing, she expelled from the vagina a typical decidua. The clots of blood above mentioned were picked away with the fingers as well as could hurriedly be done, the condition of the patient before and during the operation being extremely desperate. No washing was resorted to. as he preferred to tax her absorbents later than her recuperative power at the time.

Dr. Bovée also presented a specimen of

SOFT FIBROMA,

weighing about four pounds. removed sixteen days before from a spinster of 37 years who had become blanched from continuous uterine hemorrhage during several weeks, and which had failed to yield to his treatment persisted in during ten days. This patient was in a desperate condition, but under extreme stimulation he was enabled to remove this tumor. Upon section the entire endometrium presented no microscopical appearances of disease. During the operation the blood was noticed to be exceedingly dilute and the tissues to ooze very freely. She is still pale and anemic, but sits up, eats well, and is rapidly improving.

Dr. Fry presented a

RUPTURED TUBAL PREGNANCY.

He said clot left in the abdomen after ectopic pregnancy does harm. He had such a case develop a septic condition and die of embolism. He opened one through the vagina and was able to get out all the clots, but because of fresh hemorrhage he had to open the abdomen. He thought it was best to open through the vagina first in all cases.

Dr. Bovée said nothing was to be gained by opening the abdomen in his case. He never lost a case from blood clot; all of his fatalities were from hemorrhage. The clots are adherent and have to be removed with the fingers. He would rather trust the small clots to Nature. If there is a limiting membrane over the fetus it is proper to go through the vagina. If drainage is necessary from the pelvis he drains through the vagina.

Meeting of May 16, 1902.

The President, G. Wythe Cook, M.D., *in the Chair.*

Dr. I. S. Stone read a paper on

SOME RECENT SURGERY FOR BILIARY OBSTRUCTION.[1]

Dr. W. P. Carr said we are just beginning to realize the fre-

[1]See original article, p. 484.

-queney of gall stones and the importance of this new field of surgery. The diagnosis is doubtful unless some of the prominent symptoms are present. In many cases where pain is great there is no tenderness and jaundice is frequently absent. He has ·operated on six cases—three during the year—and in only one was there visible jaundice. All had bile in the urine. He does not operate unless there is pain present, except when malignant disease is suspected. Catarrhal jaundice may be due to duodenitis, which may last two or three weeks or months and subside. In those severely jaundiced hemorrhage is difficult to ·deal with.

A case of typhoid fever developed, after four months, pain and tenderness in the region of the gall bladder. A quart of dark fluid was let out, but no stone was found. Drainage was employed, and the next day bile appeared in the stool. There is very little chance of hernia after these operations. He does not stitch the gall bladder to the peritoneum, but uses a stiff tube with catgut.

DR. MILLER said he saw Dr. Stone's operation and was filled with consternation when he saw the hemorrhage. In thinking ·over the operation afterward he thought a phlebolith might be taken for a stone, as it has been when lying along the ureter.

DR. J. T. KELLEY said in a case which he had operated there was no jaundice. The gall bladder was filled with a clear, ·starch-like fluid, and the stones, thirty-five in number, were of a pearly white. The obstruction was in the cystic duct.

TRANSACTIONS OF THE OBSTETRICAL SOCIETY OF LONDON.

Meeting of July 2, 1902.

The President, PETER HORROCKS, M.D., *in the Chair.*

DR. R. H. BELL read a short communication on

.A CASE OF PUERPERAL ECLAMPSIA, WITH AUTOPSY AND REMARKS.

The clinical phenomena were those usually associated with ·cases of eclampsia, viz., headache, vomiting, edema, albuminuria, and finally fits and coma. It was noted, however, that the urine was little, if at all, diminished in amount, and that albumin, though always present, was never in larger proportions than one-sixth.

The presence of jaundice in the later stages of the illness was also mentioned, and reference made to other cases in which this symptom was present.

A short account followed of the autopsy and microscopical appearances of the liver and kidneys, both of which, but especially the former, showed marked degenerative changes such as have

35

been described by Pelliet and others as associated with cases of eclampsia. Their close resemblance to those seen in the early stages of acute yellow atrophy was dwelt upon, but the fact was mentioned that during life no diminution of the size of the liver was made out and that post mortem the organ weighed fifty-five ounces. The author suggested that the case was interesting as showing the close affinity of eclampsia to acute yellow atrophy occurring in a pregnant woman, the postmortem appearances being those associated with an acute toxemia.

Some experiments with regard to the toxicity of the blood, conducted by Dr. Seligmann, were then recorded. The method employed was the subcutaneous injection of serum into guinea-pigs. Control experiments were made with the blood from cases of chronic uremia in the stage of coma, and it was shown that in these cases the serum had by no means the same high degree of toxicity as existed in the case of eclampsia.

DR. CULLINGWORTH thought that there was much that was still to be elucidated both about the pathology of puerperal eclampsia and that of acute yellow atrophy of the liver, and it was quite possible that some day both might be found to be capable of being classed under one general heading. The difficulties of such a case as this would then be cleared up, and, indeed, this case might prove valuable as a sort of connecting link, all the more valuable from its having been recorded without any attempt to fit the facts on to some favorite theory. There was just one point on which he should like to ask Dr. Bell a question. The hemorrhages found in the liver were extensive and remarkable. He was not sure that their extent had been actually measured and recorded in figures, but, from his recollection, he should say the larger one had a sectional area of at least three inches by two and one-half inches. He feared he was not a sufficiently expert pathologist to be able to say whether such a condition was ever met with in puerperal eclampsia with kidney lesions only.

DR. EDEN said he thought the case, which had been so admirably reported by Dr. Bell, was a very important one. It served to support the view, now gaining much favor abroad, that it was possible to divide cases of eclampsia into two principal groups—hepatic and renal.

The morbid anatomy of eclampsia had not, perhaps, received as much attention of late as had been paid to experimental work in connection with the toxemic theory of this disorder. But the occurrence of well-defined changes in the liver, consisting chiefly of hemorrhages and degeneration of hepatic cells, was now well established, and it had of course been long recognized that marked changes might also be found in the kidneys. Dr. Bell's case appeared to belong to the hepatic class, and the relation of this class to cases of acute yellow atrophy was one of the most interesting problems connected with the subject.

DR. BELL appeared to sympathize with the view that eclampsia was produced by a toxic condition of the blood. This might be so; but toxemia, after all, was only a symptom like eclampsia, and we were therefore no nearer a satisfactory explanation of the pathology of the condition. The real problem that had to be faced was, how did the toxemia arise? Unfortunately, no answer could at present be given to this question. When physiological chemists had succeeded in separating from the blood of eclamptic women definite toxic bodies whose properties could be accurately studied, some progress might be made in settling this very difficult question.

DR. AMAND ROUTH rather doubted the diagnosis of acute yellow atrophy in this case, owing to the absence of atrophy. He saw a lady, six months pregnant, who was seized with severe vomiting, slight albuminuria, jaundice, and passage of blood per rectum. A diagnosis of acute yellow atrophy was made and the uterus emptied. The following day puerperal eclampsia ensued and she died, but no postmortem examination was allowed.

THE PRESIDENT did not think this was an ordinary case of puerperal eclampsia. On the contrary, it was a very unusual one, for, on the one hand, the urine was never loaded with albumin, and, on the other, albumin was not quite absent. Again, there was marked jaundice, which was uncommon in puerperal eclampsia. Hence, although the pathological changes in the liver and other viscera were of great interest, it did not follow that they would be found in ordinary cases. He deprecated the use of the term puerperal toxemia, for it was founded upon a still unproved theory and gave no picture of the case like the term puerperal eclampsia did.

DR. DRUMMOND ROBINSON referred to a case in which he had made some experiments with the blood serum of a patient who during her first pregnancy had developed jaundice and albuminuria. Considerable quantities of the blood serum from this case were injected into guinea-pigs without producing any effect. This patient had no fits and made a good recovery after the induction of premature labor.

DR. WILLIAMSON considered that under the term "eclampsia" we group together, at the present time, conditions which have very little in common with one another. On the one hand there is a well-marked group of cases in which the patients are the subject of chronic nephritis; in these patients what we term eclampsia is really a uremic condition, and, though modified by pregnancy, still differs in no essential from uremia occurring in a non-pregnant woman. But there is another and an entirely different class of cases in which the convulsions appear to depend upon an acute toxic poisoning, the stress of which falls more especially upon the liver, and the kidneys may almost entirely escape damage.

In support of this contention he quoted a case recently seen in which forty eclamptic fits occurred within twenty-four hours of delivery. The urine was not reduced in amount, the percentage of urea never fell below 1.6 per cent, only a slight cloud of albumin was present, and no tube casts were found. After the cessation of the fits, however, the patient became deeply jaundiced and bile was found in the urine. The patient recovered.

MR. ALBAN DORAN exhibited a

RETROPERITONEAL LIPOMA WEIGHING THIRTEEN POUNDS TWELVE OUNCES

removed from a woman aged 47. The omentum was not involved. The right kidney lay on the pelvic brim, in a lobe of the tumor, which was supplied with blood by large vessels arising close below the pancreas. The patient rallied from the operation, but died thirty-eight hours later from suppression of urine. Mr. Doran noted that surgically this kind of tumor must be distinguished from the purely omental type (Meredith and perhaps Lannander) and from lipoma of the broad ligament (Treves), varieties which allow of easy and safe removal. The results of extirpation of these absolutely retroperitoneal lipomata were very unsatisfactory. Ferrier and Guillemain question, on good grounds, whether it be justifiable to attempt their removal when their nature is recognized at an exploratory operation.

OVARIAN TUMOR OBSTRUCTING DELIVERY AT FULL TERM.

MR. J. W. TAYLOR read the notes of a case in which delivery at full term had been obstructed by the presence of an ovarian tumor in the pelvis. After considering the relative advantages of abdominal and vaginal ovariotomy, it had been decided to make a posterior vaginal section and perform ovariotomy during the progress of labor. This was successfully accomplished and then delivery had been completed by the aid of forceps without delay. The patient had made an easy and very satisfactory recovery.

THE PRESIDENT congratulated Mr. Taylor on the happy termination of his case. But he could not help feeling that he had been lucky in finding this ovarian cyst so simple and so free from adhesions. Had it been a multilocular cyst with myriads of small cysts, had there been a lot of adhesions extending to the bowel, or had the pedicle been difficult to reach, he might have been obliged to open the abdomen after all.

He related details of a case in Guy's Hospital where a tumor occupied the pelvis and obstructed labor. It was under such great pressure that it was thought to be a solid tumor. There was no fluctuation and it felt as hard as any fibroid. A needle was pushed in and pus withdrawn. Then an incision was made and a loculus emptied; a septum was punctured and another loculus emptied; and then a third one, after which it was found possible to deliver. Subsequently another loculus of this multilocular suppurating ovarian tumor opened and discharged near the navel, and the patient left the hospital and was lost sight of.

After trying operations per vaginam, he must say he preferred to tackle these tumors through the abdominal wall. One great danger was the pedicle, which sometimes tore when being pulled down in order to reach it from the vagina.

Dr. Herbert Spencer thought that abdominal ovariotomy was preferable to vaginal ovariotomy in the treatment of these cases. Mr. Taylor seemed to have chosen vaginal ovariotomy partly because he would "probably have to evacuate the pregnant uterus or do a Cesarean section before he could get at the imprisoned tumor." It could not be too strongly insisted upon that Cesarean section was quite unnecessary. In Mr. Taylor's case the tumor, which he understood contained two or three pints, would certainly have reached above the brim of the pelvis and might have been opened there possibly without much difficulty. But in any case, by enlarging the incision (and it was surprising through how small an incision the pregnant uterus would pass, if taken out one cornu first), the tumor could have been easily dealt with, and then forceps could have been applied and the uterus returned. The vaginal operation appeared to him (while having some slight advantages alluded to by Mr. Taylor) to be on the whole inferior, in that it made a wound in the vagina, but did not permit inspection of the other ovary nor allow of such careful treatment of adhesions or of the pedicle. Mr. Taylor had himself found difficulty in dealing with the pedicle, in that he had tied it by encircling it with a ligature, applied beyond a pair of forceps, and had to cut the ligature short by the sense of touch. This appeared to him to be not free from danger of slipping of the ligature.

Cases had been recorded of slipping of the ligature, and such cases showed the necessity of careful separate ligation of the ovarian vessels in the pedicle in cases of ovariotomy during pregnancy, which could only be satisfactorily performed by the abdominal operation.

Dr. Heywood Smith said that about seventeen or eighteen years ago he had a similar case under his care; he tapped the ovarian cyst per vaginam and delivered the woman. It was not till she was between three and four months pregnant again that she presented herself. He then did ovariotomy during the pregnancy; the patient did well, went her full term, and subsequently had other children.

Dr. Handfield-Jones recorded two cases of suppurating dermoid tumor which had obstructed delivery at full term. In both cases he had thought it best to open the abdomen and remove the tumors by the abdominal route. While performing these operations he had been struck by the difficulty which would have been encountered if he had endeavored to effect the removal by the vaginal route, for in both these instances the upper wall of the tumor had been densely adherent to coils of small intestine, and great risk of tearing the bowel would have arisen if an attempt had been made to withdraw the growth through an opening in the vagina. The plan of removing the tumor by the abdominal route, and then replacing the pregnant uterus and effecting delivery by the natural passages, commended itself to him as by far the safest and most scientific procedure. He thought that Mr. Taylor was to be congratulated equally on the success of his operation and the good luck which had attended it.

MR. TAYLOR, in reply, said that. while acknowledging the good fortune for which every surgeon should be grateful, he wished the Fellows to understand that the operation was deliberately chosen and that this choice was made in consequence of an experience of vaginal celiotomy, extending now over some nine or ten years, during which he had repeatedly removed small ovarian cysts, diseased tubes. small dermoid tumors, and extra-uterine pregnancies by the vaginal method.

As experience widened. one could generally judge what cases were suitable for vaginal section. and it was only in the minority of cases (possibly some five per cent) that an operation begun by the vaginal had to be finished by the abdominal route. Even when this was necessary he had found that the additional vaginal opening was no disadvantage. being often exceedingly useful for drainage. The chief difficulty of the vaginal operation was undoubtedly the comfortable securing of the pedicle, but (as a previous speaker had already stated) the surgeon could leave a pair of forceps on the stump, if necessary, with perfect safety. In addition the open method of treating the vaginal wound (with an iodoform-gauze drain) precluded the possibility of any serious hemorrhage occurring without the immediate knowledge of those in attendance.

As Dr. Spencer was describing his case—requiring a large abdominal incision, eventration of the pregnant uterus, and delivery of the child while the uterus was still outside of the abdomen—he could not help unfavorably contrasting the operation as described with the simple, direct. and comparatively easy method employed in his own case. Moreover, in his own case the patient recovered with no abdominal wound or cicatrix. In the other operation a large wound was made, and if this was closed hurriedly (a proceeding almost unavoidable under bad surroundings) a hernia of the cicatrix was extremely likely to develop later on.

Mr. Taylor said he would in no case use simple puncture or aspiration by the vagina. The danger of fouling the peritoneum by oozing from a pus sac or dermoid cyst contraindicated this practice, and in every case that recovered an operation had to be done later.

The method described to-night. Mr. Taylor believed, formed a legitimate and very useful extension of operative practice, which in suitable cases satisfied the requirements of good surgery much better than the more usual method of operation by abdominal incision.

REVIEWS.

THE PRINCIPLES AND PRACTICE OF GYNECOLOGY. For Students
and Practitioners. By E. C. DUDLEY, A.M., M.D., Professor
of Gynecology, Northwestern University Medical School;
Gynecologist to St. Luke's and Wesley Hospitals, Chicago;
Fellow of the American Gynecological Society, etc. Third
edition. Pp. 760. With 474 illustrations and 22 full-page
plates. Philadelphia and New York: Lea Brothers & Co.,
1902.

The more prominent factors leading to the success of the first
edition of Dr. Dudley's book were its straightforward, practical
style and the feeling, that grew on one as he read through its
pages, that it was the product of experience and a ripe judgment
that could safely be depended upon. These characteristics have
grown more pronounced in each succeeding edition. In the
present volume the general arrangement on pathological lines
has been retained. The subjects everywhere have been recast
and condensed. Many of the most important chapters have
been to a great extent rewritten. Everywhere throughout the
work etiology, pathology, symptomatology, physical signs, diagnosis, and differential diagnosis have been taken out of the para-
graph form, rewritten and arranged in tables and parallel columns. Many illustrations have been replaced by new ones, and
a large number of manipulations have been illustrated by new
drawings showing the procedure step by step. All of these
changes greatly increase the value of the work both for study and
for reference.

THE SURGERY OF THE RECTUM. By CHARLES B. KELSEY, A.M.,
M.D., late Professor of Pelvic and Abdominal Surgery at the
New York Post-Graduate Hospital; Professor of Rectal Sur-
gery at the University of Vermont, etc. Sixth edition. Pp.
402. With 215 illustrations. New York: William Wood &
Co., 1902.

Twenty-five years of experience and the desire that the work
shall embody all recent scientific advances have led the author
to entirely rewrite this the sixth edition of his book. He has
produced a concise, practical manual, and, while retaining those
qualities which have led to success in former editions, has eliminated much matter now out of date. In the years since the
first edition appeared the surgery of the rectum has grown and
widened, until now it reaches out to take in much that was exclusively in the province of the skilled gynecologist, and it
becomes evident that the line of division between the rectal
specialist and the abdominal and pelvic surgeon has become

broad and vague almost to the point of vanishing. Therefore
we commend the study of the subject to the gynecologist as well
as to him who would call himself a rectal specialist.

THE MEDICAL STUDENT'S MANUAL OF CHEMISTRY. By R. A.
WITTHAUS, A.M., M.D., Professor of Chemistry, Physics, and
Toxicology in Cornell University Medical College in New
York, etc. *Fifth edition.* Pp. 675. New York: William
Wood & Co., 1902.

This edition bears the marks of a very thorough revision.
The introductory section on chemical physics has been somewhat
extended, while the section on mineral chemistry has been condensed to a minimum and the philosophy and broad principles
of the science have been considered rather than the details of
isolated facts. The section on organic chemistry has been in
great part rewritten and somewhat extended. Physiological
chemistry has been given a section by itself, as its importance in
the medical curriculum undoubtedly demands. The section on
laboratory technique, contained in former editions, has wisely
been omitted.

KIRKE'S HANDBOOK OF PHYSIOLOGY. *Seventeenth American
edition.* Revised by WM. H. ROCKWELL, JR., M.D., and
CHARLES L. DANA, A.M., M.D., Professor of Diseases of the
Nervous System, Cornell University Medical College. New
York: Physician to Bellevue Hospital; Neurologist to the
Montefiore Home. Pp. 854. With 516 illustrations in black
and color. New York: William Wood & Co., 1902.

Old wine needs no bush and a seventeenth edition no introduction. The revision leading to this edition was necessary mainly
because of recent progress in physiological chemistry. The
greatest changes are noticed in the chapters on the chemical
composition of the body, on food and digestion, on metabolism
and diet, and on the blood.

THE DISEASES OF INFANCY AND CHILDHOOD. Designed for the
use of Students and Practitioners of Medicine. By HENRY
KOPLIK, M.D., Attending Physician to the Mt. Sinai Hospital,
etc. Pp. 650. With 169 illustrations in text and 30 plates
in color. New York and Philadelphia: Lea Brothers & Co.,
1902.

While based primarily upon the author's own large experience,
this book has been produced in an endeavor to unify and present
in convenient form the world's best in pediatric science. American, English, French, German, and Italian practice is fully
represented. Careful judgment has been shown throughout in
deciding between divergent views, and the ultimate result has
been the production of a well-digested, practical, and safe text
book, encyclopedic in scope. The illustrations are well chosen
and instructive, the type and presswork excellent.

THE THEORY AND PRACTICE OF INFANT FEEDING: With Notes on Development. By HENRY DWIGHT CHAPIN, A.M., M.D., Professor of Diseases of Children at the New York Post-Graduate Medical School and Hospital, etc. Pp. 326. With 97 illustrations. New York: William Wood & Co., 1902.

Dr. Chapin has produced a most acceptable book and one that will appeal not alone to the physician, but to sanitarians, dairymen, and intelligent mothers. It is essentially an exposition of the most advanced theory and practice of producing and using milk. The style is so simple and clear that any mind of ordinary intelligence should grasp the author's meaning.

The book is divided into four parts. Part I. includes a statement of the object and processes of digestion, of its chemical changes, of the processes by which the digested food is built into living tissue, of the excretion of waste and dead material, and of how and why the milk of various animals differs in its chemical and physiological properties. Part II. is devoted to the consideration of cow's milk, including its chemistry, bacteriology, preservation, marketing, and testing. There are also valuable chapters on cereal and vegetable foods and on meat and eggs. Part III., on the feeding of infants, contains most excellent and practical chapters on the selection and preparation of foods, and is the logical sequence of all the preceding sections. Part IV. is on the proper growth and development of infants.

We can safely say that the book should be in the hands of every one interested in the production and selling of milk and in the feeding of infants. Personally we have long used the methods of feeding recommended by the author, and we find them the simplest, most practical, and most successful.

PROGRESSIVE MEDICINE. A Quarterly Digest of Advances, Discoveries, and Improvements in the Medical and Surgical Sciences. Edited by HOBART AMORY HARE, M.D., Professor of Therapeutics in the Jefferson Medical College of Philadelphia, etc., assisted by H. R. M. LANDIS, M.D., Assistant Physician to the Out-Patient Department of the Jefferson Medical College Hospital. Vol. III., September, 1902. Philadelphia and New York: Lea Brothers & Co., 1902.

This volume includes the periscope on diseases of the thorax and its viscera, by William Ewart; on dermatology and syphilis, by William S. Gottheil; on diseases of the nervous system, by William G. Spiller; and on obstetrics, by Richard C. Norris.

A PHYSICIAN'S PRACTICAL GYNECOLOGY. By W. O. HENRY, M.D., Professor of Gynecology in the Creighton Medical College, Omaha, Neb. Pp. 226. With 5 plates and 61 illustrations in the text. Lincoln, Neb.: The Review Press, 1902.

This is a brief of the essentials in gynecology, intended to aid the general practitioner in treating simple cases and in quickly recognizing those conditions that demand the early attention of the specialist.

Transactions of the American Association of Obstetricians and Gynecologists. Vol. XIV. Pp. 368. Philadelphia: Wm. J. Dornan, Printer. 1902.

This volume contains the papers and discussions brought before this distinguished society at its fourteenth annual meeting, held at Cleveland, Ohio, in September, 1901. An abstract of the discussion and nearly all of the papers have appeared in this Journal.

A Brief of Necroscopy and Its Medico-Legal Relation. Arranged by Gustav Schmitt. Milwaukee. Pp. 186.

This vest-pocket volume supplies in brief form the practical facts connected with the study, diagnosis, technique, and medico-legal aspects of a postmortem examination, and will be found a useful companion when one is suddenly called upon and has no time to consult the larger works on this important subject.

BRIEF OF CURRENT LITERATURE.

OBSTETRICS.

Repeated Extrauterine Pregnancy.—Philipowicz (*Wien. klin. Woch.*, No. 13) puts on record another instance of a second extra-uterine pregnancy in the same patient. At the first operation, only the fetus and placenta were removed, the sac being very adherent. At the time of the second operation, by which the other gravid tube was excised, these adhesions had entirely disappeared.

Typhoid Fever at Term of Pregnancy.—E. Leleux (*Jour. des Sciences méd. de Lille*, Aug. 9) gives the history of a case of typhoid fever the prodromal symptoms of which came on about two weeks before labor. After labor the temperature rose from 37.6° C. to 39.6° C. The course of the disease was very mild and the puerperium absolutely normal. The diagnosis was confirmed by the Widal reaction. The patient insisted upon leaving the hospital when the symptoms diminished, and was out of her house on the seventeenth day after labor and the time of invasion of the typhoid fever.

Placenta Previa.—Franklin A. Dorman (*Med. Record*, Aug. 30) bases a paper on placenta previa upon the statistics of over 11,000 cases at the Sloane Maternity Hospital. These included 84 cases of placenta previa, or one in 133⅓ deliveries. As factors in the causation of the condition he includes any condition which would interfere with the fixation of the ovum in the uterus, such as relaxation and subinvolution of the uterus and endometritis. The causes mentioned as predisposing to such pathological states of the uterus are age, multiparity, chronic congestion from cardiac or renal disease, traumatism during de-

livery, and new growths. In the cases reviewed the ratio of
multiparæ to primiparæ is four to one, and one-half were over
30 years of age; five had albuminuria; one, fibroids. The first
symptom may be sudden severe hemorrhage independent of
exertion, but is usually slight at first, recurring, and rarely
appears before the sixth month. In three cases, however, bleeding occurred during the second month, and in five as early as the
fifth. Hemorrhage may be continuous and slight. In 50 per
cent of the cases reported the bleeding was moderate at first and
gradually increased; in 10 per cent it began moderately after
the onset of labor; in 40 per cent sudden flooding, though one-
third of these had had slight premonitory bleeding. A history
of over-exertion could rarely be obtained. In two it began while
straining at stool; in one, on rising in the morning; twice, after
vaginal examination. Diagnosis depends upon the history and
vaginal examination. The placenta is rarely felt by abdominal
palpation. In vaginal examination the intervening placenta
may make palpation of the presenting part difficult. A high-
riding head or malposition is suggestive. A patent cervix will
allow detection of a stringy or boggy tissue over the os. The
cervix is often thick and soft. Little importance is attached to
pulsation in the cervix or a bruit over the lower uterine segment.
The cases reported show a mortality of 12 per cent. Of the 10
deaths, 4 were moribund on admission; in 3 death resulted from
rupture of the uterus; 2 died of sepsis, one after rupture of the
uterus; in one there was eclampsia. Of the children, 45 per
cent were stillborn, 2 per cent of these being dead *in utero* on
admission; 12 per cent died within two weeks. The frequency
of malpresentations and malpositions is shown by the occurrence
in the 84 cases of 10 breech, 18 transverse, and 1 face. Prolapse
of the cord took place in 26 per cent. In 13 per cent the placenta
was adherent. Postpartum hemorrhage is common, from uterine
atony due to severe anemia, from cervical lacerations or tears
of the lower uterine segment. Diminished resistance on account
of anemia often favors sepsis. Expectant treatment is permis-
sible only before the seventh month, the period of viability of the
fetus. Cases are almost never fatal before that time. Labor
may be induced by a tight vaginal tampon; by a bougie if the
placenta does not entirely cover the os; but best by the Champetier de Ribes balloon, which is a perfect tampon and good
uterine stimulant. The patient must never be left until delivered, as a fatal hemorrhage might occur. If the cervix is partly
dilated a foot may be brought down and the half-breech used to
tampon the cervix by a podalic or pelvic version by the external or bipolar method. After performing the version the membranes are ruptured or the placenta quickly bored through and
a foot brought down. If the cervix is sufficiently dilated or
dilatable, a podalic version should be done by a hand *in utero*,
labor terminating naturally or by breech extraction or intermittent traction on the leg. Treatment for hemorrhage and

shock must be energetic, including intravenous infusion. Post-partum hemorrhage should be prevented by a hot intrauterine douche and controlled; if this fails, by prompt tamponade of the uterus. Shock demands free stimulation, heat externally, elevation of the foot of the bed, hot saline enemata, hypodermoclysis or saline intravenous infusion. For anemia a saline enema of one pint is given every two hours until the bulk of the blood is. restored. Fluid diet is given as soon as the stomach permits, and this is increased to a liberal diet as soon as possible. Iron is given early. From the statistics the following conclusions are' formed: that uterine relaxation and endometritis as important etiological factors are well shown; that the immense variation in the types of bleeding should warn us to look upon every bleeding at any time in pregnancy with suspicion; that the very great possibility of sepsis should cause us to employ every precaution in asepsis. The necessity for exceptional care during the breech extraction, where the cervix is not completely dilated, is apparent. The cervix in this condition is unusually vascular and soft, and tears with fatal readiness. The 4 cases of uterine rupture occurred in attempts to save the child. Moderation in the use of saline infusions is necessary, as too great dilution of the blood decreases its clotting power. Repeated small infusions are preferable. The low mortality for Cesarean section suggests its applicability to placenta previa cases.

Massage and Exercise in the Puerperium.—C. S. Bacon (*Jour. Am. Med. Assoc.*, Aug. 16) advocates the more general use of massage and exercise during the puerperium. Massage of the whole body by friction is an excellent stimulant to the general circulation and a valuable sedative. General massage with deep manipulations is a powerful circulatory stimulant and keeps up the vascular tonicity. Massage of the abdomen aids uterine contractions and stimulates intestinal peristalsis. Exercise should begin on the third day after labor, at first the extremities, and by the ninth day he has the patient flex the thighs upon the abdomen. He next has the patient flex the whole body upon the thighs. Many patients are unable to do this movement at first: it should not be attempted before the twelfth day. Bacon allows the patients to walk before he allows them to sit. They walk for two or three minutes, three or four times a day. He has his patients walking several days before they sit. As a rule a patient begins to walk on the tenth to the twelfth day.

Deciduoma Malignum.—Herbert Snow (*Brit. Gyn. Jour.,* Aug.) believes that the term "deciduoma malignum" is misleading and unscientific; that, so far, no valid evidence of the generation of malignant growths from the placental structures, whether decidual or chorionic, has yet been adduced; that the lesions described under the above title do not differ, microscopically or clinically, from the ordinary malignant diseases of the uterus.

Accidental Hemorrhage.—W. Frank Colclough (*Jour. Obst.*

and Gyn. Br. Emp., Aug.) states that rupture of the membranes is only safe when the uterus is contracting vigorously and is capable of keeping up the necessary rhythmical contractions to prevent hemorrhage. In all severe cases the danger is due to the fact that the uterus is incapable of contracting down upon its contents. The objection that plugging the vagina converts an external hemorrhage into a concealed is only valid if the uterine walls are incapable, directly or indirectly, of withstanding a pressure within them equal to the arterial pressure. If the uterine walls are so diseased that they distend as the result of intrauterine pressure, then it is claimed that the plug and binder, applied in the proper manner, render the uterus capable of withstanding the pressure of the escaping blood. The plug and binder control hemorrhage, and opportunity is given to the patient to rally, if possible. They delay the rupture of the membranes by supporting the cervix and the dilating os when dilatation commences. Delivery will be natural, for it will not take place until the uterus contracts with sufficient vigor to expel its contents. The risk of postpartum hemorrhage is done away with.

When Labor Begins.—George P. Shears *(Med. Rec.,* Aug. 23) believes the statement made in many text books that the cervix maintains its entire length during pregnancy is incorrect. The canal of the cervix does not remain closed until the beginning of labor. Usually in multiparæ, and occasionally in primiparæ, the canal, including the internal os, is dilated, to the extent of admitting one or two fingers, two or three weeks before labor begins. Dilatation of the external or internal os or of the cervical canal is not, *per se*, an indication of the beginning of labor. Dilatation of the clinical internal os, or ring of Müller, in such a manner that it begins to form a part of the uterine cavity, is at once the anatomical commencement and the diagnostic sign of true labor. Dilatation at this point is the final result of uterine distension and consequent cervical eversion. Dilatation at this point, owing to the greater resistance offered, by its effect upon the cervical ganglion and the consequent reflex awakening of effectual uterine contractions, is the physiological cause of labor.

Pregnancy after the Menopause.—Reginald G. Hann *(Jour. Obst. and Gyn. Br. Emp.,* Sept.) cites a case of pregnancy occurring in a woman 49 years old. The woman at 46 stopped menstruating and had the usual symptoms of the menopause and all sexual feeling was lost. Shortly after the last child was born the menstrual periods appeared and the sexual desire came back.

Labor in Tabes Dorsalis.—R. P. Ranken Lyle *(Jour. Obst. and Gyn. Br. Emp.,* Sept.) reports a case of pregnancy and labor in a patient with tabes dorsalis. The first intimation the patient had of her approaching confinement was the rupture of the membranes. Labor came on and was perfectly painless. The

placenta was easily expressed, and the uterus contracted normally, but with pain. Puerperium was normal. The patient
gave a history of having been pregnant nine times before, and
the previous labor was similar in every respect to the one cited
above.

Pelvic Obstruction by Fibromyomata.—T. Arthur Helme
(*Jour. Obst. and Gyn. Br. Emp.*, Sept.) reports two cases upon
which he operated for fibroid obstructing the pelvis. In one
case the woman was four months pregnant, and the fibroid was
low down in the pelvis and obstructed the vagina and caused
marked urinary troubles. Total hysterectomy was performed
with good results. In the other case the fibroids caused less
trouble, but on account of their size and position it was thought
advisable to remove the entire uterus, which was three months
pregnant. He also reports another case of fibroids complicating
pregnancy. In this case he induced abortion, which was followed by an intestino-uterine fistula. Subsequently an abscess
formed in the left iliac region and the uterine fistula closed.
The patient died some months later from the effects of this
fistula. Helme believes this case would have been saved if he
had removed the uterus instead of inducing abortion.

GYNECOLOGY AND ABDOMINAL SURGERY.

Treatment of Vaginismus.—For obstinate cases of vaginismus
Tavel (*Rev. de Chir.*, No. 2) resects the internal pudic nerve.
This is reached on each side by an antero-posterior incision in
the corresponding ischio-rectal fossa midway between the tuber-
osity of the ischium and the outer margin of the anus. The
nerve is located by the pulsation of the accompanying artery,
and is traced backward, freed from the artery, and divided. The
peripheral portion is then twisted out.

Spontaneous Healing of Wound of Ureter.—In puncturing
through the vagina a collection of pus in the pelvis, or in enlarging this opening to facilitate drainage, C. Jacobs (*Bull. de la
Soc. Belge de Gyn. et d'Obst.*, t. xiii., No. 1) injured the ureter,
as was made evident on the fourth day by a discharge of urine
through the wound. This lasted for nearly three weeks. Within
two months the vaginal wound had closed completely.

Results of Credé's Prophylaxis for Gonorrheal Ophthalmia.
—The unfavorable report of Hirsch concerning the results obtained in a number of the public maternity hospitals of Berlin induced Ernst Runge (*Berl. klin. Woch.*, No. 20) to publish those of
the Göttingen Clinic, which show a total of 1.917 cases in which
prophylactic instillations of silver nitrate solution were employed. No early, and only three late, infections were observed.
In these late cases it was not at all impossible that infection
might have occurred after birth. In the first 1,000 a two per
cent solution was employed and only one late infection was
recorded. In order to avoid the inflammatory reaction following

the use of this solution, one of one per cent was employed in the later 917 cases, and this yielded equally satisfactory results as far as early infection is concerned.

Post-operative Temperatures in Anemic Cases.—J. Henrotay *(Bull. de la Soc. Belge de Gyn. et d'Obst.,* t. xiii., No. 1) calls attention to the occurrence of irregular febrile temperatures in three anemic cases. The first was a vaginal hysterectomy for chronic uterine inversion following labor, the patient being profoundly anemic. During the entire convalescence the temperature ranged from 38° C. to 39.3° C., and the pulse from 112 to 128, but with no other symptoms—no signs of local or peritoneal sepsis or of tuberculosis, lochia odorless. The second was a vaginal hysterectomy for uterine fibroids causing severe hemorrhage. The post-operative temperature lasted eleven days. Antistreptococcic serum was given twice, the second time just before the fever began to diminish. The third was a case of removal of a portion of retained placenta which had caused serious bleeding for three weeks after delivery. The elevations of temperature occurred only during a few days after this operation. In no case could the existence of infection be proved, but the writer believes that in all operative cases a certain amount of absorption must occur, and while probably under normal conditions the natural constituents of the blood would overcome the tendency of such absorbed substances to affect the body temperature, in anemic cases the resisting power would be diminished.

Visual Examination of Abdominal Cavity with Illumination Through Vaginal Incision.—D. v. Ott *(Cent. f. Gyn.,* No. 31) places the patient in the Trendelenburg position after having made the colpotomy incision. Anterior and posterior vaginal specula retract the vaginal walls, and an electric light, with handle curved to fit within the curved surface of the anterior instrument, is introduced and illuminates the abdominal cavity, the intestines having gravitated to the upper portion. By pulling up the anterior abdominal wall by means of forceps, even the transverse colon, cecum, appendix, spleen, and lower surface of liver and gall bladder may be seen in some cases. The paper is clearly illustrated.

Primary Carcinoma of the Urethra in Women.—Hiram N. Vineberg *(Ann. of Surg.,* July) reports a case of primary flat-celled carcinoma of the urethra upon which he operated. Up to the time the case was reported there had been no recurrence, but the patient suffered from incontinence of urine due to the necessity of removing a portion of the vesical sphincter. A secondary operation was performed to relieve the incontinence, but it was only temporarily successful. When feasible, total extirpation is the only treatment worth considering. If the disease involves the nests of the bladder it is better to close the bladder below and create a suprapubic fistula.

Hemorrhage into the Spinal Cord.—Alexander Bruce *(Scot.*

Med. and Surg. Jour., Aug.) cites a case of hemorrhage into the spinal cord during pregnancy. The onset of the symptoms occurred at the fifth month of pregnancy with sudden pain in the back and trunk, with paralysis of the lower limbs and trunk muscles; paralytic retention of urine; constipation and great dyspnea; sensation lost below the xiptic sternum; disappearance of deep reflexes after six days and slight reappearance of them ten days later; rapid formation of bed-sores; painless and unconscious birth of twins at the seventh month; death from bronchitis and exhaustion. Postmortem revealed a high degree of thrombosis and dilatation of the vessels in the pia mater on the posterior aspect of the cord. Dorsal region of the cord was soft in consistence. A tubular hemorrhage extended throughout the cord from the sixth cervical to the first lumbar. Angiogliomata appeared throughout the cord and one appeared in the cerebellum. The hemorrhage was due to the angiogliomata, which had existed without giving rise to any marked symptoms.

The Pessary in the Treatment of Displacements of the Uterus.—F. H. Davenport *(Bost. Med. and Surg. Jour.*, Aug. 7) advises operation in uncomplicated cases in young women who have not had treatment. In other cases, especially where the uterus is small, where symptoms have been present but a short time, and particularly if they are associated with neurasthenia, treatment by pessary will often result in a cure. In such selected cases cure may be expected in about one-half. Even in cases where cure is not expected the pessary will relieve the symptoms and aid in restoring the general health. A patient wearing a pessary should be kept under observation and seen at regular intervals, preferably after each menstrual period.

Stricture of the Ureter.—Howard A. Kelly *(Jour. Am. Med. Assoc.*, Aug. 16), recapitulating the methods of treatment for this condition, gives the following: 1. Dilatation of the stricture by flexible or metal catheters in a graduated series, up to four or five millimetres in diameter; this is the ideal method. 2. Freeing the ureter from a bed of inflammatory tissue by dissecting it out; this is occasionally sufficient. 3. Resection of the ureter; this is rarely possible. 4. Extirpation of the entire affected side by a nephro-ureterectomy or a uretero-nephrectomy, or, as Kelly has done in one case, a nephro-uretero-cystectomy; this is the only reliable method in cases of tuberculosis, as well as of pyoureter and pyelonephrosis of long standing. 5. Amputation and implantation of the bladder; this is applicable when the stricture is low down, the opposite side diseased, and the diseased side still capable of doing work. 6. Complete division of the stricture; this plan may be of service when the stricture is unusually tight.

Fibroma of the Ovary.—John S. Fairbairn *(Jour. Obst. and Gyn. Br. Emp.*, Aug.), from a study of recorded cases of seven specimens of fibroma of the ovary which have come under his observation, finds it is possible to recognize three ways in which the growth may involve the ovary: 1. The whole ovary may be converted into a hard tumor, maintaining to some degree its original shape, but leaving no recognizable portion of its original structure. This may take place in small as well as large growths. It is difficult to understand why the pathological change should affect the whole stroma from the first, as this is more like an inflammatory fibrotic change than a new growth. 2. The growth may form a hard tumor within the ovary, which spreads over its outer surface, so that it remains more or less encapsulated within the organ. The amount of ovarian tissue remaining appears to depend rather on the position of the growth in the ovary than on the size to which the growth has attained. This variety appears to be more common than the preceding. 3. The new growth may form a pedunculated tumor attached by a pedicle to the ovary. Some of these may be growths from the ovarian ligament. The age limit for fibroma of the ovary is very wide. In none was the general health affected. Of four cases in which the tumor was large enough to form an abdominal swelling, in only one had it been noticed for any length of time. Pain was present in five of the seven cases, and in three small pelvic tumors were the symptoms which led to examination and detection of the disease. In none of the cases was any affection of the other ovary noticed.

Sarcomatous Enchondroma of the Pelvis.—Robert Jardine *(Jour. Obst. and Gyn. Br. Emp.,* Aug.) cites a case of this variety occurring in a Ipara aged 29. For two years previous to the time the growth was first noticed she had had intermittent pain in the back and thighs. During the third month of pregnancy the pains became worse, and about one month later became edematous and the edema steadily increased. The patient went to the hospital at the seventh month, when the uterus was found free from the growth and the fetus alive. The vagina was completely closed by a hard, globular mass. Cesarean section was performed on the ninth day after admission, but the child was delivered stillborn. Patient died twenty-four hours after the operation. At the autopsy the growth was found extending up to the eleventh rib. Posteriorly and externally it was continuous with the pelvic wall. Inferiorly it has incorporated practically all the ischium, pubis, and the ilium near the acetabulum. No metastatic growths were found.

Pelvic Deformity in New York.—James Clifton Edgar *(Med. Rec.,* Aug. 16) draws his conclusions from measurements upon 1,200 cases. Of these cases, 41.5 per cent were American-born women, 17.9 per cent were Irish, 10.8 per cent Russian, 8.7 per cent German, 2.5 per cent black, etc. Contracted pelves occurred in 44 cases; generally contracted pelves in 30 cases, once in 40; flattened pelves once in 85.71 cases. Twenty of the cases of pelvic contraction were American-born. Three of the con-tracted pelves occurred in black women. Special or irregular

36

forms of pelvic contraction, as osteomalacia, obliquely contracted. coxalgic, double coxalgic, spondylolisthetic, and kyphotic, fractured pelvis, are infrequent in this country. The generally contracted pelvis is the most frequent deformity met with in New York. Edgar found twice as many generally contracted as flattened pelves in his material. Private cases in New York over a period of ten years show a somewhat higher percentage than the results obtained from the 1,200 hospital cases, namely, about 5 per cent for all deformities.

Cancer of the Clitoris.—Charles E. Congdon *(Buff. Med. Jour.*, Sept.) reports a case of primary cancer of the clitoris occurring in a woman aged 60. The growth was freely removed and there has been no recurrence at the end of eleven months.

X-Ray in Cancer of the Uterus.—E. Sturer *(Cin. Lancet-Clinic,* Aug. 16) has obtained amelioration of symptoms in an advanced case of cancer of the uterus. There was arrest of the sloughing of the growth. The pain was greatly relieved and the patient gained weight. The treatment was applied daily.

Actinomycosis of the Ovary.—D. Berry Hart *(Jour. Obst. and Gyn. Br. Emp.*, Sept.) reports a case of actinomycosis of the ovary and pelvic connective tissue. The diagnosis was not made until after death, but it was thought probable that it was tubercular in character. At autopsy there were found chronic adhesions of the pelvic viscera, erosion and perforation of the rectum, septic thrombosis of the pelvic veins, and a pint of recent blood clot in the bladder. The left ovary was soft and apparently suppurative. The actinomycosis bovis was found in the ovary.

Retroperitoneal Lipoma.—Alban Doran *(Jour. Obst. and Gyn. Br. Emp.*, Sept.) removed a retroperitoneal lipoma weighing thirteen pounds twelve ounces from a woman 47 years old. Complete suppression of urine occurred and the patient died thirty-eight hours after the operation.

DISEASES OF CHILDREN.

The Artificial Feeding of Infants.—A. D. Blackader *(Montreal Med. Jour.*, July, 1902) emphasizes the following practical points: An infant fed at the breast, who suffers persistent indigestion and at the same time fails to gain in weight, should be taken from that breast. If, however, the infant gains in weight, it is better to try and correct the indigestion by treatment directed to both mother and child. To attempt artificial feeding in such a case often only adds to our troubles. In commencing artificial feeding, begin with a weak mixture and work up by frequent but slight changes to a point of tolerance. By still continuing a gradual but steady increase, never beyond the point of easy digestibility, we can in a few weeks attain to a food sufficiently nutritious in all its ingredients and yet fully digestible and assimilable. It is a serious mistake to begin on a mixture too strong, and work down, after weeks of indigestion. to the point of tolerance. The question how long an infant should be kept on a modified-milk diet is an important one. It is generally conceded that by the tenth or twelfth month a child should be able to digest almost pure milk. By this time, however, the author prefers a mixed dietary. Milk is very deficient in iron. An infant comes into the world with a high percentage of hemoglobin; this gradually diminishes so long as he is fed on milk alone. Only when a mixed diet is substituted for a pure milk diet does the percentage begin to rise again. Cereals and meat juice and broths are rich in iron. Oatmeal is among the richest in iron of the cereals, and, properly cooked, forms a useful addition to the infant's dietary. Shortly after the first twelve months, eggs, lightly cooked, may be permitted at one of the meals in the day. The great richness of the yolk in fat. lime salts, and in the organic compounds of phosphorus and iron, makes it a valuable food for the rapidly developing child. At this period, also, food involving somewhat long mastication, such as biscuits and crusts of bread, becomes necessary. The process of mastication develops the maxillary bones and the associated muscles, while disuse of the jaws starves the area supplied by the maxillary arteries, leading to their imperfect development. The bone remains small, the teeth are crowded and imperfectly nourished, and dental caries, so disastrous to the growing child, becomes inevitable.

Chronic Hypertrophy of the Faucial and Pharyngeal Lymphoid or Adenoid Tissues.—F. Marsh *(Birmingham Med. Rev.,* July, 1902) reports 1,000 cases operated on in three years; 556 of the patients were females, 444 were males; 816 were under and 184 were over 16 years of age. The youngest patient was 14 weeks old and the oldest 36 years. One-third of the 816 cases occurred in the fourth, fifth, sixth, and seventh years, the greatest number being in the fifth. Enlarged tonsils may be arranged in three groups: (1) where the hypertrophy is chiefly in the horizontal diameter—the projecting tonsil; (2) where it is chiefly in the vertical diameter—the elongated tonsil; and (3) where it is chiefly in the antero-posterior diameter—the broad sessile or flat tonsil. These types often approach each other. and are found in combination. The symptoms caused by enlarged tonsils are (1) obstructive, (2) catarrhal, (3) reflex. *Obstructive symptoms* may be due to mechanical interference, the child being able to swallow only fluids, and those with difficulty in severe cases. Buccal respiration is often impeded and the voice is thick and indistinct. In some cases the palate is pressed upward to such an extent that the action of the palatotubal muscles is impeded and deafness results from imperfect middle-ear aëration. *Catarrhal symptoms*—The crypts and recesses are suitable places for the lodgment of the catarrh microbe. The catarrh may either keep localized, causing tonsillitis, or extend to adenoids, causing adenoiditis, and from there to the middle ear or the nasal cavities, or downward to the organs of respiration and digestion. Owing to absorption of toxin generated by the catarrh microbe, or the passage of the microbe itself through the lymphatics, the lymphatic glands corresponding to the tonsils often become inflamed and enlarged. Tonsillotomy prevents these attacks, and, if promptly done at the outset, may arrest the progress toward suppuration. They are often termed tuberculous—that they are not so is usually due to treatment directed to the tonsils, not to the glands themselves. *Reflex symptoms*—The only reflex symptom to be attributed to enlarged tonsils is a short, dry, hacking cough, which may be almost constant or else spasmodic.

Operative treatment is necessary when the tonsils are so large that they mechanically cause some obstructive symptom, even if otherwise healthy; when they are the centres for frequent or prolonged catarrhal attacks or acute inflammatory attacks; when they are the cause of lymphadenitis; when the crypts and recesses are filled with caseating secretion which does not yield to treatment; when they are the probable cause of a troublesome reflex cough. The author uses Mackenzie's spade guillotine. The first step in its use is the proper engagement of the tonsil, and here care must be taken to first encircle the lower edge; the second step is to press firmly the guillotine outward; and the third to press sharply home the blade with the thumb. The causes of inefficient removal or failure are due generally to a non-recognition of the first two movements and to the use of too large a guillotine, or, more rarely, to adhesions between the tonsils and the pillars of the fauces preventing proper engagement with the guillotine. The treatment after operation is simple, its essentials being: (1) avoidance of exertion immediately afterward (a fertile cause of recurrent hemorrhage); (2) an equable temperature during the healing process, to prevent catarrhal attacks; (3) suitable diet; (4) the use of a cleansing wash.

Congenital Dislocation of Hips.—Edward H. Ochsner *(Ann. of Surgery,* August, 1902) describes the "bloodless functional weight method" of Lorenz. Reduction is accomplished by traction on the affected limb. In small children manual traction may suffice. The first important condition required is general anesthesia pushed to complete relaxation of the muscles. This accomplished, the pelvis is held firmly while even, continuous, steady traction is applied to the limb, grasping it either a little above the ankle or a little above the knee. The pulling must continue until the upper border of the great trochanter is well down to the level of Nélaton's line. In older children a tackle and windlass arrangement becomes necessary, unless one has several well-trained assistants, and even then it is to be preferred, as the amount of force applied can be more accurately gauged. The perineum is placed against a firm, well-padded support, for which purpose an inflated Barnes' bag is most satisfactory. A piece of cotton is now placed about the limb just above the ankle, and a skein of wool is tied about this with a surgical knot, so as to avoid constriction and impairment of circulation. The skein of wool is then fastened to one of the pulleys of the pulley and tackle arrangement, while the other pulley is fastened to spring scales and the scales to a fixed point in the room. The rope is fastened to the windlass, and this is now slowly set in motion. The scales are read every half-minute by one assistant, while another announces the frequency and character of the pulse every two minutes, and oftener if there is a sudden change. If the reduction is very difficult it is necessary to interrupt the traction at intervals not to exceed ten minutes. As soon as the upper border of the great trochanter is well down to Nélaton's line we may proceed to the next step, that of placing the head into the acetabulum. This is often the most difficult part of the procedure, and upon its accomplishment depends the future of the case. The chief causes of failure seem to be: (1) the shortening of the adductor muscles; (2) hourglass constriction of the capsule; (3) adhesions of the anterior portion of the capsule to the rim of the acetabulum. The first naturally interferes with abduction, which is so necessary in making the head slip over the posterior rim of the acetabulum. This difficulty is usually overcome by steady moulding manipulations. Sudden jerks must be avoided. As soon as the right degree of abduction has once been accomplished the pelvis is steadied by an assistant, the thigh is flexed to a right angle and rotated inwardly slightly. While one hand of the operator presses on the trochanter, the other hand makes strong, steady traction forward, and at the same time attempts slow abduction. The head slowly creeps up over the posterior border of the acetabulum, and suddenly slips over the rim, bounds into the acetabulum with a distinct thud which sometimes can be heard at a considerable distance, and a vibration of the patient's body which is always transmitted to the operator, and sometimes even to the table and to those who may be in contact with it. The other symptoms of an accomplished reposition are: distinct lengthening of the thigh; the development of a fulness in the groin, and the disappearance of the head on the posterior surface of the ilium, and the sudden tenseness of the hamstring tendons characterized by inability to extend the knee. The object of the inward rotation is to overcome the second and third great difficulties—namely, to loosen the capsule from the rim of the acetabulum and to utilize the head of the femur as a wedge to open up the hourglass constriction in the capsule. Reposition having been accomplished, every effort must be made to render it stable. This is secured, first, by a boring motion—the thigh is rotated outward, and with a boring motion the anterior capsule is stretched and the acetabulum deepened; second, the tense pelvifemoral and pelvicrural muscles will help to deepen and enlarge the acetabulum; and finally, third, the weight of the body in walking will greatly aid the formation of a satisfactory joint in removing the deposits in the acetabulum and securing the development of a broad cotyloid ligament. In order to fully utilize this important principle, a cast must be very carefully applied, over a pair of tightly-fitting wool trousers, including the whole thigh and the trunk to the level of the navel. In order to avoid backward dislocation until the acetabulum has had a chance to develop, the cast is applied with the thigh slightly over-extended and a degree of abduction sufficiently great to secure against the possibility of the head slipping out of the rudimentary acetabulum. Usually about ninety degrees of abduction are required. The first cast is left in place for from four to five months, when it is removed and the extremity is brought down to about forty-five degrees of abduction with slight flexion. This cast is left in place for about six to seven months, when the child can usually be allowed to go about without any appliances. During most of this time the child has been up and about. This form of ambulating treatment fulfils a threefold purpose: it develops a stable joint, secures normal motion in this joint, and during the entire course of treatment the patient will secure enough exercise to keep in a healthy condition.

Milk Idiosyncrasies in Children.—Louis Fischer (*Jour. Am. Med. Assoc.*, Aug. 2, 1902) says that physicians frequently report an intolerance of milk or its dilutions in children. It has been the milk itself or the component parts of the same that have disagreed in certain children under the treatment of the writer. Breast milk and several changes of wet-nurses gave the same distressing symptoms. Cow's milk was not tolerated and was discontinued after various dilutions. What is known as Keller's malt soup has done good service as a substitute, and is prepared as follows: Take of wheat flour 2 ounces and add to it 11 ounces of milk. Soak the flour thoroughly and rub it through a sieve or strainer. Put into a second dish 20 ounces of water, to which add 3 ounces of malt extract; dissolve the above at a temperature of about 120° F., and then add 2½ drachms of 11 per cent potassium carbonate solution. Finally mix all of the above ingredients and boil. This gives a food containing: albuminoids, 2.0 per cent; fat, 1.2 per cent; carbohydrates, 12.1 per cent. There are in this mixture 0.9 per cent of vegetable proteids. The wheat flour is necessary, as otherwise the malt soup would have a diarrheal tendency. The alkali is added to neutralize the large amount of acid generated in sick children. Biedert emphasizes the importance of giving fat, rather than reducing its quantity, in poorly-nourished children, and cites the assimilability of his cream mixture or of breast milk in underfed children as proof of his assertions. The author has used this malt soup most successfully in the treatment of athrepsia (marasmus) cases in which the children were simply starved.

Empyema in Children.—F. J. Cotton (*Boston Med. and Surg. Jour.*, July 17, 1902) draws the following conclusions from a study of 180 cases: 1. Empyema in children usually follows lobar pneumonia—after a varying interval. 2. The infection is usually with the pneumococcus. 3. Spontaneous cure, even when aided by tapping, is rare. 4. Operation should not be delayed, as time lost is strength lost, and the issue is largely one of nutrition. 5. The best form of operation is in general the subperiosteal resection of an inch of the eighth or ninth rib in the posterior axillary line, the evacuation of pus and fibrin masses, and tube drainage. 6. Irrigation at or after operation is not usually advisable. 7. The routine after-treatment in fresh cases should be tube drainage, the tube being progressively shortened, and removed when the cavity is nearly healed. 8. Where failure to heal seems to depend on failure of the lung to re-expand, treatment by valve or suction apparatus is indicated. This is especially of value in the more chronic cases. 9. The mortality is about one in seven; in small children it is much greater than in those over 5 years. The causes of mortality are, in the main, beyond our control. 10. The great majority of cases heal even when the healing is delayed for many months. Chronic empyema, in the strict sense, is rare in children. 11. The closure of the cavity depends mainly on nutrition and on adequate drainage. 12. Recurrences may occur from faulty drainage at any time, and they may occur years after apparently sound healing, without obvious cause. 13. Deformity of the chest is usually temporary and yields to treatment. 14. Long-continued discharge from the cavity is not infrequently followed by chest deformity and scoliosis of a severer type, permanent and sometimes extremely severe.

Fallacies Concerning Adenoids.—Richmond McKinney (*Memphis Med. Month.*, Aug., 1902) believes in the prevalence of adenoids and in the benefit of operation for their treatment, but he holds that these have been overstated and overrated. Moreover, certain fallacies concerning these growths exist and are continually being asserted. For instance, we are taught that the symptoms to be found are mouth-breathing, noisy respiration, a vaenous expression, distorted facies, etc. Yet many of these cases present practically no facial indications of the existence of such a condition. Frequently cases are overlooked merely because there are no objective indications of the existence of such a condition. The author states an adenoid is not always to be found where there is a purulent rhinitis. The gravest of all affections induced by adenoids are the disorders of the ears. Deafness, which is a predominant symptom among those which we are called upon to relieve, in a young child produces inattention, stupidity, and a general listless state called by Guye *aprosexia*. This condition in young children is one in which the most brilliant results follow the removal of adenoids. Another condition in which the operation is satisfactory is that of the correction of mouth-breathing. But here the author states his conviction that hypertrophied faucial tonsils are also a factor in producing mouth-breathing. Taking out of consideration the relief of ear conditions and mouth-breathing by the removal of adenoids, and the improvement in chest capacity and general physical development following the operation, McKinney holds that there is practically no other functional disorder or pathological state that is commonly benefited by this operation. In this statement he is aware that he is controverting the opinion of some prominent men of the profession. The best results in all cases are obtained in patients from 2 to 5 years of age. We are told that there is a tendency for adenoid growths, as well as hypertrophied faucial tonsils, to atrophy with the approach of puberty. The author holds that if we wait for an adenoid atrophy, which is by no means sure to occur, we are rendering the child liable to ear diseases, arch of the vault of the palate produced by insufficient respiration, poorly developed chest, etc. Another fallacy is to state that where there are hypertrophied faucial tonsils concurrently with a similar condition of the pharyngeal tonsil, removal of the latter will be followed by shrinkage of the former. This has not been the author's experience. To secure good results from operation, thoroughness of removal of the growth is absolutely necessary. Unstinted condemnation should be expressed toward the use of the finger nail alone, as it is not thorough nor aseptic. Nothing is so satisfactory as the Gottstein curette or one of its modifications.

Intussusception.—Francis Huber (*Arch. of Ped.*, July, 1902) says that injections and operative measures are rival methods of treatment. Progressive surgeons, particularly in hospital practice, favor early abdominal section. Injections, including inflation of the bowels with air or distension by hydrostatic pressure, have been advised, first, for the purpose of reducing the invagination; second, with the object of lessening the size of the tumor, and thereby limiting the field and simplifying the subsequent operation. Finally, in occasional cases, the sufferings of the patient are lessened by the use of an enema prior to operation. At present the tendency is to limit the employment of injections to the early stages—that is, not later than twelve to twenty-four hours from the onset of the symptoms. It is recognized that the longer the condition has existed the greater the dangers of pressure from within. If not successful immediately, further attempts ought to be given up and abdominal section resorted to without delay. Edmond Owen emphatically writes: "I deem it nothing less than a calamity that physicians now and then manage to chase back an intussuscepted piece of bowel by using an enema." Whether inflation by air or hydrostatic pressure be preferred, the following objections or disadvantages are apparent: 1. It is impossible to gauge the amount of pressure. 2. Except in the earliest cases, it is not possible to exclude beginning gangrene, which, as shown by the results of operation, may take place very early. 3. The reduction is not always complete. The tumor may disappear, the symptoms abate, to recur again in a few hours. There is always an element of doubt, consequently the procedure has been termed uncertain and dangerous, haphazard and therefore unscientific. When disinvagination has been successful the relief is immediate. The anxious, pallid look disappears and with it the evidences of collapse. The abdomen assumes a normal contour. Sometimes fecal movements and the escape of gas closely follow upon reduction. Relapses are not uncommon. As to subsequent treatment, the patient should be kept absolutely quiet with opium, and an abdominal bandage, just tight enough to steady the bowels, must be applied.

John F. Erdmann (ibid.) is positive that surgical interference is the only treatment when a case has passed the twelve-hour period of duration. In several cases upon which he has operated in which lacerations or ruptures of the serous coat have been found, it has seemed to him that this condition was due to hyperdistension of the bowel by water or air rather than to the distension of the gut by the intussusception. The shock present in many of these cases is not a contraindication to operation, but calls for more rapid work in reduction by surgical means. After the operation the child recovers rapidly from the shock. The operation is a simple one, requiring asepsis and expedition more than anything else during the first twenty-four hours, and rarely, except in the long-standing cases, is excision of the gut required. The position of the incision depends to a degree upon the presence of the tumor, although the author rarely finds it necessary to open except through the right rectus. and usually selects this region for the reason that the final portion of gut to be reduced is usually in the ileo-cecal region. Furthermore, all ordinary manipulations in any part of the abdomen can take place through an enlargement of this incision. In reducing the condition two things for success must be remembered: First, never pull the proximal end with the idea that reduction will be accomplished. This type of manipulation is more productive of tears of the coats of the intestines than it is of producing the end desired. Second, and the most important point to remember, is that reduction is only produced by pressure upon the apex of the mass through the gut at the distal extremity, gently guiding the proximal end. Should adhesions between the entering and the receiving gut prevent the reduction, then the passing of a blunt instrument between these portions is usually attended by success. Recovery can be assured in most cases of less than one day's standing; in cases of two days and more than one the majority recover; in cases of over two and up to three days a fair percentage recover, while in cases of over three days the prognosis is bad. From the literature to date, no case of excision of intestines in children under one year has been successful. The mortality in all cases is from 20 to 50 per cent.

Lobar Pneumonia in Infants.—In relation to the treatment of this affection, William Fitch Cheney (*American Med.*, July 26, 1902) says that it is simple, for the disease is a self-limited one. The main object is to maintain the strength until the affection runs its course. The food must be carefully and regularly administered. If the infant is nursed at the breast, let the breast continue to be used; if on the bottle, let the same food as previously given be continued at regular intervals, but diluted or peptonized if, on account of the high temperature, it is not well digested. For the fever no antipyretic drugs should be used; cold sponging or bathing of the body is far more efficacious and less depressing. For cough, if it is troublesome, or for restlessness and insomnia, Dover's powder is the most useful medicine. For symptoms of prostration, such as a pulse above 150 and tendency to stupor, brandy should be given regularly, in dose of 10 to 30 drops every two hours, well diluted; strychnine in dose of one-four-hundredth to one-two-hundredth grain, according to age, every six or four hours, and atropine in dose of one-two-thousandth to one-seven-hundredth grain at the same intervals. For the collapse that is apt to occur at crisis the best treatment is the hot mustard bath, followed by vigorous rubbing of the surface of the body.   In general it is important to remember the motto of Jacobi: *Nil nocere*—do no harm; for occasionally infants suffer more from their vigorous medication than they do from the disease that called it forth.

Local Variations in the Mortality from Summer Diarrhea.— Henry Dwight Chapin *(Arch. of Ped.,* July, 1902) says that it is certain that the great increase in the number of deaths in New York City in the summer of 1901 cannot be attributed entirely to the milk supply or to the heat, for the heavy mortality was in August, September, and part of October, and not during the excessively hot weather in the latter part of June and early July. In and around New York City there was in the summer of 1901 the greatest number of deaths for ten years, and during the same period the least number of deaths in the country.   During the previous summer there was next to the lowest number of deaths for ten years in the city district, and the greatest number for ten years in the country.   If the primary source of infection was the milk supply, the deaths in the city districts should have shown at least a proportionate increase in the summer of 1900, and the country districts should have had a large number of deaths in 1901.   It is conceded by all that the intense poisoning cases of summer diarrheas are the result of putrefactive changes in the intestinal contents, excessively foul stools accompanying high fever as a rule.   The great source of putrefactive bacteria is the *soil,* which consists of a mixture of decomposing organic matter and earth.   Dust contains great numbers of putrefactive bacteria and spores, and it is from such dust and dirt that milk becomes infected with putrefactive bacteria.   Theoretically we should expect to find a great deal of summer diarrhea in localities where soil rich in decomposing matter is being turned over and dried so that it can be carried by the wind as dust or possibly by flies.   This may account for the occasional infection of breast-fed infants.   With the removal of horse cars and with cleaner streets in Greater New York, the number of deaths from diarrheal diseases had, on the whole, been steadily declining for the past ten years, and at the same time the population had been increasing. In 1901 the Borough of Manhattan was torn up from one end to the other for the purpose of building the subway; water pipes and sewers were opened and changed, and the streets were very dusty. It is certainly a remarkable coincidence that with an unusually small number of deaths from diarrheal diseases in the remaining portion of the State, the steadily declining number of deaths from the same cause in the city district should suddenly increase 58 per cent when the streets were torn up. There can be no doubt that in preventing diarrheal diseases in summer attention must be paid to local conditions as well as to improving the milk supplies.

Purpura Fulminans following Scarlet Fever.—Hubert E. J. Biss *(The Lancet,* Aug. 2, 1902) says that hemorrhagic scarlet fever, as described in some works, is of very great rarity in England at the present time; it is doubtful, indeed, if extensive cutaneous and subcutaneous hemorrhages ever occur in the early stages of the disease; whether the cases related in those works, in fact, were not actually cases of hemorrhagic diphtheria. Hemorrhages into the skin and subcutaneous tissue are met with not very infrequently in association with obstinate suppurative lesions after scarlet fever, such as chronic suppurative lymphadenitis, suppurations in joints, and suppurations in and about the temporal bone. In the case reported by the author no such lesion obtained. The child had a very severe attack of scarlet fever, which did not present any unusual features, and convalescence appeared to be established. He still had some ulceration of the soft palate, but the other symptoms had either passed off or were much abated, the temperature was settling down, and he was bright and comfortable. At this point cutaneous hemorrhages in enormous abundance took place, accompanied by hematemesis, bloody stools, and oozing from the gums. In thirty-six hours from the appearance of the first hemorrhages he was dead. The chief feature of the postmortem examination was the state of the kidneys, which were transformed almost entirely into fat, a little blood clot being found in the calices. The change would appear to have been more in the nature of an acute degeneration than of an inflammation. The sudden occurrence of these widespread hemorrhages suggests a very acute toxemia, a blood infection due to the elaboration of some toxic substance or the supervention of some fresh organism; but what the nature of such body may have been, and what determined its appearance at this period of the disease, are speculations beyond the range of legitimate theorization.

Rheumatism in Children.—A. M. Gossage *(The Clin. Jour.,* July 23, 1902) says that in the treatment of rheumatism in the child we have rather different problems to face than in the adult. Only rarely have we urgent pain and high fever to relieve.

What is required of us is to prevent, if possible, cardiac inflammation, to prevent the valves being permanently damaged should the heart unfortunately be involved, and to prevent a recurrence of rheumatism. In this connection we must remember: (1) that rheumatism in children is specially prone to recur; (2) that it is specially prone to involve the heart, and that this liability is increased with each successive attack; (3) that a complete recovery after an attack of cardiac inflammation is, perhaps, more frequent in the child than in the adult; (4) that we are better able to prevent a patient from being attacked by rheumatism than we are able to prevent the heart being affected after a rheumatic attack has commenced. In the prevention of a recrudescence of rheumatism personal hygiene plays a very important part. Patients should avoid living in low-lying damp places, and be careful not to get their clothes wet and not to remain in wet clothes. Salicylates should be given frequently, every three to four hours, in full doses (three-quarters of a grain for every year of the child's age), until the active signs of rheumatism disappear, and then similar doses three times a day for one or two weeks. Where the heart has already been involved the main hope in promoting recovery from cardiac inflammation must lie in giving the heart as little work as possible. The patient should lie supine in bed and remain so for a lengthy period after the subsidence of the rheumatic attack, e. g., at least a month. This enforced rest may be conjoined with Dr. Caton's treatment, which consists in giving sodium iodide in appropriate doses and applying small blisters repeatedly in the lines between the middle of the clavicles and the nipples on each side.

Skin Diseases in Children.—M. E. Fitch (*The Med. Times,* Aug., 1902) emphasizes the importance of a correct diagnosis in the case of skin trouble in children. He describes *syphilitic eruptions* and advises a mercurial ointment. In the treatment of *eczema,* he says, look for rheumatic family histories, especially in children who look very healthy. Gout, too, is usually manifested as eczema in children. Heat, cold dry air, or the use of hard water or certain soaps may be the cause. The treatment depends entirely on the diagnosis. If there is deficient elimination from bowel or kidney, or digestive disturbances, find it out. Often the excessive use of farinaceous foods may be the cause of a heavy percentage of fat in the breast milk. *Erythema multiforme* frequently occurs and is a puzzling condition. The eruption consists of maculæ which vary in size and change from day to day, being irregular in distribution and pinkish in color. The child is anemic, irritable, and constipated. The existence of irritation in the eruption and the changeable character of the spots show that it is not syphilitic, while the distribution and appearance of the efflorescence show that it is not eczema. Belladonna will produce erythema, and so may strawberries, crabs, etc. A very common cause of this disturbance in children is tea. The use of iron is excellent in these cases, and the child should stop taking tea, pastry, candy, etc., and confine itself to milk, soups, and stale bread, combined with fresh air, exercise, good hours, and bathing. *Prickly heat,* or miliaria papulosa, should be avoided by the use of light clothing and plenty of bathing, and a good toilet powder such as boracic acid and starch. The bowels must be kept open and the kidneys stimulated. Powders are preferable to washes. Holt recommends the stearate or oxide of zinc, 12 parts; bismuth, 3 parts.; powdered camphor, 1 part, or simple rice flour. The diet should be fluid and easily digested. *Seborrhea* should be treated by washing the crusts with oil and removing them by the use of warm water and soap, after which a soothing ointment should be applied, such as resorcin or sulphur. *Furuncles* or *boils* require general tonics, thorough cleanliness of the skin, and incision of the furuncles which have pointed, emptying them by compression. The spots are then washed out with a solution of bichloride 1:2,000, absorbent cotton applied until bleeding stops, and then covered with a collodion dressing. *Urticaria* is almost always caused by some trouble in the digestive tract. The children should be put on a milk diet and the condition of bowels and kidneys attended to. Local causes of irritation should be sought for, such as rough underclothing, too tight bandages, etc. Local irritation can be relieved by subacetate of lead, carbolic acid solutions, or a weak dilution of vinegar. For the cure of *scabies* the child should be given a hot bath and scrubbed with soap and water for at least a half-hour. Then the body may be anointed with the ointment selected, which should be left on over night. This treatment should be repeated several nights in succession. A good ointment is: Precipitated sulphur, 1 part; balsam of Péru, 1 part; vaseline, 8 parts—or, naphthol, 15 parts; prepared chalk, 10 parts; vaseline, 100 parts. Afterward it is well to put on some soothing application.

Subcutaneous Division of the Tendo Achillis for the Relief of Equinus following Infantile Paralysis.—Russell A. Hibbs *(N. Y. Med. Jour.,* July 19, 1902) submits a report of seventeen cases studied with the distinct object in view of determining whether or not the increased length of the tendo Achillis consequent upon its subcutaneous division for the relief of equinus had any effect in modifying the action of the calf muscles. The cases are those in which the deformity was caused by infantile paralysis. The operation in each instance was that of subentaneous division of the tendo Achillis, with, in some instances, division of the plantar fascia also and immediate correction of the overdeformity. The foot was placed in a fixed dressing at an angle of 90° to the leg, and, with the patient confined in bed, was kept so from four to six weeks. Subsequently they have been under constant supervision and have worn some form of protective apparatus. In eleven cases the length of the tendon was exaggerated, it was smaller than normal, and its shape was flattened; in the next four cases the tendon was not normal in size, though it was larger than in those just mentioned, and its length less exaggerated; while in the remaining three cases it more closely resembled the normal tendon. In the eleven cases in which the function of the calf was so seriously modified, there was marked retraction of the muscle. The gait was entirely without elasticity, suggesting that of a wooden or "flail" foot, with the limp made more conspicuous by the loss of the ability to elevate the heel and thus compensate for the shortening of the limb. The fact that such serious modification of the calf as appears in these cases does not always occur after division of the tendo Achillis does not weaken the argument, because it is perfectly reasonable to suppose that in some cases the sheath is more completely divided and more seriously impaired than in others, and also that the amount of strain to which the new structure is subjected will be greater in some cases than in others, depending upon the condition of the calf muscle, which, when not seriously impaired, would exert a greater force upon it than when it was so, and thus be more likely to cause its elongation. In some cases there was no impairment of the calf from the paralysis, yet its function is now completely lost and the tendon is much smaller and exaggerated in length. Thus it would appear that the modification of the function of the calf in these patients was the result of, first, the shortening of the muscle in the production of the deformity; second, the further shortening of the muscle as a result of the lengthening of the tendo Achillis by tenotomy in the correction of the deformity; and, third, the still further shortening of the muscle as a result of the lengthening of the tendon caused by the elongation of the structure forming the bond of union between its divided ends. With what frequency such serious modification of the function of the calf will be seen as a result of the division of the tendo Achillis and the correction of equinus in this class of cases, cannot be determined from the study of so small a number, but that it does occur, and probably with greater frequency than is generally supposed, is evident.

Treatment of Summer Diarrheas.—An editorial *(Arch. of Ped.,* July, 1902) says that *principiis obsta*—"stop the beginnings"—is the golden rule for summer diarrheas. There is no such thing as a negligible diarrhea in hot weather. No excuse like teething, or delicacy of health, or supposed hereditary tendency to gastro-intestinal derangement must be allowed to make a distinct frequency of passages appear trivial to the mother, and especially to the physician. The slightest looseness of stools must be the signal for prophylactic measures. The child's food must at once be reduced in amount. If mere reduction in the diet does not modify the diarrhea favorably in twelve hours, then milk must be eliminated entirely from the dietary for a time. This seems a hard method of treatment to many, and especially to young mothers. Hence it is often delayed in the hope that improvement of symptoms will take place without such an apparently radical proceeding. Milk is, however, a most favorable culture medium for the pathogenic bacteria of the intestinal tract. To continue its use is to feed these bacteria and not the child. This idea, if put forcibly before the mother, will do more to convert her to the necessity for the complete elimination of milk from the child's food than almost any amount of direct advice or persuasion.

As to what shall replace milk in the child's food there is some difference in opinion. Egg water was popular until it was recognized that most micro-organisms causative of diarrhea will grow on it. Cereals have long been recognized as of value in preventing the growth of bacteria; they set up an acid fermentation, and acidity of the intestinal contents makes them an especially unfavorable culture medium for pathogenic bacteria. Barley gruel then, or some similar preparation, makes the best substitute for milk. The medicinal treatment of the infantile diarrheas of hot weather has become of less importance than formerly. At the beginning calomel and castor oil remove irritant material that is furnishing a soil for the growth of bacteria. Astringent drugs must be used with great caution. Only the insoluble bismuth compounds which act mechanically to prevent irritation can be recommended with confidence, and should be given in large doses—half a drachm to a drachm five or six times a day. Except for movements at short intervals accompanied by tenesmus, opium must not be employed. Irrigation of the colon is indicated only when the lower bowel is evidently the main site of the inflammatory process. The indications are foul-smelling stools containing considerable mucus. There is no specific treatment for summer diarrhea. The secret of decreased mortality from the disease is prophylaxis and early treatment by limitation of the diet.

Treatment of Results of Infantile Spinal Paralysis.—Clarence L. Starr *(Canada Lancet,* July, 1902) says that while the prevention of deformities by early application of apparatus has been advocated and practised for a long time, it is only within recent years that any attempt has been made to rearrange the attachment of active muscles so as to permit them to be used to the greatest mechanical advantage. The treatment of such deformities and disabilities is treated under four heads: I. *Cases which may be treated by mechanical support.* When, in the lower extremity, there is paralysis of all the muscles, sometimes including the adductors and glutei, producing a flail-like or uncontrollable limb, surgical procedures are not feasible. This class of cases is best treated with a mechanical support which takes somewhat the form of an artificial limb with a core of bone throughout. The support is preferably fastened to the boot and extends as a side box up each side of the leg, a leather lacing enveloping calf and thigh. The joint at the ankle may be a free joint or a stop joint, set to prevent toe dropping below the right angle. The knee joint should be an automatic lock joint, that locks itself when the patient stands and can be loosened by pressure on a spring through the clothing, so the leg can be flexed when the patient sits down. This form of support will usually enable one who has hitherto been obliged to use a pair of crutches to get about with the assistance of a cane. II. *Cases where mechanical support may be employed advantageously only after tenotomy.* The tibialis anticus and posticus muscles are frequently found permanently paralyzed. and the contraction of the unopposed peronei, together with the body weight, produces a valgus deformity of the foot. The continuous rolling over of the foot tends to bring the origin and insertion of the gastrocnemius and soleus closer together, and the tendo Achillis becomes shorter to adapt itself to the new condition. The treatment suggested is division of the tendo Achillis, and possibly the peroneal tendons, and application of a fixation dressing such as plaster of Paris after reposition of the foot. III. *Cases where the attachment of active muscles may be transposed so as to allow them to act to better mechanical advantage.* The operation for transplanting active tendons into paralyzed ones has now become established as a satisfactory plan of treatment in certain cases which would otherwise remain disabled, but where by this means function has been almost completely restored. It is applicable in any part of the body, but, on account of the less intricate arrangement of tendons, is much more useful in the lower extremities. As an example, in the thigh, where the extensor group is so frequently paralyzed, the sartorius remaining active, the sartorius can be divided at or near its insertion, and the cut end fastened into the fascial attachment of the quadriceps to the paletta. The development which takes place from the use of this muscle is often sufficient to maintain extension of the leg in walking. IV. *Cases where so little muscular tissue is left as to be useless for support and where supports are not advisable.* In cases where there is no control of extension at the knee, and continuous treatment with appliances is not feasible, the knee joint can be excised and a stiff joint secured which will allow the patient to get about without apparatus. In some cases of uncontrolled ankle movement, *arthrodesis* at the ankle may be employed, thus producing ankylosis and a stable foot producing a firm basis of support. Whitman, in such cases, does what he calls an astragalectomy, arthrodesis, tendon-shortening, and backward displacement of the foot. The astragalus is removed after division of external lateral ligaments, and this allows sufficient freedom of movement of the foot to slip it bodily backward, thus carrying the centre of gravity of the leg further forward toward the centre of the foot.

THE AMERICAN

JOURNAL OF OBSTETRICS

AND

DISEASES OF WOMEN AND CHILDREN.

VOL. XLVI.   NOVEMBER, 1902.   No. 5.

ORIGINAL COMMUNICATIONS.

THE PRESIDENT'S ADDRESS

BEFORE THE FIFTEENTH ANNUAL MEETING OF THE AMERICAN ASSOCIATION OF OBSTETRICIANS AND GYNECOLOGISTS.

OF OUR SHORTCOMINGS.

"Let us reason together."

BY

EDWIN RICKETTS, M.D.,
Cincinnati, O.

Mr. Chairman and Members of the American Association of Obstetricians and Gynecologists:

In casting a line for this paper, looking over your fourteen presidential addresses, I am profoundly impressed by the fact that they have thoroughly covered the scientific ground pertaining to our society.

It was with some timidity that I chose the above title. In doing this I was not unmindful of the fact that I was to criticise our profession in a general way in order to best consider our special shortcomings. In any or all of your discussions you have been so fair in legitimate criticism, and with it so full of forbearance, that I am encouraged to speak plainly. I fully appreciate and am thankful for the distinction you have conferred

37

on me in being honored with the Presidency of this Society of special workers. With this honor comes my first opportunity and privilege of being requested to say what I think of you, at least collectively, without fear of a reply. My position is not without responsibility, and I will make duty my only monitor. Friendly and honest criticism, offered without prejudice, càn do no harm; it may do good.

It is with pride that I call your attention to the five hundred original articles, with the one thousand pages of discussion, that stand as the result of your fourteen years' work toward erecting a monument that is to be in honor of your unselfish efforts of true special work. Your Transactions are to be read by the coming men in medicine, and it is for these that you have sowed deep and well the abdominal and gynecological seed. The work of our most worthy Secretary always speaks for itself, and does it in no uncertain sound. While it is evident that you have accomplished much, it is also as evident that you should have done better and more work. All of this goes to prove that all has not been accomplished. Such was claimed not long before this society was organized. Yòur work has surely evidenced the fallacy of such a statement.

For the study of ancient gynecology, showing that all surgical procedures were done yesterday, are done to-day and lost to-morrow, I refer you to the book recently brought out by Stewart McKay, of Sydney, Australia. In this he clearly shows and kindly points out the uneven chart lines of progress from near the time the rib was removed for the making of the first woman, that Celsus gave us his well-written observations on the anatomy of the uterus, and Galen gave his work on the dissection of the Fallopian tubes. I am yet to be convinced that anesthesia was a lost art to Galen and his followers. Our professional troubles, of so complicated a nature, began with its unfortunate marriage to the priesthood. This brought incantations and superstitions that honest efforts on lines of true philosophical reasoning have not been able to eradicate. The worst of it is that our profession is still a willing slave to the priesthood, which flatters itself that it is able to make better the chances for our future, knowing that it has rewards of present positions to extend.

Like the church, medicine is denominational. Thorough organization is not ours, and for this we lack independence and the desired highest dignity possible, which would bring greater usefulness and better work for rich and poor alike.

For the association of *our* profession with the priesthood, as coming from the many denominations, its members have had their views on practical Christianity broadened. Notwithstanding our open-handed charity, for this we have been criticised (but pills do act without ceremony, even to increasing the dose). Similar ceremonies without pills or scalpels are being taken up by many of the laity to-day. With some the patient is to recover with ceremony and without pills, while in others the recovery is to be more satisfactory if the doctor will only fail to ask for his fee; just let it be optional. Such demands were once of a more personal nature, while now they are strengthened by coming from denominational priesthood medical trusts—and no questions to be asked for the receiving.

The general practitioner of this or any other country is the backbone of medicine. It should not be otherwise. With just and co-equal considerate relations, the best interest of the physician and specialist is not to suffer. With changed relations toward the general practitioner complications are sure to arise.

Our former old-time true medical allegiance must be renewed, and in no uncertain manner. For this lack of consideration the general practitioner has been aggrieved, and he has not failed to retaliate on special lines and with a high mortality. Re-establish the better and old-desired relationship, and even a division of fees will not be requested. He sees the cases long before they are to come to you, and many times long after their return. You must have his confidence first; yours, to him, is secondary. He knows, long after your patient has returned to him, of some of your failures, when possibly you are well under the impression that they are successes. You are to be his handmaid in surgery, ready to respond to his call. Show him that he can trust you under any and all circumstances, just as so many of his families have learned to trust him—you must never forget that he has many delicate problems to overcome in order that you may be called in to any of his cases.

After Ephraim MacDowell established the fact that ovariotomy was legitimate and could be performed to save many, many lives, ovariotomy fell into dispute—not for the failures of Mac-Dowell. but for those of incompetent general surgeons; so the general practitioner decided that, for the reason of such high mortality in the hands of all operators, it should be abandoned, and it was.

It was to be taken up again after more than a third of a century—beginning with 1809—had passed; and in the meantime· thousands of women with ovarian tumors alone, not operated upon, died. Progress for the relief of these conditions ceased. For the efforts of the second generation of operators—as Dunlap, the Atlees, Sims, etc.—for the relief of ovarian tumors and for vesico-vaginal fistula, the mortality was lower than it had been in the hands of the best general surgeons for the fifty years following 1809. It remained for the Birmingham school (the third generation of special operators) to take up the scalpel in the best interests of surgical diseases of women, and to lower the mortality as never before; and with this pelvic surgery was given birth, and Lawson Tait re-established an old operation for the repair of the complete and incomplete lacerated perineum.

There is every reason to believe that abdominal surgery and gynecology, in the hands of all operators, is being accompanied with a higher mortality than is true of that done by the special workers. The work in all hands is not so thorough on conservative lines. For the "all told high mortality" the doing of abdominal surgery and gynecology undoubtedly is on the down grade; and it remains to be seen whether the brakes are to be reached, and if the general surgeon and general practitioner are the best to manipulate them. Some that have filled the demands of special workers in abdominal surgery and gynecology for a time, seem ready to join hands with the general surgeon, feeling that this and similar societies should cease to exist (notwithstanding the fact that these special efforts have made abdominal surgery and gynecology famous), and that they should become general surgeons and obstetricians—in fact, return to the doing of an amputation for gangrene to-day, a tonsillectomy to-night, with a case of erysipelas or some other infectious or contagious disease continually on hand. Under such circumstances the strictest attention to, and observation of, surgical asepsis or surgical antisepsis is to give a mortality that is to put us back fifty years. That is, the general practitioner will so judge us, and in truth.

He rendered judgment that settled the high mortality for the fifty years referred to, and it looks very much as though he will have the opportunity of doing as much again. The lowest mortality that we have ever had to record in our special work was not the result of the efforts of general surgery, for it long and loud denied, with none less than Sir Spencer Wells, that Tait had found a pus tube and pelvic surgery. The first lowest mortality came to us as the result of the arduous labors of a most trying and sacrificing personal kind, through the efforts of Tait, Bantock, Thornton, Keith, Savage, Sinclair, and others coming from England—the country (and let it be said to her great honor) that has recognized longest and with the greatest respect the true specialist.

It has been most unfortunate for the very best desired results in abdominal surgery and gynecology, and for the best financial interests of the profession at large, that those few general surgeons with wide reputations in general surgery should do abdominal surgery and gynecology as a secondary matter. Such frequently comes as the result of large and unwieldy clinics that are responsible for aiding in seductive and delusive six-weeks-touch courses called polyclinics.

It is refreshing to see and read so frank an expression as that coming from James Hawley Burtenshaw, Adjunct Professor of Gynecology in the New York Polyclinic, *New York Medical Journal,* August 30, 1902, on "Gynecology and Country Doctors." He says "that the teaching is often over the head of the average postgraduate student, and he nearly always takes it too much for granted that his listeners have been well grounded in the principles of a particular branch, and that he therefore fails to enter sufficiently into the details of his subject. This is particularly likely to be true when a large number of patients are present at the clinic, necessitating rapid and more or less cursory attention to each in order that the routine work may be completed in a specified time." He adds: "A six-weeks or three-months course at a postgraduate medical school will not serve to make of the most earnest workers a competent specialist in any branch of medical work." This is a frank and manly acknowledgment. I have purposely talked with men, East and West, who are connected with some of our best polyclinics, and they frankly admitted—in confidence—that the polyclinics are greatly at fault.

This final rapid polyclinic equipment, which is the result of the hurried and incomplete teaching, is not to bring the demanded low mortality for the work done after returning to their respective fields of general practice, general surgery, or both. For any one seeking the special field, ten years of active general practice, studying symptoms vigorously, to then spend a year working with leaders in the special surgical art, will undoubtedly accomplish more. There are no short roads to the successful general practitioner any more than there are to our special line.

There are reasons why the physician and all those engaged in the practice of the specialties should enter the political arena. He owes this to his country and to the city, town, village, or district in which he may reside. It will teach him what organization is, what and how a power can best be wielded for good. It will result in pronounced efforts for the organization of the medical profession, which in due time is to command the highest respectful consideration, as coming from the National, State, and County government. Such is to make us a free and independent profession, and to bring with it respect, as coming from church as well as state. Not well-applied commercialism is with us. I say that the medical and surgical laborer is *always* worthy of his hire; but there is a right and a wrong way of obtaining an equitable financial remuneration. Commercial agencies can be made to serve you as they do business men.

Is the number of specialists to be decreased? I would say, "Yes, for a number of years, and surely with a higher mortality." On those remaining true to the special work and their followers will be imposed the task of working on new lines— surgery of the pancreas; the earlier diagnosis of hydro- and pyosalpinx, with abdominal, vaginal, or combined drainage for restoration of function; earlier diagnosis and treatment of limited pathological lesions of one or both ovaries; stenosis, with or without fimbriated occlusion of the Fallopian tubes and their relief; the study and diagnosis of diseases of the spleen that are to be amenable to relief as coming from surgical intervention; the prophylaxis of many of the surgical diseases peculiar to women—this to be taught to the sex in the most approved way, though delicate it be; the remarriage of obstetrics to abdominal surgery and gynecology. Then we are to be in line with Germany, France, and England.

While the laity is to be the last to appreciate the importance of the lowest mortality possible, they will come along in due time, and their decision will again create desired special demands, that will be gladly catered to by a less capricious and wiser profession. With this our specialty is to be again popularized, until the general surgeon is to consider the invading of our new field, which we have made possible for the redemption of our specialty. For the reason of our pioneering, if the general surgeon cannot do the work better, in justice he should stand aside.   If he can do it better we are ready to yield to him the special surgical palm.   With medicine thoroughly organized, each specialty, along with the higher grade of merit demanded for the recognition of the surgical worker, knocking at the door, that competitive commercial spirit which now exists as one specialty against another would *not* receive the undesired recog- nition of to-day.   All other professions and trades have said of us—and not without truth—that we have no thorough organiza- tion.   Granting the truth of the assertion, the fault lies within ourselves; for the correction, we cannot expect, or ask, that others begin the work for the solution of this very important problem.

Now that women are on a co-equal footing in medicine for the same prescribed laws, State and medical, as men, it should be our duty and our pleasure to assist in the correcting of certain abuses.   For instance, the obstetrical practice, as coming from the poorer classes, should be liberated from the too oft dirty midwife and placed in the hands of the lady physician, and financially, if necessary, at the figures of the midwife.   Ten per cent added on the lines of infection comes from the deliveries at the hands of the midwife.

The true working relationship of the neurologist, as bearing on our special work, must be better and far more appreciated. He should be called into consultation oftener, and he in turn should consult with the gynecic and abdominal surgeon before sending any of his patients to an institution for partial or per- manent detention.

It is claimed by some that all men cease to be aggressive in the trades and professions at 50 years of age.   If this be true there is much food for thought as to the best interests of many of us in this society.   If this be true, then we must console our- selves with the fact that others passed from the arena as we came in.   It is with such a possible transitional state in view that we have in reserve young men who, we are sure, will plant our standard farther toward the desired pole.   In doing this, they are to prove, by their good work, all has not been accomplished.

What would come from that which we have considered?   A National Secretary of Medicine.   It would be medicine, not priesthood and medicine.   It would be medicine on its highest and broadest plane; and for this the members of the specialties would duly consider and honor each other.   It would mean dig- nity, higher regard, influence, *and an equitable financial re- muneration.*   It would be for the medical profession to assist in

making the world better. It would be for the higher education
of our boys and girls who may determine to enter the ranks of
medicine. It would be that our profession would know better
how to ask and how best to obtain that which it has so long
needed and justly deserved.

408 BROADWAY.

TRANSACTIONS OF THE AMERICAN ASSOCIATION OF OBSTETRICIANS AND GYNECOLOGISTS.

PROCEEDINGS OF THE FIFTEENTH ANNUAL MEETING,

HELD IN WASHINGTON, D. C., SEPTEMBER 16, 17, AND 18, 1902.

First Day—Morning Session.

The Association met in the Convention Hall of the Hotel
Raleigh, under the Presidency of Dr. Edwin Ricketts, of Cincinnati, Ohio.

An Address of Welcome was delivered by Surgeon-General
George M. Sternberg (retired), of Washington, D. C., which
was responded to by President Ricketts.

The first paper was on

PELVIC DISEASE IN THE YOUNG AND UNMARRIED.

BY

C. L. BONIFIELD, M.D.,
Cincinnati, O.

THE vast majority of patients who come under the care of the
gynecologist are suffering from disease due to infection either of
a gonorrheal or septic character, to the injuries incident to childbirth or abortion, or to those diseases which are prone to occur
about the time of the menopause. This paper will deal only with
those pelvic diseases or symptoms which occur in those who have
never been subjected to the disturbances of sexual intercourse
or the perils of parturition. Many of these disorders are purely
functional; others are only symptomatic of some constitutional
trouble and their treatment can safely be left to the family
physician.

An increasing number of unmarried women consult gynecologists or the family physician for gynecological troubles. Whether our young women of the present day are more prone to pelvic disease than their mothers and grandmothers were at their time of life, or whether the large number of men cultivating the gynecological field serve to attract attention to this part of the anatomy, is a question. · The modern girl would seem to take more exercise than her ancestors did and we would expect her to be stronger; but the added duties and cares of a more advanced civilization make her more nervous, and it is probable that the same disorder is felt more and heeded more than it was by her mother, as the stroke of a whip is felt more by a racehorse than by his fellow who works in a dray.

In one class of modern girls the strain on the nervous system is the struggle to compete with the stronger sex in acquiring higher education, in practising the professions, or in filling positions in commercial houses. In another it is the struggle for social prominence. The ordeal that a society girl goes through with during the season is extremely trying to the most robust and her weaker sisters are sure to break down under it. Dress reform makes slow progress; but certainly dress is now no more senseless and harmful than it was a century ago. Dancing is far from healthful exercise, indulged in, as it is, in overcrowded, superheated rooms, with tight clothing interfering with respiration; but dancing is no more injurious now than formerly. Cycling is a modern form of amusement which, fortunately, is rapidly losing popularity; it is as trying on women as the sewing machine, excepting that it is used for amusement instead of work and is used in the open air. Horseback-riding is to be commended. And golf cannot be blamed; it demands exercise, not too violent, in the open air, and the player wears rather sensible clothing. So the explanation suggested seems most plausible.

It is to call the attention of the profession to the well-known but apparently often forgotten truth that pelvic symptoms do not always mean serious organic disease of the pelvic organs, in fact that they usually do not indicate trouble of this character in the young and unmarried, and that such patients should not be subjected to local examination and treatment until reasonable effort has been made to relieve them by other methods, that this paper is written.

The journals have been saying, the last few years, that the work of the gynecologist is done; that he has taught the surgeon

how to do the operative part of his work, the obstetrician how to
recognize what should be done, and that in the future these two
worthies working together will occupy the whole field and the
gynecologist will be seen no more in the land. At the recent
meeting of the American Gynecological Society Dr. Jenks quoted
some one who had taken pains to compare the mortality of
gynecological work done by gynecologists with that of such work
done by general surgeons, and he found it to the advantage of
the gynecologist. This is as it should be. The law of ''survival
of the fittest'' is still in operation. If the gynecologist would live
he must be worthy of life. The gynecologist who graduates from
the college a specialist will perish. The gynecologist who becomes such after a six-weeks course at a postgraduate school will
fail. But the gynecologist who is first a good general practitioner, and then learns the specialty by long apprenticeship to
one of its masters, will always find a field for his efforts. It is
in diagnostic ability that the gynecologist must excel if he would
maintain his present prominent position in the profession, and
one of the best evidences of such ability is the readiness with
which he recognizes what cases do and what cases do not come
within his domain.

Among the affections that most commonly bring this class of
patients to the gynecologist may be mentioned the disorders of
menstruation, undeveloped uterus, tubercular disease of the appendages, and acute displacements.

Menstruation may be tardy in making its first appearance.
Unless there are marked local symptoms or the function is several
years behindtime, there is no necessity for pelvic examination.
But the wise physician will not dismiss the case as unworthy his
attention. He will first endeavor to find out whether the function
is really late or only apparently so. He will judge of the time it
should make its appearance by the complexion of the girl, the
latitude in which she lives, her habits of life, the menstrual history of her mother and older sisters, etc. If it is really late he
will do his best to discover the cause and remove it. Such cases
are nearly always anemic. But he will not be satisfied with having discovered that anemia exists and having prescribed iron for
it. He will investigate carefully the condition of the heart, the
lungs, and the kidneys. He will ascertain if digestion is normal
and if the diet is wholesome and nutritious. It is important that
a girl's health be as nearly perfect as possible at the time of
puberty, otherwise the proper development of uterus and ovaries

may not occur. The uterus that begins to menstruate late ceases to do so early, showing a lack of vitality.

Amenorrhea is one of the early symptoms of phthisis. When there is a gradual cessation of menstruation, unless the patient is gaining weight rapidly, this or some other grave constitutional state is to be suspected and diligently searched for. Obesity frequently lessens and sometimes stops menstruation. The treatment is dietetic and a strenuous life. Ovarian extract is sometimes of value.

It is the universal observation of the profession that the sudden cessation of menstruation in the apparently healthy is always suggestive of pregnancy, no difference what the character or social position of the individual may be. Menorrhagia, though not so common in this class of patients as in later life, is frequently present. A depraved state of the blood whereby it loses its coagulability is often its cause. Interference with circulation by disease of the heart, kidneys, or liver may also produce it. These causes should always be searched for, and corrected if found, before local measures are resorted to. Rest in bed during the period should always be enjoined. The administration of ergot or hydrastis, or a combination of the two, with a sedative for a few days before and during flow, is useful. Curettage is rarely required.

Dysmenorrhea may be of uterine, tubal, or constitutional origin. In the young and unmarried it is most apt fo be of the constitutional variety. Menstruation is preceded by a congestion of the pelvic organs. This physiological process, which so closely resembles a pathological one, readily crosses the border ground and becomes pathological and painful. Anemia, chlorosis, malaria, syphilis, and rheumatism are a few of the more common causes of constitutional conditions that make menstruation painful. The true nature of the trouble having been recognized, the treatment suggests itself, and it had best be left to the internist, to whom it legitimately belongs. If specialists were more careful to refer cases back to the family physician, they would not so often be humiliated by being asked to divide the fees.

The next most common variety is the uterine. Flexion, version, and narrow cervical canal play an important, but still subordinate, rôle in the production of dysmenorrhea. Menstruation is usually not painful from such a uterus until an endometritis develops. The endometritis is the cause of the pain; the flexion, or whatever obstruction to drainage and circulation exists, is a predisposing cause of the endometritis. Cure of the endometritis relieves the dysmenorrhea. That simple endometritis can often be cured without any local treatment has long been demonstrated. Tonics, when indicated, a nutritious and easily digested diet, fresh air, and salt baths for the anemic, a non-stimulating diet with plenty of exercise and an occasional saline purge for the plethoric, will work wonders. The society the patient keeps and the book she reads are also to be investigated. It is useless to try to relieve congestion of the pelvic organs of a girl who is spending one or more evenings every week with a lover whose endearments produce a hyperemia which her virtue prevents being relieved in a physiological way. Immoral books, suggestive plays, intimate association with other girls who habitually talk of things sexual and sensual, are harmful only in a less degree.

By proper treatment, hygienic and medicinal, a majority of these cases can be cured without resort to local measures. When examination is necessary it is usually best to administer an anesthetic; the examination will be more satisfactory to the physician and less disagreeable to the patient. Preparations should be made so that if a dilatàtion and curettage are indicated they can be done at once, avoiding a second anesthesia. Operative treatment is the only local treatment to be thought of. It is inexcusable to have such a patient coming to one's office for applications to vagina or uterus. Tubercular disease of the tubes may be the cause of dysmenorrhea. Other tubal disease practically does not occur in the class of patients under discussion.

Ovarian dysmenorrhea is not rare in such patients, though many cases are diagnosed as ovarian which are really constitutional; the pain being neuralgic in character, though referred to the ovaries, which are found upon bimanual examination to be hypersensitive but otherwise normal. Imperfectly developed ovaries, prolapsed ovaries, and ovaries having undergone cystic degeneration produce true ovarian dysmenorrhea. The prolapsed ovary may be restored to its normal position, if it be healthy, which it rarely is, and the symptoms produced by its displacement relieved; but the other two forms of disease are not amenable to treatment, and it will usually sooner or later be necessary to sacrifice the organs. I have cured ovarian dysmenorrhea by freeing the right ovary from adhesions to the appendix.

The development of the uterus may be arrested at any stage of the process, leaving the organ in a rudimentary, infantile, or pubescent state. The symptoms of undeveloped uterus are principally those connected with the menstrual function. In the rudimentary uterus menstruation is absent, but if the ovaries are not also rudimentary there will be painful efforts to establish the function. Menstruation from the infantile uterus is tardy in making its appearance, is scant and usually painful. The pubescent uterus begins to menstruate at about the usual time of puberty; menstruation is scant, but usually painless for several years or until an endometritis develops. If the effort to establish menstruation with a rudimentary uterus is sufficiently severe to justify it, the ovaries, which will often be found in a state of cystic degeneration, may be removed to stop them. With the infantile uterus efforts may be made to develop it, though they will usually meet with a small measure of success. Tonics, exercise, massage, electricity, dilatation, and curettage may all be tried. By these means the symptoms may be relieved, but it is seldom a cure will be effected; relapses are frequent, and it may be necessary to remove the ovaries to stop the menstruation. Fortunately the rudimentary and the infantile uterus are rare. The pubescent uterus is quite common. It is generally sharply anteflexed, but occasionally retroflexed, the cervix long and narrow and the body dilated. Dysmenorrhea is a prominent symptom. Treatment of the pubescent uterus is more satisfactory than of the infantile or rudimentary. Tonics, exercise, thorough dilatation and curettage, and tight packing with iodoform gauze, repeated one or more times if necessary, will develop many pubescent uteri into practically normal organs. This subject is more fully treated in a paper by the author published in the May number of THE AMERICAN JOURNAL OF OBSTETRICS for this year.

Tuberculosis of the uterine appendages occurs as a part of a general tubercular peritonitis, or they may be the only organs in the peritoneal cavity attacked. Primary tuberculosis of the appendages usually begins near the fimbriated extremity of the tube. When the appendages are the only organs involved the symptoms are those of a subacute salpingitis. The diagnosis is made by recognizing the enlarged tubes and excluding gonorrheal and streptococcic infection. The treatment is extirpation. Tubercular peritonitis is frequently mistaken for typhoid fever and occasionally for appendicitis. Painful urination and painful defecation, rigidity of abdominal walls not limited to one area, and indistinct tumor-like masses in the abdomen, in which areas of resonance are strangely mixed with areas of dulness, are some of the symptoms that will enable one to recognize tubercular peritonitis. When the general condition of the patient will permit, an abdominal section should always be made. The surgeon's judgment must be used as to what will be done after the abdomen is open. Simple section is many times followed by marvellously good results; but, as the starting point of the disease is frequently the uterine appendages, their removal is indicated when it can be accomplished without too much violence to contiguous structures.

Acute prolapse of the uterus may occur in young unmarried women as the result of a fall or heavy lifting. In a case that came under my observation it occurred as a heavy basket of marketing, which had been carried several squares, was being deposited on the floor. Like hernia, it occurs in individuals of lax fibre. Ventrofixation is probably the best treatment.

In conclusion I will repeat the statement that many young an l unmarried women suffering with pelvic symptoms require neither local examination nor treatment; when an examination is necessary anesthesia is advisable, and treatment, when possible, should be operative.

DR. L. S. McMURTRY, of Louisville, was sure that every Fellow present would indorse the teaching of this paper. While the practice of examining and treating girls and young unmarried women suffering from dysmenorrhea and similar conditions had been condemned for years in this Association, that evil had not been altogether abated. The views presented by the essayist should be indorsed in order to further emphasize the protest made from time to time. It was yet a common error on the part of many practitioners to yield to the pressure of anxious mothers and treat the uterus for menstrual disorders and vague neuroses that had no pathological connection with that organ. Such treatment too often afforded means of infection and extensive inflammatory lesions. It should be the special care of the physician to advise against such interference, and, when an examination was indicated, to anesthetize the patient for that purpose. Dilatation of the cervix, curettage, and repeated application of the tampon were the operations most commonly abused. The essayist did not advise against examination and treatment of girls and unmarried women when subjects of disease of the pelvic organs, but advised discrimination between cases of distinct and supposed disease.

DR. HERMAN E. HAYD, of Buffalo, N. Y., was inclined to believe that the essayist had endeavored to make the Fellows feel that he was more optimistic in the outlook as regards the treatment of pelvic diseases of young women than he really was. He would not for a moment wish the Fellows to believe that he (Hayd) thought they should be careless in instituting examinations in young women. nor should any unbridled license be suggested in that direction.   However, he thought practitioners erred on the other side of the question too frequently, and attributed the troubles of patients to hysteria and other reflex disturbances when in reality organic disease was at the bottom of them.   One phase of this subject he took up in a paper read last year, namely, retrodisplacements of the uterus in young and unmarried women, and also in young married women who had not borne children, or who had had miscarriages and abortions, and he was satisfied that a great many young women owed their amenorrhea, their dysmenorrhea, their hysterical and neurasthenic symptoms to an undetected retroversion of the uterus. Those who had been doing the Alexander operation frequently, and had the greatest confidence in it, realized how frequently retrodisplacements of the uterus existed in young women and in young girls and were a cause of their physical suffering.   These women were tinkered with, their uteri tamponed and painted with iodine, until they were not only injured morally, but also physically by having set up considerable tubal and ovarian mischief.   Unfortunately these young girls consulted women practitioners, who kept on treating them indefinitely, and as a result gynecologists saw the physical wrecks which came to them frequently for surgical care.

Dr. W. A. B. Sellman, of Baltimore, said there was one cause of pelvic disease which had not been mentioned by any of the speakers, it having been overlooked, doubtless, on account of the speakers being located in inland cities.   He was located in Baltimore, where very many young women went to Atlantic City, Cape May, and other seaside resorts.   They were shopgirls, typewritists, etc., who indulged in ocean bathing the day before they expected menstruation, and some of them did not hesitate to go into the surf when they were slightly sick.   He saw a great deal of pelvic disease developed because of indulgence in ocean baths when there was congestion present in the pelvis due to approaching menstruation.

In regard to the treatment of these cases, he agreed with the essayist that when there was an enlarged ovary, with general disease of the appendages, operation was the only measure to effect a cure, and tinkering by the application of glycerin tampons, swabbing out the uterus, etc., was a waste of time.   He did not deprecate operation where the appendages were involved.

Dr. James F. W. Ross, of Toronto, disagreed with the essayist relative to displacements of the uterus in young girls and unmarried women and the necessity for operation.   He had not made up his mind yet as to whether practitioners were not doing too much operating for displacements of the uterus, and he expressed some doubt as to whether displacements of the uterus caused the symptoms with which they were sometimes credited. This branch needed still further investigation.   There was no doubt that there had been great abuse of the curette in young females.   He believed, too, that there had been a great abuse of the operations of ventrosuspension and ventrofixation with shortening of the round ligaments in the same patients. When such cases came to him he preferred to do clean surgical work. He wanted to treat gross pathological lesions; he would rather let some one else deal with the neurasthenics, etc.

Teaching students to examine young girls without an anesthetic was wrong. All examinations of young unmarried women, unless they were examined by the fingers of men who were expert, and in patients who were very thin, should be carried out after the administration of an anesthetic. Furthermore, to make a thorough examination of ovaries and tubes he was frequently forced to examine through the rectum, and not through the thick tissues of the vagina, with the limbs drawn up, bladder and rectum emptied, with the uterus drawn down by volsella forceps, if necessary; then the ovaries and tubes could be mapped out and felt, so that one could say whether there *was* or *was not* disease present, and if operation was undertaken afterward one could be sure of what he would find. A case in point was given.

DR. WALTER B. CHASE, of Brooklyn, N. Y., said allusion had been made to dilatation and the use of the curette in cases of acute flexion of the uterus. He did not know what the experience of the other Fellows was, but where dilatation and curettage were done in cases of flexion, in six months patients would return with practically the same state of affairs as that which existed before those measures were undertaken. What could be done to correct the tendency to recurrence of this trouble? A professional friend gave him a hint a few years ago which was useful, namely, the use of stem pessaries. These, he thought, had a place in surgery. If one, after having dilated a uterus of that kind, introduced beyond the point of flexion a small stem pessary of glass in which there was a central channel, and tied in the tube with silkworm gut, and let it remain from one to two or three weeks, as the uterine tissues contracted there would be a straighter canal and a more patulous os.

DR. WILLIS G. MACDONALD, of Albany, N. Y., said it was a hard question to decide always just where tinkering stopped. Whether the woman practitioner or the general practitioner was guilty of all the tinkering or not was a very difficult question for him to decide. Women came to his service without any of the internal organs of generation, yet they suffered from the same symptoms which they had had previous to operation. The history of such cases was frequently not known. One surgeon would do perhaps curettage and dilatation; a second would perform an Alexander operation; and a third would remove a portion of one ovary, resort to ignipuncture of the ovary, separate adhesions; while a fourth would do a complete extirpation of everything, both ovaries and tubes, and by that time the patient was left with a hernia and all of the symptoms she had previously had. Patients were sent to surgeons impressed with the idea that the removal of their ovaries was going to cure them of all ills from which they were suffering, and it required a great deal of backbone and argument to convince them to the contrary. After a short period of treatment they drifted to other surgeons who were ever ready to operate. After operation had been done there was no relief of the symptoms and the patient suffered as much as before. It required a good deal of experience and discernment to manage this particular class of cases. Personally, he liked to see cases of real disease come in, and good-sized tumors, something which was physically palpable, in order to do surgery upon them, rather than cases in which operative intervention was more or less experimental and speculative.

Dr. Bonifield, in rebuttal, said that Dr. Ross had misunderstood him. He thoroughly agreed with Dr. Ross in regard to uterine displacements, except procidentia uteri, for which he had recommended ventrofixation. Other forms of uterine displacements in the unmarried caused very few, if any, symptoms. In the majority of cases they did not unless the ovaries were also at fault, and then the symptoms were due more to the condition of the ovaries than the uterus itself. He thought the remarks of Dr. Macdonald were appropriate. If one doctor told a patient she had serious trouble and required operative intervention, it would take six doctors to convince her to the contrary. It required a great deal of strength of character not to operate on many of these cases.

EXTIRPATION OF THE GALL BLADDER THROUGH THE LUMBAR INCISION,

WITH REPORT OF A CASE.

BY

W. P. MANTON, M.D.,
Detroit, Mich.

Mrs. G. C., aged 38, examined at the request of Dr. B. P. Brodie, April 18, 1902. She has had five children and two miscarriages, the last of which occurred about a month ago. During her pregnancies she suffered a great deal from abdominal pain and soreness, this being particularly marked while carrying her last two children. The labors were normal and she got up feeling fairly well. The family history is good. As a girl she had never been particularly robust, and the color of the skin has always been rather pale and sallow. She has, however, been able to work, and now, although rather feeble, attends to her household duties. Her present condition, she thinks, has existed for the past two years.

38

Menstruation began at 12 and was regular until the miscarriages took place. The discharge lasts five or six days and is
always profuse, the last menstruation, she states, being as "bad
as a miscarriage." At present she suffers a good deal from
sacral backache on the left side, and there is pain in both iliacs,
especially the right. On the right leg there are varicose veins
which give rise to a sensation of blood trickling down. She also
suffers from numbness in hands and feet and just below the ribs
on both sides. The head has not troubled her of late, but
formerly there was a "scalding and itching" sensation of the
scalp. There is a profuse, thick, greenish leucorrheal discharge.
She sleeps poorly and is nervous and easily worried. The appetite is poor, the bowels constipated. and she has suffered a good
deal from attacks of indigestion.

On pelvic examination there were found a slight laceration of
the perineum, relaxed vaginal walls, and a small laceration of
the cervix uteri. The uterus itself is slightly enlarged. The
ovaries and tubes are very sensitive, but not enlarged. On the
right side the appendages appear involved in slight adhesions
running up toward the appendix. The abdominal walls are well
nourished but relaxed, and there is considerable diastasis of the
recti muscles. The left kidney moves downward to the second
degree. The right kidney is enlarged to about twice its normal
size, and its lower end has a knob-like projection which extends
to an inch below the umbilicus and points downward and inward. On the outer border of the kidney a rounded projecting
edge can be felt. The organ is fairly movable and is very sensitive over all. The percussion note is dull over the kidney mass.

A diagnosis of nephroptosis with probably cystic metamorpho-
sis of the kidney was made. The patient entered Harper Hospital April 28. At this time the urine was cloudy, alkaline,
specific gravity 1020, and contained a faint trace of albumin,
but no bile or sugar. The sediment consisted of numerous pus
cells, squamous epithelia, and triple phosphates.

Operation April 30. The uterus was curetted and the cervical
laceration repaired. The patient was then turned on her face.
a large, thick roll placed beneath the abdomen, and the nephropexy incision made. When the fatty capsule of the kidney was
reached this was found surrounded by a mass of dense adhesions.
and it was evident that it was these which had given rise to the
feel of an enlarged kidney at the examination. On incising the
capsule the kidney appeared to be in good condition and of nor-

mal size. It was enucleated and delivered on to the back. The fingers then introduced through the wound below the bed of the kidney came upon a hard, rounded body embedded in adhesions, the general feel of which resembled that of the kidney. On separating the adhesions, however, a pearly-white body, traced with blood vessels, presented at the wound. A hypodermatic needle was inserted into the growth and a syringeful of turbid fluid withdrawn. The body was then gradually enucleated, the fingers following it upward to the under surface of the liver, to which it was attached. It was then seen that we were dealing with a dilated gall bladder, in the neck of which and in the dilated cystic duct gall stones were present. Separation of the adhesions about the sac was continued until the cystic duct was freed, when the stones in this were crowded back into the bladder, the duct clamped with forceps and then tied off with a double catgut ligature. A broad attachment of the fundus of the sac to an anterior linguiform process of the liver was also tied with catgut and separated, and a quantity of gauze was packed around the gall bladder and the latter cut away. The kidney capsule was then split and peeled off to just below the lateral line, four fixation sutures of silkworm gut introduced. and the kidney returned to its place. Before closing the external wound a strip of gauze was carried down to the stump of the cystic duct and allowed to protrude from the upper angle of the skin incision.

During the operation little or no bleeding occurred from the deeper structures, but an annoying oozing took place from the cut edges of the skin and muscle. The patient made an uninterrupted recovery from the operation and was in good condition when last seen.

Subsequent examination of the removed gall bladder showed it to consist of a thin-walled fibrous sac containing about four ounces of grayish fluid and nineteen gall stones the size of hazelnuts. The bacteriological examination of the fluid by the Detroit Clinical Laboratory is reported as follows: ''The fluid in the small bottle contains a bacillus having the morphology and staining properties of the colon bacillus almost in pure culture. The fluid in the large bottle shows some leucocytes and a few of the same bacilli, together with a long, large rod which retains the violet stain when stained by Gram's method. This latter may be an accidental infection. No staphylococci or streptococci were found in either examination.''

Observations.—This case presents several points of especial interest. It is, as far as I have been able to ascertain, the first instance of removal of the gall bladder through the lumbar incision; the operation was entirely extraperitoneal; and, unless we assume the gastric disturbances and the scalding and itching of the head to have arisen from the condition, there was an entire absence of symptoms pointing to disease of the biliary tract.

Several cases are on record in which the emptying of the distended gall bladder and the evacuation of stones has been done through the lumbar incision, but in most instances where disease of the gall bladder or ducts has been discovered through the nephropexy incision the operation on these parts has been completed through an anterior abdominal opening, and the kidney alone treated through the lumbar wound. Whether the extraperitoneal position of the gall bladder in this case was a congenital anomaly or the result of walling off by adhesions cannot be determined; but it is certain that the condition must have existed for a very considerable number of years, and complete occlusion of the cystic duct occurred without giving rise to noticeable symptoms.

Regarding the choice of incision in uncomplicated disorders of the bile passages, it may be said that the anatomical position of the gall bladder—its neck reaching up into the fossa vesicalis of the liver and its fundus extending to the border of the rectus muscle and abdominal wall—renders the organ of easy approach through the anterior abdominal incision, and I am quite in accord with Mayo Robson that the lumbar incision, under such circumstances, "is useful only in theory, and is surrounded by so many difficulties as to make it quite impracticable." But in the presence of a nephroptosis or a morbid condition of the kidney demanding operative intervention, together with an enlargement of the gall bladder, either from stones or fluid accumulation, I believe that the lumbar route will be found to offer certain advantages over the anterior approach. With the kidney removed and placed astride the wound after the method of Edebohls, space enough is obtained to enable the operator to work up under the peritoneum and thus complete the operation successfully.

In closing this paper I desire to pay tribute to the pioneer work of Edebohls, who has opened up a field of operation which had previously lain uncultivated.

32 Adams avenue, West.

Dr. RUFUS B. HALL, of Cincinnati, O., said there might be cases occasionally where it would be desirable to approach the diseased gall bladder through a lumbar incision, but he thought these were rare. The case narrated proved a desirable one for that method. The fact that, for practical purposes, it was extraperitoneal added to the comfort of the operator and to the safety of the patient. The extraperitoneal condition was doubtless due to some old inflammatory disease. He had had no experience in operating on gall bladders through the lumbar incision. He recalled one case that was operated on in Cincinnati a few years ago where a large number of gall stones were removed through the lumbar incision. The patient recovered with a fistulous opening. This was a case in which there was a mistake in diagnosis, the surgeon supposing that he was going to operate for an enlarged kidney.

Dr. W. E. B. DAVIS, of Birmingham, Ala., thought surgeons would be slow in accepting the lumbar incision for doing work on the gall bladder, but there was good reason for using this incision in treating other conditions of the gall ducts. His experience, however, had been, both experimentally and clinically, that drainage was satisfactory through the anterior opening, using a glass tube and gauze around it for the first twelve or twenty-four hours, at the end of which time adhesions were sufficient, so that it was no longer necessary for the gauze to drain. The duct should be treated in the majority of cases by simply incising it anteriorly and draining it. Perhaps the lumbar incision had advantages in some cases. He spoke of the advantages of hepatotomy for the relief of biliary obstruction. His own experience had been confined to the anterior incision, and he had found drainage satisfactory.

Dr. JAMES F. W. ROSS, of Toronto, said there were two benefactors to this branch of surgery: one, Dr. W. E. B. Davis, who had taught drainage from the front, and Morison, who showed what could be done by his pouch behind the liver. Of late he had been using drainage from the front and through the lumbar incision. He had two patients now in bed at home from whom he had removed stones from the common duct; he was a little afraid of the suturing on account of the friability of the duct; so he inserted his finger down to the lowest part of Morison's pouch, slipped a scissors in, made an opening, and established through-and-through drainage; there could not be such a thing as an overflow of bile over the colon into the general peritoneal cavity when this method of drainage was adopted. There was danger from drainage in front; something might happen. The drainage tube might not be attended to by a nurse or the house surgeon, and if a little bile leaked over there was danger of losing the patient. These cases could be operated on without stitching the duct. One of his patients, to whom he had referred, was over 60 years of age and was recovering rapidly. He thought it was a good thing to recommend to the profession.

Dr. L. H. Dunning, of Indianapolis, Ind., called attention to the danger in attempting to drain the gall bladder above or to the side of the kidney in such cases as the essayist had described. He thought the result was excellent in Dr. Manton's case, and it was encouraging to know that surgeons might accomplish some good by so doing, if like instances should occur. But it did seem to him that if surgeons attempted to drain the gall bladder at the side of the kidney or above it for any purpose whatever, they would endanger the perinephritic fat decidedly; it might become infected, and perhaps suppuration might take place if the bile should happen to be infected. He would be loath to drain in that way. He agreed with Dr. Ross regarding drainage by Morison's pouch and by the lumbar method.

Dr. Joseph Price, of Philadelphia, stated that all of these operations had been simplified by modern methods. Where the conditions were bad and the delivery of the stones difficult the recommendation of Drs. Davis and Ross was good. He recalled one such case which was disastrous. He believed that had posterior drainage been practised in that case the result would have been more satisfactory. Only a few days ago he had difficulty in freeing large stones which were buried in the ducts; he had to use a knife, and it was just the class of cases referred to by Drs. Davis and Ross where the question of drainage was always important. But now one could, if he used the methods of Robson, deliver the liver and ducts and work as he would in the right iliac fossa.

Dr. Miles F. Porter, of Fort Wayne, Ind., stated that one of the chief advantages in draining in the lumbar region arose from the fact that it would enable the surgeon to close the abdominal incision oftentimes and avoid hernia which would most certainly follow. Drainage in this region, when it was applicable, for that reason alone was decidedly advantageous.

Dr. Manton, in closing the discussion, said that Dr. Hall referred to an error in diagnosis, which was quite true. He would defy any man to have made a correct diagnosis from the conditions present in his case, where there was a movable mass, evidently the kidney, and the projections were due to the enlarged gall bladder, which moved with the kidney and the entire mass. He did not advocate the performance of all operations on the gall bladder through the lumbar incision. He believed, however, that where the gall bladder was enlarged, where there were stones present, the surgeon could work up under the peritoneum more easily; and if the sac was simply opened, as several French operators had done, and drained through the lumbar incision, one could more successfully do that than through the anterior incision. If the case was uncomplicated he would not go in through the lumbar incision and do the operation, because, as a rule, through the lumbar incision the kidney was much in the way and it made the working space very limited.

SUPRAPUBIC VERSUS INFRAPUBIC PROCEDURES IN THE TREATMENT OF PELVIC SUPPURATION.[1]

BY

J. J. GURNEY WILLIAMS, M.D.,
Philadelphia.

IN presenting this paper I desire very briefly to refer to what many of you have treated so fully in papers and discussions: the importance of an apprenticeship in operative gynecology. I presume most of you realize that the modern apprenticeship differs greatly from one a quarter of a century or more ago, when the specialty was being developed by men with large and varied professional and surgical experience. Again, the nature of the work in those days differed greatly from the modern. Aside from the plastic work, vesico-vaginal fistula and perineal surgery, which largely interested the specialty, ovariotomy for cystoma only was practised by the so-called masters or pioneers. The apprenticeship then was a long one, but the variety of operations small and the procedures simple. The removal of a simple cystoma in the hands of the modern operator is play or recreation compared with the great number of extensive and multiple operations done in the pelvis and throughout the abdominal cavity. We now do a variety of operations on the liver and gall bladder; the kidneys are incised, drained, and partially or wholly removed. The numerous bowel operations are about all modern. Nothing more than puncture of pelvic accumulations, serous or puriform, was practised a quarter of a century ago. Now the operations in the pelvic basin are heroic and difficult in the extreme; the removal, and clean removal, of all pelvic suppurations requires an apprenticeship and prolonged study in practice that are to be gotten only by association with some master in abdominal surgery, who educates your fingers, teaches you surgical judgment, courage, and endurance.

Observation alone was sufficient for the old apprenticeship, and that was about all many of you got. It was necessary for some of you to re-educate yourselves at large expense of time and money. Just here I want to say that the hospitals, now so common in every State and city, are not giving their resident physicians the practical education or using the great amount of material at their command for that purpose. I can speak from experience of this matter; for, after serving in two large hospitals thirty-six months, it was necessary for me to go elsewhere for my practical instruction and apprenticeship desired. All hospitals should be practical schools for the residents, and the visiting medical and surgical staff the faculty. Early in the history of pelvic suppurations antedating the present school the methods practised were conservative in nature. The contested procedures used at present are not new, as about all the evacuation or puncture methods were anciently practised. They have never been wholly rejected, but used as palliative or tentative measures, and we occasionally hear them spoken of as Jones', Brown's, or Smith's method. Many of the so-called new procedures were used in the time of Hippocrates; and it is my impression that they were better done then than now, as they used caustics and the cautery and drained through wounds that were not easily infected. The modern operator makes generous incisions or punctures, and some wriggle their fingers freely through the opening. These old procedures almost died because the modern gynecologist sought more complete methods of dealing with pathologic conditions that they had failed to relieve or cure by these ancient measures.

Should I be asked what my understanding was of conservatism in the treatment of suppuration of the uterine appendages, I would answer, that method of treatment which will remove pathologic conditions, relieve suffering, permit a woman to perform her household duties or society affairs, save her months in bed and thousands in dollars. Accepting this view, it would appear that the most conservative procedure is the most radical—i. e., remove the pathologic conditions by an abdominal section. In speaking of conservative treatment in this paper I have used it in the sense ordinarily understood as vaginal incision, suprapubic puncture, electricity, massage applications, etc. I think we all agree that in many cases the question of operation is seldom thought of in the mild, non-specific, non-puerperal inflammations of the tubes and ovaries; but there has grown up a tendency to treat pyosalpinx and ovarian abscess by conservative non-surgical and conservative surgical methods, and it is of this class of cases that I wish particularly to speak.

First let us take up the question of diagnosis. On what

patients are we to try conservative non-surgical means, on whom conservative surgical procedures? I take it that the question of what "cocci" are present is one of importance to those who treat a pus tube or ovarian abscess by non-operative means, but amounts to little to those men who wish to remove the pathologic condition and prevent reinfection, which is very likely to occur, of virulent "cocci" in a sterile pus sac. By what means can we arrive at the conclusion that an abscess contains such and such infection previous to a bacteriologic examination? Do the symptoms tell us? Sometimes, but by no means always, as I have seen pus tubes, the size of a small sweet potato, filled with gonorrheal pus, give practically no symptoms; on the other hand, I have observed a small adherent tube, containing perhaps only a drop of fluid, creating intense pelvic pain, fever, sweating, dysmenorrhea, etc., compelling the woman to give up all work and making her a chronic invalid. Again, is it always possible to differentiate between an ovarian abscess, a suppurative appendicitis, an extrauterine pregnancy, and a dermoid? This illusion is from a subjective point of view, but had you seen the cases early in the history of the disease the objective symptoms would usually make the diagnosis easy.

Taking the abscess cases, I believe 90 per cent are due to the gonorrheal virus and any conservative non-surgical or conservative surgical method is simply a waste of time and the patient's money. I have been compelled to use conservative non-surgical methods on many patients of this class, on account of their refusal of operation, and have used faithfully the various treatments, always with the same result—temporary benefit followed by relapse—and later, in some of these patients, have had the opportunity of verifying the diagnosis and counsel for early operative interference primarily advised.

That in 60 per cent of these cases the pus is sterile is a poor argument against operation, as the woman is liable to acute infection at any time, besides being a sufferer from chronic abscess, adhesions, etc. Great numbers of these sufferers have been and are being treated by vaginal massage, the rest cure, a winter in Southern France, Florida, or California, the various baths, etc., and numbers have come and will come demanding that some operation be done to relieve them. Many are anemic, nervous, worn-out, prematurely old women, penniless and hopeless. Granting that a few will be benefited by these methods, it is only temporary, and it takes little to put these patients in bed with all their old suffering; besides, each new inflammatory attack, due almost always to leakage from the tube, but adds to the adhesions and makes more difficult the removal of the pathologic conditions, which sooner or later becomes necessary to cure our patient. Dilatation, curettement, and prolonged drainage of the uterine canal for pus tube is a most unsurgical procedure. The opening of the uterine end of the tube, in the great majority of cases, is little more than a fine white wire, and even after removal of the specimen it is rare that we can squeeze out a drop of pus from the uterine end of the tube. Again, supposing the nearest pocket of the uterus be emptied, two or sometimes three distinct abscess cavities remain undrained.

To take up the question of conservative surgical means by vaginal incision and drainage is to open the road for many widely different discussions and arguments. What has driven many men to this procedure and to conservative abdominal operations? First, high mortality suprapubic—some say from 5 to 25 per cent—and, second, inability to remove the pathology, compelling them to puncture or cut away one tube, half an ovary, or abandon the operation with the excuse inoperable, congenital malformation, or indistinguishable, and then look only on the favorable symptoms which sometimes follow. Great things are claimed by the men doing vaginal incision, but, I ask, what becomes of many cases on whom they have operated? Perhaps 25 per cent is about the correct number who return for a subsequent abdominal section. A certain per cent, quite large, go to other men to be relieved of their sufferings. I sometimes wonder if these men have ever made careful post-operative examinations of specimens removed by the abdomen, and have seen the multiple pus pockets of the tube separated by strictures. Have they noticed the bowel adhesions, the adherent appendix, the fixed omentum and retroflexed uterus, or the little collections of pus due to leakage from the tubes? If so, do they drain all these pockets? Do they reconstruct, relieve adhesions, remove the appendix, and bring the uterus forward by an ever so careful vaginal incision and drainage? Who would like to treat a suppurative appendicitis by incising the vaginal vault and putting in a gauze drain, when we can open the abdomen, relieve adhesions, straighten all the S's and 8's in the bowel, remove the appendix, flush the abdomen, and drain?

To those who claim a 2 per cent mortality by vaginal incision I would answer that it should be no higher by the abdominal. As to the other objections, those of scar and hernia, the first is seldom given much thought by sufferers such as these patients are, and hernia should not occur in more than 2 per cent of cases, which is a matter of little importance when we stop to think of the results obtained. I have had, more than once, women come to me begging that something, anything, be done to relieve their suffering; and when I have explained the total removal of the abscess, they answer: "Yes, I want that done, as I would rather die under the operation than live suffering as I am." Many of these primarily relieved by punctures, later demand something more radical for their relief or cure, and all are disappointed when they learn that there is risk of reaccumulation or repuncture and that they still carry their pathology. The arguments concerning our unsexing the woman, abolishing menstruation, and compelling the patient to go through an artificial menopause are answered by the woman's being already unsexed, marital relations being unbearable, the operation at times bringing back sexual desire; besides, the menstruation is often accompanied by intense suffering, and the menopause phenomena should be slight if the patient can rest and is carefully treated. In the wealthy class the woman may elect to be a chronic invalid and go through the long treatment of rest, baths, massage, etc., but picking out the temporary good which will result and applying it to all cases is not in accordance with modern gynecology.

There has been and is to-day too much conservative treatment taught in our medical schools regarding pelvic suppuration. I mean that the young man has no practical experience in abdominal surgery; he sees some professor do a few sections on these cases, and is then taught the various conservative non-surgical methods which should be tried—the Brandt treatment, douches and applications for pathological conditions which would not be so treated at any other point of the body. The old office treatment of pelvic pathology was and is receiving money under false pretences. But few good gynecologists of to-day use their offices for more than diagnostic purposes, and seldom charge ten dollars every five days for a touch of iodine, ichthyol, or carbolic acid and a little cotton ball with a string attached. I grant that it is quite impossible to teach a student abdominal surgery while at college, but why advocate to those men who are able to operate methods which are unsatisfactory and unsurgical?

I have already said the results are largely responsible for the change of route in our surgery, but, I ask, what are the honest results, both primary and remote, of these vaginal procedures or of the conservative non-surgical methods? Good, no doubt, in some few cases, but in how many, and are they nearly so good as those obtained by abdominal section? The early reports of abdominal sections for puriform disease in the female pelvis were considered wonderfully good, and now, although vastly better, they are spoken of as unsatisfactory and poor. At the present time we hear that vaginal incision and drainage is *the* operation for brilliant results. Which are we to believe? Surely we should not accept the reports of vaginal incisions unless we are prepared to accept the early reports of abdominal sections. These papers and discussions have been demoralizing to the general practitioner; in the society meetings he listens to papers of the palliative men, the puncture and incision school, and the suprapubic school, and he naturally asks, Whom are we to believe or follow? Let me say here that while these men are talking before our county, State, and national societies about their fine results with incision and drainage, other men are doing abdominal sections on these same patients to remove the pathologic conditions. The plea that pregnancy may follow conservative surgery is to me a very poor and dangerous one. We ask a tube disintegrated by blood, pus, or water to perform its normal functions by withdrawing its contents, and we compel forty women out of every hundred to lead an invalid's life for one poor, unhealthy or ectopic baby. Joseph Price gave a very adverse judgment on this operation by saying that the vaginal puncture or incision for puriform disease or for purpose of exploration are unsurgical procedures. He states that he has never known a patient cured by this method, and considers it not only blind but incomplete. Since the publication of this opinion I have talked with him more precisely as to his opinion, and he tells me that since expressing this view he has operated upon four published cases and recorded cures previously operated upon by incision and puncture, two of these by the same author, and two of his cases remain on his list for operation. He states that he has never seen a case coming from other surgeons that he considers much benefited; they were all bent by pathology and all invalids.

Salpingostomy is unsurgical and favors the possibility of a misplaced pregnancy, as we can hardly ask the disorganized tube to regenerate. Goldspohn's method of opening up the occluded end of the tube must be a very difficult procedure, and when the tube contains pus with two or three strictures it would be a hard matter to "milk out" the contents. Fernand Henrotin reports some 250 conservative operations with 40 per cent of partial cures or failures. It is but fair to state, however, that a large number of this 40 per cent had had conservative methods used previously. Jaquet gives statistics of "3,000 postmortem examinations, in which 1,000 presented adhesions, 850 showing general matting together of the pelvic organs"; and certainly this is not encouraging to those advocating vaginal incision.

A few hours previous to writing this I saw two cases of large ovarian abscess, each the size of a fetal head, low down in the pelvis, nicely situated for a vaginal puncture. It was fortunate for the poor sufferers that this method was not chosen, as the first was a tubercular abscess strongly adherent to bladder, bowel, and pelvic wall, consisting of some twenty pockets. Any one of these, or perhaps six or eight, by careful puncturing would have been opened, leaving ten or fifteen unopened abscess cavities. The second case was a gonorrheal abscess of the right ovary fixed to large and small bowel, bladder, and appendix, general matting together of the pelvic viscera, and omental fixation to bladder. Both of these cases had been horrible sufferers for months, both had undergone conservative non-surgical treatment, and both had contracted the opium habit; what would have been accomplished by vaginal incision in these two cases (and there are hundreds similar)? Nothing but harm. I wish to report an acute case which I operated upon the first day of this month. The extent of the pathology was great pus and filth to umbilicus, big ovarian abscesses, and pus tubes all leaking and within the fifth abscess; the sigmoid lifted and carrying the pus accumulation on left side, ileum and omentum on right. The great pus cavity was evacuated, tubes and ovaries removed, toilet, drainage, and recovery. Had I punctured I should have been pleased by the evacuation of a quart or more of pus. But, for that matter, any one could have turned my patient over and through a small incision removed more than a pound of pathology, the big suppurating tubes and ovaries, and have been more pleased, and I am sure he would have had more grounds for rejoicing that he had done the right thing by his patient.

Some men are inclined to divide their patients into two classes, the well-to-do and the poor dispensary patient, and advocate radical procedure with the latter class and conservative

methods in the former. This social-status of the patient seems
to me all wrong; for if we can send a poor woman to the wash
tub, why not send one of the "400" to her opera box? Class
distinctions should not enter into the matter of giving the patient
our best; if we are able to give to the lower classes a prolonged
and happy life, should we not give to the wealthy the same?
The woman, as I have already said, may elect the invalid's life,
but that is no reason why she should be urged to do so. Again,
the influential wealthy patient is the one most needed to the
community and commands that our best be given her, as she is
the most useful citizen, the one we can least spare. I ask again,
what is the difference between the dispensary patient and the
well-to-do when it comes to relieving suffering and sending them
to their duties? I quote the following from a paper recently
published on this subject: "Thus it may be seen that, by varying our mode of treatment to conform to the ever-changing conditions, we may unquestionably carry many of our patients
through the various troubles of pyosalpinx over a period of
several years, notably relieving their sufferings during the exacerbations of the chronic ailment; when by repeated inflammatory attacks the wall of the pus sac has grown thick and the
pus has lost its virulence, a fresh attack of pelveo-peritonitis
need hardly be feared. Thus ends the tedious story of the
sufferings of these patients, for they may now be considered to
all intents and purposes cured, although there remains a little
sterile pus within a thickened sac." To this I answer that the
life history ends for the pauper in the poor house; the "tedious
story" for all classes ends with death from amyloid degeneration, renal trouble, or chronic infection. What becomes of the
ever-nagging adhesions, the many reinfections, the 28.3 per
cent of the general matting together of the pelvic organs? Do
the adhesions melt away like dew before the sun? Do we prevent reinfection by our careful method of conservatism? Surely
it is not comforting to our patient to know that the condition
of "thickened pus sac" and "sterile pus" has to be reached by
repeated inflammatory attacks with their concomitant agony
and danger.

In deciding the question of route it is well to keep in mind
the conditions which are liable to be present within the abdomen. Some of these are omental adhesions to bladder, abdominal wall, or bowel, an adherent—5 to 10 per cent of all cases—
and perhaps suppurative appendicitis, a retroflexed fixed uterus,
and small collections of pus from the tubes situated high up in

the pelvis. There may be general adhesions of large and small bowel. Can you do by the vaginal route all the reconstruction work necessary which can be done by the abdominal? Can you relieve adhesions, release a fixed uterus, bring and keep it forward, when necessary remove the appendix, control oozing, flush and dry your field of operation, and make the careful toilet necessary by the vaginal incision and drainage? It is interesting to note, in a paper before me, that of 49 vaginal incision and drainage cases, about all for puriform disease, 10, or over 20 per cent, underwent a subsequent abdominal section, 5 had a secondary incision performed, and in 6 the results are not known. Of 5 abdominal incision and drainage cases, 1 was re-operated upon for ventral hernia, and 3 underwent a subsequent abdominal section. Four of the 5 were puerperal cases.

In conclusion, so much has been said about the simplicity of puncture methods and drainage by the vaginal route, with speedy relief and recovery, that I wish to say here that, aside from the mortality, which is not small, the number of invalids leaving the hospitals is very large. The return to the same or other hospitals for reincisions or for section is large; and when one who does such work is thoroughly familiar with the post-operative conditions of both classes of cases, he is convinced by his every-day experience that the results and recovery from the suprapubic method of clean extirpation or of drainage only in the desperate cases, feeble, exhausted, and dying, with an unpleasing history of discharge of pus—I say that he is convinced that the mortality is smaller and the recoveries more pleasing by abdominal section than from any other procedure, ancient or modern, now practised. From prolonged observation and practical experience I cannot make this statement too strong. I have now in bed recovering three or four negresses, all of whom would have been considered bad subjects for abdominal surgery in most hospitals, all of whom would have been punctured. The suppuration was extensive, the involvement of surrounding viscera not less so, and the enucleation difficult. But no complication followed the procedure. You may make a mental picture of just what would have remained in the pelvis following vaginal incision or puncture in these cases.

331 SOUTH THIRTEENTH STREET.

DR. CHARLES GREENE CUMSTON, of Boston, had published several papers in which he advocated vaginal incision—not puncture, because that would be inefficient, but vaginal incision with breaking down of pus pockets and free drainage. He thought at that time he had several cases that conclusively proved that the cures were permanent following this method. But those cases had not proved so. With more experience he believed that vaginal incision and drainage was incomplete in pus cases. One could not do as clean and thorough work through the vagina as he could through the abdomen, especially with a transverse incision, for with it one obtained more working space and it facilitated matters greatly. He considered vaginal incision proper in those cases where there was a large collection of pus with a very extensive inflammatory condition within the small pelvis. In those cases he believed one would obtain a great advantage by preliminary vaginal incision, but this was by no means curative.

Dr. Howard W. Longyear, of Detroit, Mich., some twelve or fourteen years ago read a paper before the Michigan State Medical Society in which he took the ground that in cases of acute gonorrheal infection of the appendages it meant either operation or chronic invalidism to the woman. He had changed his mind since then because of increased and riper experience, as he recalled a number of women who were perfectly well, and had remained so for years, who had had acute gonorrheal infection of the appendages, whom he was able to treat from the beginning of their infection, and he now felt that there were cases in which one could bring about a complete cure. His usual plan was, in a case of acute infection of the type referred to, to use an ice bag externally during the febrile activity, hot vaginal douches, and the internal administration of urotropin, with saline laxatives, and he had succeeded in a number of cases in effecting perfect cures. As regards vaginal incision, he held that one could not cure by that method. The best way was to drain until the patient was gotten into a safe condition to operate through the abdomen. If one had a case of pyosalpinx, with high temperature, he might suspect streptococcus infection. He should endeavor to establish the correctness of the diagnosis by the use of the aspirating needle, draw off some of the pus, examine it, and if he found streptococci he should drain by the vagina first, and follow it by abdominal section when it was safe to do it. If one found the colon bacillus or staphylococcus it was safe to operate through the abdomen.

Dr. L. S. McMurtry emphasized the point that it was a good plan in some cases to make a vaginal incision, just as the last speaker had explained. In cases of advanced sepsis, where the patient was greatly emaciated and reduced to an extreme condition, many of them could be tided over or saved by vaginal incision and evacuation of a certain amount of abscess formation, built up, and afterward they could be safely submitted to thorough operation. He thought this was the extent of the value of vaginal incision, and it was becoming generally recognized that thorough work by abdominal section and removal of the sac were the only curative measures.

First Day—Afternoon Session.

ICE FOLLOWING ABDOMINAL SECTION.[1]

BY

F. F. SIMPSON, M.D.,
Pittsburg, Pa.

SCRUPULOUS cleanliness intelligently applied gives almost absolute security against bacterial peritonitis from abdominal operations in clean cases. Yet even in these cases we find, to a very limited extent, the cardinal symptoms of inflammation localized about the field of operation (and evidenced by slight pain, tenderness, disturbed function of intestines, elevation of temperature, and slight acceleration of pulse rate). This reaction is always present and is apparently due solely to traumatism. Less often it happens that a few bacteria gain entrance in spite of what seems to be a faultless technique, and a more marked inflammation of a wider area gives more decided symptoms. *Rarely* the attack is serious. The unclean cases naturally divide themselves into two groups: first, those in which the existence of a frank attack of peritonitis shows that more or less virulent organisms are present and that they have not been subdued; and, second, those in which peritonitis was present but has subsided, indicating that the bacterial invasion has been successfully resisted for the time. at least. In these cases the bacteria may be quiescent, dead, or absent. ,

Peritonitis often follows the removal of the products of inflammation from the pelvis. When bacteria are absent, dead, or depressed, the acute attack is localized, limited in degree, and usually of little significance. It may leave adhesions or an infected pedicle; usually no trace of its existence remains. While the infecting bacteria are numerous, active, and virulent, however, the danger of peritonitis is great, the attack may be severe, the results serious. If the foregoing statements fairly represent current views, the prevention or control of post-operative peritonitis, local or general, traumatic or bacterial, is a matter of practical moment, for it frequently has an associated morbidity and at times a mortality as well.

39

I believe that post-operative peritonitis may often be prevented or controlled, and its products and mortality correspondingly lessened, by the proper use of ice. This opinion is based chiefly upon clinical observations concerning its effect in several hundred cases of pelvic peritonitis due to diseased uterine appendages; upon the use of ice to relieve pain and as a prophylactic and curative agent after operation in some hundreds of cases; and upon some experiments designed to show the effects of ice when applied to the abdomen. For quite a number of years it has been our custom to employ ice in the treatment of localized peritonitis consequent upon inflammatory affections of the pelvic organs. In these cases we have usually seen—as all of you doubtless have— the local and constitutional symptoms subside very quickly. In fact, the cardinal symptoms have disappeared so speedily that the distended, tender, tense abdomen has gotten soft and flat and opiates have rarely been needed to control pain. In several hundred of these cases our mortality has hardly exceeded one per cent.

The following is typical of the more serious forms of the disease in which we have relied chiefly upon ice as a curative agent, other remedies being used to guard weak points: Mrs. P. was seen by Dr. Werder in 1899 after several attacks of pelvic peritonitis. Examination showed large pus tubes on both sides. Extirpation was advised, but declined. August 19, 1899, during Dr. Werder's absence from the city, I was asked to see her. At 2 P.M., while sitting quietly on her porch, she "felt something give way in her left side," had some pain, and went to bed. When first seen, eight hours after this attack, her abdomen was moderately distended, rigid and tender. Her pulse was 120 and temperature 102°. She was vomiting frequently and her expression gave evidence of great pain. Her surroundings and condition were such as to make an operation very hazardous. She preferred delay. Operation could not be insisted upon. Morphine was given for the pain, strychnine was ordered, and two ice bags were put upon the abdomen. Twenty hours after onset her entire abdomen was ballooned, was tender, and she suffered intensely. Peristalsis was absent. Projectile vomiting was almost continuous. Her temperature was 103°. Her pulse was 148 and small, though the heart sounds showed a fair muscle. Her condition was far from reassuring. Permission to operate was absolutely refused. It was then determined to use ice for its full effect. A pillow case was filled with it, and, when applied, the entire abdomen was covered by a layer about four or five inches thick. extending from the bed on one side to the bed on the other, and from the xiphoid to the symphysis. It was kept in this position in this way for more than five days and nights. For four days iced champagne was the only thing retained by the stomach. Vomiting was frequent. The pulse remained between 140 and 150 and the temperature varied but little. Within a few hours after ice was thus applied the abdomen was cold, red, and less tender. In forty-eight hours it was less rigid and slightly less distended. By the fourth day it was soft and she was very nearly free from pain. Though internal medication and enemata were repeatedly used, neither gas nor feces were expelled till the fourth day. The fifth day her general condition was decidedly better and her pulse rapidly dropped to about 90. A fluctuating mass surrounded by adherent intestines was found in the left iliac fossa, and wide daily variations of temperature left but little room to doubt that it contained pus. The mass grew small. The temperature and pulse came to normal and remained there. She again declined operation and was lost sight of.

After having seen many grave cases of this kind yield so favorably to this measure, and having seen a few of them die later from peritonitis following an abdominal section which removed the great bulk of filth, leaving but little behind in a fairly clean cavity, it seemed to me that, with the same infecting organisms active in large numbers before operation and in small numbers after operation, we might expect like results if the same treatment were employed in the two classes of cases: and, further, that by beginning the use of ice before peritonitis had actually developed we might succeed in preventing that complication. (No claim is made to originality in this matter, though at the time we began using it systematically I was not aware of its previous employment for the same purposes.)

The conclusion seemed rational, and we began putting bags of ice (one to five, close to the skin) on the abdomens of patients in whom we feared that peritonitis might develop. The results during the last four years have been highly satisfactory. Many patients who experienced relief from pain by the use of ice before operation have asked for it after operation. Many have complained at first of the weight of the ice, but were soon so much relieved that they felt uncomfortable while the bags were being refilled. The smooth convalescence of many patients in whom inflammatory reaction might naturally have been looked for leads me to believe that in not a few instances such attacks have been averted. The recovery of several patients who have been reclaimed from what appeared to be almost certain death forced the conclusion that it is a life-saving agent.

Though palliative measures are not advocated where grave explosive lesions, such as intestinal or appendical perforations, are threatened or have occurred, it does seem that, after the surgeon has cleansed the abdominal cavity as best he can, we have in the local use of ice a valuable remedy. It is used with good results at the beginning of inflammation everywhere else in the body. It is worthy of a more general application here. Theoretical objections have disappeared as we have become more familiar with its use. In my experience no injury to the skin has followed its use; the healing of wounds has not been retarded by it; and no depression of the general system has been observed. That cold penetrates deeply into the abdominal cavity and may produce its effect directly is shown by some careful experiments which Dr. Letive has very kindly made for me, and by observations on man made by Dr. Schlikoff and summarized by Dr. Granger, of New Orleans, in a recent article on the use of ice as a therapeutic agent. His own observations are also of interest.

In our experiments on dogs the surface and rectal temperatures were observed for more than an hour. They did not vary from 38° and 38° respectively. Another thermometer was introduced into the pelvic cavity through a small lateral incision just below the ribs. The surface temperature quickly dropped two degrees; again the surface, rectal (or vaginal), and abdominal temperatures remained stationary for more than an hour, reading 36°, 38°, 38°. Ice was then applied to the entire surface of the abdomen. The general surface temperature was not affected after some hours. The skin under the ice reached a temperature varying from 8° to 16° C. in different dogs. The thermometer close under the abdominal wall recorded 26° C., while deep in the pelvis it fell as low as 34° and remained stationary for more than an hour. The rectal (or vaginal) temperature was 2° higher (36°), though the bulbs of the two thermometers were separated only by one-eighth of an inch. Ice was removed. Within an hour all temperatures reached their ascertained normal. With another application of ice the temperatures showed the same variations as had just been recorded in the same animals. The animals were not injured.

From these experiments it would seem possible to produce, at the seat of inflammation, a degree of temperature which greatly retards the growth of pathogenic bacteria, and which contracts the blood and lymph channels, thus relieving the congested vessels and checking the serous weeping into the cavity. These results may be accomplished without effect on the general temperature and without apparent detriment to life or tissues. Practically we may conclude (and there is abundant clinical evidence to support this view) that as peritonitis subsides its cardinal symptoms grow less evident and the resulting morbidity no longer increases. Pain, which is one of the most distressing symptoms, becomes less annoying. Ice should be used for its effect, just as calomel, salts, or other remedies are. One bag on top of a thick dressing of cotton and gauze is, of course, without value. For the relief of traumatic pain one or two ice bags over a thin dressing usually suffice. But where a frank attack of peritonitis is feared or actually exists four or five bags of ice should be kept in place day and night. They should be separated from the skin only by a towel, a binder, or a very thin gauze dressing.

Contraindications.—Cold should never be used to the exclusion of other well-known medical and surgical principles and measures. Formerly I looked upon post-operative kidney lesions as contraindicating the free use of cold. But more recent experiences lead me to believe that if a serious peritonitis is feared we may use extreme cold to the abdomen, and that it will be far less harmful than the inflammation it prevents or checks. When grave post-operative peritonitis is likely to develop, or when it actually exists, I believe there is *no* contraindication to the free use of ice locally. But when merely a slight traumatic reaction exists, this measure had perhaps better be omitted in the presence of nephritis, of a tendency to catarrhal enteritis, attacks of which are precipitated by exposure to cold, and where rheumatic and bronchial attacks follow slight chilling. Not a few patients complain of greater pain soon after ice is applied. When the pain is due to a well-defined abscess with very little peritonitis, and when it is of intestinal origin, hot applications probably serve a better purpose. But when the patients complain of pain caused by the weight of the ice, that symptom points to the existence of active inflammation and constitutes the most urgent indication for more intense cold. It has been our custom to add more ice in these cases, and the results have justified the practice.

With your permission a brief report will be made of a few cases in which, it seems to me, life was saved by the local use of ice. Several others might be recorded, but their recital would be but a repetition of what follows. Simpler cases in which the morbid products of inflammation seem to have been prevented by a timely ending of the disease will be omitted for lack of time.

CASE I.—Mrs. C. had recently recovered from a sharp attack of pelvic peritonitis and cellulitis when referred to me by Dr. C. H. Hayes, of Pittsburg. The uterus was retroverted. Two pus tubes and cystic ovaries were bound firmly to the adjacent structures, the left being fixed to the pelvic wall by a rigid, mortar-like exudate. There was a positive history of gonorrhea just preceding the attack. The cellulitis indicated a mixed infection.

Vaginal hystero-salpingo-oöphorectomy was done April 30, 1901. Enucleation was difficult. Free bleeding from extensive raw surfaces could not be controlled by clamps, but was checked by firm pelvic gauze packing. She left the table with a pulse of 166. After 1,000 cubic centimetres of normal saline solution slowly given into a vein, it rapidly fell to 100 and a few hours later to 90. During the first twenty-four hours there was but little further variation of the pulse. She was very restless and suffered much pain from the tight packing. There was no vomiting whatever till the beginning of the second day. After that she vomited repeatedly, complained of tenderness, became slightly distended, and the pulse rate was 110. She was put in Fowler's position and two ice bags were applied direct to the abdomen. A slight movement from the bowels followed an enema. At the end of forty-eight hours the clamps were removed. Eight hours later the abdomen was very much distended and very tender. Peristalsis was absent. Projectile vomiting of quantities of a slightly green fluid was frequent. The pulse was 120 and not good. During the third day vomiting was almost continuous. Expulsion of gas could not be effected by medication or enemata. The abdomen was greatly distended. The pulse had grown more rapid and weak. The pelvic gauze was removed and adhesions were freed. A little bloody serous fluid escaped. During the fourth day vomiting of dark-brown fluid having a fecal odor continued at frequent intervals. All efforts failed to cause the passage of flatus from the bowels. The abdomen was still distended. The pulse was frequent, irregular, thready, and very weak. Her extremities were purple and cold. Percussion demonstrated the presence of some free fluid in the abdominal cavity. The abdomen was continuously covered with ice. To the extremities hot applications were made. The fifth day the abdomen was less distended, soft, and not tender. Peristalsis gradually returned. Vomiting gradually ceased. She retained some nourishment and bowel movements were induced. A smaller quantity of fluid was found in the abdomen. Thus far there was but little change in the character of the pulse. The sixth day the pulse grew fuller, slower, stronger, her peripheral circulation was good and her expression better. From that time on her convalescence was rapid and uninterrupted. Before leaving the hospital she was examined and no products of her severe peritonitis were found. Some months later she was in perfect health and reported that she had had no discomfort whatever. In this desperate case the ice apparently controlled the inflammation before a fatal dose of poison had been produced by it. The absence of demonstrable adhesions is more than could ordinarily have been expected.

CASE II.—Mrs. T. was sent to me by Dr. John W. Dixon, of Pittsburg. She had firmly adherent, closed tubes and cystic ovaries. They were removed by abdominal section. The operation was not especially difficult and a speedy recovery was expected. No bacteriological report from the tubes was gotten. Occasional vomiting ceased after a few hours, and at the end of the first eighteen hours nothing suggested trouble except a pulse rate which had increased about fifteen beats. After that she complained of considerable pain. The abdomen became distended and tender. Peristalsis was markedly diminished, if not quite absent. Vomiting of a light-green fluid occurred at frequent intervals. There were frequent eructations of gas, but none was expelled by the bowel. Her pulse rapidly rose to 120 and then 130, her temperature to 103°. At the end of thirty-six hours after operation the patient was put across her bed and the cul-de-sac opened without an anesthetic. About three ounces of a bloody serous fluid escaped. A rubber tube was inserted, but very little drainage occurred. At the end of twenty-four hours more it was surrounded by adhesions and was quite useless. All the abdominal dressings, except a thin layer of gauze, were removed when the probable existence of peritonitis became apparent, and several bags of ice were applied. They were kept constantly full. During the third day her pulse gained in strength and volume, the congested peripheral circulation and temperature remained unchanged. Toward the end of the day, however, the abdomen was less tender and softer. Peristalsis returned. The expulsion of some gas followed the use of enemata.

But vomiting was spontaneous and was induced by medicine, food, or drink. By the end of the fourth day the abdomen was soft, peristalsis good, food and drink were retained, and an improvement in the character of the pulse was observed. It was normal by the end of the sixth day. But the temperature did not reach normal till the eighth day. After that her progress was speedy and satisfactory. She has suffered no inconvenience from the attack of peritonitis which so seriously threatened her life. Ordinarily a post-operative peritonitis which shows so abrupt an onset and such pronounced symptoms during the first thirty-six hours, terminates fatally within a very few days. I believe the free use of ice fortified her powers of resistance and turned the balance of power in her favor.

Though the foregoing cases were most gratifying, a favorable termination in the one which follows was quite unexpected.

CASE III.—Miss L. had adherent pus tubes. November 2, 1901, vaginal hystero-salpingo-oöphorectomy was done by the clamp method. There was no especial difficulty. For twenty-four hours her condition seemed very good. About forty-eight hours after operation the clamps were removed. Her abdomen was somewhat distended and tender. Her pulse became somewhat faster and her temperature began to rise. Without effort she vomited a quantity of dark-brown fluid at frequent intervals, and at the end of the third day she was suffering considerably from distension and pain. During the fourth day the pelvic gauze was removed. Examination showed that no adhesions separated the vaginal vault from the general peritoneal cavity. Some bloody serous fluid escaped. Stimulants and enemata seemed entirely without effect. She grew decidedly worse. The fifth day numerous enemata were expelled without gas. Eructation and vomiting persisted. Her circulation was very poor, the pulse very rapid, the extremities purple and leaking. By this time the abdomen had become less distended, soft, and pressure caused no pain. The sixth day the abdomen was soft and flat, vomiting was less frequent, and some gas was expelled after enemata. But her temperature was 102°, her features were pinched, her extremities were cold, purple, and leaking. Her pulse was thready, intermittent, and could not be counted at the wrist. The carotid artery showed 172 beats to the minute. I left the hospital at 2 A.M., thinking she would be dead before morning. But fortunately the turning point was reached. She slept some the latter part of the night and at intervals during the morning. Gas was expelled voluntarily. The pulse was of better volume, less frequent, and stronger. The extremities were warmer. Five full ice bags had been kept in contact with the abdomen since the first symptoms appeared, and were continued for several days more. Her recovery was rapid and smooth. She left the hospital four weeks after operation and has been well since. In this case I believe the peritonitis was severe and that while it lasted considerable poisonous fluid collected in the abdomen; that the ice checked the inflammation, and that the production of poison practically ceased when the abdomen became soft and flat on the fifth day; that the remaining fluid continued to be absorbed and to act as a powerful depressant to the circulatory apparatus; that by the end of the sixth day this had all been absorbed, and that with its elimination the vital functions were gradually restored to the normal. It is evident that the poison was very nearly fatal and that had its production continued it would doubtless have proved so. We so rarely see so grave a peritonitis subside so unexpectedly that the ice surely stood in causal relation to this happy result.

The next case shows the value of ice as a hemostatic, as well as an antiphlogistic agent after operation.

CASE IV.—Mrs. X. was admitted to Mercy Hospital during a severe attack of pelvic peritonitis of tubal origin. Improvement was progressing rapidly when interrupted by an acute exacerbation which lasted a few days, and then by another. The abdomen was opened. Two pus tubes were freed from extensive but recent adhesions and removed without especial difficulty. The pedicles were ligated with care and were thought to be secure. She left the table with a good pulse of 84 beats to the minute. Half an hour later her pulse was 106, and when seen by me in fifteen minutes more it was 130 and much weaker, though her color was good and the veins of her forehead were distended. The foot of the bed was raised. The rate quickly dropped to 120 and the volume was better. Two ice bags were put over the dressings. In an hour more the pulse reached 146. We prepared to open the abdomen at once, but the rate had dropped to 130 by the time we were ready. A stitch was removed and a sterile glass catheter was introduced into the abdomen without trouble or pain. Free blood was found in the peritoneal cavity, but improvement was positive. Being ready to open the cavity at a moment's notice, we decided not to interfere as long as the circulation was getting better. Very nearly all the dressings were removed and two more ice bags were put on the abdomen. Eight hours after operation the pulse was 108. It remained practically the same for twelve hours more and then progressively rose to 118, 126, 130, and to 134 at the end of thirty hours. The pus in the tubes was found to contain streptococci. With the rise in pulse the abdomen became distended and tender. The stomach was not retentive and quantities of bile-stained watery fluid were thrown up at frequent intervals without nausea, retching, or even effort. Her temperature was 101°. During the second day her urine contained albumin, many granular and epithelial casts, and a few streptococci. Her abdomen was distended and tender, but some gas was expelled after enemata. The pulse rose to 138. Her features were pinched. With this condition and streptococci in the presence of a good culture medium, we feared the worst. Previous experiences with ice gave us confidence in it. For four days the four bags were kept full of ice and in direct contact with the abdomen, except just at the incision. By the beginning of the third day there was a decline in pulse rate and in the symptoms. By the end of seventy-two hours from operation her pulse was 106. This was truly an abrupt ending of what gave every indication of being a very grave condition.

In conclusion, your attention is called to the fact that in all these cases the local symptoms of inflammation subsided first, and that later the constitutional symptoms due to the absorption of poisons already produced disappeared likewise.

DR. HERMAN E. HAYD, of Buffalo, said that his attention was first called to the use of ice following abdominal section by Dr. Pryor, who made a very practical rule when he said that the more the condition was inflammatory the more he applied ice; the more severe the pain the more he used ice; and the more the pain was spasmodic—the result, for instance, of gas in the intestines—the more he applied heat. The speaker thought that the essayist had been more specific, in that he had said that the more the patient tolerated the weight of the ice the more would he continue its application. From the experience he had had with the use of ice in a limited way he had found it of great practical utility. He had never thought of applying ice to the extent the essayist had used it, where he enveloped the whole abdomen in a pillow of ice. It was a question to his mind whether the application of ice would prevent the spread of a septic peritonitis.

DR. JAMES F. BALDWIN, of Columbus, O., thought that the essayist, to make the paper more complete, should carry out the experiments upon animals presenting a fair degree of fat, with artificially induced peritonitis; then the profession would have practical demonstrations. He should at the same time conduct control experiments in other animals.

DR. HOWARD W. LONGYEAR, of Detroit, had not used ice in as thorough a manner as the essayist, but he had used it enough to look upon it as an important factor of treatment. He had been specially pleased with the manner in which the ice had relieved pain. Patients would ask for the ice if pain returned. He usually depended upon the body temperature as an indication for its discontinuance or use again. If the temperature declined to nearly normal, he directed the nurse to remove the ice and to apply it again if the temperature arose. Where the circulation was poor it was necessary to protect the skin by the application of gauze. This was necessary because if one applied a rubber ice bag directly to the skin he was liable to produce a slough.

DR. CHARLES GREENE CUMSTON remarked that it used to be the routine practice of the advocates of vaginal hysterectomy to apply an ice bag immediately on putting the patient to bed, for the first forty-eight hours, keeping it there to prevent elevation of temperature and distension of the abdomen. There was one point that occurred to him in regard to applying ice to the abdomen, namely, if it was pushed too far a certain amount of danger might accrue. He believed where it was applied in cases of local inflammation, as in appendicitis, if its application was continued for too long a time, there might be sloughing of the appendix, although one would not get it had the patient been let alone without the ice-bag treatment. For a long time he had applied ice after vaginal hysterectomies, but had abandoned it, as he could not see that it made any difference in the termination of the case.

DR. C. L. BONIFIELD commended the paper because its author had followed out painstaking, careful investigations. It was a question whether ice was really of value in these cases. The application of ice was of inestimable value in cases where operative intervention was very limited, or in cases of appendicitis, for instance, that had not been operated upon, or in cases of tubal suppuration where it was desirable to prevent the extension of the local inflammation. But in a case where the abdomen had been opened, the intestines and abdominal contents having been generally handled, he believed that the thorough application of ice would interfere with the digestive function of the peritoneum and retard efforts at purgation, and in that way do more harm than good.

DR. SIMPSON, in closing the discussion, said that it was only in rare cases he had used a large amount of ice, where the patient was going from bad to worse, where the peritonitis was spreading as the hours went by, and at times he had seen it do good in such instances. Of course one could not tell positively whether the ice accomplished this good or not. In all cases where a considerable amount of ice had been used the general temperature had been kept up by hot bottles applied to other parts of the body. The temperature had never been reduced below normal by the local use of ice.

With regard to the fact that ice had been generally used for a long period of time in cases of vaginal hysterectomy, etc., the speaker said that there was no effort on his part to claim anything original, but that he had simply presented a clinical report of the application of a well-known remedy.

As to whether ice did more harm than good, in a considerable series of cases he had before the use of ice, contrasted with a like number of cases he had observed since its use, he believed that the patients had gotten along better with it than without it. In short, the mortality had been lower with it than without it.

TWO FATAL CASES OF TETANUS FOLLOWING ABDOMINAL SECTION, DUE TO INFECTED LIGATURES, WITH A PLEA FOR THE ANGIOTRIBE IN ABDOMINAL SURGERY.

BY

WALTER B. DORSETT, M.D.,

St. Louis, Mo.

BOTH of these cases were in women upon whom I had made ventrofixations of the uterus. The choice of the operation was made on account of adhesions of the uterus to surrounding tissues, due to previous inflammatory conditions. The suture material used was, for fastening the uterus to the anterior abdominal wall, kangaroo tendon of a little above the average size; for closing the abdominal peritoneum, catgut, sizes Nos. 1 and 2; and for the through-and-through abdominal sutures, silkworm gut. The catgut and kangaroo tendon were taken from the hermetically sealed tubes. The silkworm gut was obtained from a local firm and was in skein, but was antisepticized by a thorough boiling immediately before being used. The catgut and kangaroo tendon were the same brand I had repeatedly used before, and were prepared and put up by one of the best-known manufacturing firms of this country.

CASE I.—Mrs. S., aged 25 years, married only a few months, consulted me May 1 on account of a badly retroverted uterus which was firmly adherent to the posterior wall of the cul-de-sac of Douglas. An incision in linea alba was made May 3, 1902. The uterus, after being freed from adhesions, was brought up, and the anterior face a little below the fundus was attached to the anterior abdominal wall with three medium-size strands of kangaroo tendon. The peritoneum was closed by means of No. 2 catgut, and the abdominal wall brought together with silkworm gut.

The patient suffered from no appreciable shock, and did well until May 7, when she complained of some rigidity about the lower jaw when she would attempt to take nourishment. Later in the day there appeared a good deal of rigidity of the masseter muscle, and the case became clearly one of tetanus. At 2 o'clock on May 8, 10 cubic centimetres of antitetanic serum were injected subcutaneously, and 8 grains of chloral hydrate were given by the mouth, and repeated every hour until some sleep was produced. Later in the forenoon she complained of some discomfort between the shoulders, when, upon examination, a bright-red spot about the size of the palm of the hand was seen. This blush had an abrupt margin, and in the centre were two abrasions which were supposed to be due to scratches inflicted by the finger nails of patient's own fingers. At 12 o'clock noon 10 cubic centimetres of antitoxin were given. Marked convulsions came on, and nourishment by the mouth became impossible and rectal nutritive injections had to be resorted to. At 4 P.M. of the same day 10 cubic centimetres of cerebro-spinal fluid were withdrawn, and 10 cubic centimetres of antitetanic serum were injected into the spinal canal. Chloral to the extent of 30 grains per dose every three hours was given by the rectum, but produced little effect upon the convulsions, which increased in severity and frequency until from thirty to seventy occurred per hour. The body was bathed with perspiration, and throughout the entire illness the temperature did not rise above 100° F. May 10, morphia sulphate in quarter-grain doses was combined with the chloral to produce sleep and to quiet the nervous system. Later in the day it was decided to transfuse her with normal salt solution and a vein was opened for this purpose, and while in the act of throwing the salt solution into the vein a violent convulsion came on, which ended the scene, patient dying on the third day after the disease was recognized.

During the entire treatment there were given 500 grains of chloral by mouth and rectum, frequent hypodermatic injections of morphine, and 80 cubic centimetres of antitoxin. None of these remedies had the least effect beyond the occasional hypnotic effect produced by the chloral and morphine.

The abdominal sutures were removed on the second day after the onset of the disease, and the secretions were given to the bacteriologist; so also were the scabs from the abrasions on the back, as well as the scrapings from beneath the nails, and the 6 or 7 ounces of cerebro-spinal fluid that was withdrawn by lumbar puncture, all given to the bacteriologist, with the following result:

No. 1. *Scab from Skin under the Left Scapula.*—The material was rubbed with normal salt solution and the emulsion was injected into mice subcutaneously. *Mouse No. 1:* Weight, 15 grammes. Amount injected, 1.5 cubic centimetres. Time of injection, May 8 at 3 P.M. Result: May 9, very slight scoliosis; May 10, scoliosis marked; May 11, marked scoliosis, and contraction of the left hind leg; spasm; May 12, dead. *Mouse No. 2:* Weight, 13 grammes. Amount injected, 1 cubic centimetre. Injection made May 8, 3 P.M. Result: May 9, possibly slight scoliosis; May 10, scoliosis distinct; May 11, scoliosis marked; May 12, much progressed; May 13, found dead at 11 A.M. Both of these mice died of typical tetanus.

The area of subcutaneous tissue into which, in mouse No. 2, the injection of the emulsion was made, was excised and utilized for cultures. From these cultures a pure growth of tetanus was obtained May 19.

No. 2. *Three Scrapings from Finger Nails.*—These were emulsified with 1.5 cubic centimetres of sterile physiologic salt solution and injected into a mouse designated as *Mouse No. 3.* Weight, 16 grammes. Amount injected subcutaneously, 1.5 cubic centimetres. Time, May 8, 4 P.M. The mouse remained well and showed no signs of tetanus.

No. 3. *Cerebro-spinal Fluid.*—*Mouse No. 4:* Weight, 12 grammes. Amount of cerebro-spinal fluid injected, 1 cubic centimetre. Time of inoculation, May 9, 9 A.M. The mouse showed no signs of tetanus. *Mouse No. 5:* Weight, 16 grammes. Time of inoculation, May 9, 9 A.M. No result. *Mouse No. 6:* Weight, 14 grammes. Injected 1 cubic centimetre of cerebro-spinal fluid plus 0.1 cubic centimetre of serum from a horse that died of tetanus (0.1 cubic centimetre being the fatal dose of a mouse of that weight). Time of inoculation, May 11, 4 P.M. Result: May 12, possibly slight scoliosis; May 13, appears well; and May 14, seemed to be all right, and did not die.

(Signed) C. FISCH.

CASE II.—Mrs. P.. aged 45, mother of several children. History of several attacks of pelvic inflammation. On examination uterine retroversion with fixation was discovered. The previous history of this case was one that clearly demanded surgical interference, and on May 26. after a thorough preparation, the patient was anesthetized and the same operation as in the preceding case was performed. No unusual shock followed the operation. and the patient did as well as could be expected till June 1, at 4 P.M., patient complained of a soreness about the angle of the jaws, and she became very restless and was unable to sleep. Nausea came on and she was unable to retain nourishment. Slight rigidity about the masseter and trapezius muscles now became apparent. This condition gradually extended down the back and convulsions finally set in, and she died of tetanus June 4, or three days after the first symptoms were manifested. The treatment of this case was about the same as was followed in Case 1, except the intraspinous injection of antitetanic serum and the intravenous transfusion of normal saline solution were not practised.

Summary of Treatment in Both Cases.—Chloral in from 10 to 30 grain doses per rectum was given from every two to four hours; occasionally with this one-fourth to one-half grain of morphine was combined with the chloral; ten cubic centimetres of antitetanic serum hypodermatically every six hours, and one-half per cent solution of carbolic acid hypodermatically. An attempt at reducing the violence of the convulsions was made with inhalations of chloroform, but toward the last the convulsions were so frequent that it was impossible to continue the chloroform without producing chloroform narcosis.

Immediately after the death of Case 2 all of the sutures were removed from the wound. The catgut used in uniting the peritoneum were found to be partially dissolved. The kangaroo tendons used to hold the uterus forward were somewhat macerated. The silkworm gut used for closing the abdominal wound were unaffected by their presence in the tissues. All of these, together with secretions in and about the wound. were given to a very competent bacteriologist for a thorough investigation. Having been impressed with the fact that the cause of infection was present in the suture material, the entire unused stock of suture material that had been purchased some time before. and from which the material used in these cases was taken at random, was turned over to the bacteriologist with instructions that it should also be examined.   The result of these examinations is here given.

INVESTIGATIONS INTO THE ORIGIN OF THE TETANUS INFECTION IN MRS. P.'S CASE.

June 2, 1902.—On removing the dressing a large amount of pus was found, which was removed with sterile cotton and preserved, so also were the catgut sutures, and were placed in a sterile container and sealed.   Upon examination microscopically, a few bacteria were found in the pus, among them bacilli of the size, shape, and staining qualities of tetanus bacilli.   Only one spore-forming bacillus could be found.   The cotton was soaked in bouillon for twenty-four hours and incubated at 37° C.   After this time the fluid was drained off and used for animal injections.   The catgut sutures were cut into small pieces and incubated with bouillon in the same way.   With the fluids thus obtained the following experiments upon mice were made.

June 3, 1902, 3 P.M.—*Mouse No. 1:*   Received subcutaneously 10 cubic centimetres of the pus bouillon (twenty-four hours); died of typical tetanus June 7.   *Mouse No. 2:*   Subcutaneously 1 cubic centimetre of same material; died of tetanus during the night of June 8.   *Mouse No. 3:*   Subcutaneously 1 cubic centimetre of the suture bouillon (twenty-four hours); died of tetanus June 9.   *Mouse No. 4:*   Subcutaneously 0.5 cubic centimetre of the same material as in No. 3; showed no symptoms, except slightest degree of scoliosis on the second day after injection. Cultures from the pus yielded in one tube tetanus bacilli; and on hydrocele-agar typical gonococci could be cultivated.[1]

On June 3 I received from Dr. Sibley the kangaroo tendon by which the uterus had been fixed during the operation.   It was treated like the catgut sutures before mentioned.

June 4, 4 P.M.—*Mouse No. 5:*   Subcutaneously 1 cubic centimetre of the tendon bouillon; death from typical tetanus June 9. *Mouse No. 6:*   Subcutaneously 1 cubic centimetre of the same material as in No. 5; death from tetanus June 11.   The examination of the tissues removed at autopsy revealed nothing that could be used for the question under discussion.

[1] It will be noticed in the history of this patient that she had had several attacks of inflammatory trouble of the appendages; one, at least, may have been due to the gonococcus, though no direct history was obtained.

EXAMINATION OF THE DIFFERENT KINDS OF SUTURING MATERIAL
USED IN MRS. P.'S CASE.

For my experiments Dr. Dorsett and a member of the firm from which the suture material had been obtained put at my disposal samples of the following sutures: (1) sterilized catgut No. 2, two tubes; (2) sterilized catgut No. 1, from the same firm, two tubes; (3) sterilized kangaroo tendon, from the same firm, four tubes.

This material was utilized in the following way: After sterilizing the outside of the tubes for twenty-four hours by putting them into a 1:500 $HgCl_2$ solution, the tubes were opened and the sutures were extracted with sterile forceps and put into sterile Petri dishes, which were allowed to remain at incubation temperature for some hours. After the evaporation of the alcohol, pieces of varying length were cut out from them (some from ends, and others from middle) and carefully inserted into small incisions in the skin made on guinea-pigs and mice. The wounds of the animals were thoroughly closed with collodion. In some cases the pieces of sutures were dipped into sterile agar and thus introduced. The results obtained were:

I. *Sterilized Catgut, Size No. 2.*—June 8, tube No. 1: No. 1*a*, guinea-pig, 5 centimetres of the gut, no symptoms, no suppuration, animal well June 30; No. 1*b*, mouse, 2 centimetres of the gut, no symptoms, animal well. June 14, tube No. 2: No. 2*a*, guinea-pig, 5 centimetres of the gut, no symptoms, animal well June 30; No. 2*b*, mouse, 2 centimetres of the gut, no symptoms, animal well June 30.

II. *Sterilized Catgut No. 1.*—June 14, tube No. 1: No. 3*a*, guinea-pig, 5 centimetres of the gut, no symptoms, animal well June 30; No. 3*b*, mouse, 2 centimetres of the gut, no symptoms, animal well June 30. June 16, tube No. 2: No. 4*a*, guinea-pig, 5 centimetres of the gut dipped in agar; suppuration, no tetanus; animal died with multiple abscesses.

III. *Sterilized Kangaroo Tendon.*—June 8, tube No. 1: (*a*) guinea-pig, 7 centimetres of the tendon, no symptoms, animal well June 30; (*b*) mouse, 2 centimetres of the gut, same as in (*a*); (*c*) mouse, 2 centimetres, result as in (*a*) and (*b*). June 16, tube No. 2: (*a*) guinea-pig, 5 centimetres of the tendon, first tetanic symptoms June 18, death from tetanus June 21; (*b*) mouse, 2 centimetres of the tendon, scoliosis June 19, death from tetanus June 22. June 20, tube No. 2—this time the pieces were cut from places far distant from those where the

40

material for the experiment of June 16, with the same tube, was taken: (c) mouse, 3 centimetres of the tendon, scoliosis June 19, death from tetanus June 22; (d) mouse, 1 centimetre of the tendon, no symptoms, well June 30; (e) mouse, 1 centimetre of the tendon, death from tetanus June 25; (f) mouse, 2 centimetres of the tendon, no symptoms until June 24 slight scoliosis (?) on this day, suppuration at point of injection, tendon expelled from wound June 22, recovery. June 12, tube No. 3: (a) guinea-pig, 5 centimetres of tendon, no symptoms, well June 30; (b) mouse, 1 centimetre of the tendon, no symptoms, well June 30; (c) mouse, 2 centimetres of the tendon, no symptoms, well June 30. June 16, tube No. 4: (a) guinea-pig, 7 centimetres of the tendon dipped in agar, suppuration but no tetanus, tendon expelled on third day; (b) mouse, 2 centimetres of the tendon, scoliosis June 19, death from tetanus June 21; (c) mouse, 2 centimetres of the tendon, no symptoms, well June 30.

Result.—While the catgut material (Nos. 1 and 2) was found to be sterile, two of the kangaroo tendons examined contained undoubtedly spores of the tetanus bacillus.

(Signed) C. Fisch.

It will be observed that tetanic symptoms were noticed in the first case three days after the operation, and in the second case five days. The period of incubation is by no means a fixed period, as is shown by a careful study of the literature, although most authors claim that it is seven days or longer. Senn, however, claims that in rare instances twenty-four hours only may be required to produce toxic symptoms. In Case 1, so short a time (three days) having elapsed after the operation, and the presence of inflamed area between the scapulæ, pointed to a probable infection from the patient's finger nails prior to the operation, and while in the act of scratching; hence the reason of a bacteriological examination of the scab taken from this point, as well as the examination of the scrapings from beneath the nails. However, after the investigation of the suture material from the unused tubes, which was the same used in both cases, it was shown conclusively that the source of infection lay in the kangaroo tendon. There is no doubt that the fatal result in both cases was due to the tetanus bacillus in the tendon. Tendons from this same stock were used in a number of cases, which were anxiously watched for some weeks afterward, but, as no symptoms of tetanus appeared, the conclusions were that in the other cases, fortunately, sterile tendons were used, and, while some of these tendons were sterile, some certainly contained the tetanus bacilli.

The bacteriological literature of the tetanus bacillus shows that it is anaerobic in nature and is abundant in the soil. This fact demonstrates the cause of its activity in punctured wounds (caused by infected objects, as "the rusty nail") where there is but little chance for drainage.

In the above reported cases there was no chance for drainage in the closely coaptated abdominal incision, hence the greater chance for general intoxication.

When once the disease has manifested itself, even an early opening of the wound will do no good, as the rigidity of the muscular system is always a clear indication that the intoxication is already general. However, this was not overlooked, and they were opened and cauterized.

Tetanus following abdominal section is rare. H. C. Coe, in the *Gynecological and Obstetrical Journal,* December, 1901, page 500, reports two fatal cases, one following operation for pus tube, and one following operation for cystic ovary and fibroid of the uterus. In one case symptoms developed sixteen days after the operation, and in the other ten days were required before the disease manifested itself. In the *Philadelphia Medical Journal,* February 16, 1901, James B. Bissel reported two fatal cases following laparatomy, in one of which tetanus developed fourteen days after operation, and in the other nine days after operation. The source of infection in these two reports, if found, was not given, nor is there any mention made of the suture material used. Thompson, of Hull (*London Lancet,* June 20, 1900), reports a fatal case following nephropexy. Source here also not given. It appears from the above quotations that the infections in these cases were not ascertained, or were at least obscure. This may have been the reason for not giving the source, but they were certainly operations in which animal ligatures are generally used.

Experiments have shown that tetanus spores are among the most resistant of all germs. They will retain their vitality after three hours' soaking in a solution of 1:1000 bichloride of mercury. A 10 per cent solution of carbolic will not affect them. An exposure of 80° C. has also no effect. An immersion of an animal ligature in a 50 per cent solution of alcohol will not be sufficient for a thorough penetration into the substance of the structure, particularly the kangaroo tendon generally used in surgery, as the alcohol will quickly coagulate the albumen contained in the surface of the ligature, and goes no further. Formol or formalin will not answer, as it so hardens the tendon as to render it unfit for use. Heating by boiling an hermetically sealed tube of kangaroo tendon produces such shrinkage of the tendon as to render it unfit for use. So it appears that the safest ligature to-day is some material that can be thoroughly boiled immediately before being put to use. So far silk is the only suture we can use in the abdomen with any degree of safety. But the silk, when it can be supplanted in the ligation of stumps by the angiotribe, should be discarded.

So far I have used successfully the angiotribe twenty-five times, as follows: Abdominal hysterectomy, ten times; pus tubes, five times; hemorrhoids, once; extrauterine pregnancy, four times; dermoid cyst, once; ovariotomies, three times; and once in a vaginal hysterectomy, and my observations are:

1. Patients upon whom it has been tried suffer less post-operative pain.

2. No adhesions to stumps have followed its application.

3. No secondary hemorrhages have followed its application.

4. It can be applied, when two instruments are used, alternately by the operator and the assistant without the fear that is incident to the slipping of a ligature knot, and in less time.

Why not use it?

3941 WEST BELLE PLACE.

DR. HOWARD W. LONGYEAR said the paper emphasized the importance and necessity of the use of sterilized animal ligatures. Surgeons had to depend upon some unknown person to sterilize ligatures for their use, and personally he had always felt great hesitancy in accepting these ligatures from any source. In the last ten years he had prepared his own ligatures; he had not bought a ligature which he had to bury. He had not buried a single animal ligature that was not prepared by himself. He relied upon boiling the ligature in alcohol at a sufficiently high temperature to kill the tetanus spores. He had had no trouble with tetanus following any of his operations. Sometimes, when he had not used gloves, he had observed a mild form of infection which he believed was from his hands. Since the use of rubber gloves he had had no trouble.

DR. A. GOLDSPOHN, of Chicago, said that if the angiotribe could take the place of all ligatures, then there would be a strong reason for its use. But all surgeons knew that it could not.

Ligatures operators must have, because the angiotribe took the place of ligatures only as far as pedicles were concerned. The liability of the occurrence of tetanus following surgical operations was extremely rare. The objections of the essayist to the use of absorbable ligatures were not well taken, because he had not referred to the proper, potent antiseptic preparation of absorbable ligatures. Hardly any one now depended on the use of chemical antiseptics, particularly not on alcohol alone or bichloride of mercury alone. There were other, better agents than those in the domain of chemical antiseptics. But he did not use chemical antiseptics; he used heat and water moisture combined, not alcohol boiled. Germs had been boiled in absolute alcohol in an autoclave at 212° for an hour and still they grew. He referred now to the anthrax bacillus. Pure alcohol, or commercial alcohol, was not the most destructive form of alcohol. The most germicidal alcohol was one that contained from about 55 to 60 per cent of water, because of the softening, disintegrating effect of the water. The alcoholic solutions of any antiseptic were far inferior to its watery solution. All of these absorbable ligatures could be hardened by formalin, so that they could not shrink, and could be boiled satisfactorily.

As to the use of the angiotribe without any supplementary ligature and without getting secondary hemorrhage, he thought the essayist stood alone in such experience, because all men who had used the angiotribe considerably, and those whom he had observed, had used supplementary ligatures. They had used the angiotribe simply to compress the tissues, and then used ligatures. Several of these men had had secondary hemorrhage.

DR. WILLIS G. MACDONALD, of Albany, N. Y., said the surgeon could not depend upon manufacturers for the sterilization of his surgical material, particularly ligatures. However competent they apparently were, there came a time when their material led to unfortunate results.

In relation to animal ligatures, particularly the kangaroo tendon and gut of the size larger than so-called No. 3, he did not believe, after several years of experience, that there was any way that one could effectually and always make it sterile. He did not use kangaroo tendon, but had finally fallen back upon the use of the cumol method, carrying out the boiling of the cumol for a longer period than was recommended by Dr. Kelly or Dr. Clarke. He spoke very highly of the use of fine silk. The smaller the ligature one used the better would his cases do; and he had within the last year used 00 silk in his cases, applying as many as one hundred and fifty or two hundred ligatures in the wide opening of tissues, and he had not seen any consequences from it, cutting them off short, using fine ligatures, and not taking up large masses of tissue.

With relation to the angiotribe, he had done more than one hundred hysterectomies with it, or with the modified instrument of Newman, of Chicago, and he had not had a single unfortunate result. He then did a hysterectomy and his patient died of secondary hemorrhage. He had not applied the angiotribe for the absolute control of hemorrhage since; but he used it largely to crush tissue, make small pedicles which can be ligated much better by the use of silk particularly.

DR. WASHINGTON H. BAKER, of Philadelphia, said it occurred to him that in these operations the surgeon might start with sterile tendon and his hands be practically sterile; but after working the hands vigorously for ten or fifteen minutes, the sepsis, being situated a little deeper in the skin, might become dislodged and come to the surface, and the previously sterile tendon might become infected. He thought probably that some of the instances mentioned, where the ligatures seemed to have been sterile and others unaccountably infected, might be viewed in that light and considered as a possible factor in the infection.

DR. CHARLES GREENE CUMSTON had used cumol catgut for buried sutures in the abdominal wall almost entirely, and had not had a single case go wrong. He had never purchased his sutures from manufacturers. Every bit of catgut or kangaroo tendon used by him was either sterilized by himself or by his operating nurse. He had used the dry method. His use of the animal preparations had been entirely with buried sutures, but there was a ligature now which possessed many virtues that silk did not. This was celluloid thread. The finest size, number 00, was extremely small. It had this advantage, that the longer it was boiled the stronger it became, and for gastro-intestinal work or for ligatures he thought there was nothing that equalled it.

DR. WALTER P. MANTON did not like silk. He had used it for a number of years, and then gave it up. If one abandoned the use of the animal ligature it left him to use the angiotribe. He believed he was the first practitioner in Michigan to publish a series of cases in which the angiotribe was used. He had used it for about a year, then gave it up. He did not have a single case of secondary hemorrhage, although he had used it in vaginal hysterectomies and operations through the abdomen; nevertheless he came to the conclusion that the angiotribe was a dangerous instrument, and that sooner or later he would meet his Waterloo. After publishing a series of cases he received several letters, one in particular, urging him not to use the angiotribe on account of secondary hemorrhage. He found himself gradually using the angiotribe and ligature, so that finally he abandoned the angiotribe entirely and relied on ligatures alone. He had used kangaroo tendon extensively and did not recall having any serious trouble with it. Occasionally there would be suppuration, but not often. For a number of years he had used only catgut prepared after the method advocated by Dr. Carstens. Last spring, however, after returning from the meeting of the American Medical Association, he began to use catgut, prepared in the same manner and he presumed by the same operator's nurse, but had ten successive cases of suppuration of the abdominal wound. He dropped this catgut immediately and bought some outside, prepared by one of the manufacturers, and since then he had not had any trouble.

DR. DORSETT did not believe surgeons were ready to give up the animal ligature, and he did not believe that there was any absolute way of thoroughly antisepticizing animal ligatures.

With reference to the remarks of Dr. Goldspohn as to boiling kangaroo tendon in absolute alcohol, bacteriologists would tell us that absolute alcohol will not penetrate kangaroo tendon as deeply as a fifty per cent solution. Even then it simply coagulated the albumen on the outside of the ligature and did not penetrate the centre.

The objection to the angiotribe offered by Dr. Macdonald was justifiable, yet it must be remembered that even silk ligatures would slip. Any kind of ligature would slip occasionally.

DR. WALTER B. CHASE, of Brooklyn, N. Y., read a paper on

SOME PROBLEMS IN EXPLORATORY LAPARATOMY.

DR. A. GOLDSPOHN said that in abdominal surgery, outside of the female pelvis, instances would always be rather frequent in which an exploratory abdominal section was necessary, where the diagnosis without it could not be even approximately made. Neoplasms of the pancreas, the liver, the bile ducts, the gall bladder, kidneys, and anomalous conditions about the stomach, mechanical ileus, etc., would leave surgeons in such a degree of doubt as to make an exploratory abdominal section the proper thing. But he contended for the female pelvis that an exploratory abdominal section was not often necessary. He believed that a number of men who operated on the female pelvis did not qualify themselves in bimanual palpation and did not attempt to make sufficiently approximate diagnoses. His standard in regard to gynecology was that practitioners needed to practise bimanual palpation in order to become even approximate normal workers as gynecologists, just as much as one would have to practise on the piano, not to become an expert, but an ordinary player on that instrument. Practitioners had no right to do gynecological work until they had thoroughly drilled themselves, had schooled their fingers also. If practitioners schooled themselves in bimanual palpation as they should, and as they could if they limited themselves to the female pelvis, they could acquire that degree of skill and ability which would enable them to exclude such errors as had been made from time to time.

DR. CHASE, in closing the discussion, said that the standard which the last speaker had set was a very fine one, and one to which all desired to attain. Great skill in abdominal palpation would doubtless enable a practitioner to determine with reasonable certainty in most cases whether there was disease in the pelvic cavity or not. However, in the case of a woman with a fat abdomen, thick abdominal walls, a large amount of exudate, and the neoplasms glued together by adhesions, he confessed that he had in certain instances not been able to make a satisfactory diagnosis. In such instances, if one was in doubt, it was best to make a frank statement to the patient and proceed. If a mistake had been made the diagnosis could be corrected after opening the peritoneal cavity.

The following papers were read, after which they were discussed jointly:

GENERAL CONSIDERATION OF DRAINAGE IN ABDOMINAL AND PELVIC SURGERY.[1]

BY

JOSEPH PRICE, M.D.,
Philadelphia, Pa.

THE great Keith said in one of his last valuable productions: "After all, where would we be without drainage?" We have been playing battledore and shuttlecock with drainage for many years, but few of us have practised it with unvarying confidence from the beginning of our trying and painful experience in pelvic surgery. Early in the history of ovariotomy, in the hands of about all the ovariotomists, while using the clamp and pins for closure of the incision with harelip sutures, the method was so crude that it favored drainage in a good number of cases. In the ligature method the ligatures were large and numerous and were drained through the lower angle of the incision. The more progressive and successful specialist, doing painstaking operations in every detail, where filth and complications or adhesions were found to exist, practised most extensive sponge packing or operative drainage. The modern operator does the same operative drainage, by his gauze pack or the dry operation. The same operator, in many instances, also uses gauze, or some form of tubular drainage, both local and general, and his results are so good, his mortality so low, that it would be difficult for him to tell you just why he attains such results. The English and Continental operators of prominence, with long series of operations with low or *nil* mortality, have all practised one or more methods of drainage; they have all recognized that, aside from the pleasing primary results, they have minimized post-operative complications. About all the repeated operations are coming from operators in hospitals opposing drainage or practising it only when they are compelled to; and it is curious that these same men favor drainage when they abandon procedures or practise incomplete ones. You find they commonly say, "I stopped and put in a drain." Such an apology always reminds me of men who puncture or stab, thrust in a drain, and run.

My confidence in drainage has always been progressive. I fortunately recognized the value of it early in my experience; and as my work was then, and is now, largely for suppurative forms of pelvic diseases, and the results so good in a class of cases many of whom would have died without it, that I have never regretted its use. As the operative field was extended and broadened, drains placed in the renal regions after a variety of operations there, in the pelvic region after extensive and heroic operations in that cavity, I always felt like thanking the drain for the very valuable assistance and support it was giving me in what was commonly called bold or aggressive surgery, as surely without the drain our hands would have been tied.

A good number of operators, doing fairly good work by the suprapubic route, condemned or partially rejected drainage. Some of them never learned, and never will learn, how to handle drainage well. Some of them will unfortunately die without knowing how to drain. After abandoning the suprapubic route they were placed in the uncomfortable position of admitting that drainage was doing what they had refused to do by suprapubic surgery.

The operators doing suprapubic surgery in pelvic suppurations and in all forms of appendicitis must possess thirty-three vertebræ. It is hard and complicated work; it requires and demands prolonged apprenticeship, as the surgery is extensive, the toilet important, and drainage always vital. You can save about everything with drainage, and your mortality will be large without it. Nothing has pleased me more in the last few years than the knowledge of the fact that the young school of surgeons in about every instance are using drainage with great success and skill, in spite of the fact that they have been under the instruction of that class of men about the country and in the hospitals condemning it. Only recently a brilliant young surgeon connected with the Bryn Mawr Hospital opened two bad subjects in two places, made a careful toilet, and drained, saving both cases. The first was done for a gangrenous appendix and general peritonitis, the second for a lacerated

spleen. He put a gauze overcoat about the mutilated spleen.
One of his colleagues, about the same time, drained a lacerated
kidney and saved his patient.

DR. CHARLES GREENE CUMSTON, of Boston, reported four cases
of

RUPTURED PUS TUBES,

with special reference to the treatment of perforation into the
bladder.

TREATMENT OF PELVIC ABSCESS.

BY

HERMAN E. HAYD, M.D., M.R.C.S.,
Buffalo, N. Y.

THE pathology of pelvic disease was given to us by Goupil and
Bernutz, and their teachings have been amplified and embellished
by the assistance of modern bacteriology. They demonstrated
that inflammatory processes travel by continuity of tissue from
the endometrium to the tubes and ovaries and peritoneum, and
also, by way of the lymphatics of the cervix and body of the
uterus, along the lymph channels of the broad ligament and the
lymph vessels between the bladder and uterus to the peritoneum
and to the ovary, and even to the tube secondarily. The gonococcus travels by the route of the mucous membrane only, while the
streptococcus and staphylococcus—which are the ordinary pus-
producing organisms—may take either channel. Consequently
we may have pus in the pelvis as the result of an extension of a
gonorrheal infection, of post-abortum and post-puerperal processes, of traumas and injuries of the cervix and body of the
uterus resulting from accidents occurring during labor, and of
careless surgical   interference and intrauterine manipulations.
These infections may produce a primary tubal and ovarian abscess with secondary localized purulent peritonitis, or, by way of
the lymphatics, suppurating foci in the broad ligament, or even
an abscess between its folds or in the lymphatic network between
the vagina and bladder, or it may extend to the peritoneum and
produce a collection of pus in the free pelvis, or an ovarian abscess, or even a secondary tubal abscess.

A pure gonorrheal infection is not common; in fact, the pathology is usually the result of a mixed infection. Latent intraliga-

mentary cysts, ovarian tumors, dermoid cysts, and other adventitious growths are often brought into pernicious activity, and acute suppuration takes place in them very suddenly as the result of the irritation of these infecting organisms. It is surprising, in studying these cases, to see how diverse and many-sided the complications can be. In some where the infection is not severe gross lesions often result, and yet resolution of the organ to healthy function takes place; at all events, opportunities for careful and conservative surgery come when least expected. In one case the tube and ovary may be distended with pus, and yet there will be no intraperitoneal collection; while, on the other hand, the infection seems to leave the tube and involve the peritoneum, producing a large pelvic abscess, yet the tube wall may be simply thickened from exudate and the ovaries comparatively healthy; and even in these cases the infection must have travelled by the mucous membrane, because the broad ligament and structures which contain the lymphatic vessels are not involved. The contrary we occasionally see—tubes and ovaries healthy, and yet the broad ligament a huge phlegmon. There is evidently some susceptibility on the part of the individual tissues and structures which explains these different expressions of infection. Nature, by her beautiful protective processes, shields herself from the approach of pus by making dense barriers of adhesions, and, as a rule, confines the suppuration to certain definite areas. If it were possible to locate these different points and to establish free drainage through the vagina, the acute trouble would soon subside and reparative processes begin. But, unfortunately, these pus cavities are often not located; some are drained, while others are left unopened, and others are lined with a secreting membrane and will continue to cause trouble and discharge pus so long as these membranes are left *in situ*. Therefore, in many of these cases, a cure cannot be effected unless the diseased organ be eradicated; and if it is intensely bound down to important organs, irreparable mischief will follow unless the greatest care be exercised in the delivery. Of course there are other avenues of infection, as through the blood stream, as in tuberculosis of the peritoneum; or by an extension of a tubercular process from intervisceral ulcerations; or directly through the healthy bowel wall, as the colon bacillus infection—this possibility can alone explain the adhesions which take place in a virgin retroverted uterus; or again by way of the ureters and pelvis of the kidney.

The advocates of the vaginal method of operating attack all

these cases, with but few limitations, from below, and they presuppose a diagnostic ability which we all know none of them possess. For example, so good a man as Pryor, and one whom I respect most highly for all that he has taught us in vaginal work, says: "I would always consider that the vaginal is the operation of election in all cases of pelvic suppuration where the vermiform appendix did not require removal, and where there was no fistulous opening between a coil of small bowel and a pus sac." We all know that it is impossible to say in a given case of pelvic suppuration that in this patient the appendix is adherent to the pelvic mass and is diseased and requires removal, while in another such a complication need not be expected. I have frequently delivered a large pus tube or ovarian abscess and found that I had torn away or stripped off the peritoneal coat from the appendix—in fact, so mutilated the organ that I had to resect it close to the cecum and close up the bowel opening. And if this experience were confined to right-sided disease alone, there would be some excuse for his sweeping classification;; but sometimes I have found the appendix long and adherent to the left tube or ovary, and its coats so infiltrated that it was necessary to resect it close to the bowel attachment. So with fistulous tracts; and although they most frequently exist between the pus tube or ovarian abscess and the sigmoid flexure or rectum, yet it is impossible to make such a diagnosis, and if there existed other openings into the small bowel and they were left uncared for death would probably follow. Kelly reports a number of satisfactory experiences in connection with vaginal puncture in localized tube and ovarian pus collections. Not only did these cases recover from the operation, but the tubes and ovaries got well and functionated. I must confess that I have had no such good luck, and beg to say that in every case that I operated through the vagina and drained an appreciable amount of pus through the cul-de-sac, later, in some within a few weeks and in others within two years, an abdominal section was necessary to relieve these patients of their suffering and chronic invalidism, due to adhesions between ovary, tube, or uterus and pelvic cavity, and bowel and omentum and bladder, or to recurrent collections of pus, with fever and the usual accompanying constitutional symptoms.

However, there is a class of cases—and it is this class that I wish to bring out particularly in this paper—where vaginal drainage, supplemented with curettage when indicated, should be first employed to get rid of the free pus, and then later an abdominal section should be made to cure the patient of her suffering when the danger and risks associated with such an undertaking are reduced to the minimum. All of you will agree that a large collection of pus low down in the pelvis, in a moribund woman, should be evacuated through the vagina, and nothing more undertaken unless some grave complication sets in. But to this weak and dying class of patients I am not calling your attention in this paper, but to the strong women who are suffering from acute, active streptococcic infection, who are running a high temperature with great pain and tenderness, who are in splendid physical condition and, under ordinary circumstances, ready to undertake capital operations, and in whom there can be felt an acutely tender mass low down in the pelvis on one or both sides, and even filling up the cul-de-sac, and in whom we are positive there exists pus, which is easily determined by a large aspirating needle passed through the vault of the vagina. In this class I strongly recommend an early vaginal incision for the purpose of draining off all the free pus, and, if necessary, extend the incision to one or both sides and evacuate a tubal and ovarian abscess, if easily reached. This procedure is without danger, and instead of increasing the difficulties of future operations they are very much simplified. The size of the mass is diminished; the immediate dangers of rupture into the bowel and bladder or peritoneum are lessened; the pain and constitutional symptoms subside; and the pus organisms are no doubt lessened in their virulence, and the whole clinical picture of the case is improved and changed.

Of course it is possible that even such a case may get well without any further interference, and it is so claimed by many good men, but on that point I have expressed my doubts; but the experience with a number of successful cases of this kind has satisfied me that this course of treatment I am advocating should be very generally adopted. For a number of years I have felt an increasing anxiety in operating upon acutely sick women, with high temperature and marked constitutional disturbances, by abdominal section, and if it is possible for me, with ease and without danger to surrounding organs, to first drain off the pus through the vagina and in this way to lessen the possible danger of contaminating the peritoneal cavity at the time the abdominal section is performed, I attempt to do so. If one or more pus cavities are opened and the pus has freely escaped, the temperature usually falls and the general condition of the patient improves very much; the local signs and symptoms of the disease are relieved; and then in the course of a few weeks, when the section is done, not only is there no free pus encountered, but I am satisfied the micro-organisms have lost most of their virulence and consequently the dangers of the operation are very much lessened. If, however, the temperature continues high I should not hesitate to act promptly and operate from above, because I should then assume that higher up there must be another collection of pus, and to make any further attempts to locate it from below would be unwise, because such manipulations are blind and perhaps would be dangerous procedures. Unfortunately these patients are not cured by vaginal drainage, and sooner or later, often within the first few weeks, the diseased organs must be removed by laparatomy or through the vagina; and it is surprising to see how easily the various structures are separated, and if the vagina has been properly prepared and the abscess cavity thoroughly washed out with peroxide and copious irrigations of water or weak bichloride solution, the dangers of infection are practically *nil.*

Last winter I had an interesting run of these cases, having operated upon three in two months, and I was impressed more strongly with the wisdom of the practice, although for a number of years I have been carrying out this course of treatment. All the women made splendid recoveries and are well and happy. These three cases practically presented the same history. All had suffered for years from womb trouble, but not seriously, and none had had children for a number of years. So far as I could make out, in none had there been recent gonorrhea or a history of abortion. All were suddenly taken ill with great pain and high fever and marked constitutional disturbances. In all, huge abscesses had been drained through the cul-de-sac—one of the patients Dr. Crockett operated upon twice through the vagina and evacuated a large collection of pus each time. A low fever continued for three weeks; the evening temperature would run to 101°, with exacerbations of acute pain; and when it was evident that no cure could result without further interference, the abdominal section was performed. All the operations were surprisingly easy; the adhesions were very general, but easily separated. No free pus was met, and, other than thickened tubes and enlarged ovaries, nothing was found, although the ampullar end of one tube contained pus, but the broad ligaments were not especially involved. These cases were, therefore, the result of mixed infection and took the route of the tubes and had a complicating purulent peritonitis; and it was this pus collection which we drained per vaginam, and had we not done so before performing the section I am sure a large mortality would have resulted. All pus in the pelvis is fortunately not dangerous—in fact, most old collections are sterile; and it does not matter whether the bowels are bathed in it as the result of a rupture at the time of operation, little harm results. But active, virulent pus, as indicated by high fever and marked systemic disturbance, is not so benignant. Many of you will claim that the accomplished surgeon can protect the peritoneal cavity by gauze towels and do away with the necessity of previous vaginal drainage. Others of you will say that with copious irrigation and a properly placed drainage tube the peritoneum will take care of itself. But this is not always true, as all these precautions have been carefully and thoroughly attended to by myself, yet too many of my cases have gone on nicely for thirty-six to forty-eight hours, and, when hope was high, quickly died of septic peritonitis. Through the opening in the cul-de-sac a piece of iodoform gauze was loosely packed and served for drainage. The vaginal-hysterectomist has to remove the uterus in order to deliver satisfactorily the pelvic masses, but he also claims that the uterus without tubes and ovaries has no value in the physical economy. Moreover, he says it is a menace to the woman's future wellbeing, because cancer is so easily engrafted upon it. These are also sweeping statements and will not bear the crucial test of experience. True, cancer may develop in a womb without tubes or ovaries, and a womb without tubes or ovaries may be the source of future annoyance and suffering and may have to be removed; but that is no reason why every uterus should be sacrificed when it appears healthy and is free from erosions and cervical tears. Moreover, it is impossible to always tell what the condition of the tube and ovary is when a pelvic abscess exists, because one tube or ovary could have caused this complication and the other be quite healthy or, at all events, capable of being restored to future usefulness. In one of the three women I recently operated I did the laparatomy later to relieve a retroverted uterus which I did not know existed when the big abscess was opened, and I found one tube and ovary practically healthy. I then did a ventral fixation, and since then the woman has menstruated regularly and may at any time conceive and beget a family. Such possibilities are denied women when every uterus

is removed, because we conclude upon a vaginal examination
that with a big pelvic abscess surely both tubes and ovaries can
be no good. Moreover, it was not possible in this case to tell what
condition the tube and ovary were in until they were inspected
from above. From below it was, impossible, because the tube
and ovary were adherent high up on the roof of the pelvic abscess, and could not be distinguished from other tissues. The objections to opening the abdomen are very serious, and the least
of them is that a scar results. The great danger and serious
drawback is that an adhesive inflammation is set up in many persons, and as a result adhesions between omentum and bowel and
abdominal wall are made possible, with all their future dangerous complications. Three times I have operated for obstruction
of the bowels coming on some years after a simple laparatomy.
In two of the cases I did a simple ventral suspension, because I
did not then know how to always successfully perform an Alexander operation, and from the third woman I removed a small
ovarian cyst. Each life was sacrificed, as they were *in extremis*
before I saw them; but they showed what possibilities may follow a simple abdominal section. The mere opening of the abdomen is not a serious matter, so far as the immediate mortality is
concerned, but it is the dangers from remote complications which
would make the vaginal route preferable, providing we could establish a satisfactory diagnosis and be able to work with assurance and confidence. But this is impossible, and there must,
therefore, always be cases best attacked per abdominem, and
others best reached per vaginam, backed up by the individual
qualifications of the operator.

493 DELAWARE AVENUE.

THE VAGINAL ROUTE FOR OPERATIONS ON THE UTERUS AND APPENDAGES; WITH CASES.

BY

J. H. BRANHAM, M.D.,
Baltimore, Md.

IN contributing this paper to the Society my object is simply
to give my personal experience in operating on the uterus and
its appendages by the vaginal route, deducing therefrom some

conclusions which I hope may be of interest. In doing this I shall try to bring out the advantages of this method, and also note its limitations. To study more carefully the results of this method, I shall take up the various conditions in which it is used and consider each separately.

1. *Pelvic Inflammation.*—The most common condition threatening the life of our gynecological patients, caused by gonorrhea, abortion, tuberculosis, and other conditions not always discernible, and often requiring prompt action to save life. Here the vaginal method of treatment makes its best showing. Even before the appearance of Henrotin's timely paper I had begun to use the method of vaginal drainage in treating these cases. A few operations by the abdominal route with uphill drainage through a glass tube, resulting in sacrifice of organs, abdominal hernia, and slow or incomplete cure, convinced me that opening and draining the abscess through the vagina was the more rational method.

The operation is, briefly, as follows: After carefully cleaning the vulva and vagina, the uterus is curetted and packed with sterile gauze saturated with a solution of carbolic acid and iodine (20 per cent) in glycerin. A small incision is made through the mucous membrane back of the cervix; then a pair of forceps is forced into Douglas' pouch, the blades separated so as to admit the fingers. This opening can be dilated to almost any extent. The pelvis is now thoroughly flushed with salt solution, after which the organs are carefully explored; usually one or both tubes and ovaries must be opened. If the ovaries are entirely destroyed they can be readily enucleated and removed. In such cases it is sometimes best to bring down the tubes, and, if they are necrotic, to excise them, either tying or clamping the stump. In most cases, however, it is best to simply open thoroughly all the cavities, cleanse them, and drain with iodoform gauze.

Results.—I have operated on more than one hundred cases by this method, with three deaths. The first fatal case was the result of general septicemia, due to forcing a sponge tent through the uterine wall in an attempted abortion. The tent was removed from the pelvic peritoneal cavity, the patient dying a few hours later. A hopeless case, operated on in a dying condition. The next case died from shock, probably due to the use of a bichloride solution which was employed by the nurse instead of salt solution as had been directed. The third death followed an exploratory incision in a case of general plastic peritonitis

41

caused by the use of a strong solution of mercuric chloride in the bladder of a woman for gonorrhea. This treatment was ordered by her husband (a mechanic) without consulting a physician. In this, as in the first case, the operation was done in a hopeless condition, had nothing to do with the fatal result.

More important than the mortality is the condition of these patients after operation. The acute case in which the toxic agent is gonococcus or other germ of moderate virulence often entirely recovers, and many women who have had salpingitis of this type afterward become pregnant. In others the results are not so favorable and recurrent or chronic inflammatory conditions may require secondary operations. As a rule, however, even the severer cases gradually improve; and although the functions of the ovaries and tubes may not be restored, still the lot of these patients is happier than that of the many women who have undergone castration.

In a few cases the organs may be so thoroughly diseased, especially the trouble due to tuberculosis, that complete removal of the uterus and appendages becomes necessary. In chronic cases various conservative measures may be employed, adhesions broken up, tubes and ovaries freed; the former may be straightened or even resected. By opening Douglas' pouch great assistance can be gained in doing Alexander's operation when the organs are bound down by chronic adhesion.

Vaginal drainage is the method usually used in the treatment of pelvic abscess at the present time. Current literature, however, shows that many operators still employ the abdominal section in pyosalpinx with ovarian or pelvic abscess, often removing tubes and ovaries. In view of the greatly lessened danger and far more conservative and better results from vaginal drainage, the grave operation should at least be limited to those cases where the infected tubes are situated very high in the pelvis, or after the acute symptoms have passed.

CASE I.—Miss A., aged 16, school-girl, was seized, June 1, 1902, with severe abdominal pain accompanied by a chill and vomiting. I saw her June 2 at 10 A.M.; found her condition as follows: Great tenderness over the entire abdomen, with exaggerated sensitiveness over the right inguinal region; temperature 103°, pulse 126. Ordered calomel purge and hot fomentation to the abdomen. June 3, 10 A.M., temperature 102½°, pulse 128, general condition little changed. After consultation at 1 P.M. with Prof. C. U. Smith and Dr. B. K. Stumburg—the latter of whom made a blood count, finding marked leucocytosis —diagnosis of internal abscess, probably due to appendicitis, was made. Patient was removed to the Franklin Square Hospital and at 8 P.M. was anesthetized. Examination now showed that the abscess was on the right side and was confined to the pelvis. The patient's condition at this time was very bad; temperature 105° and pulse more than 150. Vagina dilated and an opening made into the pelvic peritoneum. A large quantity of foul-smelling pus escaped. After thorough flushing the right ovary was found to be thoroughly necrotic and was enucleated. The abscess was limited to the pelvis and no evidence of appendicitis could be discovered. Patient made a rapid recovery and returned to her home entirely well in three weeks. Bacteriological examination showed the presence of colon bacillus and a staphylococcus. The vagina, vulva, and uterus were all small and entirely free from any indication of infection, so that the source of the contagion must have been internal.

Neoplasms.—Vaginal hysterectomy for carcinomata. The advantages of this method for operation on uterine cancer are the greater ease and rapidity with which it can be done; the more complete control of the involved area, which lessens the danger of operative transplantation; the more thorough removal of the danger zone in the vagina and lower pelvic plane; and the lessened mortality. In cases where the lateral pelvic tissues and glands are involved abdominal section should be made in order that the diseased tissue may be more thoroughly resected.

Myomata. In cases of small multiple myomata where tumors are very numerous, vaginal hysterectomy is easily done and in my experience has proved a very safe and satisfactory operation. Vaginal myomectomy is advisable when the growth is in the lower posterior segment of the uterus and is single. Under these conditions the operation is not difficult.

CASE II.—Mrs. C., aged 40, white, widow; operated September 20, 1900. Examination showed a small myoma situated in the lower segment of the uterus posteriorly. On opening into Douglas' pouch and exploring the organ, growth was found to be single and about the size of a hen's egg. It was drawn into the incision and enucleated; the uterus was carefully sutured by catgut. The patient made an uninterrupted recovery and is still in excellent health.

CASE III.—Mrs. W., aged 39, white, married; operation January 10, 1901. This growth was smaller than in the previous case and was complicated by chronic pelvic inflammation and purulent endometritis. After uterine curettement an operation similar to the above was done. In this case acute pelvic inflammation followed the operation, and patient was quite ill for several days; afterward her convalescence was slow. She was recently examined by me and is entirely free from pelvic symptoms and enjoying excellent health.

Extrauterine Pregnancy.—I have operated in four cases of this nature by the vaginal route; it has been especially advantageous in cases of some days' standing where elevated temperature indicates infection. The danger of infecting the general peritoneum is avoided by this method. All my cases have done well, and one is of sufficient interest to deserve relating:

CASE IV.—Mrs. V., aged 21, white, married, mother of one child 8 months old, complained of severe uterine cramp for several days, which was accompanied by slight bloody discharge from the vagina. On November 30, 1897, she was seized with great pain and symptoms of collapse, followed by intense uterine and rectal tenesmus. Examination showed pelvis filled with fluid and clotted blood. Extrauterine pregnancy was diagnosticated. As soon as the patient could be prepared, opening was made in Douglas' pouch, large quantity of fluid and clotted blood washed out. The left tube was brought into the incision; a recent rupture was found near its fimbriated end. When the adherent clots were removed a vessel began to bleed; this hemorrhage was controlled by a clamp which was left on for twenty-four hours. The pelvis was packed with iodoform gauze, which was removed on the third day. The patient's recovery was uneventful; she became pregnant and gave birth to a healthy child about seventeen months after the operation.

Conclusions.—Vaginal drainage is the natural method; it is far more effective and safer. Extensive pelvic inflammation associated with pus formation rapidly walls off the general peritoneum; this wall should not be broken through and cannot be interfered with without danger of general peritonitis. Opening through the vagina is associated with a minimum amount of shock and hemorrhage, and is thus indicated in extreme cases associated with severe toxic symptoms.

While freer dissection in the lateral pelvic plane for infiltration complicating uterine cancer through the abdominal route can be made, yet the less thorough dissection of the surrounding vaginal wall, and the greater danger of operative transplantation with increased mortality due to shock and infection by it, render vaginal hysterectomy the safer operation and the one to be advised in most cases.

DR. WALTER B. DORSETT stated in reference to vaginal incision, not vaginal puncture, that in recent cases of pus collection, not confined to the tube, but free in the cul-de-sac of Douglas, his experience had been more favorable than that of Dr. Hayd, inasmuch as he had two cases that he had reported in which pelvic abscesses were evacuated through the vagina through the cul-de-sac of Douglas, and one of these women had borne a child since, while the other had had two children, showing that the ovaries and tubes were functionating. They were perfectly well to-day. If one had an acute inflammation to deal with, whether it was a streptococcus, a staphylococcus, or a gonorrheal infection, the case was almost always more serious when a laparatomy was undertaken, and, as he had stated in a paper read before the Assoelation at its meeting in Toronto, incision in the posterior vaginal fornix was for the purpose of expediency, not for a moment dismissing the patient, taking care of the patient when the pus was virulent, with the intention of doing a laparatomy at some future time. He had saved some patients by vaginal incision and drainage through the cul-de-sac of Douglas, taking out the ovaries at a subsequent time. In a case of ovarian abscess he would not think of going through the posterior cul-de-sac with a view of removing the ovaries or tubes in that way.

As to extrauterine pregnancy, spoken of by Dr. Branham, he had opened the cul-de-sac of Douglas in two or three cases, drained, and gotten the fetus out in that way; but where the afterbirth was attached to the omentum, the intestine, or the end of the tube, it was an extremely hazardous undertaking. If the afterbirth was loose and could be gotten at, this was the better way to accomplish it.

DR. C. L. BONIFIELD, of Cincinnati, said there were three questions which occurred to him. First, were palliative operations for pus in the pelvis ever indicated? Second, shall radical operations be done through the abdomen or through the vagina? Third, shall gynecologists employ drainage or not after these operations?

Briefly, as to the first question, he thoroughly agreed with everything Dr. Hayd had said, and disagreed with the paper which was read at the morning session which stated that palliative measures were never indicated and that drainage of pus through the vagina was unsurgical. He could not regard it as such. Any one who had taken pains to drain these cases to see whether they improved or not could be convinced of the good effect of drainage. He did not claim it would cure many cases, but the great majority of cases would be benefited by it, after which operation was much easier. Oftentimes the incision could be made above Poupart's ligament; occasionally in the median line. It did not matter very much whether the infection was gonorrheal, streptococcic, or tubercular; if the accumulation of pus was large an operation would be rendered easier if drainage was previously established. He cited one case of tubercular inflammation. The right tube was distended above the umbilicus. He made an incision in the median line below the umbilicus, drained off a gallon of pus, and when he came to do a radical operation the tube was scarcely larger than his two fingers. Its removal was very easy. The same was true of infection after delivery. Any one who operated on these cases during the acute attack took unnecessary risk. There might be a few men who were sufficiently skilful to operate with a comparatively low mortality, but the average practitioner who operated for pus in the pelvis when the temperature was high, with the pus scattered, would have a high mortality. He had been incising and draining these cases for more than twelve years. He had seen patients within the last two months that were drained six years ago, and they were as well as those patients who had been subjected to the most radical operations. He admitted that these results were only obtained in a minority of cases. He was an advocate of the abdominal route because the operator could see what he was doing and it enabled him to do more thorough and complete work.

As to whether drainage should be instituted after abdominal operations, it depended on whether pus had been spilled, or whether the operator was able to cover up raw surfaces, and whether there was any oozing when he had finished. If the surgeon could do ideal surgery drainage was not necessary.

Dr. JOSEPH PRICE, of Philadelphia, stated that one or two of the papers were a surprise to him on account of their teachings. If the surgeon could arrest infection he would save life, it made no difference how it was done. For instance, an acute appendicitis, taking it as the type of a murderous disease, was infectious from its inception. All over this country at present there was scarcely a railroad which was not carrying children, men, or women who were dying of appendicitis. He thought that this simply meant that surgeons were not as yet fully prepared to meet the demands of the laity. No one would dare to tell him that he should not operate upon cases of acute virulent pelvic peritonitis and do so in the midst of the flames, so to speak. He had no hesitation in saying that he had saved such cases by the hundreds, and there was scarcely a member present who had not seen him wash away pus and filth in large quantities, the accumulation of only a few hours or days.

Speaking of vaginal work, he said he was satisfied that it was largely practised because it was easy. However, there was a great deal the operator did not know and never would know when he resorted to the vaginal route, except to ascertain his ignorance at the postmortem examination. Extirpation of the uterus by the vagina was regarded by him as one of the easy operations in surgery. In Jacobs' seventy-two cases of bilateral suppuration of the appendages, he had nine visceral lesions of the large and small bowel, bladder, etc. Jacobs and Ségond had both abandoned the vaginal route. They came to America on a missionary trip, but admitted later that they had been enlightened and re-educated. He knew perfectly well that suprapubic work was trying and difficult because it was complete work. Vaginal work, on the other hand, was easy because it was imperfect.

If one would read the ancient literature before advocating vaginal incision and drainage, he would find that vaginal drainage was an old procedure. In advocating vaginal puncture or incision surgeons were giving to ignorant general practitioners without experience a method with which they might do serious damage or mischief. They would resort to vaginal puncture when they would not go in by the suprapubic route and do an up-to-date operation with both eyes open.

Dr. A. Goldspohn had practised vaginal incision and drainage in more than one hundred cases, making an incision transversely of never less than two inches in length, and three inches oftentimes, made preferably with the Paquelin cautery, so that hemorrhage could be controlled whether the blood came from the vaginal folds or the structures from above. The cellular tissues were then broken down and the cavity entered with the finger. If it be an ovarian abscess and not a pelvic cellulitis abscess, the finger could find its way into it and break down the meshes, making one cavity out of a honeycomb, then packing the cavity thoroughly with gauze, so that permanent or long-continued drainage would be possible. In the class of cases referred to by Dr. Price he feared that if they were attacked by the suprapubic route probably one out of ten would die. These patients were nearly dead when subjected to operation, and were in no condition to stand such a radical operation as an abdominal section. The majority of patients whom he had treated by vaginal incision and drainage did not require a secondary operation, and many of them had borne children since the operation. Of course in some of them it became necessary to do a secondary operation, but, contrary to his expectations, the majority of them had recovered and did not require a secondary operative procedure.

Dr. John B. Murphy, of Chicago, said he did not think the Fellows were so far apart in their views as the discussion would seem to indicate. Furthermore, he thought it was their duty to come together, to know what they were talking about, and the Association had no right to permit its proceedings to go out in a loose and haphazard way. We must have definite conditions and a definite understanding. Pelvic inflammation, in his opinion, had no right in surgical literature. It should be expunged. We had in the pelvis definite types of pathology due to definite types of infection which went through definite and classical courses, and until the pathology of the pelvis was first discussed there could be no rational agreement as to what method of operation should be resorted to. He spoke of pelvic infection and of the conditions under which it came on, mentioning postpartum, post-abortum, gonorrheal, or appendical infection. If pelvic infection was considered in that way, then the members would have a clear idea of what it meant. Pelvic infection meant, first, an infection of the pelvic cellular tissue, if that term was admissible. and it should be confined to that alone. We had in the pelvis other tissues, as the uterus, which might become infected, or we might have a uterine phlebitis. We had the tubes and ovaries. which might become infected; also the cul-de-sac of Douglas. which might be the receptacle of infective material. If the infection was gonorrheal the practitioner would start from the history and make a diagnosis. If the infection involved the mucosa of the tube or tubes, naturally the mucosa should be removed. A typical pus tube, in his opinion, meant not alone an infection of the mucosa, but the tube was either strictured or occluded. What good would it do to simply drain the infected mucosa and allow the stricture of the tube to remain? The tube would have to be taken out sooner or later, no matter how frequently one drained. It was an entirely different proposition when the infection was due to the streptococcus or staphylococcus. If the tubal infection was of the streptococcic variety, as soon as the tube was drained the tendency was for the tube or mucosa to return to its normal condition.

He then alluded to ovarian abscess of the mixed type. The ovary might have an epithelial or a connective-tissue lining; and if it was the former and the infection was gonorrheal, the rule was that that ovary must be removed to cure the disease. When one had an infected mucosa to deal with the conditions were different and the treatment should be radical. He did not resort to the vaginal route for any other than infections of the connective-tissue type. All of the other pathological conditions, including abscess of the ovary, he thought could better be treated through the abdominal route.

Dr. J. H. CARSTENS, of Detroit, said there was a vast difference between a pelvic abscess and an abscess in the cellular tissue following confinement. He maintained that it was good practice to incise such an abscess, as healing would take place rapidly. If, however, he had a case of large pus tube, situated deep in the cul-de-sac, adherent, the patient lying on her back for weeks suffering from inanition and indigestion, also septicemia, he would incise it and let out the pus, and when the woman had recovered from this conservative operation subsequently he would remove the pus tube. If a woman was brought to him with a lot of fibroid tumors of the uterus which were causing a great deal of trouble, he would not hesitate to remove the uterus. If he could take it out through the vagina, lessen the danger, shorten the convalescence, prevent an abdominal hernia, get the woman on her feet in eight or ten days, he held that this was good practice, anybody else to the contrary notwithstanding. There were cases suitable for the vaginal operation; there were also cases which it were better to attack through the abdomen.

DR. RUFUS B. HALL, of Cincinnati, did not believe that all gynecologists who resorted to vaginal incision and drainage occasionally should be relegated to the scrap pile, as railroad men would say. He thought that Dr. Price saw cases that the average operator could save by incision and drainage temporarily, whereas the same operator would probably lose patients if he did a radical operation. He believed it was the duty of the gynecologist to practise vaginal incision and drainage in desperate cases, tiding them over for a subsequent radical operation. Cases in point were cited.

DR. L. H. DUNNING, of Indianapolis, said that vaginal incision in many cases was a life-saving measure, and it should not be discarded *in toto*. He began this procedure some thirteen years ago, and it had yielded such splendid results that he had continued to resort to it up to the present time. Out of one hundred and fifty cases in which he resorted to vaginal incision, he could say that only one died as the result of the operation. He had not been called upon to do a secondary operation more than four times. There were a few indications that were clear and distinct to him for the operation from below. One is that it shall be a large abscess; it shall be situated behind the uterus; it shall push the uterus forward or to one side; and it shall be immovable. He would not attempt to incise a large abscess through the pelvis that was freely movable. He would remove it by the supravaginal method. Vaginal incision was life-saving, and gynecologists must resort to it in extreme cases if they desired to do the best for their patients.

DR. JAMES F. BALDWIN said that if in a case the pelvic inflammation was limited to the connective tissue the patient would get well, and he would no more think of opening the abdomen in such a case than of amputating a man's arm because he had a boil on it. If the abscess was limited, as many of them were, to the cul-de-sac, surrounded by peritoneum, the tubes not involved, the case would get well if the surgeon opened through the vagina and drained. When, however, the tube was involved, it was a doubtful question whether the patient would get well with vaginal incision and drainage, but occasionally such patients did recover. There might be destruction of the mucous membrane of the tube. If so, it got well. But if it was not destroyed, then there would probably be an abscess remaining; the incision closed up, there was a recurrence of the trouble, and the patient did not get well until the tube was removed. Not all cases of pus tubes by any means came to operation. There were prostitutes in all cities by the thousand who had pus tubes, but who had never been operated upon, and yet they were symptomatically well. There were masses on each side, and if one operated on them he would find hydrosalpinx. Nature took care of the pus under many conditions without surgical intervention. He narrated such cases.

Dr. Howard W. Longyear, of Detroit, in speaking of drainage in abdominal section, said that he drained less and less because he was differentiating the kind of pus he had to deal with. If possible, a pathological or microscopical examination was made beforehand. If he had a case in which there had been high fever of long standing, he concluded that he had a streptococcus infection, and in that case he would drain. If he did not drain in a case in which such pus had been spilled over the cavity, he knew the patient would die, and if he did drain he thought she would die sooner, but he would drain just the same. As to infection by the colon bacillus, the staphylococcus and gonococcus, the peritoneum would take care of it, in his experience. He recalled cases in which pus filled the pelvis from rupture of a tubal abscess, in the pus were found the colon bacillus and staphylococcus, and yet those patients recovered without drainage. In these cases he said he washed out the cavity thoroughly with several gallons of normal salt solution, then closed the abdomen.

In regard to vaginal incision and drainage for pus in the pelvis, he agreed with Dr. Hayd in his conclusions.

The discussion was closed by the essayists.

Second Day—Morning Session.

A RÉSUMÉ OF THE RATIONALE AND THE TECHNIQUE OF BI-INGUINAL CELIOTOMY FOR COMPLICATED ASEPTIC RETROVERSIONS OF THE UTERUS;

AND A FURTHER REPORT OF ITS REMOTE RESULTS.

BY

A. GOLDSPOHN, M.S., M.D.,

Professor of Gynecology in the Post-Graduate Medical School; Attending Gynecologist to the German, Post-Graduate, and the Charity Hospitals of Chicago.

Rationale.—1. The reasons for surgical treatment of retroversio-flexion of the uterus without very formidable complications, constitute merely an *indicatio quoad valetudinem* and never an *indicatio quoad vitam.* Therefore the service which is thereby rendered the patient is relatively small or inferior in degree and does not warrant the surgical risk, worry, loss of time and expense incident to a major operation, unless such operation be not merely innocent of harmful results to future gestation and labor, but yield also a lifetime service to the patient in not permitting a return of the displacement after subsequent parturition.

2. The one only operation which has been proved to stand this double test of pregnancy, practically without exception, in a large number of cases, and to yield the more ideal results which this test implies, is that in which the round ligaments of the uterus are correctly traced, liberated, shortened, and anchored in an anatomically correct and thorough manner via their natural channels from without (not the operation or technique of Alexander, Kellog, or Longyear). This operation has no real competitor, ten operators alone having eighty cases which have passed the crucial test of subsequent normal pregnancy without a return of displacement of the uterus in any, except two cases in which it was to be expected for good reasons. But a beginning in this the right direction was made by Wertheim (Vienna), who, after shortening round ligaments via the vagina, had seven out of eight cases pass the crucial test suc- · cessfully, but he had 20.7 per cent of recurrences of displacements otherwise independent of pregnancy; and the tenfold greater number of ventrosuspension operators have recorded only an aggregate of seven cases of this kind, examined after subsequent mature delivery, and four of them are failures.

3. The reason why the round ligaments of the uterus only, and none of the improvised artificial ligaments, can render the required service is because, while the latter can stretch to accommodate the maturely pregnant uterus, they cannot retract, but must remain long and therefore useless after labor; and that these idle pathological bands are not innocent is shown by at least fifteen cases of ileus, usually fatal, that were directly caused by those bands. The round ligaments, on the contrary, being a part of the muscular apparatus of the uterus itself, not only grow with it during every gestation, so that they become palpable through the abdominal wall at term, but they also undergo involution with the uterus after labor and thus resume their former function. Several German observers have noted that when normal gestation and delivery follows in a case of inguinal shortening of the round ligaments, they become rather shorter and stronger, probably through the incidental muscular activity *(Arbeitshypertrophie)*; and observation of my eleven cases of that kind tends to confirm that opinion.

4. The reasons for choosing the inguinal route, specifically, to operate upon these ligaments, are that their weakest spots, where the stretching occurs, are at their insertion in the abdominal wall, where they are often very slender and soon become frayed

out in the inguinal canals. A useful shortening of these ligaments, .one that at the same time strengthens them, implies an
elimination of these weakest portions, and that can be done only
by the inguinal canals from without; because the vulnerable
parts are not accessible via the vaginal and ventral routes, and
all shortening of these ligaments by doubling-up of their thicker
and proximal portions is both irrational and unstable.

5. The greatly superior results of this operation indicate that
it should be chosen not merely for the small number of unimportant cases of uncomplicated retroversion, but that the much
larger number of aseptic cases with adhesions or degenerate
conditions of the appendages should also be given the benefit of
this procedure. For there is a large class of retroversions
with complications which are the result of an inflammatory pro-
·cess in which the infectious agent has died out. Adhesions thus
resulting are commonly liberated, by all considerate operators,
through a small incision by touch alone, without sight, by both
the vaginal and ventral routes. After the adnexa have been
thus liberated by those routes, they are drawn near to or into
the entrance wound, if necessary, and inspected, resected, or removed. The same thing can be done as intelligently and thoroughly by bi-inguinal celiotomy via the inguinal canals and the
dilated lateral femoral rings, without cutting any tissues, aside
from the skin and subcutaneous fat down to the aponeurosis of
the external abdominal oblique muscle. These inguinal rings
are readily found by following the round ligaments, and they
usually admit one finger very readily and can be stretched
enough for two fingers. But, as the normal location of the ovary
and ampulla of the tube beneath or back of it is nearly on a
line running directly backward from the ring and not far from
it, it is clear that the respective ovary and tube can be drawn into
a smaller opening and treated, in that part of the abdominal
wall, than would be required near the linea alba or via the
vagina to make the same organs equally accessible for the same
treatment.

6. Introduction of an index finger through the lateral inguinal
ring on each side should be practised as an important supplementary act in connectión with every so-called Alexander operation, in all supposedly simple cases: (a) To detect obscure adhesions of appendages, chiefly, that were not discovered previously. (b) To find out degenerate conditions of these parts,
such as closed tubes, follicle cysts, or cirrhotic portions of ovaries,

which cannot be certainly recognized by bimanual palpation, and which if not corrected would greatly reduce the good which the operation might otherwise have done. (c) To be able to know whether the round ligament in each wound has been sufficiently liberated from the broad ligament, so that traction upon it imparts a direct forward impulse to the fundus uteri or pulls upon the broad ligament at a variable distance from the uterus, without directly influencing the latter at all. The latter condition is the case in about every fourth or fifth individual wound, even in simple uncomplicated retroversions after the round ligament has been apparently drawn out as far as it can be made to come by extraperitoneal traction and dissection. It is clear that by merely pulling upon the broad ligament at some distance away from the uterus, the shortened round ligament cannot very well prevent a return of retroversion when the fundus uteri is heavy or is bent over backward. It is only by introducing the index finger through the ring against the uterus and then pulling upon the round ligament that this condition can be detected, and also corrected by carefully freeing the round ligament sufficiently from the broad ligament and then testing again, so that thorough work and not merely a blind sham may be produced—such as has resulted in very discreditable recurrences of retroversion in cases treated upon the ephemeral design and shallow technique that are advocated and practised on this subject by Kellog and a few others. In a thorough operation the round ligaments are given a most positive and useful function by being thus really shortened (with the incidental elimination of their useless weaker portion) and by being changed in their course from a more lateral to a nearly forward direction. Whether they have previously had or have exercised any similar function or not in any given case is of no significance whatsoever. The supervention of hernia is positively prevented by the application of a reasonable degree of care and common sense to the abundance of normal tissues which are always available for the very freest use to that end.

Technique.—An incision varying from five to seven centimetres in length, according to the amount of adipose tissue, is made one centimetre above and parallel to Poupart's ligament, beginning near to the pubic spine, and down to but never into the aponeurosis of the external abdominal oblique muscle. The median or superficial inguinal ring is very carefully exposed, best by rubbing with a gauze sponge toward the median line.

Sometimes this ring is obscure and other similar and adjacent triangular clefts in the aponeurosis, emitting vessels and nerves, are easily mistaken for it. When this occurs it is a particular misfortune, because the correct or actual ring, and particularly the bunch of fat protruding from it mostly in conjunction with the ileo-inguinal nerve, practically always contains the terminal portions of the round ligament and should be carefully caught in a small forceps. With or without cutting a few crossing fibres at the lateral acute angle of this ring, the aponeurosis is split from that angle outward about four to five centimetres, entirely without cutting, and its edges are held apart, together with those of the superficial tissues, by retractors. From the floor of the inguinal canal thus exposed, the round ligament is gathered up, beginning with the bunch of fat caught in the forceps. It is seen first as a slender band of muscle tissue containing some vessels. Further inward, nearer the peritoneal investment, it usually has a slender tendinous appearance, especially when drawn upon. Its attachments to the internal oblique and transversalis muscles are severed very carefully until the apex of the peritoneal investment appears drawn up into the wound. This it is best to incise on the lateral side, not too near the liga- ment, with scissors, in order to obtain clean-cut edges into the peritoneum for the finger to follow, which otherwise easily passes in between the layers of the broad ligament instead of into the peritoneal cavity. With the ligament constantly drawn upon, the peritoneum (broad ligament) is now, by cutting and by traction, severed from the round ligament at a variable distance from it, so as to leave a strip of the most firmly attached peritoneum to reinforce the round ligament, which in that manner can always be developed strongly enough to serve the de- sired purpose. An index finger is now inserted into the poste- rior cul-de-sac to sever adhesions of the uterus whenever there are any. And from there it is passed along the upper or pos- terior surface of the broad ligament, and behind the ovarian ligament and the tube outward, until the ovary and ampulla of the tube are reached and liberated from adhesions which occur there chiefly. Both uterus, and tube and ovary of one side at least, being now free, come forward readily; the tube appears in the wound almost voluntarily, and, after drawing out its end, the ovary usually follows soon. Rarely its attachments will re- quire to be drawn upon, or the ring to be stretched a little, in order to allow the ovary to pass out; and when it tends to slip back it is readily held by a curved pedicle forceps caught upon the tendinous utero-ovarian ligament. Enucleation of the follicle cysts, or resection of the ovary, or salpingostomy, is then more conveniently performed than from any other approach to the parts,[1] and when their joint lateral support allows them to hang too low it will also allow them to advance equally far out of the wound, and can be shortened by uniting the edge of the web that extends from the ovary toward the end of the tube, at about its middle, by one or two silk sutures to the side or edge of the infundibulo-pelvic ligament where this emerges from the wound while stretched.

Each wound is closed carefully in four layers of sutures and after the general plan of the Bassini hernia operation. The first layer consists of a pursestring suture that catches the edge of the round ligament drawn out *ad maximum* and the edges of the ring with the peritoneum. The second tier of sutures is the most important of all. In it the internal oblique and transversalis muscles are in part drawn down into the inguinal canal and sutured to the posterior surface of Poupart's ligament, and the round ligament is sandwiched in between these two, for a distance of four to six centimetres, by the same sutures. To do this the posterior surface of Poupart's ligament is made accessible for this suturing by turning the lower edge of the split wound in the aponeurosis of the external oblique muscle down, or down and forward, by means of a broad-mouthed pedicle forceps. A continuous double thread is used in this important layer, and before the round ligament itself is caught two or three good rolls of muscle, from the muscles mentioned, are drawn down over the closed ring and anchored laterally from the round ligament. After that the round ligament is caught upon the needle in the four to six succeeding stitches, but never without a good roll of vascular and elastic muscle tissue being first hooked upon the needle to prevent excessive constriction of the ligament. At about every second stitch the needle is passed under the thread to prevent unfastening and to secure even tension. Thus three important things are secured in this layer of sutures: (1) firm closure of the inguinal canal; (2) a broad attachment of the round ligament to an unyielding fixation point; (3) a guarantee against cutting off the necessary circulation in the ligament,

[1] For my indications and technique of salpingostomy and resection of ovaries see Jour. Amer. Med. Assoc., August 24, 1901, and AMERICAN JOURNAL OF OBSTETRICS. vol. xliv., No. 5, 1901, and vol. xlvi., No. 4.

which would certainly occur if the ligament were caught alone in the sutures. The third tier of sutures consists simply in coaptating the edges of the aponeurosis, formerly split open. These fall together as they are liberated, and demonstrate nicely that all structures which have a holding capacity have been preserved for use to guard against hernia.. For these three tiers of buried sutures catgut only is used. In the fourth layer the skin and subcutaneous fat are united by silkworm gut, either continuously or interruptedly. Drainage is never needed, as the several tiers of sutures are united to each other enough to prevent accumulation of serum or blood between them.

Cases.—The present collection of my cases of 1900 and 1901 not heretofore reported comprise 34 which could be traced, and have each been carefully examined by myself or by one of three other gynecologists. Seven cases were not available for examination, and they have been therefore omitted entirely, although 4 of them are known to be in good health. The dates of operation and examination are given, together with the anatomical findings at both times in each case, and the subjective status. The average length of time between operation and examination is 16⅝ months. Of these 34 cases, 9 presented adhesions of both uterus and ovaries, and 11 others had such of the adnexa alone of one or both sides. In two cases of severe fixation two fingers were introduced on one side, and in one of these a thick curved dilating sound was introduced into the uterus to steady it during its liberation. In 10 cases both ovaries were resected. In 12 others the right ovary was resected and the left one removed along with the tube. Resection of the left ovary and removal of the right one was done in 3 cases. Resection of the right ovary alone was done in 3 cases, and removal of the right ovary alone in 2 cases; while removal of the left one alone occurred once. Suspension of one ovary was made once and of both ovaries also once. Salpingostomy was performed on one tube in two instances, and on both tubes in one case. There was not one simple case, uncomplicated by either adhesions or degenerate conditions in adnexa, that did not require intraperitoneal treatment. The Schröder operation for pathologic cervix was performed in 5 cases and the Emmet operation once. My intrapelvic, infravaginal perineorrhaphy was performed in 10 cases. and hemorrhoids were removed by thermo-cautery twice. In one case a small parovarian cyst was extirpated through the dilated inguinal ring without difficulty. Among these 34 patients no childbirth has occurred during the period of time they have so far been observed; 9 were single and remained so at the time of the reviewing examination. Of these 34 patients, 29 are now in good pelvic and general health, but in two of them hysterectomy has been performed because of insufficient relief afforded by the previous conservative operation. Two others required intrauterine irrigation, iodine and local galvanic treatment of tender ovaries, before getting well. The remaining 7 cases are able to attend to their regular duties most of the time, but are somewhat ailing, some of them from endometritis, due in 3 cases to a reinfection, others from chronic parametritis and one from renal insufficiency.

I have heretofore made a report, similar to this one, of 49 cases before the International Congress of Obstetricians and Gynecologists at Amsterdam in 1899,[1] and of 22 cases before the meeting of this Association at Louisville, Ky., in 1900.[2] In this aggregation of 105 cases one death has occurred that is ascribable to the bi-inguinal operation. In one single instance a return of retroversion was found of sufficient degree to require the use of a pessary. This has never been advised in any other case after the operation. *No hernia occurred in any case,* aside from a weakness or predisposition to one in one case that slid down an entire icy stairway on her buttocks five weeks after operation.

The operation has certainly been innocent of unfavorable effects upon gestation and labor. Seventeen cases of conception are known to me among my cases. Only four abortions have become known in these 105 cases during the time they were under observation, and three of these were confessedly induced, leaving only one as spontaneous. Eleven cases went to term normally, and all had normal deliveries, except one with a breech presentation. In every one of these a uterus well involuted and in pronounced anteversion was retained. Two other cases are near the end of an uneventful gestation period.

519 CLEVELAND AVENUE.

[1]AMERICAN JOURNAL OF OBSTETRICS, vol. xlii., No. 5, 1900.
[2]Ibid., vol. xlii., No. 5, 1900.

42

Case number. Age. Para (?). OCCupation.	AnatomiCal diagnosis at time of operation.	Operations performed in addition to shortening and anChoring the round ligaments via the inguinal Canals. Date of same.
1. 24 years. Nullipara and abortion Laboring housewife.	Puerperal endometritis and metritis. Mobile retroversion. Large cystic descended ovaries.	January 18, 1900. Curettement. Bilateral. inguinal celiotomy. Resection of both ovaries.
2. 33 years old. Multipara. Widow. Runs grocery store.	Metritic. retroverted uterus. Both ovaries cystic. Right hydrosalpinx. All densely adherent. Lacerated perineum.	January 19, 1900. Curettement. Intrapelvic, infravaginal perineorrhaphy. Bilateral inguinal celiotomy. Liberation of uterus and left adnexa. Removal of right ovary. Resection of left ovary.
3. 22 years old. Multipara. Barber's wife.	Retroverted, metritic uterus. Multicystic adherent ovaries.	February 1, 1900. Curettement. Bilateral inguinal celiotomy. Liberation and resection of both ovaries.
4. 35 years old. Single. Nullipara. Dressmaker.	Extreme retroversion. Movable cystic and cirrhotic ovaries markedly descended. Endometritis	April 9, 1900. Curettement. Bilateral inguinal celiotomy. Removal of left ovary. Resection of right ovary.
5. Age 24 years. Multipara. Working housewife.	Mobile retroversion. Endometritis. Cystic ovaries Adnexa adherent.	April 12, 1900. Curettement. Bilateral inguinal celiotomy. Removal of left ovary and tube. Resection and liberation of right ovary.
6. Age 35 years. Multipara. Working housewife.	Severely adherent and metritic uterus. Ovaries walled over by extensive adhesions to rectum and cul-de-sac.	April 17, 1900. Curettement. Bilateral inguinal celiotomy. Difficult but complete liberation of uterus and appendages, assisted by thick, curved sound in the uterus and use of two fingers in one of the inguinal wounds. Removal of right ovary and tube.

Nature of ConValesCenCe after operation.	Date of last examination. Position and Condition of pelViC organs, objeCtiVely considered.	Patient's subjeCtiVe Condition, and treatment reCeiVed.	Other conComitant disorders, and remarks.
Uneventful. Complete primary union.	August 6, 1902. Uterus and ovaries in good normal position, but endometritis and dysmenorrhea since a reinfection. Curettement needed.	Patient suffering from new gonorrheal infection and rheumatic conditions.	Peculiar ridges of cicatricial tissues in line of inguinal scars, said to be tender and sometimes painful.
Normal, and primary union complete.	August 17, 1902. Uterus normally anteverted and in healthy condition. Both ovarian regions negative and painless. Little relaxation of pelvic floor, drawing cervix toward vulva.	Menses normal, with little pain first day. Some dyspepsia. Is strong and working hard in her own grocery daily.	
Some temperature, but otherwise normal. Primary union.	August 15, 1902 Normal uterus and adnexa in ideal position.	Menses normal and painless. Great gain in weight. General health very good. Working hard.	
Smooth. Complete primary union.	August 6, 1902 Uterus and ovary in condition. No pain.	Menses sometimes delayed and then profuse. General health good. Gained weight from 117 to 140 pounds.	Patient required several intrauterine applications of chloride of zinc a couple of months after operation, to control menorrhagia.
Uneventful. Primary union.	August 10, 1902. Ideal condition and position of all organs.	Menses painless and normal. General health perfect.	Patient also received several extrauterine applications of tincture of iodine.
With considerable temperature for several days. and slight suppuration in one wound.	January 31, 1901. Abdominal total hysterectomy. and with removal of left pyosalpinx and ovarian abscess (free pus) on account of a reinfection. Subsequently vaginal extirpation of broad-ligament cyst.	Patient had recovered fair health previous to reinfection, and now is in good health, after third operation.	

Case number Age. Para (?). Occupation.	Anatomical diagnosis at time of operation.	Operations performed in addition to shortening and anchoring the round ligaments via the inguinal Canals. Date of same.
7. Age 30 years IIIpara + two abortions Laboring housewife.	Mobile retroversion, with severe endometritis Both ovaries cystic and much descended. Lacerated perineum.	June 4, 1900. Curettement. Bilateral inguinal celiotomy. Resection of both ovaries. Intrapelvic, infravaginal perineorrhaphy.
8. Age 24 years Virgin. Nurse.	Extreme retroversion and endometritis. Cystic ovaries. Anemia and renal insufficiency.	July 5, 1900. Curettement (without cauterization). Bilateral inguinal celiotomy. Resection of both ovaries, right one slightly.
9. Age 38 years. Multipara. Laborer's wife.	Adherent retroversion. Endometritis. Left ovary cirrhotic; right ovary cystic. Lacerated perineum.	August 4, 1900. Curettement. Bilateral inguinal celiotomy. Removal of left tube and ovary. Resection and liberation of right ovary. Intrapelvic, infravaginal perineorrhaphy.
10. Age 29 years. IVpara + one abortion. Working housewife.	Extreme retroversion. movable. Endometritis. Severe menorrhagia. Right ovary cystic and adherent with tube; left ovary cirrhotic. movable. Lacerated perineum.	September 24. 1900. Curettement. Bilateral inguinal celiotomy. Left ovary and tube removed, right ovary resected and liberated Intrapelvic. infravaginal perineorrhaphy.
11. Age 27 years Virgin. Domestic.	Uterus large; in marked retroversion; mobile. Excoriated external os. Left ovary normal, but a parovarian cyst size of walnut near it; right ovary with corpus luteum and other cysts.	September 24, 1900. Curettement. Bilateral inguinal celiotomy. Resection of right ovary. Removal of left parovarian cyst.
12. Age 32 years. Vpara. Working housewife.	Subinvoluted, large, friable uterus in extreme retroversion. Left ovary cirrhotic; right ovary with large corpus luteum and other cysts.	October 9, 1900. Curettement Bilateral inguinal celiotomy. Removal of left ovary and tube. Resection of right ovary.

Nature of ConValesCenCe after operation.	Date of last examination. Position and Condition of pelViC organs, objeCtiVely considered.	Patient's subjeCtiVe condition, and treatment reCeiVed.	Other Concomitant disorders, and remarks.
Primary union, but much nervousness	August 6, 1902. Uterus and ovaries in good position; the latter normal and pain less, but uterus large and tender	Menses painful and exCessive. Curettement needed.	Has also some dyspepsia, anemia, and neurasthenic status.
Primary union, but some temperature. Much spinal and occipital pain, and later hysterical symptoms.	June 1, 1902. Uterus and ovaries in normal position, but uterus and left ovary quite tender.	Menses exCessive, with pain in left ovary. Leucorrhea constantly. Needs another curettement.	Has decided renal insufficiency, with seVere periodical headaches and fainting spells, but has gained in weight and works hard as trained nurse most of time.
Stitch abscess on one wound. Otherwise normal recovery.	July 30, 1902. Position and condition of uterus ideal. Adnexa sensitive.	Amenorrhea since last six months. General health exCellent. and working hard.	
Hysterical first day. Afebrile course. Perfect primary union.	July 30, 1902. Position and condition of ovaries very good Perineum a little relaxed again.	Menses sCant but painless. Complains of general nervousness.	
Normal. Primary union.	August 4, 1902. Normal position and condition of uterus and adnexa.	Occasional intercostal neuralgia. Menses scant but painless Gain in flesh Good general health.	
Uneventful until nineteenth day. Patient sat up and walked. Felt sudden pain in pelvis; fainted, and slight chill. Pulse rapid and temperature 102°. Painful swelling and induration. deep in both wounds, from secondary hemorrhage from some stump. Wounds opened, and healing by granulation. Anteversion of uterus retained.	May 11, 1901. Normal position and condition of right ovary. No tenderness.	Some occasional pain and tenderness on left side from stump of removed adnexa. Great improvement in general nutrition. Menses three days and normal.	

Case number. Age. Para (?). Occupation.	Anatomical diagnosis at time of operation.	Operations performed in addition to shortening and anchoring the round ligaments via the inguinal Canals. Date of same.
13. Age 20 years. Virgin. Domestic.	Small catarrhal uterus in mobile retroversion. Narrow, contracted vagina. Left ovary large, cystic, and adherent; very low down. Compression excites her. Constant lumbar and sciatic pain.	October 20, 1900 Curettement. Bilateral inguinal celiotomy. Resection of both ovaries after liberation of left ovary.
14. Age 33 years. Nullipara. Dressmaker.	Extreme retroversion, movable. Catarrhal endometritis. Left ovary cirrhotic: right ovary follicular cystic. Neurasthenic. Severely hysterical. Drug habit.	November 11, 1900. Curettement. Bilateral inguinal celiotomy. Removal of left ovary and tube. Resection of right ovary. Round ligaments firmly held in broad ligaments
15. Age 37 years. IIIpara + five abortions. Working housewife.	Severely metric uterus extremely retroverted Right ovary cystic; left ovary cirrhotic Lacerated perineum. Cf. "treatment received" column.	December 11, 1900. Curettement. Bilateral inguinal celiotomy. Removal of left tube and ovary. Resection of right ovary. Intrapelvic, infravaginal perineorrhaphy.
16. Age 24 years. IIpara + two abortions. Working housewife. . .	Metric, retroverted uterus. Left ovary cirrhotic, descended, very adherent and tender; right ovary cystic. Lacerated perineum. Valvular heart lesions.	January 12, 1901. Curettement. Bilateral inguinal celiotomy. Removal of left tube and ovary. Resection of right ovary. Intrapelvic, infravaginal perineorrhaphy.
17. Age 36 years Ipara. Lady housewife.	Large metric uterus, extremely retroflexed and severely adherent, along with extremely descended right ovary and ampulla of tube against cervix. Right ovary composed of serous and bloody cysts chiefly. Left tube and ovary also adherent and cirrhotic. Lacerated perineum.	February 4, 1901. Curettement. Bilateral inguinal celiotomy. Difficult but perfect freeing of uterus and appendages. Removal of right tube and ovary. Inspection of left ovary and tube. Intrapelvic, infravaginal perineorrhaphy.
18. Age 20 years. Virgin. Schoolgirl. .	Extremely retroverted uterus, movable. Descended cystic left ovary. Hematoma of right ovary, size of hen's egg Catarrhal endometritis	March 1, 1901. Curettement. Bilateral inguinal celiotomy. Resection of both ovaries and suspension of right ovary.

Nature of conValesCenCe after operation.	Date of last examination. Position and condition of pelvic organs, objeCtiVelY considered.	Patient's subjeCtiVe condition, and treatment reCeiVed	Other concomitan- disorders, and ret marks.
Smooth. Primary union.	August 18, 1902 (Dr. R. N. Rice) Uterus anteverted. Some tenderness on left side.	Menses scant, with some dysmenorrhea. General health good.	
Afebrile. Primary union. Some nervousness.	May 21, 1902. Uterus still large and tender. Right ovary tender. Both in very good position. Marked tenderness of left stumps	Complains of pain there. Has continued former drug habits. Is markedly hysterical and neurasthenic	Abdominal total hysterectomy. Drug habit stopped in hospital, and subjectively well when dismissed.
Afebrile. Perfect primary union. Little bladder irritation.	July 29, 1902. Large metritic, tender uterus in complete anteversion, not descended. Ovary negative.	Excessive menses, with pain in uterus. Much intercostal neuralgia and paroxysms of pain in region of solar plexus, but has gained in weight. Patient had elsewhere curettement and trachelorrhaphy five months previously without noticeable benefit.	
Complete primary union. Some bronchitis.	September 12, 1902. Uterus and ovaries in good condition, aside from a little cervical catarrh.	Nervousness at menstrual periods. General health good.	
Afebrile course. Perfect primary union. Was up in twelve days and home in seventeen days.	August 12, 1902 (Dr. Barnard.) Normal position and condition of uterus and ovary.	Menses regular and painless. Leucorrhea at times. No other symptoms. Good general health and increase in weight.	
Primary union. Afebrile, but much nervousness.	July 25, 1902. Position and condition of organs ideal.	Menses two days; painless. General health good.	But was feeble and quite hysterical for a year after operation.

Case number. Age. Para (?). OCCupation.	Anatomical diagnosis at time of operation.	Operations performed in addition to shortening and anchoring the round ligaments via the inguinal Canals. Date of same.
19. Age 30 years. Ipara. Teamster's wife.	Endometritis and metritis. Uterus retroverted and very tender. Right ovary enlarged, descended and cystic; left ovary cirrhotic. Pathological cervix.	March 4, 1901. Curettement. Bilateral inguinal celiotomy. Removal of left ovary. Resection of right ovary. Schröder cervix amputation.
20. Age 31 years. Ipara. Barber's wife.	Adherent, retroverted, metritic uterus, with pathologic laceration of cervix. Right ovary cystic, tender, and painful; left ovary less so. Hemorrhoids.	April 3, 1901. Curettement. Schröder cervix amputation Bilateral inguinal celiotomy. Liberation of uterus. Removal of right ovary and tube Resection of left ovary. Removed three hemorrhoids by cautery.
21. Age 19 years Virgin. Telephone operator.	Extreme retroversion. Movable catarrhal cervix. Cystic, descended, and tender ovaries.	April 15, 1901. Curettement. Bilateral inguinal celiotomy. Resection of both ovaries.
22. Age 22 years. Virgin. Domestic.	Catarrhal endometritis. Movable retroversion. Left subacute salpingitis and ovaritis. Parts very adherent.	April 20, 1901. Curettement. Bilateral inguinal celiotomy. Removal of left tube and ovary with difficulty. Parts extremely adherent.

Nature of ConValesCenCe after operation.	Date of last examination Position and Condition of pelvic organs, objectiVely considered.	Patient's subjeCtiVe condition. and treatment reCeiVed.	Other concomitant disorders, and remarks.
Extremely smooth course. Perfect primary union.	September 6, 1902 Uterus reduced in size, not tender. In excellent position. Adnexa negative.	Menses normal and painless. Best of general health. Gained much in weight.	
Afebrile course. Complete primary union.	September 1, 1902. Uterus in good position, and now also small and not tender. Left resected ovary likewise.	Is now in good health, but was treated for lingering metritis and persistent tenderness of left ovary and parametritis for six months with galvanism, massage, and glycerin tamponade.	
Afebrile after twenty-four hours. Primary union throughout. Almost no pain.	August 8, 1902. Uterus and ovaries in excellent position and normal condition physically.	Occasional pain in left ovarian region during her constant sitting employment at telephone. Menses normal, general health good.	
Patient in good condition four and a half hours, then signs of internal hemorrhage. Secondary laparatomy. Evacuated much blood. Clamped bleeding left broad ligament and ligated same by mass sutures, stopping hemorrhage. Patient rallied upon much stimulation, but pulse and temperature rose rapidly until death occurred, twenty hours after operation. as from acute sepsis. Bleeding occurred from slipping of ligature from stump, owing to inclusion of tissues from parietal wound in the ligature of stump.			

Case number. Age. Para (?). Occupation.	Anatomical diagnosis at time of operation.	Operations performed in addition to shortening and anchoring the round ligaments via the inguinal canals. Date of same.
23. Age 23 years. Virgin. Seamstress.	Mobile retroversion and descensus of uterus Large cystic ovaries. Endometritis. Dyspeptic, emaciated, and nervous. Severe dysmenorrhea.	April 28, 1901 Curettement. Bilateral inguinal celiotomy. Resection of both ovaries.
24. Age 30 years IIpara + one abortion. Laborer's wife.	Endometritis. Uterus retroverted and retracted. Adnexa adherent. Lacerated perineum.	June 28, 1901. Curettement. Bilateral inguinal celiotomy. Liberation of adnexa. Removal of left tube and ovary. Resection of right ovary. Intrapelvic, infravaginal perineorrhaphy.
25. Age 35 years. Ipara. Housewife.	Mobile retroversion. Metritis. Pathologic cervix. Lacerated perineum. Cystic ovaries.	July 11, 1901. Curettement. Bilateral inguinal celiotomy. Resection of both ovaries. Both tubes and ovaries distinctly adherent. Some fluid in pelvic cavity. Schröder's cervix amputation Intrapelvic, infravaginal perineorrhaphy.
26. Age 22 years. Nullipara. Laboring housewife.	Severely adherent retroversion. Adherent right ovary and tube. Extreme descensus of left ovary. Menorrhagia. Sterility.	July 16, 1901. Curettement. Bilateral inguinal celiotomy. Difficult but complete liberation of all parts by two fingers in one side. Removal of left tube and ovary. Left salpingostomy. Free bleeding from raw surfaces. Packing short time.
27. Age 34 years. IIpara + two abortions. Widow. Washwoman.	Severe metritis. Lacerated cervix. Adherent retroversion. Cystic ovaries.	August 30, 1901. Curettement. Bilateral inguinal celiotomy. Liberation of uterus. Resection of right ovary. Emmet cervix operation. Removal of left tube and ovary.
28. Age 36 years. Ipara + two abortions. Housewife.	Severe chronic metritis (fibrosis uteri). Adherent retroversion. Severe fixation of adnexa.	October 25, 1901. Curettement. Amputation of cervix. Bilateral inguinal celiotomy. Complete liberation of all parts. Opening of both tube ostia out of very firm adhesions. Resection of both ovaries.

Nature of ConValesCenCe after operation.	Date of last examination. Position and Condition of pelViC organs, objeCtiVely considered.	Patient's subjeCtiVe Condition, and treatment reCeiVed.	Other ConComitant disorders, and remarks.
Afebrile. Comfortable and perfeCt primary union.	August 18, 1902. Position and condition of uterus and oVaries now normal.	Slight dysmenorrhea still General health and strength good, but patient required five or six intrauterine applications Tincture of iodine to overcome dysmenorrhea since operation.	
Nearly afebrile course. Entire primary union.	June 1, 1902. (Dr. Barnard.) Position and condition of organs very good.	Menses normal, painless. Good general health.	
Smooth, complete primary union.	July 31, 1902. Uterus and adnexa in normal position and condition.	Menses little, scant, but painless. Robust general health.	
Maximum temperature 102°. Slow pulse. Primary union.	August 15, 1902. (Dr. Barnard.) Position and condition of organs normal.	Menses regular and without discomfort. Perfect general health.	
Comfortable. Normal. Perfect primary union.	August 1, 1902. Uterus remains large, but in good position. Marked metritis Left femoral hernia has veloped.	Menses profuse and painful. August 1, 1902, curettement. High amputation of cervix and femoral hernia operation	
Smooth course. Good primary union. Very comfortable.	August 10, 1902. (Dr. Barnard.) Position and condition of organs normal on. careful examination.	Has intervals of four or five months amenorrhea without discomfort. General health good.	

Case number. Age. Para (?) OCCupation.	Anatomical diagnosis at time of operation.	Operations performed in addition to shortening and anchoring the round ligaments via the inguinal Canals. Date of same.
29. Age 22 years. Nullipara. Clerk.	Endometritis. Retroversion. Left ovary cystic, size of small hen's egg; right ovary normal, but adherent. Right floating kidney.	November 19, 1901. Curettement. Bilateral inguinal celiotomy. Resection of left ovary and suspension of same. Right ovary liberated.
30. Age 32 years. IIIpara + three abortions. Laborer's wife.	Metritis. Retroversion. Pathologic cervix. Ovaries normal, but adherent. Lacerated perineum.	November 19, 1901. Curettement. Amputation of cervix. Intrapelvic, infravaginal perineorrhaphy. Bilateral inguinal celiotomy. Liberation of adnexa.
31. Age 27 years Vpara. Laborer's wife.	Large metritic uterus. Adherent retroversion. Both tubes and ovaries adherent. Left ovary sclerocystic, right ovary cystic. Lacerated perineum. Hemorrhoids.	December 2, 1901. Curettement. Intrapelvic, infravaginal perineorrhaphy. Bilateral inguinal celiotomy. Liberation of organs. Removal of left tube and ovary. Resection of right ovary. Removal (by cautery) of three hemorrhoids.
32. Age 25 years Nullipara. Housewife.	Anteflexed uterus in mobile retroversion. Retracted posterior vaginal wall. Cystic left ovary.	December 9, 1901. Curettement. Bilateral inguinal celiotomy. Resection of left ovary.
33. Age 24 years. IIpara. Housewife.	Endometritis, metritis. Retroversion. Left ovary large. Corpus luteum cyst.	December 16, 1901. Curettement. Bilateral inguinal celiotomy. Resection of left ovary.
34. Age 32 years. Ipara. Housewife.	Metritic, retroverted uterus. Appendages severely adherent. Left tube a hydrosalpinx. Cystic ovaries. Movable right kidney.	December 6, 1901. Curettement. Bilateral inguinal celiotomy. Liberation of adnexa. Resection of left ovary. Amputation and salpingostomy on left tube stump. Removal of right ovary and tube.

Nature of ConValesCenCe after operation.	Date of last examination. Position and Condition of pelViC organs, objeCtiVely considered.	Patient's subjeCtiVe condition, and treatment reCeiVed.	Other conComitant disorders, and remarks.
Normal. Primary union.	August 19, 1902. Position and condition of uterus and ovaries normal. Has extreme descensus of both kidneys.	Menses regular, but somewhat scant. and painful one to two hours before flow appears. August 26, 1902: Bilateral nephrorrhaphy.	
Uneventful. Primary union.	June 1, 1902. (Dr Barnard.) Position and condition of organs normal.	Menses regular and painless. Occasional bladder symptoms General health much improved; good now.	
Aseptic primary union. Normal course.	June 1, 1902. Uterus in good position, but too tender bimanually. Right ovary tender, source of right-side pain most of time.	Patient anemic and neurotic.	
Very smooth, afebrile. Primary union.	September 1, 1902. Uterus and left ovary in normal position and condition.	Recently pain in right ovary. Subsided after four applications of Vaginal galvanism. General health good. Menses normal and nearly always painless.	
Afebrile, but much nervousness. Primary union.	September 1, 1902. All organs in good position. Little tenderness of one ovary	Little pain at menses. Some nervousness, but fair general health.	
Some temperature and stitch abscess. Otherwise normal.	August 8, 1902. (Dr Barnard.) Position and condition of uterus and ovary normal.	Menses regular. painless. Has occasional symptoms from right kidney. Otherwise in good health. Working regularly.	

DR. HERMAN E. HAYD thought the ground of the essayist was untenable. All were agreed that there were simple, uncomplicated cases of retroversion of the uterus; there were likwise complicated cases where the uterus was either fixed or bound down, with or without tubal and ovarian mischief—appendicitis, intraligamentary cysts, dermoid cysts, or any complication which might exist in the pelvis. The Alexander operation was intended for use in uncomplicated retrodeviations of the uterus, where the organ was freely movable and the ovaries and tubes healthy. Was it possible to make a diagnosis of a simple, uncomplicated retroversion of the uterus? It was. If it was, the Alexander operation was simple, without mortality, without danger, and easily done. If, however, after having operated upon one of these patients, there was complaint, the explanation was not that the Alexander operation was to blame for the condition which existed, but there was latent tubal and ovarian mischief, so slight that the operator did not recognize it, and by pulling the ligaments he had lighted it up in the cavity. Having put the uterus into its normal anteverted position, if pain and suffering continned and the patient desired relief, one could operate through the median line, which would enable him to do better work than the essayist could through the route advocated by him. If the first test of the Alexander operation was taken as to whether the patients were subjected to the possibilities of pregnancy and had remained cured after the operation, he agreed with the essayist thoroughly, and he could report 128 cases, of which he had confined 26 women, and in every one of them the uterus had remained where he had placed it from three to ten years ago.

DR. HOWARD W. LONGYEAR said that, after listening to the essayist's description of his operation, he thought it must be looked upon largely as a surgical curiosity, excepting possibly in his hands. Undoubtedly it was possible for an expert anatomist to accomplish it. As far as he could judge, the essayist made a hernia, and did a Bassini operation, which of itself was a long procedure. Where there were adhesions and it was necessary to go into the abdomen, by going in the median line, breaking up adhesions, doing what was necessary, and afterward shortening the round ligaments externally, he contended that any operator half as expert as Dr. Goldsphon could do both in less time than it took him (Dr. Goldsphon) to do the two tedious operations he had outlined in his paper. The speaker had not done the operation of Dr. Goldsphon for the reason that it did not appeal to him. He shortened the round ligaments by a modified Alexander operation which he had found satisfactory in 60 cases.

DR. JOHN B. DEAVER, of Philadelphia, had never found it necessary to open the peritoneal cavity in stripping the round ligament. He had opened it accidentally, but he did not think there was a good reason why it should be opened. It was easy to strip the peritoneum back, but if one was in a hurry he might open the peritoneal cavity. He had in the majority of instances in doing this operation avoided opening the peritoneal cavity. He spoke of this from an anatomical standpoint, saying that it could be done without opening this cavity. He questioned if it was a more simple matter to find the ligament in the inguinal canal than at the external abdominal ring.

DR. JOSEPH PRICE said that most of the members were familiar with the evils or disasters of ventrofixation. and operators were willing to accept procedures that were more scientific. The Alexander operation, as practised years ago, was very much lauded, and at that time it seemed a very successful operation. At present the so-called Alexander operation in the hands of a number of operators was a positive failure. He did not see the necessity of doing two operations where one ought to be sufficient, as in the method advocated by the essayist. The method of the essayist was complicated. The tendency in these days was to simplify all surgical procedures.

DR. GOLDSPOHN, in closing the discussion, said that the Alexander operation was for simple cases. This fact was recognized by the men who did the Alexander operation to the best effect and most frequently: they did so because it was anatomically the right thing; and not only that, because it cured the displacement, which no one could say of his operation who did anything but the inguinal shortening of the round ligaments. If this was true, why not give a much larger class of patients the benefit of this permanent cure? Where we had one simple case of retroversion of the uterus we had three complicated cases in which the infection had died out. Why, he asked, should he not give these three cases the benefit of a permanent operative procedure, which he could do by extending a simple procedure, rather than cure a simple case that did not require an operation perhaps, but which could be treated by means of a pessary?

DR. LONGYEAR asked whether the essayist had had suppuration in any of his cases, to which DR. GOLDSPOHN replied that in his table were two cases in which stitch-hole abscess had occurred.

THE IRRATIONAL STARVATION TREATMENT OF APPENDICITIS.

BY

JOHN B. DEAVER, M.D.,
Surgeon-in-Chief, German Hospital,
Philadelphia, Pa.

ACUTE appendicitis is dangerous in that it excites septic peritonitis, the gravity of the appendical inflammation depending upon the severity of the peritoneal infection. In my experience, based upon several thousand cases, this infection is progressive, and in order to stop the invading process the source of infection must be removed. We must then admit that the early removal of the appendix is the only treatment which promises a low mortality. Furthermore, if the appendix is taken out in the pre-inflammatory stage, that of appendical colic, with aseptic surgery, and barring accidents, there should be no mortality.

Were it possible to be as cock-sure of the degree and bacteriological type of the peritoneal inflammation as we are of the good results following the early removal of the appendix, then, and then only, might there be ground for arguing in favor of delay. To claim to foresee the degree, type, and extent of the peritoneal inflammation is, to say the least, absurd. It is the privilege of the gentlemen who make these pretensions to claim so great knowledge, but to possess this knowledge I do not think any sane mortal will admit. I have no sympathy for those deceiving themselves in this way, but great sympathy for the poor sufferers who unfortunately come under their care.

We claim to be able to recognize a grave type of peritonitis, but beyond this we make no pretensions and have but little confidence in statements made as to the degree, type, and extent of the peritoneal infection. Bearing this in mind, we wish to sound a note of warning against the advocates of the so-called "rest" or starvation treatment of appendicitis, not, however, against the practice in certain cases of washing out the stomach and giving of all nourishment per rectum. For this method it is claimed that, by withdrawing all nourishment and cathartics by the mouth, by rectal feeding, gastric lavage, and the use of small doses of opium and local antiphlogistics, particularly antiphlogistine (whatever that may be), which I have seen used, the extension of the peritoneal inflammation in the presence of a gangrenous and perforative appendicitis will "regularly" remain circumscribed. It is further claimed that these patients, recovering, come to the operating table with their abdominal cavities practically in a normal condition, except occasionally a small abscess at the site of the origin of the trouble, or the presence of adhesions. Lastly, it is claimed that by the use of this method of treatment the mortality of acute appendicitis may be markedly reduced.

Against these statements it is the object of this paper to protest and to make a firm stand against any form of treatment, other than early operation, aiming to restore the peritoneal cavity to the condition which exists in the early hours of an appendical inflammation.

The author's experience for the past two and a half months has furnished the lesson from which the objection to the rest treatment is drawn. From June 15 to September 1 there were operated upon in the German Hospital 98 cases of appendicitis, not including the cases occurring in children. (These statistics were compiled by my Senior House Surgeon, Dr. Müller.) Twenty-seven cases were of the type called chronic, and all recovered. The remainder, 71, were acute in character and 12 died, a mortality of 16.9 per cent. A detailed study of these cases reveals the following points of interest: Thirty-two patients suffering from acute appendicitis were sent to the hospital early in the course of the disease, and in whom the infective process was limited to the appendix or to the tissues immediately contiguous. These cases were operated upon immediately, after cleansing the digestive tract with a gentle cathartic or after the giving of an enema. They were typical of the acute type of appendicitis, with the sudden onset, the usual symptoms, and a swollen, edematous, and congested appendix, sometimes with exudate or a local peritonitis about the diseased organ; in a few cases there was a small abscess immediately about a necrotic focus in the appendix. With the exception of one case, they all made a nice and uneventful recovery—a mortality of 3.1 per cent. The single death was a man 64 years of age, whose appendix was removed twelve hours after the onset of the attack. His abdomen was closed with silk tier sutures and he made a good recovery from the effects of operation. Nine days later he collapsed and suddenly died from cardiac dilatation. Autopsy showed a healthy peritoneum and the wound in the cecum healed and in good condition.

The remaining 39 cases were those unfortunate patients in whom the infective process was allowed to proceed until the diseased appendix had perforated and become necrotic. About this organ, and sometimes extending into the pelvis or upward toward the liver, an abscess existed. They were suffering from systemic poisoning induced by the presence of this highly infectious pus, and an examination of the condition of the abdomen revealed a grave peritonitis from leakage. From their symptoms we knew that they had had an acute attack of appendicitis: from their appearance we knew that they were suffering from grave peritonitis; but beyond this we made no pretensions. Owing, in most instances, to the wishes of the attending physician or to the

43

patient himself, operation was performed within thirty-six hours on 22 of these patients. Five died, a mortality of 22.7 per cent.

In every case there was bilateral rigidity, slight distension, and a more or less well-defined mass. At operation an abscess was found, usually behind the cecum and surrounding the necrotic and perforated appendix. There was but little difficulty in protecting uninfected peritoneum with gauze pads. The abscess was opened, evacuated, the cavity thoroughly cleansed and drained after removing the appendix or its remains. At operation three of the cases were found to have free pus throughout the abdominal cavity. These all died twenty-four to forty-eight hours after operation, and the autopsy revealed general purulent peritonitis.

A fourth death was that of a patient with a large abscess, well walled off, but suffering from the absorption of septic products. The operation further weakened the resisting power and death ensued in a few days. Autopsy revealed gangrene of the cecum, local adhesive peritonitis, with the remaining peritoneum apparently healthy.

The fifth case was one that had been treated for gastritis for six weeks before admission; she was confined to bed and given minute quantities of nourishment by mouth and with occasional rectal alimentation—a sort of modified "rest" treatment. She slowly became more and more septic and was operated upon in twenty-four hours after admission. A large mass of adhesions was present. There was pus about a badly diseased appendix in the pelvis, and an infected tube on the right side. Patient died five days after operation, and the autopsy showed a gangrenous cecum with a local peritonitis. It is hardly fair to class this case among these deaths because of the closeness with which her attending physician followed the starvation treatment for so many weeks.

The remaining 17 cases were treated by the "rest" or starvation treatment as practised by Dr. Ochsner. These patients were admitted on an average of five days after the onset of the attack. Fifteen cases had marked bilateral rigidity. In 2 cases right-sided rigidity alone was present. In every case distension was present in greater or less degree. There was fever, a rapid pulse. and tenderness over the entire abdomen. In 9 cases a mass could be palpated. In 8 cases none was present. The leucocytes numbered from 15,000 to 30,000, with a polynuclear increase indicating pus. The stomach was well washed out and all food and catharsis by mouth was withdrawn. Rectal feeding every four to six hours was resorted to, and either ice or warm fomentations applied to the abdomen. The progress of the case was then carefully watched. We found that the distension lessened in 13 of the cases and that the rigidity became less pronounced in these cases. In the other 4 there was no improvement noticed after from four to seven days of treatment.

In those cases where a mass existed on admission we found a slow and steady increase in the size of this tumor. It never decreased in the slightest extent. Of the 8 cases in which a mass was absent on the first examination, in 4 a mass promptly appeared a few days after the inauguration of the rest treatment and was accompanied by agonizing pain. In 3 cases there never was a mass, and these were those cases where a small abscess was found about the appendix with a mass of adhesions in the right iliac fossa. One of them died five days after operation. This patient was admitted seven days after the onset of the attack, with marked abdominal distension, pain, and tenderness, most marked on the left side. No distinct mass could be determined. There was a leucocytosis of 17,600. The patient was slightly septic. The starvation treatment was inaugurated and continued for nine days. During the first few days of this treatment the condition seemed to improve—that is, the condition of the abdomen—but the patient slowly weakened and about the fifth day after admission relapsed, the abdomen once more distending. There was slight delirium for a few hours. Again an improvement began and operation was performed. About the appendix a small abscess was found, with the organ on the brim of the pelvis and adherent to the cecum, which was soft and friable. The right side of the abdominal cavity was a mass of adhesions, which were more highly organized about the site of the appendix and more recent toward the middle line. The appendix was removed and the pelvis and right iliac fossa were drained. On the second day after operation the patient began to show the characteristic signs of septic peritonitis and died on the fifth day. An autopsy revealed a general adhesive peritonitis, with collections of pus in the pelvis and among the coils of intestine, and a gangrenous cecum. It is evident, in my mind, that an early operation would have saved this case—one performed before the advancing peritonitis had sapped the resistance of the patient until operation was too late to prevent death.

The eighth case was one in which the diagnosis grossly exaggerated the gravity of the intraperitoneal lesion. After fifteen days of "rest" treatment the appendix was found thickened and nearly occluded and adherent to the floor of the iliac fossa; very few adhesions were present. A microscopical examination revealed an interstitial appendicitis of long standing.

The course of the 13 cases with large abscess formation was that of a steady progressing toward increase in size of the mass and sooner or later the absorption of its septic products. When the symptoms of pyemia began operation was performed. It was then found that, instead of the nearly normal peritoneum, the entire right side was a mass of adhesions, with a large abscess about the infecting appendix, in several cases extending from the pelvis to the liver. The amount of pus in some of these cases was too enormous for description and was very malodorous. In 2 fatal cases the entire pelvis was a huge abscess extending up to the right iliac fossa. In 6 cases no attempt was made to find the appendix; we were satisfied with opening and draining the abscess, so terrible was the condition of affairs found. In one case the appendix had sloughed off. Two cases were opened by reflecting the peritoneum and going into the abscess from the outside.

The cases were all well drained and left unsutured.

Six of these 17 cases died, a mortality of 35.3 per cent. Where, then, is the reduction in the mortality? Five of these 6 patients were distinctly made worse by waiting, and some of them would probably have recovered had they been operated upon earlier. It was observed that even the etherization of these cases was more difficult than usual, and I have frequently remarked to my students that the way a patient takes ether is often an index as to the gravity of the intraperitoneal lesion. After opening the abdomen it was a serious problem how to dispose gauze pads before opening the abscess; there were so many adhesions, not so complete as to effectually wall off the pus, but enough to interfere with the placing of the gauze. It was also found that the infected coils of intestine were so friable that the breaking of any adhesions would cause the serous coat to peel off. The latter remark might suggest that in the presence of a walled-off abscess the peritoneal cavity should not be opened; but it is impossible to gain access to these abscesses in any other way, situate as they are behind the cecum and colon and well to the median line side of the flank.

The autopsies revealed a general purulent peritonitis in 4 cases.

a general adhesive peritonitis in 2 cases, with pockets of pus among the coils of bowel and in the pelvis. The cecum was gangrenous in 5 of the autopsies.

The cases recovering were discharged on an average of thirty-two days after operation, while 5 of the cases are at date of writing still in the hospital, one of them with a large fecal fistula twenty-nine days after operation. In a second case a secondary pus collection was evacuated a few days ago.

What are the lessons we draw from these cases?

1. That an early operation, preferably in the stage of appendical colic, is the only rational procedure and is the only treatment which will reduce the mortality in acute appendicitis to insignificant figures.

2· That the so-called "rest" treatment of appendicitis fails to check peritoneal inflammation and will in the majority of instances harm the patient.

The figures presented in this paper bear their statements out to the letter. In the cases where there was no active inflammation, no infection, the mortality was *nil.* In the cases operated upon before the peritoneal inflammation had become extensive. or in those where the appendix alone was involved, the mortality was 3.1, and that mortality due to a late complication. In those cases suffering from advanced peritonitis with abscess formation and operated upon immediately the mortality rose to 22.7 per cent, while the "rest" treatment, for which it is claimed that the mortality is greatly reduced, gave 35.3 per cent of deaths.

It is evident that the gentlemen who make these claims have either been deceived, in that they have encountered a different class of cases than we have, or that they have misjudged their cases. I believe that teaching the "rest" or starvation treatment has and will raise the mortality of the disease under discussion, in that it cannot benefit nor improve the serious cases where the intraperitoneal lesion is extensive; that it defeats the cause of early operation; and last, but by no means least, it gives the attending medical man as well as the friends of the patient a false hope. It gives them something apparently tangible to cling to as against the teaching of operation immediately following the making of an early diagnosis. In my own experience I find that a septic process once inaugurated continues to play havoc so long as it lasts. and no treatment other than early operation will stay that process.

Those cases of appendicitis brought to the operating table

several days after the onset of the disease, where the starvation treatment has been carried out and a local abscess or a mass of exudate and adhesions is found, do not by any means convince me that those patients would not have been better off by operation earlier. In my experience these cases do not give a high mortality from operation. To attempt to foretell what the intraperitoneal condition is, or what it will be a few days or weeks later, is assuming a graver responsibility than is justifiable. Such a prediction is never made by those whose experience with the disease would justify such a confidence.

I have never had cause to regret the removal of a healthy appendix, if there is such a thing, and I have not yet seen any influence, except for the worse, exerted upon the progress of peritoneal inflammation following acute appendicitis by the use of the "rest" treatment. I am willing to grant that operation in the presence of an acutely inflamed general peritonitis is attended by great risk to life, and therefore it is often wise to defer operation in the hope that the inflammatory process will become localized. This is often my practice; but I flatly deny that the starvation plan of treatment promises more in these cases than the more common practice of abstaining absolutely from giving opium, keeping the bowels freely open by solid cathartics. giving nourishment by the rectum when the stomach is intolerant, and using ice or heat locally in the shape of poultices or hot turpentine stupes.

Dr. L. S. McMurtry thought that there were some cases presented by the essayist which should not have been operated on. He referred particularly to cases of general suppurative peritonitis. the patients being almost in a dying condition, and when operated upon tended to throw discredit upon surgical intervention in appendicitis and deterred and delayed others that might be saved by prompt operations. He had seen such cases. and he did not believe surgeons were able to save patients by operation who were dying of general suppurative peritonitis.

An important point to discriminate between in the discussion was as to the influence of rest and delay as separated from starvation and opium. In his judgment there was nothing to be gained by the administration of opium in appendicitis. In a large experience extending over a number of years, seeing and operating on every variety of case that had been mentioned. he had never seen an instance in which opium had any place whatever in the successful therapy of this disease. In the next place, all of his experience had been a protest against delay. He was satisfied that Dr. Deaver had presented some, cases where an operation was practically hopeless, but the man was not living who was able before operation to make an accurate diagnosis and separate the hopeless cases from those that might be successfully operated upon.

DR. RUFUS B. HALL said that every patient with an abscess in the side, who was not dying, should have the chance offered by surgery. He believed all cases should be operated upon as soon as possible, and patients should understand how little chance they have from delayed operations. They should be operated upon because they would die if they were not so treated.

DR. F. D. THOMPSON, of Fort Worth, Texas, said that operation should always be done, if possible, in the first twenty-four to thirty-six hours, and when so treated such patients got well. He had never seen a case that had been operated upon in the interval that did not get well. What should be done with those cases of appendicitis that ran over and the surgeon did not hear of them for three or four or possibly five days? In such cases there was great distension of the abdomen, with a pulse of 150 or 160, with well-marked general peritonitis. He had quit operating on those cases. In his early experience he made a small opening and drained, and the patients died; he made a larger opening, drained, and they died; he made an opening on both sides, drained, and still they died—so that he had given up operating on patients with general suppurative peritonitis.

DR. BROOKS F. BEEBEE, of Cincinnati, O., had become a convert from the medical to the surgical treatment of appendicitis, and this change had come about because of his own personal experience.

DR. MILES F. PORTER said that Dr. Ochsner believed in the early removal of the appendix, and that he would not starve some of the cases that had been mentioned. He said that Ochsner likewise believed in the removal of appendices in the interval. He treated by the starvation method only those cases that had been described by Dr. McMurtry as inoperable, and by Dr. Hall as the patients that die, and by the gentleman from Texas as the ones that died whether operated upon or whether they were let alone. It did not occur to him that it was good surgery to let any man die with his belly full of pus. It was a good plan to let out pus, and not treat it with the respect of an ordinary funeral. Not every case with distended abdomen, with a pulse of 150, would die if let alone. Not every patient with a cold, clammy skin, rapid pulse, and distended belly had peritonitis. He might have a limited virulent peritonitis, but he had a load of toxic material in his blood. Such a patient would undoubtedly get better, so that he could be operated upon in the interval if the surgeon had a chance to do it. This kind of cases could be dealt with successfully by the starvation treatment and operated upon in the interval, provided any man living could tell that kind of case from one that had the abdomen full of pus. Was there any such man? He had never seen him.

DR. C. L. BONIFIELD stated that there were few operators at the present time who did not agree with Dr. Deaver that every case of appendicitis should, if the diagnosis can be made and the patient can have a skilled operator to do the work, be operated upon within the first twenty-four hours. What shall be done with those cases that are not seen at that time or that the surgeon did not have an opportunity to operate upon? He prefaced his remarks with that statement because he tried to prove that the Ochsner treatment was not irrational in that class of cases.

As to the uselessness of opium, he called attention to the fact that many years ago Alonzo Clark brought forward the opium treatment of peritonitis, which was accepted for a number of years. While the opium treatment had grave objections, and personally he never resorted to it, yet he believed it was founded on a little sense, and it was this: The peritoneum, in attempting to limit inflammation, welds together the bowels to make a dam. The only good effect opium had was to stop peristalsis, and in that regard it was good; but it had the disadvantage of obscuring symptoms, blocking up the secretions, and its disadvantages outweighed its advantages. A peritonitis arising from appendicitis or from salpingitis was an entirely different state of affairs. When one operated on such a patient he disseminated more or less infection over the peritoneal cavity; while Nature's method of treating peritonitis was to limit it as much as possible. Now, if the surgeon could help Nature to limit peritonitis without the disadvantages of opium, he was helping to treat the disease, and this was all the treatment Ochsner claimed to do. By keeping the stomach absolutely empty peristalsis was arrested, and he thought in many of these cases it was better to abstain from rectal feeding.

Dr. John B. Murphy said that the Ochsner treatment was founded on two conditions. First, that by withdrawing food peristalsis was arrested. Second, by not allowing food it prevented decomposition above the site of inflammation and the absorption of the decomposing contents of the intestinal tract. The first condition obtained under physiological, but it was absolutely false under pathological, conditions. He contended that peristalsis could not be produced in the presence of a general suppurative peritonitis with abrasions, he did not care whether calomel or food was given. In the sero-purulent type of peritonitis, where there was a quart or more of fluid in the cavity, where the intestine was not blistered, he looked upon the case as favorable for recovery, and he did not recall a single patient with that type of peritonitis who had died after operation.

The next condition was with reference to stopping the decomposition above the site of inflammation, etc. This had a deleterious influence. He believed that it depressed the patient mentally the same as the decomposition above the point of obstruction in a case of mechanical ileus where there was no strangulation, especially where obstruction had existed for four or five days.

Should the surgeon operate on every case when he saw it, taking the desperate with the favorable cases, and would the results justify him in waiting weeks. thinking that he could tell what the subsequent pathological course would be. and going ahead in others, thinking that he could not? He believed, first, that no one could estimate what the subsequent pathological course of the case was going to be. Second, while many cases looked as though they were a general suppurative peritonitis, where one would imagine there was a large quantity of pus, yet at the operation nothing but a deep retrocecal cellulitis and a circumscribed inflammation were found, and the paralysis of peristalsis. which was believed to be due to a general peritonitis, was the paralysis of peristalsis from the intense infection which occurred.

The public generally were being educated in regard to appendicitis, and he thought if they were educated in other subjects as much as they were in appendicitis there would be a greater decrease in the mortality from this disease than now.

Dr. JOSEPH PRICE lamented the publication of the paper of Dr. Ochsner in reference to the starvation treatment of this disease. It would take a long time to get at the large number of practitioners who had heard his paper with a view to counteracting the influence it had produced over 48 States. He said there were 400 deaths recorded in Chicago alone from appendicitis. and this was not one-fourth of the deaths said to be due to and recorded as cholera infantum, cholera morbus, inflammation of the bowels, etc. Many deaths could be attributed to the use of calomel, Rochelle salts, and procrastination.

Dr. J. H. CARSTENS agreed with Dr. Deaver in everything he had said. The objection he had to the Ochsner treatment was not the manner in which he had qualified it since, but in his original statement he (Dr. Ochsner) never said anything about operative intervention the first and second days. This was an afterthought. He now came around and said that he would operate in the first forty-eight hours, and if he could not operate then he would wait. This idea of the Ochsner treatment had gone out and general practitioners had made use of it, and some of them had told the speaker that they could practise it just as well on the first and second days, and they did not call in a surgeon. It was here that the harm came in. A good deal depended on the men who operated for appendicitis. He thought a great many practitioners were trying to do too much. Some of them tried to remove the appendix from amongst a mass of adhesions. If they did like Deaver and others, simply open the abscess, drain, and give the *vis medicatrix naturæ* a chance, the patients would recover; but many of them fished around for the appendix, spread pus over the peritoneal cavity, and the patients died.

Dr. WILLIS G. MACDONALD said every method of treatment. the starvation treatment, or whatever it might be, which involved delay in undertaking an operation, was a bad thing. He was satisfied that if every case of appendicitis in the United States, regardless of the character of the operator, was operated upon under the best local conditions that could be obtained, the mor-

tality on the whole would be less than it was now.   Appendicitis
had become a local question in a good many neighborhoods, and
in a certain territory there was a very small mortality from this
disease, because the general practitioners and surgeons were
educated up to the point that this disease was not one to speculate
about.   It demanded immediate action.

Dr. Deaver, in closing the discussion, said that the principal
object of his paper was to impress the importance of early operation as against the abominable treatment of starvation in cases
of appendicitis.

SURGICAL RELATIONS THAT THE REGION OF THE APPENDIX BEARS TO PELVIC SUPPURATION AND OPERATIVE COMPLICATIONS.

BY

JOSEPH PRICE, M.D.,
Philadelphia, Pa.

THE title of this paper takes up a simple discussion of the
important complications found and dealt with surgically by
removal of pathologic conditions of the right tube and ovary—a
complication occurring in at least 10 per cent of suppurative
forms of tube and ovary on the right side and occasionally on
the left.   In bilateral pelvic suppurations we occasionally find
the appendix on the left side, fixed to tube, ovary, bowel, or
epiploic appendages.   I have several times found it on the left
side or situated in the middle of the pelvis in a tangle of adhesions; and, again, in post-operative complications, in operations
done for pus tube or a hysterectomy, have seen the appendix in
many anomalous places.   Only recently I found a large appendix
lying across the stump of a supravaginal hysterectomy; it was
strongly adherent and strictured, 'and constantly tugging at
the cecum.   It is well to be prepared for finding and dealing
with anomalous positions and conditions of this character, now
that we have so many operations to repeat.

In a good number of cases normal topographical or anatomical
landmarks do not exist.   Freeing the tangled bowel, relieving
all adhesions, repairing all surrounding lesions, and removing
the appendix ends the complications.   In suppurative forms of
pelvic disease in the female the appendix is often removed,
as it is quite commonly found strongly adherent, much enlarged,
and occasionally disorganized.   I have repeatedly tied off the
tube and ovary, and then the appendix, without freeing the

adhesions between them. The fusion of appendix to tube and ovary, all disorganized and in the midst of filth, occurred in this city, a few years ago, in the daughter of a prominent Government official. The removal of the diseased tube, ovary, and appendix, cleansing and draining of pelvis and groin, resulted in speedy recovery. The operative complications are quite familiar to all of you.

The importance of removing the appendix when the slightest complication exists, and the adoption of the rule of removal whenever the patient's abdomen is opened, is a good one. I have repeatedly had patients ask me to remove the appendix while the abdomen was opened for some other purpose. The danger is so slight, the operation so simple, so little time and surgery are required for the safe and clean removal of a very common offender, that I am strongly inclined to urge its removal in all cases while doing pelvic surgery. Again, we see a good number of patients complaining of obscure symptoms and pelvic pain, general ill health, abdominal colic, and intestinal disorders, coming from general practitioners for treatment or operation on the pelvic organs. In a good number of these cases the appendix is the cause, its removal speedily relieving the patient of all symptoms.

The symptoms are so conspicuous, the diagnostician so cocksure, in the male, that they are operated upon in great numbers. What a number of cases we must be overlooking in the female! I find the profession are making a more careful study of this important subject. Teachers, authors, and prominent operators have strongly advocated conservative or non-operative methods of treatment until they lost one or more of their own children or were driven to operative interference after some delay or the loss of a dear friend or relative.

The operation cannot be too early in the acute attack. It is fire department work. If done the first day, they all recover. Positive arrest of the peritoneal infection is secured, as is beautifully demonstrated in the cases operated upon on the verge of perforation. The mortality increases with the number of days of the illness. In fulminating cases it is always high after the fourth or fifth day; yet even in these eleventh-hour operations there ought not to be 16 or 20 per cent mortality, if toilet and drainage are complete in general. Exceptionally few recover spontaneously; the recurring and well-to-do cases go to health resorts or travel with an abscess in their right groin or beneath their cecum, and often die with a recurrence away from home.

The operation is often charged with the death. Not so; these cases are really dying during their second or third recurrence, and should have been operated upon on the first day of their first attack; or it may be the procedure was an incomplete one, as the Willard Parker operation. Large numbers who have been treated medically are reported as cures after they are dead and buried, by the man who saw them in their first attack. Large numbers remain chronically ill, the precise nature of their trouble not being recognized by their attendant. Our present precise knowledge of the acute and chronic pathology are the results of the operations done in both conditions.

Operations upon nurses and resident physicians in hospitals demonstrate beautifully the value of early interference; most are done on the first day. One nurse in every six in my private hospital, and in two public hospitals with which I am connected, has been operated upon for appendicitis—all early operations, without a death, and with pleasing recoveries. All of them have continued their profession in better health than their associates. The same is the history of the operations on the resident physicians. The mortality in students in the same school or college hospital is high, the operation being commonly done two or three days later than on the residents. Treves continues to teach conservative treatment and discourages prompt surgical interference, while he publishes a large number of internal operations with a low mortality—and it should be *nil* in such a group of cases, the death of any only due to error in diagnosis or overlooking diseased conditions of the heart or some other important organ. He makes the remarkable statement that if none were operated upon, 5 per cent only would die. If this were true, I am satisfied most prominent, successful operators would weed out the five cases for operative interference and the ninety-five for non-operative interference, and in all probability save the five operated upon. The diagnosis is so easy, the symptoms so prominent, that it would be not difficult to exclude the ninety-five that ought to recover without operation.

To illustrate what I mean I will cite a recent experience. I was called to Rochester, N. Y., to see a Yale student on the fourth day of his illness, dying of appendicitis; it was a midnight operation and a number of good clinicians and surgeons were present. While washing for the operation I alluded to Mr. Treves' statement and remarked that the young man belonged to the 5 per cent group; that I was satisfied all of them felt that nothing short of operative interference could save him; if let alone or tinkered with he would surely die—with which opinion they all agreed. He was greatly distended and vomiting almost continuously. A gangrenous and perforated appendix was quickly and easily removed and the dirty groin carefully cleansed. Just at this point in the operation I remarked that the procedure seemed complete, but that the general surgeon's inflammatory wall was rarely complete at either end, and that to have stopped there the operation had just as well not have been done. I then pushed two fingers over the ilio-pectineal line into the pelvic cavity, and a gush of dirty fluid flooded the field of operation. Probably twenty inches of adherent ileum was freed and cleansed of all lymph, the peritoneal cavity washed and drained. He will go back and finish his college course.

While speaking of the general surgeon's inflammatory wall I must call your attention to the remarkable series of four cases of appendicitis reported by Senn from the Berlin Clinic:

CASE I.—Diffuse peritonitis following appendicitis. First attack; had lasted two weeks previous to operative interference, although "the symptoms had been strong from the beginning." Vomiting and distension of abdomen were suspicious of pus in the right iliac fossa. Long incision was followed by large quantities of fetid pus. Diffuse peritonitis was present, with no tendency to limitation. The inflamed appendix was ligated and removed. There was no gangrene or perforation. The extent of the disease was mentioned as a contraindication to irrigation.

CASE II.—Perforative appendicitis recognized on the ninth day. Pain, vomiting, and frequent eructations, accompanied by tympany and pain in right iliac fossa. The initial symptoms were mild. Large quantities of pus followed the incision; the peritoneal cavity generally dirty, and no attempt was made to cleanse it. The tissues were so much disorganized that they would not hold a ligature.

CASE III.—In this case there was doubt as to the diagnosis, the physical signs indicating an accumulation of pus in the left iliac region. Almost the entire linea alba was incised. with negative results. Then a transverse incision was made over the pubes and left Poupart's ligament, and a large quantity of extremely offensive pus was evacuated. Careful search failed to ascertain the cause, but an abnormally situated appendix was suspected as the starting point of the infection.

CASE IV.—"Fetid empyema following rupture of an appendical abscess into the left pleural cavity. This case was an extremely obscure one. The patient, a young man of 16, when admitted into the hospital presented all the indications of empyema. The early history of the case was obscure. A segment
of the seventh rib was excised in the axillary line, and a large
quantity of very fetid pus was liberated. The patient not improving as was expected, the opening in the chest wall was enlarged by resection of the adjacent lower rib. As the suppuration and septic condition persisted, it was finally decided to follow the abscess cavity its entire length in a downward direction.
The remaining lower ribs were excised and a perforation was
found in the diaphragm. The abscess cavity was followed by
extending the incision downward as far as the crest of the ilium.
From this time the patient improved rapidly, and at the present
time the enormous wound is granulating satisfactorily and promises to heal in a short time. It is believed that an appendicitis
was the cause of abscess formation, and that the secondary suppurative pleuritis resulted from the entrance of pus into the
pleural cavity through a perforation in the diaphragm."

I have briefly abstracted the first three and quoted entire
the fourth of the Berlin cases to illustrate the rapidly destructive nature of the disease, and demonstrate, in a series of four
cases, how incomplete or wholly absent is the general surgeon's
inflammatory wall. In the series this point is not referred
to. Our distinguished friend, Deaver, at a very late hour in his
life, gives us a good paper on the general surgeon's "walled-off."
My Yale student's operation demonstrates very beautifully how
incomplete the wall was below, Senn's fourth case how incomplete above, and there are numerous cases quoted in papers and
discussions of similar nature, one recently reported by Dr.
La Place. In the cases reported by Senn we see beautifully
illustrated the progressive nature of an appendical inflammation
and of how speedily the general peritoneal cavity or remote
points of the body may be involved. Again, we see that they
are not operating sufficiently early on the Continent, as three
of the four reported cases were about destroyed by the disease,
as the diagnosis in each case was of obscure and doubtful origin.

We have referred pointedly to the ease and facility of diagnosis in appendicitis early in the disease. This reference is
made to demonstrate how little importance the teachers and
authors place upon the necessity of an early diagnosis. The
general peritonitis, the partial destruction of important organs,

and the invasion of other cavities would never occur if practitioners were all good, wide-awake diagnosticians and could be more speedily convinced of the importance of early operative interference.

DR. HERMAN E. HAYD said the most important area in the physical makeup of either man or woman was the lower right quadrant of the abdomen, and it was surprising to see how much trouble could quickly occur in that area. The question of diagnosis largely depended upon one's environment, how he had been educated. For instance, the general surgeon assumed that everything in that territory of a pathological character was appendicitis, while the man who had devoted himself to the diseases of women found that this was not true; consequently, although Dr. Price considered the diagnosis was ordinarily easy in these cases, yet there occurred cases from time to time where the difficulties in diagnosis were great. In this area there could be either an appendicitis with localized abscess, a tubal or ovarian abscess, or a suppurating extrauterine pregnancy in woman, and really it was very difficult at times to make a differential diagnosis.

If he found tubal or ovarian trouble complicated with appendicitis, he favored operating through a median incision. If he did not encounter pus he did not drain, but sewed up the wound. All such cases invariably recovered. If, however, he found pus, he protected the abdominal cavity from the infection or rupture of a possible abscess; then he dug out the appendix, broke up adhesions, and drained both in front and to the side.

The next thing in order was the President's address, which was delivered by Dr. Edwin Ricketts, of Cincinnati, Ohio. Dr. Ricketts selected for his subject

OUR SHORTCOMINGS: LET US REASON TOGETHER.[1]

Second Day—Afternoon Session.

SOME UNUSUAL CASES OF APPENDICITIS AND THE LESSONS THEY TEACH.

BY

MILES F. PORTER, M.D.,

Professor of Surgery, Clinical Surgery, and Gynecology, Fort Wayne College of Medicine, Fort Wayne, Ind.

CASE I.—Mrs. S., æt. 27, was taken with cramps and vomiting during a menstrual period when 15 years of age, and up to the time of operation had had numerous attacks of typical appendi-

[1] See address, p. 577.

citis. For four months prior to operation the tenderness and pain were constant. She had been in bed several weeks. On opening the abdomen the adhesions between the cecum. ileum, parietal peritoneum, and omentum were found to be dense. Attached to the cecum was a small stump, closed, which was all of the appendix which could be found. Behind this and under the iliac fossa was a small abscess, which was drained. Immediate relief followed the operation, and she was discharged January 25, twenty-five days after, with a small sinus. Six months later I learned that she had been having some pain and that the wound had again opened, but I have not seen her. Possibly the distal end of the appendix or a fecal concretion was left behind and caused the trouble to recur.

That this is probable is proved by

CASE II.—Master J. J. was operated by me on June 17 last for frequently-recurring attacks of pain, tenderness, etc., following a simple drainage operation for appendical abscess done eleven months before. While the sinus was open he was free from pain. Shortly after it would close an attack would come on, to be relieved by spontaneous opening of the abscess. On opening the belly there was found in the centre of an abscess cavity a large fecal concretion and the appendix, the latter free from all connection either to bowel or meso-appendix.

In these cases of long standing the operator should search as thoroughly as consistent for fecal concretions, and, in cases of detachment of the appendix from the cecum, for the appendix, and, finding either neither or both, should provide ample drainage and not be in haste to secure closure of the external wound.

The appendix may become separated from the cecum and become surrounded by adhesions in a position quite removed from its normal position, as is illustrated by a case referred to me by Dr. Cook, of Bluffton, Ind.

CASE III.—The patient had presented the usual symptoms of recurrent appendicitis, save that in the last attack the pain and tenderness were widespread at first, but when I saw him several days after the onset the tenderness was very slight, as determined by abdominal palpation, and located centrally. By rectal palpation a very tender mass was found low down in the pelvis between rectum and bladder. Through the open belly this mass proved to be composed of intestine, bladder, and the rectum bound by adhesions enclosing a small, yellowish-white mass of necrotic tissue which in no way resembled an appendix to the naked eye, but which was declared to be a necrotic appendix by

Dr. Rhamy, who examined it for me. The cecum, released from adhesions, showed a cicatrix marking former attachment of appendix.

CASE IV.—The next case I have to report emphasizes the more remote dangers incurred by delay in operating in appendicitis. I found the boy with an abscess of appendical origin occupying the lower right fourth of the abdomen. His general condition was extremely bad and a simple drainage operation was done. From this he rallied and did well for two weeks, when another abscess formed in the opposite quadrant and was opened. From this he recovered completely and was enjoying the ordinary pleasures of boys of his age, when, at the supper table at the close of a hearty meal, he was taken with pain in the belly, which three days later was known to be due to bowel obstruction. The point of obstruction was located above the umbilicus. Incision was accordingly made here in the mid-line, and the obstruction, due to peritoneal adhesions, was relieved. To get the bowels back in the abdomen it was necessary to empty them through a hole cut with the scissors. His recovery was uneventful and he enjoyed good health for five years, when he had several attacks of belly pain accompanied by obstinate constipation. These attacks grew more severe, frequent, and obstinate, until finally an attack came on which failed to respond to the usual measures. A celiotomy was done, and only after nearly three hours of patient and hard work were the adherent bowels released and the obstruction overcome. It is now three years since the last operation; the boy, now a young man, is in perfect health.

CASE V.—The only case I have ever seen of what seemed to me to be appendical colic—i.e., pain in the appendix without inflammation—was that of a farmer referred to me by Dr. Hackerdorn, of Antwerp, O. The pain was extreme, but the constitutional symptoms practically nil. The tenderness was marked only upon rather severe pressure over a space not larger than a silver quarter. On removal the appendix seemed healthy, but contained a seed, of a kind unknown to me, which was triangular in shape with exceedingly sharp corners. The seed had produced several wounds in the mucosa of the appendix. Appendectomy was followed by complete relief. Prof. Schultze, of the Fort Wayne High School, examined the foreign body and pronounced it a seed, but could not tell the kind.

CASE VI.—I have many times found the lumen of the appendix obliterated partially at the distal end, and have often met with

44

strictures, but never saw but one example of complete obliteration of the lumen. The patient was an elderly lady referred to me
by Dr. Sprowl, of Warren, Ind. Celiotomy was done for diagnostic purposes. There was a history of attacks earlier in life
that were thought might have been attacks of appendicitis. At
the time of operation there were no signs of appendicitis, save a
complaint of pain over the whole right side of the abdomen. On
opening the abdomen the appendix was found considerably adherent, exceedingly firm to feel, and not larger than three-six-
teenths of an inch in diameter. On examination after removal
it was found to have no lumen, but was merely a solid cord of
what seemed connective tissue covered with peritoneum. No
microscopical examination was made. Whether this appendix
was simply a deformed one, or whether its condition at the time
of operation was the result of previous inflammatory attacks, I
cannot say. That the latter is true seems not improbable from the
history and the adhesions found.

CASE VII.—I was called by Dr. Harrold, of Roll, Ind., to operate on an elderly lady for an appendicitis of a week's duration.
The case presented no unusual feature, save that the tumor was
very prominent to sight (the belly was rather flat, flabby, and
thin), and on palpation was found to be almost spherical and so
freely movable as to permit of its being pushed to the left of the
median line. This condition was easily understood after the
belly was opened. There was a long meso-appendix and a long
meso-cecum. The inflamed appendix was found wrapped in the
omentum, but there were no adhesions to surrounding structures.
This case is reported because of its rarity, and because of the
possible difficulty in diagnosis which such cases might present,
especially if not seen until all active inflammation had subsided.
I know of no similar case on record, but Dr. Ochsner, of Chicago,
told me of a similar case which occurred in his practice and
which was considered by him to be a malignant tumor until the
operation had progressed until the infected appendix was un-
covered.

CASE VIII. *Cancer of the Ileo-cecal Valve mistaken for Appendicitis.*—This case came to me for operation after having the
diagnosis of chronic appendicitis confirmed by several physicians,
among whom was Dr. Nancrede, of Ann Arbor. I also confirmed
the diagnosis, but on opening the belly found the trouble to be
cancer of the ileo-cecal valve with adhesions in the region denot-
ing peritoneal inflammation. The tenderness, pain, etc., due to
the latter condition led to the diagnosis of appendicitis. As I look

back upon this case I can find some features in the case which might help me to a correct diagnosis were a similar case presented to me in the future. They were as follows: 1. The pain was too great for the tenderness. 2. There was too much loss of flesh and too much anemia to be accounted for on the ground of sepsis. The patient could get up and move about the next day after an attack of pain. So far as I could learn, there never had been any but very mild symptoms of sepsis, and yet, as indicated above, the man had lost quite a good deal of weight and was anemic—in a word, was showing the cachexia of cancer.

CASE IX.—Ethel B., æt. 11 years. Referred by Dr. Webber, of Warsaw, Ind. She gave a history of three previous attacks of pain in the appendix region, all of which had come on suddenly and disappeared suddenly after a few hours' duration at the most. One of the three had disappeared immediately after a warm rectal injection; the others had disappeared spontaneously. In neither attack was there any tenderness after the pain left, although it was present and well marked while the pain lasted. The child had never menstruated, nor did her development indicate a near approach to menstrual activity. She was of constipated habit. When I saw her, forty-eight hours after the attack came on, there was an elevation of one degree in temperature, the pulse was 100, there was some pain and exquisite tenderness in the right iliac region, with an exquisitely sensitive tumor just above Poupart's ligament. It was remarked at the time that the tenderness and tumor were both rather low for the appendix. A digital examination per rectum, made without the aid of an anesthetic, was negative. I told the parents that I thought the case was one of appendicitis, but that I might be mistaken in this. However, I was positive that there was something there causing a peritonitis and that the proper course to pursue was to operate and remove, if possible, the cause of the trouble. A vertical incision through the right rectus muscle revealed a right ovarian cyst the size of a small egg, with a pedicle tightly twisted by three complete turns, and gangrene commencing. It is but right to say that disease of the uterine adnexa was thought of before the operation, and ruled out. The child made a prompt recovery. This case is interesting for other reasons, but is reported here for the purpose of emphasizing the importance of tenderness disassociated with pain in differentiating between inflammatory and non-inflammatory lesions.

CASE X.—Miss H. was seen by me at the request of Dr. Deming, of our city, on the second day of a very mild attack of appendicitis. It was the first attack. On the next day the symptoms were practically gone, save localized tenderness which was not very marked. The belly was opened and the appendix was removed. Near the distal end was a cyst the size of a large pea, with walls not thicker than the normal peritoneum. The contents were clear. It was, in my opinion, a retention cyst following inflammatory occlusion of the lumen of the appendix.

CASE XI.—This case, the last I shall report, is one of many similar ones I have had and is in no way unique, but, for reasons which will appear later, I deem it worthy of consideration. Mr. Q., a middle-aged man, was seen by me at the request of Dr. Harrod, of our city, forty-eight hours after the onset of his first attack of appendicitis. There was slight tympany, frequent vomiting, great pain and tenderness, with some hardness in the appendix region. The pain and tenderness were spreading over a greater area. Pulse was 84, temperature was 101°. He was moved to Hope Hospital and operated on at once. Some muddy serum was free in the peritoneal cavity. The appendix was gangrenous and perforated; it was removed and drainage provided for. The man made a prompt recovery. Here was a case in which the infection was already spreading, the infectious material was free in the peritoneal cavity. Had this case been put under the starvation treatment what would have been the result? As stated above, this is but one of many (perhaps 200) similar cases that have occurred in my practice in which there was infectious material free in the peritoneal cavity, the symptoms and appearances inside the belly indicating a widespread and rapidly-spreading virulent infection. Will any mode of treatment give these patients as good a chance to recover as will the operative treatment? Can any treatment corral germs distributed over a large part or the whole of the peritoneum, and pen them up in a small corner and keep them there? No one doubts that the majority of cases of suppurating appendicitis will result in circumscribed abscess if properly treated, but is there any medical treatment which will lead to this result in all cases? Can those which can be made to yield this happy result be differentiated from those which cannot be made thus to yield?

As for myself, I want the truth, and am free to confess that my own experience is perhaps not sufficient to base conclusions upon: but I am of the opinion that the case last narrated would have ended fatally had it not been promptly operated: that the sooner a case of appendicitis which is growing progressively worse is operated the better; that no man can tell in a given case the pathologic changes that have taken place until he sees them.

207 WEST WAYNE STREET.

DR. WASHINGTON H. BAKER, of Philadelphia, would like to answer yes to the question which was asked in the paper, and he was thankful to be supplied with such a beautiful illustration as the first case mentioned. In that case the pain was not in the appendix; it was due to reflex symptoms; the irritation was transmitted from the appendix to the intestine reflexly and produced intestinal colic. The indication was not an operation, but to help the great effort Nature was making to get rid of some irritating influence there. The great indication was to him, whenever the system made a decided effort in any direction, to further that effort all he could, and he felt that he was proceeding naturally and to the great advantage of the patient, and he would not institute any operative procedure in opposition to that until his efforts had entirely failed. Nature gave the physician an intimation in these cases, and what he should do was to endeavor to supply what was wanting. The physician should not force Nature, but aid her in these cases.

DR. JOHN C. SEXTON, of Rushville, Ind., said he believed it was the sense of the Association that it would be a backward step to delay operative intervention in cases of appendicitis after making the diagnosis, and he thought it would be a retrogressive step if the so-called starvation or waiting plan was generally adopted. As to fulminating appendicitis, the surgeon might open the abdomen and find a large amount of dirty brown, watery fluid, with no pus or rupture, yet, on account of the epithelial plate being stripped off, absorption would rapidly take place and the patients would die. On the other hand, if the abscess had not broken down into a dirty brown, watery fluid there would still be a chance to save the life of the patient, for the reason that the epithelial plate had not been removed. He believed it was the duty of practitioners to continue along the old line, namely, to operate upon every case of appendicitis as soon as the surgeon got to it.

FOUR CASES ILLUSTRATING THE DIFFICULTIES OF DIAGNOSTICATING APPENDICITIS.

BY

WILLIAM WOTKYNS SEYMOUR, M.D.,
Troy, N. Y.

MY excuse for presenting a paper founded upon so few cases is that they are to be taken as the text of my remarks and to elicit discussion.

For some years I have been greatly impressed, on listening to and reading society discussions, with the apparently current opinion that appendicitis was one of the easiest of diseases to diagnosticate. While this has been my experience in most cases, yet there is also a considerable percentage of cases which in their very inception simulate very closely appendicitis of such severity as ordinarily to require operation. These cases of simulated appendicitis may be divided into two great classes—those actually of the right iliac fossa, arising from inflammation of other organs than the appendix, and those more misleading cases, from the purely diagnostic standpoint, in which severe symptoms of abdominal trouble appear and yet the actual disease is an effusion in the chest or an inflammation of the lung of the same or even opposite side, without any actual implication of the appendix. If Richardson, with a personal experience of between two and three thousand cases, can be mistaken in diagnosticating as acute appendicitis a case of inflammation of the right pleura, it seems that every one dealing with appendicitis should have burned into his memory the existence of such treacherous cases of mimicry. Unless this is done, sooner or later our preconceived opinions, distorting our judgment, will lead us into the temptation of doing an operation for appendicitis where none exists and where no operation is needed.

CASE I.—Mrs. Florence A., aged 19 years, Armenian, 4 feet 6½ inches in height, weight 90 pounds, was delivered by a colleague of a dead child, after a severe labor, on December 26, 1900, by high forceps. The hospital records give no details of the delivery or the condition of the fetus. On January 4 she was transferred to my care and almost immediately had a chill and high temperature; my colleague who delivered her said she had already had a sudden elevation of temperature with an equally sudden fall, and regarded this as due to nervous excitement. He having just examined the patient, I refrained from so doing. The next day the temperature was 103.5° and pulse 120; marked tenderness under McBurney's point, no dulness, some muscular spasm. Vaginal examination negative, save the womb was tender on elevating the cervix and the pain referred to the right side. My diagnosis was septic infection, probably of tube and ovary of right side, with a possible involvement of appendix. Immediate operation disclosed absolutely normal tubes and ovaries, no involvement of the appendix, but a sloughing, gangrenous fibroid, the size of an English walnut, in the right anterior wall of the uterus below the attachment of the round ligament. This I enucleated, and, after cleaning out its bed and stitching it over, I drained with gauze drains and the patient made a good recovery, to require at my hands an operation for post-operative hernia in March of this year and an elective Cesarean section for a conjugate of less than eight centimetres in July. Mother and son are now well.

CASE II.—Lottie B., married, aged 23 years. Four months after delivery was operated upon by a colleague for an abscess of the right iliac fossa with the ante-operation diagnosis of appendicular abscess. A large abscess was evacuated and drained, but no appendix found, and the post-operative diagnosis appendicular or tubal abscess from infection made. Four months later the patient entered my service because a sinus in the scar was still discharging and annoyed her. She had no pain, but a soreness, and wished to be relieved of the sinus. She was up and around the wards during my visits, so I missed her for a few days, and then had my attention called to her for intense pain in the right iliac fossa, tenderness under McBurney's point, rigidity of rectus muscle, and an extensive mass immediately beneath the cicatrix of the former operation. I believed I had to deal with a recrudescence of the appendicular abscess. At 11:30 A.M. her temperature was 103° and pulse 120, and I appointed 3 o'clock P.M. for operation. At 2:30 P.M. I was telephoned that her temperature was 107° and pulse 180, and was asked what I intended to do. My reply was that if at 3 o'clock she was living I would operate. A 3 P.M. the temperature, taken with three thermometers, was still 107° and pulse from 180 to *nil*. After a hypodermatic of morphine and atropine, an oblique incision was made parallel to the former scar, but internal to it, and the belly entered and walled off with gauze. After evacuating several ounces of offensive pus I enucleated a solid suppurating tumor of the right ovary the size of my closed fist. Gauze drainage was used and the patient made a good recovery. The operation was completed in nineteen minutes from start to finish, and the patient's condition was actually better on leaving the operating room than when she entered. Never before have I seen such a temperature in a surgical case, and I felt that on thorough, rapid work her future depended.

CASE III.—I was asked by a very accurate friend, practising in the country eleven miles from Troy, to see with him a case of appendicitis and to come prepared to operate. The patient, a young woman of 25, who always had had pain and distress at her periods, had been unwell ten days before my visit and the period had lasted the usual time. Five days before my visit she was taken with a severe pain in the *left* side which lasted several hours and was only quieted with morphine. Three days later she had a similar attack, but not so severe. The pain then was referred to the *right* side, which was tender and rigid. The day before my visit a distinct mass was to be felt in the right iliac fossa and there was marked tenderness under McBurney's point. At times the pain was paroxysmal and severe and referred to the right side, but at the time of my visit the pain was slight, although the tenderness was marked under McBurney's point and there was some rigidity of the muscles. The temperature, however, was normal and pulse 80. A mass, however, as large as my closed fist, lay in the right iliac fossa. This the attendant declared to be twice the size which it was at the visit the previous day. This statement, together with its apparently close connection with the uterus, its closely following upon the usual painful period, the absence of chills and temperature, led to the probable diagnosis of ovarian tumor with twisted pedicle. The patient's house and circumstances precluding a satisfactory operation and care so far from medical attendants, I advised her removal to the Samaritan Hospital in Troy, where two days later, October 17, 1901, I did a celiotomy, which disclosed an ovarian cyst of deep claret color, flecked with black, holding nearly a quart. The pedicle was twisted one and one-half times. The tumor was the left ovary, and the torsion of the pedicle had led also to a torsion of the uterus, so that the right border of the uterus was directed against the anterior vaginal wall. The removal was very simple and the recovery prompt.

CASE IV.—June 14, 1902, I was asked to see Miss B., 20 years, single, whose previous medical history, apart from irregular menstruation, had been excellent. Her periods came every four or five weeks and usually lasted four days, with neither marked discomfort nor flow. Her last period, several days ahead of time, lasted six days, with considerable flow, and ended June 7, 1902. June 8, the day after the period ceased, she began to have general pains, not merely in the joints of the extremities, but also the abdomen. Bowels and bladder acted normally. At the time of my visit the temperature was 101°, pulse 120, respiration 18; there was no nausea nor vomiting, but great complaint of constant pain in the right iliac fossa, with paroxysms of epigastric pain. The liver and spleen were normal and no tenderness over the region of the gall bladder. McBurney's point was exquisitely tender, and the immediate neighborhood also tender but in a less degree. There was no muscular spasm and no tumor could be made out by gentle percussion or palpation. The rest of the abdomen was free from sensitiveness. Examination of the lungs disclosed no dulness anywhere, but at the base of the *left* lung behind there was an increased vocal resonance to both spoken and whispered voice and an occasional sibilant râle. The uterus was normal and no evidence of ovarian or tubal trouble nor exudate. I could not believe the case to be one of appendicitis. On my evening visit I found the temperature 102°, pulse 120, respiration 20. The abdominal tenderness, however, was somewhat diminished. Some sibilant râles were to be heard over both backs. June 15: The abdominal tenderness vastly less, no muscular spasm, sibilant râles over both chests, front and back, on deep inspiration, no dulness nor vomiting. June 16 the temperature, pulse, and respiration were normal and all tenderness about McBurney's point had disappeared. Now there was cough, but without expectoration, and a few sibilant râles in each chest. Some tenderness continued along the descending colon and sigmoid flexure, which, however, disappeared after a copious enema. From this on the restoration to health was rapid.

Was the pain in the appendicular region in this case to be referred to the action of some toxin similar to that of the so-called rheumatic cases of appendicitis, or was it mimicry pure and simple by reason of the usual localization of pains which at first had been articular? So strong an impression did the case make upon me at my first visit—especially as I had only a few days before read Maurice Richardson's article from the *Boston Medical and Surgical Journal* of April 17, 1902—that I saw the patient several times that day, for fear that I might, in my hesitancy, be caught napping by a case of appendicitis requiring prompt operation. The other three cases all called imperatively for operation, although in none of the three was the appendix involved. Apart from the high temperature, 107°, in Case 2, which I have never before seen in an operative case, there was nothing very remarkable. Yet each of the three cases furnished conditions in the right iliac fossa easily confused with appendicitis, but at the same time imperatively requiring operation for the dangerous condition existing. Time and again I have been in grave doubt whether I had to deal with a stone in the right ureter at the pelvic brim or a case of chronic appendicitis, and I cannot believe that the diagnosis of appendicitis is as simple as many of the discussions would imply.

The investigations of Arthur Keith, undertaken at the request of Sir Frederick Treves, as to the anatomical relations of Mc-Burney's point,[1] show that this point is far from indicating the location of the base of the appendix, as has been claimed. but that in most cases it corresponds to the site of the ileo-cecal valve. Tenderness of this point is found in many other conditions than appendicitis. A wise scepticism is well to inculcate regarding this very generally cherished symptom. Far be it from me, believing as I do in early operations, to inculcate timidity or hesitancy in operation. However, I believe that if we are as a profession to progress, we must from time to time take soundings to learn whether our accepted landmarks give us the true range by which to pilot our ship into a safe harbor.

DR. H. HOWITT, of Guelph, Ontario, called attention to the temperature and pulse in appendicitis. He looked upon those cases in which there was a high pulse and low temperature as desperate, and the mortality was usually high. With a temperature of 105°-107° the chances for recovery were much better than when the temperature was low with a high pulse.

DR. JAMES F. BALDWIN said that in the beginning of an attack of appendicitis pain was almost invariably felt by the patient in the pit of the stomach, and the patient's physician. if not accustomed to seeing these cases, regarded the case as one of colic. He had had within the last year two cases illustrating that point. One patient, a very intelligent man, had had several attacks of severe pain in the abdomen, which he located to the left of the umbilicus. The physician had made a diagnosis of appendicitis and sent the patient to him. The symptoms had then subsided. but he was able to feel on the right side a nodule about the size of a walnut. After getting a history of the symptoms in the case and examining the patient, he agreed with the diagnosis, cut down, and found a gangrenous appendix with a mass of adhesions. It was removed and the patient recovered. A second similar case was narrated.

DR. W. E. B. DAVIS said that from the discussion this morning one would conclude that the diagnosis of the disease was a very simple matter in all cases; and while he admitted that this was true in many instances, in others it was exceedingly difficult. Inflammation of the gall bladder had given him not a little trouble in some cases in differentiating it from appendicitis, but in some of them he had made his incision sufficiently high so that he could reach either of them. In gall-bladder cases, however, there was not the same amount of rigidity of the abdominal muscles as in

[1] British Medical Journal, June 28, 1902.

appendicitis, and in making a diagnosis between a stone of the kidney and appendicitis, or any intrapelvic or abdominal inflammation, this was a very important point. In the severe cases— speaking now of the desperate ones—in which a question arose as to whether one had peritonitis, appendicitis, or obstruction of the bowel, he did not believe that it was usually difficult to make the differential diagnosis. The surgeon who had seen many cases of mechanical obstruction of the bowel would have very little difficulty in making a differential diagnosis of the conditions. In mild cases of appendicitis he believed that a blood examination was of great assistance. In a case of appendicitis of any consequence one would always get considerable leucocytosis, and this would lead him to operate in some cases of mild appendicitis where he might not get the patient's consent to operate. If he found a marked leucocytosis he would urge operation more energetically.

DR. J. H. CARSTENS spoke of the difficulty of diagnosticating some cases. For instance, during last year he had operated on two patients in whom a diagnosis had been made of kidney stone, and yet both proved to be appendicitis. He was called now and then by general practitioners to operate for intestinal obstruction, and found the cases to be plain appendicitis. The general practitioner had diagnosticated obstruction of the bowels, but the obstruction was secondary to peritonitis. He was called to other cases to operate for appendicitis, and found it was not appendicitis at all. The patient had been overeating and loading up the bowels, or there had been constipation with resulting absorption of excrementitious matter, producing toxemia which simulated appendicitis.

DR. WASHINGTON H. BAKER discussed the methods of diagnosticating appendicitis, and said that if the physician felt that he could not do anything for the case medically, he should not delay surgical interference an instant.

DR. WALTER B. CHASE said that while the diagnosis of appendicitis was comparatively easy in some cases, the physician should be on his guard and not make a superficial examination, thereby reaching the conclusion that there was nothing serious present. He was sure that physicians and surgeons were surprised at times in not detecting evidences which later on were indicative of serious trouble, and then they felt it was largely due to lack of proper investigation on their part.

One of the speakers referred to rigidity of the abdominal muscles indicating trouble underneath. He thought there was a great deal of force in that remark. If the right or left ovary was involved, the rectus muscle on the corresponding side was sufficiently rigid to prevent the production of pain.

DR. MILES F. PORTER admitted that an accurate, scientific diagnosis was impossible in many cases. As a rule, however, the diagnosis of appendicitis was comparatively easy. A diagnosis sufficiently accurate for a working basis could usually be made.

It did not make much difference if a diagnosis of appendicitis was made and the surgeon cut down and found tubal trouble on that side, for the reason that the latter would need operation anyhow. It was nice to make a positive diagnosis, but this was only easy with one class of men, namely, those who had never seen the inside of the belly more than two or three times.

His observation concerning cases of mechanical obstruction of the bowels had been that when the patient came to him the case may have progressed sufficiently far to make an accurate diagnosis impossible. But cases of mechanical intestinal obstruction gave a history of intense colicky pains coming on periodically at intervals of hours, unaccompanied for some time by tenderness on pressure, and this was the history in nine-tenths of the cases of mechanical intestinal obstruction.

DR. L. H. DUNNING and DR. JAMES F. BALDWIN related interesting cases illustrating the difficulty attending the diagnosis of appendicitis in some cases.

DR. WALTER P. MANTON said that McBurney's point was not reliable for diagnostic purposes, and the general practitioner, if he did not find pain at this point, was very apt to conclude that the patient did not have appendicitis. In many cases where the pain was most severe there was absolutely no tumor to be felt. There were perhaps numerous adhesions binding the appendix down and causing the patient to suffer intensely.

INTRAUTERINE FIBROIDS COMPLICATING PREGNANCY, AND RETAINED PLACENTA ASSOCIATED WITH INTRAUTERINE FIBROIDS COMPLICATING PREGNANCY.

CASES AND TREATMENT.

BY

MAGNUS A. TATE, M.D.,

CinCinnati, O.

A PERUSAL of the literature at my command on the subject of intrauterine fibroids complicating pregnancy reveals two things: first, that I am dealing with an extremely rare condition; and, second, that the literature on this subject is very meagre. I am unable to state the frequency of intrauterine fibroids complicating pregnancy, but that I am dealing with a great rarity when the case is further complicated by the placenta being retained is shown by my inability to find more than two cases besides the two that I report. Intrauterine fibroids complicating pregnancy may give rise to hemorrhage before, and often to alarming hemorrhage after, the birth of child and placenta, as some of the cases reported will show. It is reasonable to suppose that the presence of a foreign body in the uterus, such as a fibroid, will naturally interfere in many cases with the child assuming the normal position, and that the breech may present nearly as often as the vertex. This is mentioned by Lefour in his thesis, where he places abnormal presentations in the following ratio: vertex 50.58 per cent to breech 32.25 per cent. It is also reasonable to suppose that an intrauterine polypus (and especially if it be of any size) will be a prime factor in the causation of an interruption of pregnancy, and this is shown in the history of some of the cases mentioned; but, on the contrary, Lefour (who is quoted by Budin) shows that pregnancy is frequently not interfered with, however profuse the hemorrhage. If hemorrhage does occur it often corresponds to the menstrual epoch, and, unless excessive, simulates menstruation, and in this way is misleading. Hence a proper diagnosis is not made (if at all) until after an abortion, late in pregnancy, or after birth of child and placenta. In cases where pregnancy has gone to full time it is surprising to note that so many of the labors were normal, the polypus not being discovered until after the birth of the placenta, when one would expect that labor would not only be difficult and prolonged, but that there would be a further complication, namely, that of improper contraction of uterine muscle. Whenever involution is interfered with a secondary hemorrhage is a common sequel. The results of feeble contraction of uterus during labor, and improper involution afterward, may be contaminated blood clots and a gangrenous polypus (especially if there has been any injury during labor), and these in turn followed by sepsis. If added to this the placenta in part or whole be retained, the patient is indeed a fortunate woman if she escapes with her life from severe septic poisoning. When there is much disturbance of pelvic circulation, it is followed by a serous infiltration which gives rise not only to a slight enlargement and softening of the polypus, but the uterus becomes heavy, boggy, and flaccid, and so does not contract properly to any form of treatment; and this explains why the patient succumbs to uncontrollable hemorrhage. In a few cases the tumor extrudes spontaneously from the uterine cavity, and then it becomes a simple one to manage. Ligate and cut off the pedicle. If the os is not yielding and the growth remains in the uterus, it is very difficult, if not impossible, to remove it. Here the wisest course is to let it alone and not resort to any surgical measure. The placenta remaining in a uterus which contains an intrauterine fibroid is a serious menace, for the longer it remains the greater the danger, primarily of hemorrhage and secondarily of sepsis. Hence the sooner the placenta is removed the less the danger, the better the treatment, the easier the patient's mind, and the surer the chance of recovery.

Queries which are of much interest to science are: Does the existence of pregnancy originate polypi, or were the polypi minute growths existing before pregnancy and then developed rapidly with the advance of gestation?

The following cases I take from the paper written by J. Halliday Croom. (1) Ramsey: Submucous pediculated fibroid; hemorrhage; expelled spontaneously, although gangrenous, on the tenth day; recovery. (2) Sedgwick, (3) Maunvoury, (4) Ashwell: Reported cases. (5) Tarnier, (6) Fallin, (7) Oldham, (8) Priestley, (9) Valtorta: Tumor expelled by simple uterine contraction without either being gangrenous or decomposed. (10) Martin, (11) Horwitz: Tumors became gangrenous, gave rise to septicemia, with a fatal result. (12) Kuchenmeister: Tumor expelled the fourth day post partum, after giving rise to a high fever from suppuration. (13) J. Halliday Croom:[1] Fetus expelled at the fifth month, followed by profuse hemorrhage; tumor removed by evulsion; on the fourth day the discharge became very offensive, and patient died on the eighth day of septicemia; the septicemia due to either gangrene of stump of tumor or a second polypus becoming gangrenous through admission of air. (14) J. Halliday Croom: Case seen in consultation with Dr. Playfair; followed a normal labor; profuse hemorrhage on fifth day, due to a uterine polypus, which was removed by twisting, and a perfect recovery followed. (14) Senderling, (15) Yeld, (16) Kiwisch: Reported cases. (17) Wynn Williams: Case of difficult labor, and in trying to break up the child a large submucous tumor obstructed, which was enucleated, and recovery of patient followed. (18) Duncan reported a case. (19) Weber: Child had to be turned to be born, from the presence of a tumor, which polypus was removed at the same time with placenta. (20) Simpson, (21) Underhill: Reported cases.

These 21 cases were grouped by Croom as follows, he also making the statement that the above were all of the cases reported that he could find to date (1885): (1) Non-gangrenous

[1] Edinburgh Med. Journal, 1886.

cases, in which a healthy tumor expelled without any artificial aid, 5; (2) gangrenous, 6; (3) gangrenous or non-gangrenous removed artificially with hand or instrument, 10—total, 21.

I have collected the following cases.

1. D. Macgibbon:[1] Labor on December 24 was normal and recovery satisfactory. Patient was up and attending to household duties. January 3, had an attack of measles; recovery. January 21, had a uterine hemorrhage. February 3, passed a small uterine polypus; recovery.

2. Budin:[2] Great difficulty in removing child; had to be done by separating arm from body with scissors. An intrauterine fibroid was discovered, but patient left hospital, not allowing tumor to be removed.

3. T. Gaillard Thomas:[3] (1) Case of repeated abortions due to fibrous polypus, which was removed by twisting off pedicle, and case recovered. Attention was called to the sanguineous flow after supposed recovery. (2) Large submucous fibroid discovered after delivery. All efforts to stop hemorrhage by two praetitioners were of no avail and patient died.

5. T. Reber:[4] (1) Patient aged 34, multipara, aborted at fifth month; fetus softened and discolored. Following placenta, a dangerous flooding. Upon introducing hand two submucous fibroids were found which had a broad base. Long-continned efforts, internal and external, such as cold and ergot, produced partial contraction and arrest of hemorrhage. (2) Patient aged 30, primipara. Small submucous fibroid existed before marriage and grew rapidly after marriage, but, under treatment of iodides and ergot, diminished. Patient became pregnant and at the seventh month gave birth to child which lived a few hours. Life of woman was endangered by profuse hemorrhage following the delivery of placenta, but after several hours hemorrhage was controlled. Patient's recovery was slow but complete. The same patient became pregnant again, went to full time, gave birth to twins (breech presentations) with little difficulty. It was now found that the tumor had grown and involved a large part of the uterus. The placenta was not removed for one hour, and when removed a most fearful hemorrhage followed. This resulted in patient passing into a state of collapse and uncon-

[1] New Orleans Med. and Surg. Jour., 1852-3.
[2] AMERICAN JOURNAL OF OBSTETRICS, 1884.
[3] Ibid., 1875.
[4] Transactions of Illinois State Medical Society, 1881.

sciousness. Whiskey and ergot injected hypodermatically, vinegar cloths were put into uterus,. and patient slowly revived. On the third day puerperal mania set in, followed by septicemia, but the patient eventually recovered. (3) Labor natural, hemorrhages, and on examination polypus was found, but its removal was found to be impossible. Later on patient had a very hard bearing-down expulsive pain and the polypus was discharged into the vagina. (4) Patient had a very easy labor, followed by profuse hemorrhage. On examination polypus was found and the placenta retained. The hand of the operator was passed into the uterus and the tumor and placenta were delivered without any difficulty.

9. Dr. Fergusson, of Kings College: (1) Polypus was mistaken for the child's head and forceps applied, and tumor was drawn down and delivered. Child was extracted dead. Patient succumbed to peritonitis. (2) Felt a small tumor, which at first was thought to be the scrotum of the unborn child, but later it was made out to be a polypus. Child was born alive. Frightful hemorrhage followed delivery of placenta and the patient was rescued with great difficulty. Patient afterward would not allow tumor to be removed.

11. Dr. Ramsbotham: Patient 30 years old. Labor was normal. Three weeks after labor patient had slight irregular hemorrhages. Dr. Ramsbotham was called in consultation by Dr. Morn, of Tottenham. Upon examination uterus was found as large as a six-months pregnant uterus, tender, os soft, and Dr. Ramsbotham could just get a finger in and thought that there was a large coagulum or a secondary fetus. Ergot was given. Following day the nurse found something protruding from the os. Dr. Morn introduced his hand and grasped the mass, attached by something like the funis to the fundus. He embraced the stem firmly, and under strong uterine contractions his hand and the tumor, size of a large ostrich egg, were expelled together. Patient recovered.

12. Crisp: Attended a lady aged 36, with her sixth child. Had had three miscarriages. During the last month or six weeks of her present pregnancy she had been subject to frequent small discharges of blood from the uterus. Birth of child was normal. Placenta was retained, and, after waiting nearly an hour, he introduced his hand and removed it. In withdrawing his hand he thought he felt another child enclosed within its membranes, and endeavored to pull away from the side of the

uterus what he thought was the placenta, but failed, and then desisted from further interference. Drs. Clowne and Mr. Bristowe, being called to case, discovered that there was a large polypoid growth within the womb, causing violent expulsive pains which greatly exhausted the patient. This energetic action of the uterus forced the polypus so low down in the vagina as to interfere with the passage of the catheter. Patient died of collapse, worn out with constant uterine action, though it was unattended with hemorrhage.

13. M. Guyot relates a case seen five hours after delivery; removed the polypus without any history of loss of blood. Patient recovered.

14. Churchill: (1) Case where labor was natural. In a short time after delivery flooding came on, resisting all treatment, and patient died in ten hours. A polypus was found. (2) Flooding came on ten days after labor. Uterus was larger than natural and a polypus could be felt. Hemorrhage arrested; but when Dr. Churchill would have tied the polypus it was beyond reach, though the end could be felt. There was no further bleeding and the patient did well.

15. Dr. Radford: (1) Natural labor. A fortnight after, a profuse hemorrhage frequently came on in gushes, with paroxysms of violent pain and bearing-down sensations. No benefit from treatment given and patient succumbed. On postmortem a polypus within the uterus was found. (2) Natural labor, but hemorrhages the following day. Upon examination a small polypus was found within the os. It was removed and patient recovered.

16. J. C. Reeve:[1] Multipara. Labor normal. One week after delivery a parade of militia, passing in front of patient's house, fired a volley which frightened her, and she was immediately taken with severe pains and flooding. On examination os uteri was found to be patulous and a ragged mass was found in uterine cavity, much firmer than placental tissue. A part was detached, and upon further exploration of uterus a pedicle was found attached to mass. This polypoid tumor was removed and patient made an uninterrupted recovery.

17. Magnus A. Tate: (1) Patient aged 20, in my service at the Ohio Maternity Hospital. First and second stages of labor normal. Child lived ten days. Placenta could not be born even after repeated efforts with Credé method, and, as there was little

or no hemorrhage, patient was allowed to rest. In two hours the nurse called interne's attention to a slight hemorrhage. I was immediately summoned and found patient had had another flooding spell (much more severe than the first) just before my arrival. The placenta was still in the uterine cavity, and as two hemorrhages had occurred, the last one quite severe, the time for temporizing had passed, and so I proceeded to deliver placenta. Patient was prepared for operation, and as the anes-thetic was being given bleeding commenced, and almost simul-taneously and following this bleeding a terrific gush of blood poured out from the uterine cavity. As I began to introduce my hand the anesthetist told me that patient was dead and ceased the chloroform, but this proved to be a false alarm. I proceeded with the operation, but did not administer any more chloroform. Partly blocking the os was a hard, round mass which felt at that time like a premature fetal head, and at its side was an enormous clot of blood. Cleaning out the blood clot, I was able to introduce fingers and then hand into the uterus, and then I found out that I was dealing with a polypus half the size of a fetal head, and at its base was the placenta encircling it. By this time patient began to rally, and as she did so another violent hemorrhage took place, so I forced my whole hand into the uterus, grasped polypus and placenta, and delivered by twisting the whole mass. Patient gave one scream that she was dying and passed into a deep faint. Polypus and placenta were delivered, but nearly at the cost of woman's life. Hemorrhage at this time was so fright-ful that it was almost indescribable, but at last the uterus was packed with plain gauze, patient given hypodermatics of strychnia and whiskey, salt solution injected, head lowered, feet elevated, and heat applied externally. Pulse was imperceptible, but heart could be felt to beat in an irregular and feeble man-ner. Outlook was anything but encouraging, but she slowly rallied, and in three hours pulse could be felt at the wrist. For two days patient slowly but steadily improved, and on the third morning I attempted to remove the gauze packing. As I did so another hemorrhage took place, so I ceased, and it was not until the tenth day that I could remove all of the gauze. The temper-ature and pulse steadily increased from the third to the seventh day, when the temperature was 105° and pulse 140. For the next six weeks temperature ranged from 103° to 105° and pulse 120 to 150, and patient had a very offensive discharge from the uterus. Temperature and pulse began to decline the seventh week, and at the end of twelfth week patient left the hospital, temperature and pulse normal, but she was very weak and emaciated. Three weeks after leaving hospital I was summoned to her house and found patient with a temperature of 105° and a pulse of 140. Diagnosis was now malaria, which was confirmed by Dr. B. K. Rachford, who saw case with me. This illness lasted four weeks, but recovery at last followed.

18. Magnus A. Tate: (2) Patient, aged 29, had been pregnant twice, had had two miscarriages, and was now pregnant for the third time. First miscarriage two years ago, in which no difficulty was encountered, but during the second one, some ten months afterward, there was quite a loss of blood and a retained placenta, which was extracted, and this was followed by a long spell of fever. At this the third miscarriage child was about six and a half months old and the placenta could not be expelled. Dr. Dunlap, who was in charge of the case, made repeated attempts at delivery, but was unsuccessful, and, as there were no untoward symptoms, placenta was allowed to remain in the uterus with the hope that Nature would accomplish what external manipulation could not do, namely, expel the placenta. For ten days the placenta remained within the uterus and no symptoms developed; woman seemingly apparently well. On the morning of the eleventh day pulse was 100 and temperature 100°, and then I saw patient for the first time. I, like Dr. Dunlap, tried external means to deliver, but could not do so, and, after preparation, I operated. Chloroform was administered. Os would not allow more than the introduction of one finger at first, but by perseverance I was able to insert three fingers into the uterus. Finger tip came in contact with a hard mass the size of an orange, and back and partly around it I felt the placenta. Finding that I would be unable to deliver with fingers, I inserted placental forceps and delivered polypus and placenta piecemeal. Having removed all of the mass that I could feel, and as the hemorrhage was quite profuse, I hurriedly packed uterine cavity with plain gauze. The second day after delivery, and the thirteenth day after beginning of miscarriage, temperature was 102° and pulse 110, following day each 100, and from that time on pulse ranged from 90 to 70, temperature 99½° to normal. Three weeks after that both were normal. During these three weeks patient had a discharge composed of a mixture of blood, pus, masses of placental tissue, and portions of polypus, and it was so offensive that it polluted the bedding and carpet so that

both had to be burned after patient's recovery. Such an offensive discharge I never smelled, and with such a condition (barring the odor) patient was comparatively comfortable and temperature and pulse good, the former never above 102° nor the latter more than 110. Under treatment discharge gradually decreased and odor lessened, and in one month patient was able to do light housework.

Analyzing the above 41 cases, the histories of which, as a whole, are not complete, I note the following: In 9 cases only the names of reporters are given, without any mention of history of case. In 6 cases the tumor became gangrenous. Hemorrhage was the prominent symptom, it occurring in 18 cases. Three polyps were expelled spontaneously. Seventeen polyps were removed. In 10 cases the labor was normal. In 4 cases labor was difficult; in 2 the child had to be destroyed, one was a case of turning, and the other a breech. In 3 cases the polyp was not removed. In 4 cases the tumor was discovered before, in all of the rest after, labor. Four cases reported where labor set in before time; 2 were at the fifth and 2 at the seventh month.

Following are complications reported: septicemia, 8; measles, 1; puerperal mania, 1; retained placenta, 4 cases. Treatments mentioned: cold applications, ergot, iodides, whiskey, vinegar cloths in uterus, packing of uterus with gauze, and removal of tumor. Causes of death: sepsis, 3; hemorrhage, 3; peritonitis, 1; and collapse, 1, making in all 8 cases. If all of the other cases, including the 9 without histories, recovered, we have 33 recoveries and 8 deaths, a mortality of 19½ per cent.

DR. L. H. DUNNING reported a case which occurred seven or eight years ago. The woman had been delivered four days before he saw her. He came into the case accidentally. There had been no suspicion of trouble of any kind. Her convalescence was normal until suddenly one afternoon she was seized with a violent hemorrhage. The family physician was out of town and he was called to see the case. On reaching the bedside he supposed the placenta had been retained. He made a digital examination. The os was patulous; he inserted his fingers into the uterus readily and found quite a large submucous fibroid tumor.. It was as large as an orange, and the pedicle was attached near the fundus of the uterus. Fortunately he had with him a pair of long forceps, introduced it into the uterus, twisted the pedicle of the tumor off, washed out the uterus, and the patient made an excellent recovery.

DR. J. H. CARSTENS said that cases of multiple fibroids where the placenta could not be removed were rare. He saw one case about a year ago. He made strenuous efforts to remove the placenta. The attending physicians had tried to remove the fibroids, but could not do so. They called him, and he did an abdominal hysterectomy. He had been unable to find a case where an abdominal hysterectomy had been done for the purpose of removing a retained placenta.

DR. JAMES F. BALDWIN reported three cases, one of them very much like that of the essayist. In the first the woman had miscarried repeatedly and had a distinct submucous fibroid tumor. She would not consent to its removal. She went to full term, when the fibroid disappeared.

The second case was a woman who miscarried at six months. She was in labor for twenty-four hours. The attending physician tried to deliver the afterbirth, but was unable to do so. The speaker was called and made an abdominal hysterectomy with recovery of the patient. He narrated a third case.

DR. WALTER P. MANTON said he had delivered a good many women with fibroids in different positions of the uterus. Subserous fibroids, unless they were of large size, rarely, if ever, complicated pregnancy. He did not recall ever having seen a case of interstitial, mural, or submucous fibroid of any considerable size where pregnancy had gone on to term. He had seen but one case in which a large cervical mural fibroid interfered with delivery, and he was obliged to remove the fibroid before the woman could be delivered.

DR. C. L. BONIFIELD reported two cases of fibroid tumors complicating pregnancy. The first one he saw in consultation within a year after he had graduated. The pedicle was twisted, cut off, and there was no further trouble.

In the other case the patient had been pregnant about six months. She was the wife of a physician; had miscarried, and there was a retained placenta. He was summoned without being told what the condition was. He found her in an extremely bad condition. Her temperature was 105°, pulse could scarcely be counted, and he was hardly prepared to do the work necessary. He tried to remove the placenta and a submucous fibroid as large as a cocoanut, which he succeeded in doing as the patient expired.

DR. L. S. MCMURTRY asked the essayist to state whether or not, as the result of his studies of the subject, he did not think that in cases of retained placenta and a sessile intrauterine fibroid tumor it would not be good practice to do an abdominal hysterectomy.

DR. WILLIAM D. PORTER, of Cincinnati, O., had never seen a case of submucous fibroid tumor where pregnancy had gone on to term. He saw a case once in consultation in which there was a polypus as large as a fetal head in the vagina. This came on three months after the beginning of pregnancy following an abortion. The diagnosis made was that of an inverted uterus, but investigation showed it was a sloughing mass, which was readily removed.

DR. EDWARD T. ABRAMS, of Dollar Bay, Mich., reported a case that came under his observation six months ago where a uterine fibroid complicated pregnancy. His assistant went and delivered the woman, but there was a profuse hemorrhage. Immediately after this the speaker was sent for. When he arrived he discovered a large uterine fibroid, and after considerable trouble he delivered both the placenta and fibroid. The woman made a good recovery.

DR. MONTGOMERY LINVILLE, of Newcastle, Pa., met with a case of intrauterine fibroid complicating pregnancy about two years ago. The woman had aborted at four months. She was attended by a colleague, who did not succeed in removing the afterbirth for twenty-four hours. The uterus was so large that it reached the umbilicus. The patient had severe pain, which continued for a week or ten days, so that it became necessary to keep her under the influence of anodynes to relieve it. She likewise had a profuse hemorrhage, which continued off and on for five or six days. He was finally called in consultation, at which time her temperature reached 107°, pulse 150. Her condition was such that he thought a suprapubic hysterectomy was impossible. He excised the vaginal portion of the uterus and found a fibroid which occupied the upper two-thirds of the uterus. He succeeded in removing the fibroid tumor by morcellation, although it was exceedingly difficult to do so. Patient improved after the operation and recovered. In two weeks he closed the wounds in the cervix, and at the end of three weeks she had entirely recovered.

DR. TATE, in closing the discussion, said it was surprising how cases of this character, with such a frightful and profuse hemorrhage, could rally and get well. Another thing that surprised him in looking up the literature was how these women could go to term with large polyps within the uterine cavity. If the patient was in a good condition and did not lose too much blood, if he should encounter another such case as he had reported, he would do abdominal hysterectomy. But the feature of losing so much blood was so prominent that he did not know whether it would be wise to do abdominal hysterectomy or not.

DR. J. H. CARSTENS, of Detroit, Mich., read a paper on

ABDOMINAL SECTION DURING PREGNANCY.[1]

DR. EDWIN RICKETTS said it had been his good fortune to meet a number of cases of appendicitis in connection with the puerperal state, and on his way to attend this meeting he did three operations for appendicitis complicating pregnancy.

The statement had been made that appendicitis did not occur so frequently in the female as in the male. He thought if gynecologists were able to differentiate the puerperal conditions

[1] Will appear in a succeeding number of the JOURNAL.

and recognize their association with appendicitis, it would result in the profession changing their minds in regard to appendicitis appearing as frequently in the female as in the male.

In regard to fibroid tumors complicating pregnancy, some eight years ago a patient consulted him in whom a fibroid was present in the left fornix. He succeeded in delivering this woman at full term, but the hemorrhage was profuse, and it was with great difficulty that he was able to save the patient.

He had a case recently in which an attack of appendicitis came on during the third month of pregnancy. The attending physician, however, had made a diagnosis of involvement of the right ovary. Upon careful examination appendicitis was diagnosticated, the abdomen opened, and a catarrhal appendix found filled with concretions.

DR. WILLIAM J. GILETTE, of Toledo, O., about three months ago was called to see a woman who had been pregnant about five months, the pregnancy being complicated by a large interstitial fibroid tumor. The tumor was about the size of a cocoanut and impacted in the pelvis. He suggested hysterectomy, but on opening the abdomen found he could get it out above the pelvic brim. An important point that had interested him was, could he have enucleated this tumor in a pregnant uterus without producing a miscarriage? He would like to know whether it was possible to remove a fibroid tumor as large as a cocoanut from the wall of the uterus and have pregnancy go on to term.

DR. MILES F. PORTER said he reported a case before the Western Surgical and Gynecological Association which really answered the question of Dr. Gilette. This case negatived the statement made by Dr. Carstens, i.e., the size of the tumor itself did not call for operation in cases of pregnancy. In his case the operation was done and the tumor removed for the express purpose of allowing the woman, who was 30 years of age, to carry her child to term. The tumor was attached to the right side of the fundus; the woman was four months pregnant.

DR. L. S. McMURTRY said that the case reported by Dr. Porter ought not to be taken as a universal justification for operative intervention in fibroid tumors complicating pregnancy, the same as in treating fibroid tumors of the uterus that were not complicated by pregnancy. He thought it would be very unjust to have it go forth from the Association that operations for the removal of fibroid tumors complicated by pregnancy should be undertaken with the same aggressive spirit as was done in cases of fibroid tumors disassociated with pregnancy.

DR. CARSTENS, in closing the discussion, said that if an operation was indicated in a case of pregnancy either for appendicitis, gall stones, or any other septic or acute condition, it should be done. In those cases where the fibroid tumor or tumors were situated above the pelvic brim and did not interfere with labor, operation was not necessary. He had emphasized that point in his paper.

DECIDUOMA MALIGNUM,

WITH REPORT OF A CASE.

BY

LEWIS S. McMURTRY, A.M., M.D.,

Louisville, Ky.

(With one illustration.)

In 1888 Prof. Sänger reported to the Obstetrical Society of Leipzig two cases of malignant disease of the uterus presenting distinctive pathologic characteristics and which had not been previously recognized. The growth appears upon the mucous lining of the uterine corpus following abortion or ordinary labor, with profuse bleeding, and is succeeded by bloody and offensive discharges. Metastatic deposits in the lungs, vagina, and other organs are very common, and progress to a fatal result is rapid. The cachexia is marked, and the progress of the disease, if uninterfered with, is so rapid that the time from the first symptoms to the death of the patient occupies only a few weeks or months. The diagnosis of the disease is not especially difficult, and the treatment is encompassed by a single decisive surgical procedure —early and complete extirpation of the uterus.

The greatest difficulties centre about the pathogenesis and true pathological classification of the disease. Sänger believed the growth originated from decidua cells, and accordingly gave it the name of deciduoma malignum.[1] Pfeiffer, in 1889, reported a case and proposed the same name.[2] The theory advanced by both Sänger and Pfeiffer attributed the growth to malignant changes in the decidua cells. In his second paper, in 1893, Sänger submitted a review of his case and a study of eleven additional cases reported, and suggested another name, more accurately in accord with his interpretation of the pathology as revealed by more extensive investigation, suggesting ''sarcoma uteri deciduo-cellulare.''[3] His conception of the pathology was that of sarcoma originating from the products of conception.

Gottschalk reported a case and proposed the name ''sarcoma chorio-cellulare,'' believing the disease to consist in 'malignant degeneration of the stroma of the chorionic villi.[4]

---

[1] Centralbl. f. Gyn., 1889.   [2] Präger Wochen., 1890.
[3] Archiv. f. Gyn., 1893.   [4] Ibid., 1894.

In 1895 Marchand first published his studies upon this subject, and in 1898 made additions to his valuable contribution. These important investigations were exhaustive and have done more than any other toward the elucidation of the subject.[1] He demonstrated the epithelial character of the growth and claims that it springs from the two kinds of tissue composing the epithelial covering of the villi. The tumor, in accordance with Marchand's views, arises from the syncytium and Langhans cells, which undergo malignant degeneration and proliferation. He believes that metastases obtain by way of the blood vessels. Fränkel and Gebhard have confirmed Marchand's observations, and German investigators generally concur that the growth is epithelial in character, growing from the epithelial layers covering the chorionic villi—that is, an epithelioma.

This view has been accepted in America; and, while our English cousins maintained for a time that the disease was sarcoma and not necessarily associated with pregnancy, they, too, have become converted to Marchand's teachings. But with this important pathological basis established, the origin of the syncytium (a structure composed of epithelial cells lying between the decidua and chorionic villi over the layer of Langhans) and Langhans cell layer (the epithelial covering of the chorionic villi) is not settled; thus Gottschalk and other observers claim that both are derived from the fetal ectoderm, while others believe that the syncytium is derived from the surface epithelium of the uterus. The result of this difference is that it remains unsettled whether the growth we call deciduoma malignum has its origin in fetal or maternal structures, or in both. For clinical purposes, however, this term, originally proposed by Sänger, is quite sufficient to indicate the present state of our knowledge. An interesting feature of the pathology is the frequency with which the disease follows hydatid-mole pregnancy.

The area of active growth is situated superficially upon the uterine mucosa and forms a tumor bulging into the uterine cavity. The macroscopic appearance resembles placental tissue, but microscopic examination shows granular masses and large nucleated cells derived from the syncytium and Langhans layer, and, beneath this, chorionic villi whose epithelium is in active proliferation.

Clinically the disease presents a distinct history. Hemorrhage is invariably the first and most persistent symptom. Cu-

[1] Monatsch. f. Geb. u. Gyn., 1895.

rettage does not control the hemorrhage. The flow is at first red, but later, as the disease reaches an advanced stage, it becomes dark and offensive. Pain here, as in other forms of malignant disease of the uterus, is not a constant symptom. The uterus is usually found to be enlarged and soft, with the os patulous.

A conspicuous and distinctive characteristic of this disease is the marked tendency to early metastasis. The metastatic growths consist of the same elements as the primary tumor, but usually exceed the primary growth in extent and activity. The lungs and vagina are the most frequent loci of metastasis. Cough and bloody expectoration are in some cases the first symptoms to bring the patient to the physician, and in some instances the vaginal metastasis has been treated for the primary disease and the intrauterine tumor only discovered post mortem. The brain, spleen, ovary, broad ligament, kidney, and liver may be invaded by metastatic deposits. Since our German colleagues called attention to this insidious and rapidly fatal form of malignant disease, numerous cases have been reported. Ladinski[1] has recently collected 132 authentic cases from the medical literature of the world. There is reason to believe that it is more frequent than is now supposed, and I doubt not that many unrecognized cases terminate fatally, or, if recognized, treatment is instituted too late. As the only means of cure consists in early and complete extirpation of the uterus, all suspicious cases of persistent hemorrhage following abortion and labor, especially after mole pregnancy, should be subjected to intrauterine exploration and microscopic examination of scrapings from the uterus. Early diagnosis and prompt operation are essential to successful treatment.

The following case, both in clinical history and objective symptoms, affords a typical illustration óf the disease:

Mrs. L. E. W., aged 35 years; mother of six children, the youngest child 3 years old. In May, 1902, she missed her menstrual period, which was due on the fifth day of that month. On June 9 she observed hemorrhage from the uterus, which, though not excessive, was persistent. For several months beforehand she had suffered with pain in the deep pelvis and had received treatment from her physician for pelvic inflammation. She came under my care on June 18, presenting a letter from her family physician. The hemorrhage had been so profuse,

[1] AMERICAN JOURNAL OF OBSTETRICS. April, 1902.

with clots. that she was believed to have miscarried. Upon examination the uterus was found displaced backward and fixed, with a distinct inflammatory mass (tubo-ovarian) on the left side. The temperature rose to 102° F. every day and she had several rigors. The hemorrhage persisted and was not controlled by curettage under antiseptic precautions. The bloody discharge continued and was quite offensive, and six days after curettage was more profuse than ever. On June 27 I did abdominal section and found a pyosalpinx on the left side, with the usual accompanying adhesions. The uterus was slightly enlarged and its walls were thickened and congested. The persistent bloody and offensive discharge had so impressed me

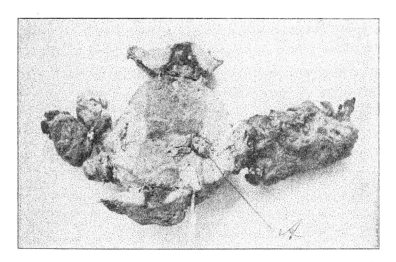

Bilateral section of uterus exposing endometrium : growth shown at point *A*.

with the probability of malignant disease that I decided to remove the entire uterus, as well as the diseased adnexa. This was done. and the abdomen closed, with gauze drainage per vaginam as usually applied in such cases. Convalescence was easy and uncomplicated, and the patient sat up at the end of two weeks, and left the hospital at the end of the fourth week in excellent condition. She has now regained her color, strength, and flesh, and is quite well.

A bilateral section of the uterus disclosed a distinct elevated nodule on the posterior wall near the left cornu. This nodule was so closely attached to the mucous surface and wall of the uterus that it appeared as if it were a projection of the uterine muscularis through a hole in the endometrium. It was friable, bled freely when touched. and evidently was not placental structure. Its structure evidently was not that of a uterine myofibroma. In view of the clinical history, and especially the persistent hemorrhage and offensive discharge after miscarriage and curettage, I was convinced that the case was one of deciduoma malignum.

The specimen was submitted to careful microscopic examination by Dr. James Vance, Director of the Pathological Laboratory of the Hospital College of Medicine. Dr. Vance found the histological structure of the growth typical of deciduoma malignum, both syncytium and Langhans cells participating.

Microscopic sections of the growth have been submitted to other competent observers. who have in every instance confirmed these observations.

Dr. James F. Baldwin stated that six or eight months ago he was called to remove a cancer of the uterus, this being the diagnosis of the attending physician. He found the woman had been delivered at full term without difficulty six or eight weeks previous to his visit. The afterbirth was delivered by itself, and, so far as the attending physician knew, it was normal. Two weeks later, trouble continuing, another physician was sent for, who examined her and found a piece of afterbirth, which he removed, curetted, and supposed there would be no further trouble. Criticism was indulged in and a suit for malpractice was in the air. The second physician, two or three weeks later, in examining the woman, found more afterbirth. Dr. Baldwin again examined the woman carefully and found malignant disease, and told the physician it was deciduoma malignum. Vaginal hysterectomy was made. There was no involvement of the vagina. He was careful, however, to pull down the omentum, and found a secondary nodule as large as the end of his finger. He ligated above. Recovery was satisfactory, but a few weeks later the woman developed cachexia and died. He believed he had seen half a dozen such cases in his practice.

Dr. John B. Murphy, of Chicago, read a paper entitled

PERFORATING ULCER OF THE DUODENUM.[1]

---

[1] Will appear in a succeeding number of the Journal.

REPORT OF A NUMBER OF CASES OF OPERATION FOR PERITONEAL TUBERCULOSIS,

WITH REMARKS.

BY

RUFUS B. HALL, M.D.,

Cincinnati, O

In presenting this short report it is not the intention of the writer to enter into a discussion of the etiology or pathology of tuberculosis as it invades the various regions of the human body, but rather to confine his remarks to clinical phases of the disease as it invades the peritoneum, especially in the female.

Peritoneal tuberculosis in women is not a rare disease. It occurs often enough to make it necessary to consider it in the diagnosis of all obscure diseases in the pelvis and abdomen. In a large majority of the cases of peritoneal tuberculosis coming under the writer's observation there were no appreciable manifestations of the disease in other parts of the body. In a few cases there were unmistakable symptoms of the disease either in the lungs or other parts of the body, as enlarged glands in various regions or necrosis of bone. The symptoms of the disease vary so much in different cases that many other diseases in the abdomen or pelvis may be simulated so accurately by tuberculosis that it requires patient and careful study in each case to differentiate one from the other.

A very perplexing condition which is often met is tuberculosis with agglutination of the intestines, due to the localized inflammation, forming a distinct mass in the region of the appendix. These patients have repeated attacks of inflammation so closely resembling the recurrent attack of catarrhal appendicitis that a correct diagnosis is next to impossible before the abdomen is opened. The writer has operated a number of times for relief of recurrent attacks of appendicitis, the attacks recurring at irregular intervals of from three to six months, confining the patient to bed for from ten to twenty days at each attack. The patients all have a temperature of from 101° to 102½° for a day or two at the commencement of the attack, and a distinct tumor in the region of the appendix, which disappears in three or four weeks. One may suspect tuberculosis, but in the absence of any of the usual symptoms of that disease in other parts of the body he cannot always confirm his suspicion until after the abdomen has been opened.

The following case will serve as an illustration of this group: Miss N., aged 27, a highly-educated and refined woman, had been the subject of recurrent attacks of appendicitis for three years, during which time she had suffered from five severe attacks, each attack confining her to bed for a period varying from ten days to three weeks. After each illness there remained a distinct mass in the region of the appendix for from ten to twenty days, and the soreness remained for several weeks. At the time of the operation, which was made in the interval, a small, distinct, hard mass, which appeared as large as a man's thumb and two inches long, could be felt in the region of the appendix. There were no symptoms nor manifestations of tuberculosis in any part of the body, but his past experience made the writer suspect tuberculosis as the cause. The operation revealed the most extensive ravages of tuberculosis. The appendix was enlarged and thickened, with no accumulation in it, yet the removal of the appendix cured the attacks. The patient recovered, has since married, and is enjoying most excellent health.

Peritoneal tuberculosis often resembles a small fibroid of the uterus associated with tubo-ovarian disease. In both conditions the patients have the excessive loss of blood at the menstrual periods, which are prolonged and more frequent and are accompanied by the pain which is so frequent in fibroids. They also have recurrent attacks of inflammation at irregular intervals, just as the patients do who have fibroid tumors with tubo-ovarian disease.

An illustrative case is Mrs. H., aged 36, mother of three children, the youngest 10 years old. She has been a widow eight years. She entered my service at the Presbyterian Hospital October 10, 1898. She has always worked hard and enjoyed good health until five months ago. Since that time the menstrual periods have been very excessive, amounting almost to a hemorrhage, and accompanied by a good deal of pain. On two occasions at her periods she was obliged to call a physician and remain in bed for three days on account of pain in the abdomen. When she entered the hospital she had been bleeding for ten days. She had the appearance of a strong and vigorous woman. Vaginal examination revealed the pelvic cavity filled with a mass extending for three inches above the pubic arch. The whole mass was not unlike a small fibroid of the uterus with old tubal disease passing through an acute attack of inflammation. The patient was kept under observation for a week, with quiet in bed, and there was a change for the better in the local condition. The tumor was not so large. The bleeding stopped. By vaginal examination a distinct mass, separate from the uterus, could be made out to one side of the pelvis. The upper border of the mass could not be clearly defined, as is usual in a small fibroid tumor. A positive diagnosis was not made, but an operation was advised and accepted. When the abdomen was opened the disease proved to be tubercular, with a large abscess at the side of the pelvis involving the tube, which was removed. The patient recovered.

There are cases of encysted dropsy, due to peritoneal tuberculosis, in which the most careful examination may fail to reveal the true condition. The following case illustrates this point: Mrs. H., aged 30, mother of two children, the younger 2 years old, had always enjoyed unusually good health previous to the present illness. The patient was in her usual flesh, felt perfectly well, and had the appearance of a strong, vigorous woman. She never required the attention of a physician except in her confinements, which were normal. Seven weeks before the operation she consulted her physician, complaining of pain in the lower part of the abdomen, which disappeared in a day or two. An examination at that time revealed an enlargement in the pelvis and abdomen as large as a cocoanut, which was supposed to be ovarian. Upon close questioning the patient admitted that she had observed some vague discomfort in the pelvis and abdomen for five or six weeks. She was informed that she had a tumor and it should be removed early. She went to visit a friend in the country, and four weeks later had a sharp attack of pain in the abdomen and was confined to her bed three or four days. After that time the abdomen remained sore and tender to the touch. It enlarged rapidly up to the time she entered the hospital, seven weeks after her first knowledge of the disease. At that time the abdomen was as large as at full term of gestation. The physical examination and clinical history simulated ovarian cyst so perfectly that one might easily have made an error and pronounced it ovarian. But by careful examination the upper boundary of the supposed tumor could not be accurately defined, as it can always be in ovarian cyst. The condition was such as always exists in encysted dropsy due to tuberculosis. By vaginal examination the uterus was found to be fixed, and there was marked tenderness with distinct hardness upon both sides of the uterus—very unusual in ovarian cysts and quite the rule in encysted dropsy. The general appearance of the patient was that of a strong, robust woman, except the abdominal enlargement. Operation was advised and made.

When the abdomen was opened fully two gallons of encysted fluid were evacuated, revealing very extensive ravages of tuberculosis. The pelvis was filled by the enlarged uterus and diseased tubes, which were apparently the focus of infection. Both tubes were the seat of large abscesses, and were removed. After cleansing the cavity a drainage tube was placed and the patient put to bed. She had a slow and tedious convalescence, but recovered and is enjoying excellent health at this time, five years after the operation.

While there are many conditions in the pelvis and abdomen, due to other causes, which are very difficult to differentiate from tuberculosis, the diagnosis of that disease is not impossible in most instances. There may be nothing in the appearance of the patient, the clinical history, or the pelvic or abdominal conditions to even suggest the tubercular condition. But by a little patient, careful observation we may, if the case is one of tuberculosis, set the whole matter at rest or make a provisional diagnosis of tuberculosis by the temperature chart. The temperature should be registered every three or four hours for ten or fifteen days. In no other condition do we have the exact regularity of afternoon rise of temperature as in this disease.

That certain phases of peritoneal tuberculosis call for surgical interference there can be no doubt. In all cases where there is an encysted dropsy or an accumulation of pus, the abdomen should be opened, the fluid or pus evacuated, and, after the necessary surgical repair has been completed, free drainage should be established. The experience of surgeons in this class of cases is that the remote results are exceedingly gratifying. The writer has made abdominal sections for the relief of tubercular conditions upon 110 patients: for appendicitis, male 4 times, female 8 times—12 times; other conditions (female), 98 times; total sections, 110.

CASE I.—One patient died apparently from shock the day of the operation.

CASE II.—One patient died from septic peritonitis the third day after operation.

CASE III.—One patient died of meningitis on the seventeenth day after the operation. For fifteen days this patient's convalescence was perfectly satisfactory in every way. She was a girl 11 years of age. On the morning of the sixteenth day she complained of pain in the head and in one hour was delirious.

CASE IV.—One patient died of general dissemination while yet in the hospital, six weeks after operation.

CASE V.—One patient died of general dissemination while yet in the hospital, ten weeks after the operation.

CASE VI.—One patient, a woman aged 26, made an easy and smooth convalescence and left the hospital at the end of the fourth week. She was able to go out for a drive on two or three occasions. She died of meningitis at the end of the sixth week, after a three days' illness, two weeks after she left the hospital.

CASE VII.—One patient recovered and left the hospital at the middle of the fourth week, and died of general dissemination thirteen weeks after the operation. This patient was a man, operated for appendicitis. He had suffered from several attacks extending over a year or more. There was a distinct lump in the region of the appendix, and he was operated on in the interval. The appendix did not contain any foreign body, yet it was removed after great difficulty in separating the adhesions.

Early in my work in peritoneal surgery a number of cases were operated upon for tuberculosis in which no fluid, either serum or pus, was evacuated. If a diagnosis of tuberculosis could be made, the dictum of the day was to operate. If no diagnosis could be made, the dictum was to explore for a diagnosis. The writer has long since abandoned both of these dicta. He has not made an exploration for diagnostic purposes for years. Neither has he knowingly operated for eight years for peritoneal tuberculosis where fluid was not believed to be present.

In studying these cases and following the after-results, the writer has been very forcibly impressed by the fact that in the cases operated in which there was fluid to be evacuated, either pus or serum, the ultimate results were very much more favorable than in those cases in which the enlarged mass proved to be an agglutination of the abdominal viscera and where no focus of infection was removed or fluid was evacuated. The first class of cases, which were by far the largest majority, were greatly relieved at once following the operation. Convalescence was established early, and as a rule the cases made satisfactory prog-

46

ress. In the latter cases the operation did not seem to have exerted the marked beneficial results noted in the former. They did not regain their strength so rapidly, convalescence was more prolonged, and other manifestations of the disease were more likely to be noted within a year. This group comprises 11 cases of the 110 referred to in this paper. Of these 11, one died the third day following the operation (Case 2), previously referred to. Of the remaining 10, 6 have died of tuberculosis in from fourteen months to three years after the operation, and 4 are now apparently well, without any other manifestation of the disease. Of the remaining 94 cases, one died three and a half years after her operation, from tuberculosis of the lungs. This case remained apparently well two and a half years after operation. One case died four and a half years after her operation, from laryngeal tuberculosis, after an illness extending over nearly three years. Two cases are now suffering from advanced pulmonary tuberculosis and will probably die within a year. The remaining 90 are symptomatically well. A few of these cases have been operated so recently that no conclusions can be drawn from them.

Taking these cases as a whole, the results are certainly gratifying beyond expectation. A large per cent of the cases are enjoying the best of health, and from their appearance one would never suspect that they have had tubercular disease.

The only complication to mar the otherwise most gratifying convalescence in not a few of the cases was the persistence of the fistulous opening at the site of the abdominal drainage. For several years the silk used for ligatures was given all the blame for the persistence of the fistulæ, some of which remained for a year or more. Finally catgut was substituted in all cases, but the fistulæ came just as often and remained just as long. It is not the fistula itself that is the greatest objection to its presence or long continuance, notwithstanding the great annoyance and, at times, pain to the patient, but the ventral hernia that always follows in cases in which a sinus remains for a long period of time. We will not discuss its treatment nor dilate upon its danger. You are all familiar with them. I would rather suggest a method to avoid the fistula and the subsequent hernia. In all cases in which the subject is a female this is avoided by substituting vaginal for the abdominal drainage. The writer has used it in sixteen cases, and his experience has been most gratifying.

Dr. John B. Murphy said that, with one single exception, he had never seen a case of tubercular peritonitis in the female without involvement of the tubes, and this led him to ask the question, Does the peritonitis occur from the tubal disease, or is the tubal disease a sequence of the peritonitis?

Speaking of the differential diagnosis between peritoneal tuberculósis and appendicitis, he said it was difficult, and the only real assistance was obtained from an examination of the pelvic organs through the rectum, rather than through the vagina, because these cases occurred in children, nulliparæ, and virgins, and examination through the rectum revealed induration and thickening of the lower portion of the cul-de-sac of Douglas. Another point in the clinical history of the disease in the virgin was a discharge from the vagina and an erosion of the cervix. In girls from 10 to 16 and from that age on he had not succeeded in finding tubercle bacilli in the vaginal discharge.

Dr. J. H. Carstens said, if the peritoneal tuberculosis had existed for a long time, secondary deposits could usually be found in the lungs; and if this were the case he did not operate on them, because invariably they died of general tuberculosis. If he got a case of peritoneal tuberculosis, and was convinced there was no secondary deposit in the lungs, he would operate. The site of the focus of the disease would govern him largely with reference to doing an operation. If the focus of disease was around the appendix, he removed the appendix invariably; if, however, it was around the tubes, he did not remove the tubes. He only removed tubes which were occluded and contained pus and there was a septic condition probably from mixed infection.

Dr. Walter B. Dorsett said there were different types of tubercular peritonitis. There was the dry variety, which was entirely different from that he had heard spoken of to-day. We had ascending tuberculosis, where the tube or tubes were involved.

As to drainage, where we had a dry peritoneal tuberculosis, where the intestines were agglutinated to each other but still no fluid in the abdominal cavity, there was no question about the advisability of sewing the wound up without drainage; but where there was serum, it should be washed out with normal salt solution and the wound sewed up. Where pus was present, it was a different matter; drainage should be established by the vagina or through the median line.

Dr. Miles F. Porter said, in looking over the whole field, his results had been better where drainage was not resorted to, unless mixed infection had made it plainly necessary. He disagreed with Dr. Carstens when he said in case he found secondary deposits in the lungs he would not operate. He (Dr. Porter) believed this was wrong. There were certain cases where secondary deposits were in favor of rather than against operative intervention. Here he was supported not only by his own experience, which was small, but a careful study of the literature showed that it was a good rule not to avoid operation on these cases, even though there were secondary deposits in the lungs and elsewhere.

DR. JAMES F. BALDWIN reported a case in which he had an opportunity to reopen. He had operated for encysted ascites, the woman having a tumor about the size of an eight-months pregnancy. The case was sent to him as one of ovarian cyst, but he changed his diagnosis to encysted ascites of tubercular origin. He found a large cavity containing fluid, surrounded on all sides by firm adhesions involving the intestines, large and small. He made no attempt to break up the adhesions. He drained. The patient recovered, but with a fistula due to infection, which remained for three or four years, when patient returned to him to have it dissected out. He opened the abdomen and was amazed at its appearance. The intestines, mesentery, and mesocolon were normal. It was a revelation to him of what Nature could do. He dissected out the fistula, which was a blind tube running down into the pelvis, and she made a prompt recovery. He reported this case to show that we could have a good deal of confidence in the *vis medicatrix naturæ* in very many instances.

DR. C. L. BONIFIELD said that some five or six years ago a girl, 17 years of age, was admitted to the Good Samaritan Hospital and operated on by Dr. Joseph Ransohoff for appendicitis. She recovered from this operation. Subsequently she went to the medical service of the late Prof. Whitaker for tuberculosis and was injected with tuberculin. Whether Dr. Whitaker based his diagnosis on what was found in the appendix or lungs, he was not prepared to say. After she had been under his (Whitaker's) care for six or eight weeks, and still not getting better, the main symptoms she complained of being persistent tympanites and indigestion, she was referred to Dr. Bonifield's service. He opened her abdomen and removed her appendages for tuberculosis. They contained no pus; but the adhesions between the coils of intestines in the pelvis were very firm, as were the adhesions of the appendages. The removal of the appendages resulted in a complete cure, as far as he could judge without reopening the abdomen. He saw her on the street within a year, the picture of health. The point he desired to make was that in these cases it was good practice to remove as much of the tubercular trouble as possible. If there were large nodules in the omentum, which could be removed, it should be done. If the appendages were markedly tubercular they should be removed, and if there were indications of tuberculosis of the appendix he would remove that organ.

DR. WALTER B. CHASE could not refrain from expressing the belief, from his own observations and what he had learned clinically, that there was good and sufficient reason why we should not drain in the majority of cases of tuberculosis of the peri-

toneum, as the recuperative power of Nature was very pronounced and in excess of that, perhaps, in any other organ.
He thought it was hardly necessary to drain except in cases
of mixed infection.

DR. HALL, in closing the discussion, speaking of the mode of
infection in women, said it was not probably through the
general system, but through the vagina, uterus, and tubes, as
it was in ascending gonorrhea. The more he saw and did of this
work, the more he was convinced that some one would rise up
and demonstrate that positively by original investigation, and
prove that those were the principal sources of infection in
women, and served as an explanation why tubercular disease
existed in women more frequently than in men. He had not
classified his cases, but in a large majority of them it was plain
that the nidus of infection was in the tube or both tubes, so
that he had almost universally, when he opened the abdomen,
removed the tubes. In young women, for the last eight or nine
years, he had universally tried to save an ovary or both and had
r' moved the tubes. He had cut them off into the uterus to get
rid of the nidus there, leaving the ovaries and uterus, so that
the woman could menstruate.

As to drainage, the dry cases should not be drained. The
serum cases recovered more easily without drainage; but take
the class of cases of mixed infection, if they were not drained
they would die, or the surgeon would have to reopen the abdomen on the second or third day. If one drained by the abdomen
the patient was likely to have a hernia; he had drained by the
vagina, the drainage being kept up for a considerable time.

DR. L. H. DUNNING, of Indianapolis, Ind., read a paper on

CARCINOMA OF THE CERVIX UTERI: A SUMMARY REPORT OF THE
AUTHOR'S SIXTY-TWO CASES OPERATED UPON BY
HYSTERECTOMY, WITH REMARKS.[1]

DR. HENRY HOWITT, of Guelph, Ontario, followed with a paper
entitled

SURGICAL TREATMENT OF PERFORATED GASTRIC ULCER, WITH GEN-
ERAL INFECTION OF THE PERITONEAL CAVITY; NOTES
OF A SECOND SUCCESSFUL CASE.[1]

The following officers were elected: *President*, Dr. L. H.
Dunning, Indianapolis, Ind.; *First Vice-President*, Dr. Marcus
Rosenwasser, Cleveland, O.; *Second Vice-President*, Dr. Herman
E. Hayd, Buffalo, N. Y.; *Secretary*, Dr. William Warren Potter,
Buffalo, N. Y., re-elected; *Treasurer*, Dr. X. O. Werder, Pitts-
burg, Pa.

Chicago, Ill., was selected as the place for holding the next
annual meeting; time to be fixed by the Executive Council.

[1] Will appear in a succeeding number of the JOURNAL.

BRIEF OF CURRENT LITERATURE.

DISEASES OF CHILDREN.

Chronic Joint Disease in Children.—Henry Ling Taylor *(Med. News,* Aug. 16, 1902) says that chronic joint disease in children in nine cases out of ten, probably oftener, means tuberculosis. Statistics of over 13,000 cases show, as to the distribution of the disease, that rather more than two-fifths are vertebral, somewhat less than two-fifths are situated in the hip, and about one-fifth in all the other joints; of this remaining fifth the knee claims more than half. One of the most marked characteristics of tuberculous joint disease is its insidiousness. The symptoms vary, but the most characteristic one is stiffness or limitation of motion due to peculiar spasmodic contraction of the muscles. In vertebral disease the location of the pain varies; it is found in the neck, shoulders, and back of the head in cervical disease; at the sides or front of the chest and in the abdomen in dorsal disease; in the loins, lower back, lower abdomen, through the hips or down the thighs, or even in knee, leg, ankle, or foot, in lumbar disease. The medical student clings with as desperate tenacity to the knee pain of hip disease as a pathognomonic symptom as does the school-boy to the date of the discovery of America as the key to all history. It is well to know that disease of the lumbar spine, knee disease, and other affections may cause pain in the knee, and that it is frequently absent in hip disease. The endeavor to elicit pain in the suspected hip by forced movements, pounding on the heel, or otherwise, is perfectly useless and may prove injurious. One should, on the contrary, seek to demonstrate and define the limitation of motion and the involuntary, spasmodic muscular contractions without pain to the patient. The limitation of hyperextension at the hip is the earliest and most delicate test. In knee disease the joint very early becomes flexed and causes limping, which may be intermittent. There seems to be an antagonism between rheumatism and gout and tuberculous joint disease; also between rickets and joint tuberculosis. There are probably few chronic diseases in which correct early treatment is so beneficial, and in which the results of delay are so serious, as the chronic joint diseases of children.

Treatment of Tubercular Joint Affections by Apparatus.— G. G. Davis *(Inter. Med. Mag.,* July, 1902) says that to attempt extension in Pott's disease is practically impossible when the patients ambulate, and it must therefore be applied in the recumbent position, and in those cases in which it is required the patients must be put to bed. Immobilization combined with extension is the most efficient means of treating tubercular joint disease; of these two the first is the best and extension is an added resource. When, therefore, we find a case which either becomes worse or is not improved, we resort to all possible measures which will help us to check the progress of the disease. We must in such cases discard braces and insist on absolute rest in bed, with extension applied to the head. Extension in general is merely a tentative measure, designed simply to relieve partly the excess of weight above the lesion and to procure a certain degree of immobility; for in a flexible column such as the spine the two go hand in hand. When the trouble is situated low down, extension cannot be accomplished by suspension. except to a limited degree. The principles involved in the application of a brace when the lesion is situated low down are of two kinds: (1) direct support by the crutches, and (2) a lever using the kyphosis as a point of support. The power is represented by the parts above and the weight by the pelvis below. When we come to the question of the hip we find, as in the case of the spine, that the necessity for immobility overbalances the importance of extension. By means of adhesive plasters the lower point of fixation can be obtained as long as the plaster strips can be borne by the patient. For the upper joint a perineal band on which the patient sits makes a more secure upper support than is otherwise obtainable. To prevent tilting of the pelvis a pelvic band is needed. If lateral support is desired it can be had by drawing the hip outward against the outer iron bar by a strap encircling them both. To apply extension at the knee the apparatus of Thomas is the most efficient, but it is desirable to so modify the appliance as to fasten the foot to the lower end of the apparatus to prevent a rotary motion of the tibia. The question of rotation in ankle disease is not considered, because a certain amount of immobility is obtained by the means used for fixation, provided crutches. and a high shoe on the other side, be used. In the elbow and wrist extension is seldom considered; it is necessary to rely chiefly on the rest secured by fixation and such other measures as may be indicated by the condition of the patient.

Hip Disease, the Diagnosis of.—Robert W. Lovett *(Boston Med. and Surg. Jour.,* Aug. 14, 1902) gives an analysis of 95 cases, and in conclusion says that it is obvious that the signs ordinarily taken to be diagnostic of tuberculous hip disease are not characteristic of it, but are also present in cases which rapidly recover, and in other forms of chronic joint inflammation than the tuberculous. It is therefore obvious that some diagnostic criterion must be sought more accurate than the presence of one or all of the signs—muscular spasm, atrophy, night-cries, gluteal wasting, and sensitiveness of the joint. It seems probable that this work will lie in the closer study of these signs. and their grouping along with the development of the facts to be learned by careful palpation of the parts about the joint. Of all the signs given, "thickening of the trochanter" proved to be the most reliable. The X-ray is of great value in early diagnosis.

B. Brindley Eads *(Inter. Med. Mag.,* July, 1902) says that a limp in a child is immediately suggestive, and should never be regarded as a trifling affair.   The early limp is due to sensitiveness, and by comparison with the opposite joint it is not difficult to detect restriction of function.   Lay the child upon its back, upon a solid supporting surface, and examine the well side first; place the hand upon the limb and roll it from side to side, note the degree of resistance with muscles relaxed, and then test the side in which the disease is suspected for limitation of motion occasioned by muscular spasm.   Grasp the ankle, flex the leg upon the thigh, the thigh upon the pelvis at right angle, then for purpose of comparison it becomes plainly evident that more force is required to execute the movement than upon the sound side.   This important test is one of the earliest indications, and combines with placing the child upon its face testing the degree of extension, which, if less than ten degrees, is one of the earliest signs of approaching deformity.   Stiffness in the joint probably precedes the limp.   Pain is an early symptom and is usually situated remote from the actual seat of the disease, within the knee, or on the inner side of the knee joint.

The Present Position of the Surgical Treatment of Hip Disease in Children.—G. A. Wright *(Practitioner,* July, 1892) reviews the subject and concludes that no very radical change has taken place in the treatment of hip disease in the last few years.   Rest, extension, and fixation by one or other form of splint, of which the varieties are many, and none better, once the limb is in good position, than Thomas'; intra-articular and peri-articular injections of iodoform—a preventive more trusted on the Continent than in this country; extirpation of "abscesses," or in some cases aspiration and injection of iodoform; excision where the disease is progressive in spite of treatment, and amputation when a useless limb and pelvic disease render recovery hopeless, constitute the main features of present-day treatment. Certain variations in the details of treatment are, as has been already said, employed in different countries or by individual surgeons.   Thus traction and immobilization are throughout the whole period of active disease obtained largely in America by a splint such as the Davis-Taylor long traction apparatus.   The importance of traction in the axis of deformity is insisted upon by some writers; another lays stress upon traction in the axis of the neck of the bone.   Immobilization without extension is largely used in this country, unless there is marked malposition.   As regards operative treatment, excision by anterior incision is preferred by some surgeons; others have used the flap operation; others still employ the old posterior incision.   Probably all are now agreed that excision, if performed, should be done before sinuses and therefore advanced mixed infection exist—late excision is worse than useless.   After removal of the bone some surgeons keep up extension to separate the bony surfaces; others abduct the limb to keep the stump applied to the acetabulum.

Diphtheria.—A. Kuyvett Gordon *(The Med. Chronicle,* May, 1902) says that the chief element in the prognosis of a case of tracheotomy, as in other forms of diphtheria, is the length of time that has elapsed between the onset of the disease and the administration of antitoxin. With regard to the latter, it must be remembered that if a case is seen early, on the first or second day, there is every possibility that the normal dose of the serum—about 4,000 units—may effect a cure; the object of a larger dose than this is to endeavor to compensate for the failure to give the early normal dose. Within certain limits there is reason to think this is possible. We know, however, that the occasional ill effects of antitoxic serum do not depend on the amount used; incidentally they are by far the more frequent in adults, in whom laryngeal diphtheria is a very rare disease. The chief sign that a case of tracheotomy is going wrong is a change in the character of the secretion through the tube: instead of being thin and watery it becomes viscid and scanty, and in some cases almost like glue. There may be no gross obstruction, but ultimately the child dies of suffocation; it is getting air in, but it is unable to use that air. The author has never seen this symptom occur when serum had been given before the third day. Before the days of antitoxin it used to be a common mode of death. The thing to do when the secretion becomes scanty is to raise the foot of the bed, in order that the expulsion of the contents of the trachea may be assisted by the force of gravity; but when the condition is far advanced there is no way to prevent the blocking of the lungs. Since the introduction of antitoxin the mortality of tracheotomy has fallen from about 80 per cent to about half that number. The author wonders whether some of this improvement is due to the fact that the increased attention drawn to the disease by the introduction of that remedy has taught us better technique.

Rötheln (Rubella, or German Measles).—R. W. Marsden *(The Med. Chronicle,* May, 1902) says that the diagnosis of this affection is to be made upon a mild infectious disease with a long incubation period, extending usually to two weeks or more, without sudden onset, the rash being often the first indication of illness. Occasionally the patient may previously complain of stiffness in the neck behind the sterno-mastoid, or general malaise, or have one or more attacks of sneezing. The rash appears as discrete pink spots (usually slightly raised, of variable size, and less punctate than in scarlet fever), most frequently on the face, including the circumoral ring, and spreads over the rest of the body. At its full development the spots often coalesce in certain areas. It does not, as a rule, last longer than four days, and is not seen developed over the body at any stage, but is fading or faded in the area of its origin before full development is attained in the area last to be attacked. At the same time there is slight conjunctivitis, slight sore throat or dryness of the throat, with some congestion (though occasionally no evident change), and very rarely ulceration. The glands in the posterior cervical triangle are also frequently enlarged, shotty, and somewhat tender. The associated pyrexia is very slight and evanescent, and the patients seldom very ill. It is customary to isolate for three weeks those who have been exposed to infection and for a like period those suffering from the disease. The author thinks such a period for isolation certainly errs on the side of liberality, and holds that there is no risk of conveying contagion during the twelve days succeeding exposure, and that not only is the disease most infectious at the beginning, but that the infectiousness seems to disappear very rapidly. Special treatment is usually quite unnecessary. Demulcent drinks for the soreness or the dryness of the throat, and symptomatic treatment of any of the occasional complications, is all that is called for.

Summer Diarrhea of Infants.—W. Cecil Bosanquet *(Practitioner,* Aug., 1892) says that: 1. It is easier in this disease, as in others, to prevent infection than to cure the patient when it has occurred. 2. There is no "average baby," and no one method of treatment avails in all cases. The disease may vary in severity in different countries, so that methods of treatment found successful in England may be ineffectual in Australia or in the United States. 3. Whether the disease be due to an extrinsically formed poison which is taken into the alimentary canal or to toxins formed by bacteria within the body, it is equally evident that the first indication is to assist Nature in expelling the offending material. The diarrhea is, therefore, not in itself harmful or to be rashly interfered with by drugs. It has indeed been said that it would be no worse practice to seal up an abscess cavity and prevent the escape of the pus than to prevent the peristaltic action of the bowels in gastro-enteritis and thus aid the absorption of toxins from the intestine. 4. Since there is little doubt that the poison or infective organism is conveyed by means of milk, it seems advisable in all severe cases temporarily to suspend the use of this food. But as milk is the natural diet of infants—and it may be remembered that in adults suffering from diarrhea a milk diet is usually insisted upon—it is advisable to resume its administration as soon as possible, with due precautions against further infection. 5. After the offending materials have been expelled from the body, attention must be directed to maintaining the alimentary canal, as far as possible, in an aseptic condition, and soothing any remaining irritability of the mucous membrane. 6. The prominent clinical phenomena suggest the necessity of supplying, if possible, the fluid lost to the body; of reducing the temperature when it is excessive, and supplying heat when the extremities are cold and collapse imminent; and of aiding the failing heart by stimulants.

In treating of the *Public Health Aspects of Summer Diarrhea* Arthur Newsholme (ibid.) says that: A. Epidemic diarrhea is chiefly a disease of urban life. B. As a fatal disease it is a disease of the artisan, and still more of the lower laboring classes, to a preponderant extent. C. Towns which have adopted the water-carriage system of sewerage have, as a rule, much less diarrhea than those retaining other methods of removal of excrement. D. Towns with the most perfect scavenging arrangements have the least epidemic diarrhea. E. The influence of soil is a decided one. Where the dwelling houses of a place have as their foundation solid rock, with little or no superincumbent loose material, the diarrheal mortality is, notwithstanding other unfavorable conditions and surroundings, low. On the other hand, a loose soil is a soil on which diarrheal mortality is apt to be high. Steep gradients are mostly associated with low diarrheal mortality. F. Towns with a high temperature and a deficient rainfall, especially in the third quarter of the year, suffer severely from diarrhea. In conclusion, the fundamental condition favoring epidemic diarrhea is *an unclean soil, the particular poison from which infects the air, and is swallowed, most commonly with food, especially milk.*

M. H. Gordon (ibid.), studying into the *Bacteriology of Epidemic Diarrhea,* concludes that while great progress has been made of recent years, much remains to be settled. From an examination of the literature of the subject one fact comes out very clearly. It is that a more precise knowledge of the relative abundance and the attributes of bacteria occurring in the *normal* intestine would be of great value in enabling us to attach their due relative significance to many of the observations that have been made in cases of diarrhea. Again, the relative abundance of the pathogenic organisms that have been found .to occur in the dejeeta in diarrhea is a subject about which too little is known. Yet such knowledge might prove of the greatest use. For instance, did we know exactly the nature of the micro-organisms that occur in one-ten-millionth gramme of normal feces, and their attributes, we should then, on analyzing a similar quantity of fecal material from the intestine in a diseased state, be in a position to see at once what alteration had occurred. By means of the dilution method it is a comparatively simple matter to make accurate observations of this kind, and their value promises to be great, especially if a large number of cases are examined. More exact methods are bound to bring more exact information. A further subject about which accurate information would be welcome is with regard to the exact relationship of various pathogenic members of the great coli-typhoid family. Hitherto most attention has been paid to bacillus coli communis and to bacillus typhosus, but as our knowledge increases the pathogenic importance of other members of this large family of bacteria becomes more plain. Enteritis as a whole seems to be often intimately associated with various members of it, and further knowledge **of** their relations and characters may result in more accurate perceptions both of their effects and of the ways to counteract them.

Margaret Taylor Shutt *(Jour. A. M. A.,* Aug. 2, 1902) says that in every case, but especially where there are other children, and in institutions, the care-taker must be impressed with the fact that the disease is an infectious one, and that the discharges must be disinfected, the napkins boiled before using again, and hands that have come in contact with the discharges thoroughly cleansed. The after-treatment of these cases is of great importance. The chief necessity is an outline of diet. and in difficult cases the ingenuity of the physician may be taxed to the utmost. In some instances it seems almost impossible for the child to return to a milk diet until the onset of cool weather. In some of these cases the proprietary foods are of value temporarily. In other cases a modified milk. partly or completely peptonized, may succeed when the undigested milk mixture cannot be used at all. In most cases the child can in a few days return to a milk diet, but it must be made very weak at first and be given in small quantities, gradually working up to the usual strength and amount.

C. H. Johnston *(Memphis Med. Month.,* Aug., 1902) says that if vomiting is present neither castor oil nor calomel should be given until the vomiting has been controlled by stomach-washing, which consists in the introduction of water into the stomach through a flexible catheter or stomach tube and then siphoning it out. The apparatus for stomach-washing is very simple. There are required a soft-rubber catheter, size 16—one with a large eye is preferred—a glass funnel holding four to six ounces. two feet of rubber tubing, and a few inches of glass tubing to join this to the catheter. The child should be held in a sitting posture, the body protected by a rubber sheet with a pan conveniently near. The catheter should be moistened. While the tongue is depressed with the forefinger of the left hand, the catheter is passed rapidly back into the pharynx and down the esophagus into the stomach. The first part of the introduction should be as rapid as possible, for if the child begins to gag from the pharyngeal irritation the introduction of the tube may be quite difficult; no resistance is ordinarily encountered after the tube reaches the esophagus. About ten inches of the catheter should be passed beyond the child's lips. When it has reached the stomach the funnel should be raised as high as possible to allow the escape of gas almost invariably present, and from two to four ounces of water poured into the funnel from a pitcher. The funnel is then lowered and the water is siphoned out; this is to be repeated several times until the fluid comes back perfectly clean. Various solutions have been advised for stomach-washing, but the author uses only boiled water at a temperature of 100° to 110° F., the higher temperature being used when the gastric irritation is very great.

M. A. Auerbach *(Buff. Med. Jour.,* Aug., 1892) considers three forms: acute dyspeptic diarrhea, cholera infantum, and acute enterocolitis. The first is chiefly due to errors in diet, sometimes to dentition and the extreme heat of summer. A prescription which has given the author splendid results, in conjunction with a carefully restricted diet, is the following:

℞ Bismuthi subnitratis.................... .... ℨ i.
 Tincturæ opii deodoratæ.......... .... ℩x.
 Glyco-thymolin................................. .... ℨ ij.
 Aquæ rosam...................... ....ad q s. ℥ iv.
 M. et Sig.: One drachm every three hours (for child 1 year of age).

For cholera infantum the fever should be combated by a bath containing some glyco-thymolin, at about 80° F., reduced by adding small pieces of ice to 70° or 65°. Pain should be controlled by one-hundredth grain of morphine sulphate, then stimulation with strychnia hypodermatically, iced champagne to prevent vomiting, and other stimulants. The large intestine may be irrigated with a pint or so of warm water containing 25 per cent of glyco-thymolin. Acute enterocolitis is an affection of an inflammatory nature, chiefly of the ileum and colon, affecting especially the lymph follicles. Anodynes are imperatively demanded for the great suffering, and depletion may be needed in the beginning by salines, but the child's strength must be watched. The colon should be flushed with a 25 per cent solution of glyco-thymolin, and may be made with iced water. The gums should be scarified, if necessary.

I. H. Mason Knox *(Johns Hopkins Hosp. Bull.,* July, 1902) writing of the leucocyte count in the summer diarrheas of children, thus summarizes his conclusions: 1. A differential count of leucocytes in the blood of well children under 2 years of age, when compared with the blood of adults, shows that there is a relative increase in the small mononuclear elements and a decrease in the number of polymorphonuclear cells. 2. In the summer diarrheas of infants the number of leucocytes in the blood is usually increased, but the count of the white cells varies within such wide limits, even in the milder forms of the affection, that a high or low leucocytosis cannot be regarded as of diagnostic value. 3. In the simple dyspepsias of childhood a differential count of the leucocytes does not show any marked variation from that of a healthy infant, but as the cases become more severe in type there is apparently a progressive increase in the polymorphonuclear neutrophile cells, and a decrease in those of the small mononuclear variety, thus presenting a picture more like that of adult blood. 4. As pointed out by Japha, the polymorphonuclear leucocytosis is an indication of an intoxication with decomposition products in the intestine or of the toxins of pathological bacteria—*i.e.,* it takes place both in the cases of acute intestinal poisoning and in the more severe forms of ileocolitis. 5. The cases of simple infantile atrophy present a nearly normal differential leucocyte count, but it would seem that an increase of the polymorphonuclear cells may indicate the setting-in of an inflammatory intestinal complication.

James H. McKee *(Phil. Med. Jour.,* July 26, 1902) says that when a laxative must be given several times during the course of the disease, unscientific as it appears in theory, calomel or gray powder may be combined efficiently with an astringent:

    ℞ Hydrargyri cum Creta . ... gr. ⅛.
       Salol. ....gr. i.
       Bismuthi subnitratis................................. gr. v.
       Sacchari lactis........ ....gr. v.
    One dose.

Or when there is much tenesmus, castor oil may be combined in a somewhat similar way:

    ℞ Olei caryophylli.................... ... . ℳij.
       Olei menthæ piperitæ.......... ....,........ ....ℳij
       Olei ricini. .... ℳx.
       Bismuthi subnitratis.................................. gr. v.
       Mucilaginis acaciæ,
       Aquæ..q. s. ad fl. ℥ i.
    One dose.

The author always uses salol to decrease putrefactive changes. To an infant aged 1 year the dose is one grain, given every two or three hours, and preferably before feedings. Such dosage has never in his experience led to symptoms of salol poisoning. *Enteroclysis,* while it has been overdone, is valuable: 1. When irritating material still remains within the bowel, and is giving rise to mechanical or bacterial disturbance. 2. When, in acute cases, fever and foul-smelling discharges persist for several days. 3. In cholera infantum, when it should be supplemented by lavage. Early in the attack, when the temperature is high, iced saline solution is valuable; but when prostration has supervened and the temperature is low, hot solutions (110°) are preferable. 4. In acute cases, only the sodium chloride solution is needed. 5. Except in cholera infantum, enteroclysis should rarely be used more than twice daily, and seldom more than once. 6. In chronic ileocolitis tannic acid or silver nitrate injections, given once daily, may prove more valuable than any drugs given by the mouth. *Hypodermoclysis* is a most effectual measure in the treatment of cholera infantum or the condition seen in ileocolitis which has been styled hydrocephaloid. The sterile salt solution should be higher in temperature than the body temperature, and only two to four ounces should be introduced.

Thompson S. Westcott (ibid.) states that an often unrecognized cause of deterioration of milk in the household may be traced to a rather common habit of heating the night bottle quite hot just before the parents retire, and keeping it warm in a cozy or in the bed itself until such time as the baby wakes for its feeding. No more favorable conditions for producing rapid souring of milk could be desired, and the writer has proved by experiment the startling rapidity with which bacteria may increase in a milk mixture thus kept. Another precaution that may be helpful in very hot weather is to give no milk that has been kept over night from the supply of the day before. If a fresh supply cannot be obtained before the first morning bottle is due, a bottle of albumen water or of condensed milk mixture may be given. Again, it will often be advantageous to weaken the strength of a baby's food mixture slightly during the hot weather. In many instances the danger of serious milk poisoning may be avoided if, at the slightest sign of disturbance of the stomach or bowels, the mother has been previously instructed to stop milk-feeding at once and give a good dose of castor oil, followed, when there is greenness or curdiness of stools, by small doses of calomel, say one-twentieth of a grain, three or four times a day for two or three days.

W. L. Harris (ibid.) says that the only thing in the line of drugs that he has found useful is bismuth in some form—either the subnitrate or subgallate. He uses the former in doses of ten to twenty grains every two or three hours, and the latter in doses from three to ten grains every two or three hours, in emulsion always. If there is much tenesmus he gives paregoric, but only when it is strongly indicated, and alone—not in diarrhea mixtures to be given after each action. The importance of fresh air cannot be overestimated, but neither mountain nor sea air will cure a case so long as the patient is improperly fed or treated by drugs.

Maurice Ostheimer (ibid.) holds that the first and most important treatment of summer diarrhea is absolute withdrawal of food, no matter what the infant is taking. All milk and other foods are to be stopped and a diet of barley water ordered, to be given every three hours for children over 3 months. In the case of older or of large, healthy children, stop all food except milk, which, if the child particularly wants it, may be given every three or four hours with lime water, if vomiting does not persist. Should it persist, a return to absolute barley-water diet will be necessary. This method has proved successful, a normal condition reappearing after a few doses of calomel. In young infants, or those who are severely prostrated, panopeptone or liquid peptonoids, in doses of fifteen to thirty drops added to the barley water, acts as an excellent stimulant. From forty-eight hours to four days after its withdrawal milk with lime water can usually be given again. Fresh air is a necessity, and in severe cases is often life-saving.

Spontaneous Reduction of Acute Intussusception.—W. Gifford Nash (July 25, 1902) reports the case of a child of 11 months which was seized with abdominal pain that caused screaming and great collapse. Vomiting occurred. On examining the abdomen a swelling could be seen passing from the region of the cecum obliquely upward toward the epigastrium. On palpation a firm, sausage-shaped tumor three or four inches in length could be felt. The author concluded that intussusception was present and made preparations for immediate operation. Hot bottles were applied to the extremities and hot flannels to the abdomen. Three hours later the child was looking much better, having had a sleep. The hump could still be seen and felt, but was evidently smaller, and during manipulation suddenly entirely disappeared. There was a history of looseness of the bowels on the previous evening. The author is positive as to his diagnosis and thinks that the reasons why the intussusception was reduced were: (1) the manipulations necessary to form a diagnosis acting on a very recent intussusception; (2) the occurrence of fainting and vomiting leading to relaxation of muscular spasm; (3) the application of heat to the abdomen acting in the same way.

Recurrent Vomiting.—Charles W. Larned (*Amer. Med.*, Aug. 16, 1902) describes two cases in children, and gives a history of the affection gathered from the literature. As to the clinical manifestations, vomiting, as a rule, ushers in the attack. It is at first forcible, but toward the end of the attack, when exhaustion becomes marked, is unaccompanied by much effort. The vomitus at first consists of the stomach contents, and later of a little water mixed with mucus; as the retching becomes intense it is not uncommon for both blood and bile to be ejected. Constipation is most obstinate, there is an absence of abdominal pain, the pulse becomes rapid as prostration increases, the respiration is rapid and sighing. Convulsions occurred in a case reported by Snow; itching of the skin was present in two of Griffith's cases. The duration of attacks is variable, even in the same individual. In neither of the author's cases did the attacks last over eighty-six hours, and usually by the end of forty-eight hours the patient had entered upon convalescence. His observations have led him to the conclusion that the condition is certainly due to some toxic substance, its nature and origin as yet remaining to be satisfactorily demonstrated. It may be an autointoxication, with the intestinal canal as the offending focus, or it may be due to some failure on the part of the excretory organs to eliminate certain poisonous substances which accumulate in the organism and produce toxemia. The stomach is probably not primarily at fault. The prognosis has always been considered good, but Marcy has published two fatal cases. As to treatment, nothing has as yet been found that will cut the attack short, but certain measures seem to alleviate the suffering of the patient. The first indication is to stop all food and drugs by the mouth. Morphine and normal salt solution through the skin, predigested food, salt solution, and opium by the rectum, are useful. Flushing out the lower bowel once daily with a copious high injection of normal salt solution seems of some benefit. With the subsidence of the vomiting a calomel purge is indicated. Between attacks the child should lead an out-of-door life, should not be subjected to over-fatigue or excitement, should have its bowels carefully regulated, and, most important of all, should be made to drink a good deal of water.

THE AMERICAN
JOURNAL OF OBSTETRICS

AND

DISEASES OF WOMEN AND CHILDREN.

| Vol. XLVI. | DECEMBER, 1902. | No. 6. |

ORIGINAL COMMUNICATIONS.

PERFORATING ULCERS OF THE DUODENUM.[1]

BY

JOHN B. MURPHY, A.M., M.D.,

AND

J. M. NEFF, M.D.,

Chicago, Ill.

THE subject of duodenal ulcerations is always an interesting one, both on account of the extreme rarity of the disease and the many difficulties which attend an accurate diagnosis. Although a number of articles have appeared within the past few years, the literature is still meagre. Dr. Robert F. Weir, in his address before the American Surgical Association in 1900, gave us the masterpiece on the subject of duodenal perforations. He brought the literature up to date (April, 1900), and recorded all cases operated on for acute perforation previous to that time.

The purpose of this article is to review briefly the salient points in the etiology, pathology, and diagnosis of duodenal ulcers, and to consider especially the surgical treatment of perforations. We have collected from the literature nineteen ad-

[1] Read at the meeting of the American Association of Obstetricians and Gynecologists, Washington, D. C., September 16, 17, and 18, 1902.

47

ditional cases, including one of our own, in which operations were performed for this complication.

FREQUENCY.—The relative frequency of duodenal ulcer as a cause of death is given by Weir[1] from collected statistics as two-tenths per cent. Kinnicutt,[2] from an analysis of 30,000 postmortem records, gives it as four-tenths per cent; Perry and Shaw's figures are practically the same. Krug gives the proportion as forty-four-hundredths. Von Wyl found three duodenal ulcers in 12,806 postmortem examinations. The ratio of gastric to duodenal ulcers, given by Burwinkel (Weir), is 12 to 1.

AGE.—Duodenal ulcerations occur at all ages. Collin's statistics for the different decades is as follows, in descending order of frequency: (1) 30 to 40 years; (2) 40 to 50 years; (3) 20 to 30 years; (4) under 10 years; (5) 50 to 60 years; (6) 60 to 80 years; (7) 10 to 20 years. Hahn[6] records a case in a child 1½ days old, in which there was a duodenal ulcer close to the pylorus and a second one lower down. These must have been formed before any food reached the stomach. Vanderpoel Adriance[3] reports, in an infant of 10 months, an ulcer on the posterior wall of the duodenum just below the pylorus, and Oppenheimer has collected 15 cases of melena neonatorum resulting from duodenal ulcer. Chvostek (Moynihan)[4] found the ulcers in children from a few hours to a few weeks old. Von Wyl (Laspèyres)[5] states that of all cases under 10 years of age, fully half are in the first year and many in the first few days after birth. He states that the latter are not due to intrauterine causes, as some have supposed, but rather, in all probability, to thrombosis of the umbilical vein with embolism of the vessels of the small intestine.

Thrombosis of the mesenteric veins from this source is possible, as a branch of the umbilical vein communicates with the portal; the thrombus may extend into and occlude the latter, thus producing necrosis of the intestinal wall by venous stasis. We cannot, however, understand how an embolus from this thrombus, passing through the general circulation, could be arrested in the duodenal arteries. While the embolus might be arrested in these vessels in fetal life, as there is no pulmonary circulation, it would be impossible for this to occur postnatal, as then the ductus arteriosus is obliterated and the embolus would be arrested in the lung. If portal thrombosis were an important factor in the production of the ulcerations, it would seem that they should be more frequent in pylephlebitis. This, however, is not the case, as they are not mentioned by Bryant (Guy's Hospital Reports, 1897) in any of the 20 cases of pylephlebitis analyzed by him. In one case it was thought that a duodenal ulcer was the cause of the thrombosis, but in none were ulcerations found as a sequence.

As regards the other extreme of life, Krammhals observed a case in a woman 79 years old, and Merkel found an ulcer in the duodenum of an old woman of 94 years (Moynihan).

SEX.—The great majority of duodenal ulcers are found in males. Laspèyres says that men are affected two or three times oftener than women, and quotes from the various authorities the following ratios: Krauss, in 64 cases, found the ratio in men to women as ten to one; Lebert, in 39 cases, four to one; Trier, in 54 cases, five to one; Chvostek, in 61 cases, three to one; Oppenheimer, in 71 cases, two and a half to one; Collin, in 257 cases, four to one.

Of Weir's cases, 176 in number, 144 were in men and 30 in women. Dr. Lee Dickinson (Clarke and Franklin)[1] maintains that the women in whom duodenal ulcers occur are not young, but in two cases reported by them they were under 20 years of age.

COINCIDENT LESIONS.—1. *Burns:* That duodenal ulcerations are frequently associated with extensive burns is well known. In Collin's 297 cases burns were the cause of the ulcers in 38 instances. Holmes says that the ulcers appear in from seven to fourteen days after the burns; they may be much earlier (Weir). Probably the correct explanation in these cases is that a septic infarct has been produced by the lodgment of an embolus which entered the circulation at the site of the burn. The theory of toxic products in the bile (Hunter) is not so plausible as the embolic. Neither of these theories has a good pathologic basis. Paget believed that nervous influences played an important rôle in the production of the ulcers after burns.

2. *Kidney Disease,* especially the various forms of chronic nephritis, is very frequently associated with ulcerations in the duodenum. The reasons for this are not clear, and so far no satisfactory explanation has been offered to account for the association, although a number of theories have been advanced.

Boas claims that the necrotizing effect of urea or its derivative, ammonium carbonate, circulating in the blood, is the active agent, but it is more likely that the presence of sclerosed vessels in the duodenal wall, with the consequent malnutrition of certain areas, is the real cause (Kinnicutt).

Poynton[8] observed one case which presented no symptoms during life, but in which, after death, there were found duodenal ulcers associated with cirrhotic kidneys.

3. *Pulmonary Tuberculosis:* In some of the cases associated with advanced pulmonary tuberculosis, the duodenal lesion was probably originally a cheesy degeneration of a solitary follicle, with secondary digestion of the caseous material by the gastric juice. Satterthwaite[9] reports a case of tubercular enteritis in which there were ulcers in the duodenum. He believes that tuberculosis is an important factor in the etiology. A family history of tuberculosis is sometimes obtainable, as in four out of five cases reported by Burwinkel.[10]

4. *Trichinosis* and duodenal ulcer have been reported by Ebstein and Klob. Duodenal ulcer is also occasionally found as a complication in heart and liver diseases, carcinoma, extensive internal suppurations, frostbites, erysipelas, septicemia, and pemphigus. Bolton Carter[11] thinks that in some of his cases the ulcerations in the stomach and duodenum might have followed the septic condition of the peritoneum. The hemorrhage from the stomach and duodenum which sometimes follows operations, not necessarily on the abdomen, may be from fresh ulcerations (Clarke and Franklin). Eiselsberg recorded seven cases of hematemesis following laparatomies in which fresh ulcers were found in the stomach and duodenum. Ladevèze[12] thinks that there is often a relationship between previously existing infectious diseases and duodenal ulcers. Duodenal and gastric ulcers are frequently found together, so frequently, in fact, that many writers suppose their etiology is identical. Röschmann reported three cases of duodenal ulcers associated with ulcers of the esophagus.

THEORIES OF CAUSATION.—These are almost as numerous and varied as the number of observers who have studied the condition. The most rational, and at the same time the most widely accepted, theory is that duodenal ulcerations are due to the same cause as gastric—namely, the effect of the gastric juice on a circumscribed portion of the mucosa, the vitality of which has been impaired. This view is held by Virchow and has been proven experimentally (Laspèyres).

According to Riegel, hyperchlorhydria is an essential factor, and he believes that many of the corrosive ulcerations follow primary hemorrhagic erosions. Lenbe says that hyperchlorhydria is frequently present in duodenal ulcers, and Koch and

Ewald have produced the ulcers by giving to animals hydrochloric acid in 5:1000 solutions. The duodenum is not protected from the acidity of the gastric juice above the papilla, through which empty the alkaline secretions of the pancreas and liver, and it is in this first portion that the great majority of the ulcers occur.

Talma believes that they are due to spasmodic contractions of the pylorus, which produce an anemia of the adjacent parts, closure of the blood vessels, and hemorrhage. He thinks this view is strengthened by the fact that the majority of the ulcerations are near the pylorus. We cannot understand how such a condition could possibly be caused by spasms of the pylorus, as contraction of this portion is part of its normal function and could not interfere with the blood supply to such an extent as to bring about hemorrhage and necrosis, especially as the blood supply for the duodenum does not come through the pylorus.

Box[13] favors the infectious theory because the ulcers many times appear opposite to each other, or in close proximity, and present a surrounding zone of inflamed and softened tissue. He also calls attention to the fact that most of the intestinal ulcerations below the duodenum are conceded to be of infectious origin.

Zimnitski[14] determined, by a series of experiments on animals, that there was an etiological relation between retention of bile and ulcers of the duodenum. He thinks that the same conditions which are essential to the development of the ulcers are present in biliary retention from any cause. These are hypersecretion, local circulatory disturbances, stasis—dependent upon changes in the liver—and anemia or hydremia with decrease in the alkalinity of the blood.

Boas believes that rough food, alcohol, and tobacco are factors in the etiology. Laspèyres says that the lesion is frequently found in habitual drunkards. Alvazzi, in three cases of chronic lead poisoning, found round ulcers of the duodenum. Foreign bodies which have been swallowed, as in certain cases of dementia, may produce ulcers by pressure (Pittiet and Deny)

From an analysis of the clinical histories reported, and consideration of the various theories on the genesis of duodenal ulcers, it appears to us that the causes may be grouped in the order of their importance, as follows: (1) hyperchlorhydria, (2) local infection, (3) embolism or thrombosis. (4) foreign bodies. We are, however, forcefully impressed with the close relationship between duodenal ulcerations and diseases of the organs of elimination, as the skin in burns, pemphigus, and erysipelas; the kidney in various diseases compromising elimination; and the lung in tuberculosis. We believe the defective elimination has an important etiological relation.

PATHOLOGY.—Moynihan divides duodenal ulcers into acute and chronic—acute when there is rapid destruction tending to perforation; chronic when the symptoms are latent and the pathologic processes passive. He says that the acute ulcer may be but an early stage of the chronic.

The ulcerations are usually single, though they may be multiple, in which case they are often grouped in the first portion of the duodenum. Occasionally two ulcers are opposed to each other, suggesting an infectious cause. An acute perforating ulcer may be found with a chronic one.

In Collin's 253 cases, 195 (83.6 per cent) were solitary. In 26 cases there were two ulcers; in 3, three ulcers; and in 4, five ulcers.

SITUATION.—Perry and Shaw, in 149 cases, found the first portion of the duodenum involved 123 times, the second portion 16 times, the third and fourth portions twice.

In 8 cases the ulcers were scattered (Laspèyres).

Weir gives the analysis of Collin's statistics for perforating ulcers as follows: In 119 cases the lesion was in the first portion. Of these, 68 were in the anterior wall, 39 in the posterior, 10 in the superior, and 1 in the inferior. Of 8 cases involving the second portion, 5 were on the internal wall, 2 on the posterior, and 1 on the external. Of 4 cases affecting the third portion, 3 were on the anterior and superior walls and 1 on the posterior.

Of the perforating ulcers collected by Perry and Shaw, 48 were in the first division, 2 in the second, and 1 on the border line between the first and second. In 28 cases the location on the wall was not mentioned; in 19 the anterior wall was affected; in 6, the posterior; and in 3, both.

Wanach says the ulcers most frequently perforate the anterior wall of the horizontal upper portion. In Oppenheimer's cases the perforation was 34 times in the transverse portion and 3 times in the descending. In 19 of the 34 cases the wall was not mentioned. In the other 15 the anterior wall was involved 11 times, the posterior 3 times, and the superior once. Nothnagel says: "There is little or no difference in the frequency of **per-foration** of the anterior and posterior walls."

DESCRIPTION OF THE ULCERS.—They may be circular or ellip-tical in shape, and, if the latter, are frequently situated trans-verse to the long axis of the bowel. They are often cone-shaped, with the apex of the cone toward the peritoneum (Marocco). The margins and base are commonly very tough and dense and exhibit but feeble attempts at repair. If large, the borders may become irregular, but usually they possess a sharply-cut, punched-out appearance. In old cases the edges are apt to be much thickened. The floor of the ulcer is usually clean and may be formed by any of the coats of the bowel or by adherent organs. Dr. Poynton, in necropsies on 8 cases of chronic duodenal ulcers, found that in all of them new floors had been formed by ad-hesions to neighboring structures.

In size they vary from one to three and a half centimetres in diameter—or from the size of a lentil to that of a dollar. If perforation takes place, the opening is usually much smaller than the ulcer itself, being rarely larger than a quarter of an inch in diameter and having comparatively thin edges.

PERFORATION.—Laspèyres gives the following statistics as to the frequency of perforation: Chvostek, in 63 cases, noted it 27 times—42 per cent; Collin, in 262 cases, 181 times—69 per cent; Oppenheimer, in 79 cases, 38 times—48 per cent.

Perforation may take place into the general peritoneal cavity or into the retroperitoneal tissue. Of Bolton's 5 cases, 3 per-forated into the general peritoneal cavity, 1 behind the peri-toneum, and 1 toward the under surface of the liver, to which it was adherent. Aside from the usual sites of perforation, ad-hesions may form between the duodenum and the surrounding viscera, and perforation take place into any of them. Weir records cases where the gall bladder, aorta, vena cava, portal vein, superior mesenteric vein, and hepatic artery have been perforated. A gastro-duodenal fistula has never been found the result of the perforation of a duodenal ulcer.

If perforation takes place into the free peritoneal cavity before adhesions have formed, a general septic peritonitis is the result. In these cases, where the perforation is in the first or upper half of the second portion, the fluid is usually discharged on to the upper surface of the mesocolon and follows the ascending meso-colon to the right iliac fossa, before the diffusion becomes general. It is for this reason that a perforative appendicitis is so often simulated. If perforation takes place slowly, giving time for adhesions to form, a localized abscess may result, the situation of which will depend upon the position of the perforation. If this be in the superior wall of the upper portion, the abscess is frequently subphrenic and always to the right of the falciform ligament. Nowak collected 58 cases of subphrenic abscess, 6 of which were due to perforating ulcers of the duodenum. Seven similar cases were reported in Maydl's monograph. In some instances the abscess forms beneath the liver and does not invade the subphrenic space. After the formation of the abscess it may burst in any direction—back into the duodenum or the other hollow viscera in the neighborhood, upward into the pleural or pericardial cavities, or even externally, as in a case recorded by Lumeau and Buoquoy. Planchard reports one case in which the rupture of a localized abscess led to a general peritonitis.

That duodenal ulcers heal spontaneously is proven by the findings post mortem. Perry and Shaw found evidences of repair in 50 per cent of their cases (70 autopsies), in some of which the cicatrices had produced narrowing of the bowel. Krug, in 1,220 autopsies, saw 30 cases of cicatricial healing. Laspèyres says that very few completely cicatrized ulcers have been observed, and that stenosis, with obstruction to the common bile duct, often results after healing. Dilatation of the duodenum on the proximal side of the contraction has been observed, and in some cases has been so great as to necessitate gastroenterostomy.

The tendency to development of carcinoma in the scars is not nearly so great as in gastric ulcer.

From the absence of manifestations of tissue reaction in the margins of many perforating ulcers, it would seem probable that the pathologic process was an extremely rapid one, such as might be expected from the action of the digestive secretions. In the case observed by us there was not the slightest inflammatory reaction in the margin of the opening, no evidence of tissue proliferation, and no effort at adhesions. The margin was perfectly smooth and there was no vascular injection at the periphery.

SYMPTOMS.—The symptomatology of duodenal ulceration is notoriously uncertain and inconstant. In some cases (more than half in which the lesions are found in necropsy) there had been no symptoms indicating the disease. In many the symptoms are indefinite, and often so mild that the patient does not think it necessary to consult a physician; while, again, in others they are well marked and severe. The symptoms are much like those observed in gastric ulcer, and Moynihan believes the two are often associated.

The three cardinal symptoms, in the order of their importance, are: (1) pain, (2) melena or hematemesis, (3) vomiting. They may be single or combined and any one predominate.

Pain: In general, the pain may be said to resemble that of gastric ulcer, but is usually much less severe, because the duodenum is more fixed and the stomach contents are less irritating. In some cases it is merely a sense of discomfort, while in others it is severe and intolerable. Its character is burning, or "boring," and it may radiate downward and to the sides. Boas says that it rarely goes through to the back, and Riegel and Burwinkel state that it never radiates in this direction. Marocco, on the other hand, says the pain is usually situated in the right upper quadrant of the abdomen and radiates to the shoulder and tenth and twelfth dorsal vertebræ. Schwartz has also noted the right shoulder pain. The situation of the pain is in the right hypochondriac region, about two centimetres below the gall bladder in the right parasternal line, though it may be in the epigastric or umbilical region. It comes on from one-half to six hours after a meal, but is characteristic when it makes its appearance from two to four hours after the ingestion of food. Moynihan says that the nearer the ulcer is to the cardia the earlier is the onset of pain after eating. In some cases the pain has been sudden in its onset and colicky in character. Rarely it has been observed in the left hypochondriac region, as in the case recorded by Lissjansky,[15] where it came on in this region in severe paroxysms, the right side not being even very sensitive to pressure. In a case reported by Poynton the severity and long duration of the pain were important features, and it resembled that due to erosion of the vertebræ, or abdominal aneurism. He also cites an instance in which the pain was excessive at night. Pressure to the right of the twelfth thoracic vertebra occasionally elicits pain, but tenderness, if it be present at all, is usually found on deep pressure over the duodenum.

Hemorrhage may manifest itself either through the stomach or bowels, and is caused by the erosion of a blood vessel. In some cases it is the first symptom to attract the patient's attention. Weir states that it is present in one-third of the cases of non-perforating ulcer, and the blood may be dark and "tarry" or, more rarely, bright red in color. The hemorrhage may come from any of the blood vessels in the neighborhood, but most often from the pancreatico-duodenalis, the gastro-epiploica dextra, and the pancreatic arteries.

Ladevèze divides the cases of hemorrhage into three classes: (1) the fulminating form, which speedily ends in death; (2) the acute form, in which hemorrhages of less intensity are frequently repeated and finally exhaust the patient; (3) the chronic form, in which they are continuous and persistent, but often unperceived.

In Perry and Shaw's 60 cases which presented symptoms, hematemesis was noted fourteen times and melena nine times. In Oppenheimer's 34 cases of hemorrhage, 8 were from the stomach, 10 from the bowels, and 16 from both. The patient may become extremely anemic and even bleed to death before the blood is passed or vomited. Repeated small hemorrhages may cause death from cachexia, but this may be due, in some measure at least, to the vomiting which is often present.

Vomiting is relatively rare in duodenal ulceration. It occurs in about 17 per cent of the cases (Oppenheimer), and is not usually characteristic, unless it comes on from two to four hours after a meal. It often takes place at the height of the painful paroxysm, and is not always dependent upon taking food. The vomitus may contain bile and partly-digested food, with or without an admixture of blood. The vomiting may relieve the pain.

Very little has been done in the examination of the stomach contents. Leube and Reckmann each had a case of subacidity, and Devic and Roux described one of hyperchlorhydria (Laspèyres).

Icterus is rare. Collin mentioned it but nine times in 262 cases. When present it may be due to tumefaction of the mucous membrane of the common bile duct in the cases of active ulceration, or to cicatricial contraction in those of long standing.

Other symptoms, which have been described by various observers, are: (a) Digestive disorders, usually resembling hyperchlorhydria, or less frequently chronic gastric catarrh. (b) Paroxysmal dyspnea, the origin of which, although not certain, is probably reflex. (c) Neuralgias, also reflex, affecting various portions of the abdomen and chest. (d) Palpitation of the heart.

It is rarely possible to palpate a tumor mass in case of a duodenal ulcer. When present it is due to a localized peritonitis or secondary enlargement of the head of the pancreas.

The course of the great majority of cases is essentially chronic and seldom tends toward spontaneous recovery. It is often marked by exacerbations of the symptoms, followed by intervals of good health. Chvostek has recorded a case in which the symptoms had been present off and on for thirty-nine years. This chronic course, however, is not taken by all of the cases, for in some the first symptom may be a profuse or even fatal hemorrhage, or the sudden development of a general peritonitis due to the perforation of an ulcer.

PERFORATION.—As mentioned above, many of the cases of perforating ulcer present no symptoms whatever prior to the onset of those due to the perforation. Weir states that in 20 out of 25 instances of perforation analyzed by Schwartz the patients were in good health previously, and in only 5 cases had there been gastric symptoms. In his own collection of 51 cases treated by operation, gastric symptoms formerly existed in 25 out of 34. Of Perry and Shaw's 151 cases, 91 presented no symptoms until perforation or hemorrhage appeared. The symptoms due to perforation are usually sudden and violent in their onset, often coming on when the patient is at work, frequently after the ingestion of a full meal. The reason for this is probably an increased tension within the duodenum, caused by the contraction of the abdominal muscles, which press upon the stomach and force its contents out through the pylorus.

The first symptom of perforation is pain, which is very severe and usually referred to the epigastrium or right hypochondrium, although in rare cases it may be in the centre of the abdomen or to the left. The pain may be so intense as to prostrate the patient and produce rapid collapse resembling that of fat necrosis. Stevens (Weir) records a case in which death occurred twenty-one hours after the onset of symptoms of perforation. Moynihan did not observe that there was any tendency toward primary localization of pain in the right hypochondrium, although in many cases, after a few hours, the symptoms all point toward a lesion in the right iliac fossa. This is explained by the fact that the fluid gravitates into that region along the ascending mesocolon. In the cases collected by Schwartz the pain after perforation was seven times in the right side below the false ribs, five times in the epigastrium, four times in the left side, and twelve times in the region of the right costal border. The pain soon became general (Laspèyres).

Following the pain the other symptoms of general peritonitis rapidly make their appearance. These are: vomiting, elevation of temperature, abdominal tenderness (which at first may be localized to the right hypochondriac and right iliac regions, but soon becomes general), tympanites, coprostasis, and often shock.

On percussion of the abdomen, if several hours have elapsed since perforation took place, there is usually flatness in right flank, with tympany above. Liver dulness may be obliterated. The line of dulness, laterally, may shift with the change of position of the patient, because of the gravitation of the fluid which has escaped from the duodenum.

The peritonitis, instead of becoming general, may localize, if previous adhesions have formed, as a subphrenic or subhepatic abscess, which may secondarily rupture into any of the neighboring viscera or occasionally into the free peritoneal cavity. If the opening is retroperitoneal or in the superior wall of the upper portion, a subphrenic abscess containing pus and gas is likely to be formed, the symptoms and physical signs of which are much the same as in a similar condition from any other cause. It is important to remember, however, that in the cases resulting from duodenal perforation the abscess is always to the right of the falciform ligament, and not to the left of it as after gastric perforations.

In the cases of perforation there is, primarily, an acute leucocytosis. In our case, eight hours after perforation there were 23,400 leucocytes per cubic millimetre, showing a pronounced reaction of the peritoneum to the irritation and toxicity of the escaped fluid. The leucocytosis is quite in contrast to that of fat necrosis of the pancreas and omentum, the other symptoms of which so closely resemble duodenal perforation.

DIAGNOSIS.—I. *Non-perforating Ulcer.* The diagnosis of this lesion is extremely difficult, especially in the absence of hemorrhage, and can be made only by careful attention to the various symptoms presented and the exclusion of all other probable disorders. At best the diagnosis must be a provisional one, as the symptom complex is rarely classic. Even when the hemorrhage is present Jackson says that it is not of much value in the diagnosis, as hemorrhage secondary to cirrhosis of the liver is often simulated.

Ladevèze gives as important symptoms in diagnosis the following: 1. Sudden intestinal hemorrhage occurring in the midst of apparently perfect health, repeated for many days, and producing a profound anemia. Hematemesis may come on before, or simultaneous with, the melena. 2. Pain to the right of the median line, appearing usually two to four hours after the ingestion of food. 3. Absence of gastric phenomena.

Differential Diagnosis.—1. *Gastric ulcer.* Of the diseases which must be considered in making a diagnosis, this stands first, and Von Wyl says in 90 per cent of the cases it is impossible to distinguish between the two. He gives the important points of differentiation of each as follows:

Gastric Ulcer.	Duodenal Ulcer.
1. Usually in women 20 to 35 years of age.	1. Most frequent in men.
2. Pain comes on soon after eating.	2. Pain two to four hours after eating and located in right hypochondrium.
3. Pain lessened by vomiting.	3. Vomiting does not relieve pain.
4. Vomitus contains mucus, food remnants, and often blood.	4. Vomiting more rare than in gastric ulcer and does not often contain blood.
5. Severe dyspeptic symptoms usually present.	5. Dyspeptic symptoms slight.
6. Melena rare.	6. Melena comparatively frequent.

2. *Irregular cholelithiasis,* with or without cholecystitis or cholangitis, may be difficult of exclusion, as in this condition the pain is referred to the duodenal region and intestinal hemorrhage may occur (Laspèyres). We have never observed an intestinal hemorrhage in cholelithiasis except with extreme cholemia. In cholelithiasis, if the pain be colicky, it is usually referred to the right shoulder, and there is a tender point just beneath the tip of the ninth costal cartilage, on the right side, at the end of deep inspiration. In about 400 cases operated by us for cholelithiasis in which gall stones were found, icterus, at any time in the course of the disease, was present in only 16 per cent of the cases, showing that icterus has but little value as a negative symptom in duodenal ulcers.

3. *Hyperacidity* without gastric ulcer may cause confusion in the diagnosis, according to Laspèyres. Both may give the same symptoms, especially pain which comes on several hours after eating, and sensitiveness in the pyloric region.

4. *Acute fat necrosis* is the most difficult disease in which to make a differential diagnosis from perforation of the duodenum.

The pain in both is intense; the collapse or immediate depression is more pronounced in fat necrosis than in perforation. The vomiting is more persistent and severe in the early hours of fat necrosis (up to twelve or fifteen) than in perforation; the vomiting in the second twenty-four hours is less frequent in fat necrosis than in perforation. The collapse of the second twenty-four hours in fat necrosis is less pronounced than in perforation. Superficial or piano percussion note is resonant in fat necrosis, flat in perforation (in the right hypochondrium). Pain and tympany are the same in both. There is an absence of leucocytosis in fat necrosis, and a pronounced leucocytosis in perforation of acute ulcers. This is the most important differential diagnostic manifestation. In fat necrosis there is rarely a primary elevation of temperature; in perforation there is usually a primary elevation of temperature.

5. *Intestinal obstruction* (mechanic ileus) may be mistaken for perforation. In obstruction the pain is usually of a colicky character; in perforation it is constant. In obstruction the vomiting increases in frequency with time; the same with perforation. In obstruction there is pronounced increase in the intestinal peristalsis; in perforation there is an absence of peristalsis. In intestinal obstruction there is never a primary elevation of temperature; in perforation there is a primary elevation of temperature. With intestinal obstruction there is no leucocytosis; in perforation there is a pronounced leucocytosis. With both there is a coprostasis; in obstruction it is due to mechanical causes, in perforation it is due to the paralysis of peristalsis induced by the peritonitis.

Other conditions which may cause difficulty in diagnosis are: (*a*) pancreatitis and suppurations in the liver (Bolton), and (*b*) tabes dorsalis (two cases by Box).

II. *Perforating Ulcer.* In only 2 of the 51 cases collected by Moynihan was a correct diagnosis of perforating duodenal ulcer made—one by himself, and another case by Perkins and Wallace.

The clinical picture of perforative appendicitis is so accurately copied in cases of perforating duodenal ulcer that in 49 of those reported by Moynihan 18 were operated upon for appendicitis.

After the primary shock has passed, the course of the peritonitis differs from that following gastric perforation. In the latter general peritoneal infection rapidly develops, while in the former there is an earlier involvement of the peritoneum in the right iliac fossa. The reason for this is given under Pathology. In the majority of cases it will be possible to make only a general diagnosis of perforative peritonitis, as previous symptoms which point to the duodenum have not *usually* been present. This was done in our case.

PROGNOSIS.—It is probable that the majority of duodenal ulcers will perforate the intestinal wall sooner or later, and the prognosis is therefore most grave (Bolton). Reckmann states that one-half of the cases result fatally from perforation into the peritoneal cavity (Weir). In 262 cases collected by Collin diffuse and fatal peritonitis occurred 135 times, or 51 per cent.

The prognosis in the cases of perforation will depend largely upon the length of time which has elapsed between the perforation and the operation. In Moynihan's collection of 51 operated cases of acute perforating ulcer there were 8 recoveries. Of these, 2 were operated on thirty hours after perforation; 1, twenty-eight hours after perforation; 1, twenty-five hours after perforation; 1, fifteen hours after perforation; 1, twelve hours after perforation; 2, ten hours after perforation. The average time of operation after onset of symptoms was twenty hours in the cases that recovered.

In 20 cases of perforation treated by operation collected by Darras, 17 died and 3 recovered—a mortality of 85 per cent. Bolton Carter collected 59 published cases of perforating duodenal ulcer. Of these, 27 died without operation, the lesion being found post mortem. The remaining 32 cases were operated on, with 11 recoveries—a mortality of 68.5 per cent.

Lennander says that the statistics so far published (1898) show that from one-fourth to one-third of the cases of perforating ulcer of the stomach and duodenum operated on are saved, and that the prognosis depends on the time of operation after perforation and on the quantity and quality of the fluid found in the peritoneal cavity.

Laspèyres gives the following statistics of the results of surgical treatment for the general peritonitis following duodenal perforations: Of 18 cases in which the exudate was drained only, 17 resulted fatally and 1 died four months later of general peritonitis. Of 15 cases in which the perforations were found and closed, 5 recovered—$33\frac{1}{3}$ per cent. In 79 cases collected by Weir and Foote, the mortality was 71 per cent. In the 51 cases collected by Weir, 25 had the opening closed by suture. Thirteen of these were operated upon thirty hours after the onset of symptoms, and all resulted fatally. In 12 others, less than thirty hours had elapsed, and of these 8 survived—a mortality of 33⅓ per cent. Pagenstecher gives the mortality as 60 per cent for perforations that have been found and sutured. In our collection, the length of time that had elapsed was given in only 4 cases—not a sufficient number from which to make deductions of value.

SURGICAL TREATMENT.—We shall concern ourselves with the surgical treatment of the perforations only, and not consider the various operations, such as gastroenterostomy, excision, and the like, which have been advocated for the non-perforating ulcers.

The cases in which perforation has taken place should be submitted to operation at the earliest possible moment, as all statistics show that the earlier the operation the greater are the chances of recovery. The abdomen should be opened, as recommended by Weir, through an incision four to six inches in length, in or along the outer edge of the right rectus muscle. The transverse incision is rarely necessary, as ample room is secured without it.

In most cases the diagnosis of perforative appendicitis will have been made, and this organ is the first to be examined. The gall bladder is next inspected, and, after determining that it is not the seat of perforation, the region of the duodenum is explored. When the opening is found, it is closed with a double or triple row of interrupted silk sutures of the Lembert type, taking care to bring large areas of serous surface in apposition without tension. Lennander says: "If it is not possible to close the opening in this way, the edges should be brought together as well as possible and the line of suture covered with omentum." This method should never be resorted to; it is insufficient and dangerous. There is a well-recognized rule governing the closure of intestinal fistulæ wherever situated, viz.: where the intestinal wall is indurated and adherent to neighboring tissues, it must first be sufficiently liberated and freed to admit of an easy apposition of its convex surfaces with two rows of sutures. The failure to free the intestine from neighboring structures is the most common cause of failure of union. The line of suture should usually be transverse to the long axis of the bowel, in order to avoid constriction when healing is complete, and the line of suture should always be supplemented with an *omental* support.

After closure of the perforation the peritoneal cavity is thoroughly cleansed by sponging or irrigation, and the abdominal wound closed, with or without drainage, depending upon the pathologic condition of the peritoneum at the time of operation.

It is not best to attempt to excise the ulcer, as the danger is greatly increased by this procedure. Bolton, however, recommends excision and closure by Czerny-Lembert sutures, as in pyloroplasty. For cleansing he advocates irrigations with saline solution, through the Chamberlain tube, until the fluid returns clear; and afterward sponges the peritoneum dry. He puts in a gauze drain down to the line of suture. Some surgeons recommend the use of glass drainage tubes, inserted into the pelvis through a separate incision above the pubes. Peritoneal irrigation should not be resorted to, except where there is a pronounced exfoliation or destruction of the endothelial covering of the intestines. This destruction is recognized by the absence of peritoneal gloss and the presence of a roughened or blistered serosa. We have taught as a result of our experiments, since 1892, that the peritoneum is not a lymph sac, as physiologists would have us believe. Under normal physiologic conditions the peritoneum absorbs, like the skin, only small quantities. When it becomes blistered or eroded, like the skin, it becomes a rapidly absorbing surface. Its endothelium is more easily removed, abraded, or destroyed than the epithelium of the skin, and therefore requires more respect and more delicate treatment. Where the peritoneum is not eroded it should not be irrigated. When it is eroded irrigation may be of service. In our practice we have used solutions in the peritoneal cavity only fourteen times since 1889, and believe that better results can be secured by delicate swabbing and extensive tubular and gauze drainage.

After operation the patient should always be put into the sitting posture, so that all fluids may gravitate into the pelvis, as it is well known that the pelvic peritoneum can take care of a large quantity of infectious material, as absorption takes place *slowly* and the patient is not immediately overwhelmed with the toxic products.

Periduodenal abscesses are to be opened through the abdominal wall in front, and subphrenic abscesses through the anterior or lateral walls of the abdomen or in the low intercostal space posteriorly.

The following is the history of a case which we recently operated on at Mercy Hospital: F. K., laborer, aged 24 years.

48

Family history: Negative.   Personal history: Had always been well and worked hard; appetite had been good and bowels regular; no previous illnesses; claims that prior to onset of present illness he was perfectly well and had had absolutely no gastric or intestinal symptoms.   Admitted to Mercy Hospital May 22, 1902, at 6 A.M.

Illness began at half-past 2 on the morning of admission, with sudden and severe cramping pain in abdomen.   Patient had been working on night shift at the time of onset, but had to stop his work on account of the severity of the pain.   In a few moments the pain subsided, but returned shortly afterward and continued until his admission to the hospital.   It was diffuse over the abdomen at first, but soon became more intense, and at the time of admission was localized in the right side. He walked several blocks to the hospital.   The abdomen was very tender on pressure, especially on the right side.   About 5 A.M., before coming to the hospital, he swallowed a little coffee, which caused nausea and vomiting.   On examination of patient abdomen was found uniformly distended and motionless during respiration.   It was very sensitive all over, but more so on the right than on the left side.   Over the entire right side there was dulness on light piano percussion, resonance on deep percussion.   The right abdominal muscles were very tense and would not permit deep palpation.   On admission pulse was 68 per minute, and temperature per axilla 98° F.   At 8 A.M. temperature by mouth was 100° F. and pulse 74 per minute.   A leucocyte count was made and 23,400 per cubic millimetre found. A diagnosis of perforative peritonitis was made, probably of appendical origin.   The patient was at once prepared for operation.   His depression was not sufficiently marked to consider it a case of fat necrosis.

Operation (eight hours after the onset of symptoms).—Incision was made through the outer border of the right rectus muscle, as for appendicitis.   When peritoneum was opened there was an immediate escape of viscid green fluid, which was odorless and clear with the exception of some white flakes floating in it. The fluid appeared to be tinged with bile.   The peritoneal covering of the intestine was considerably congested and reddened; an adherent fibrinous exudate was present in patches here and there.   The endothelial covering, however, was not blistered or eroded; it seemed to be intact throughout.

The caput coli was easily brought into the field.   The appendix was examined; it was thickened and adherent to the under surface of the caput coli, showing that it had been the seat of previous inflammation; as there was no acute inflammation and no perforation at this point, it was not the cause of the present trouble. The peritoneal cavity continued to fill with fluid as rapidly as it was sponged out, and this fluid seemed to come from the direction of the gall bladder. The caput coli was replaced and the incision was extended upward toward the costal arch. The gall bladder was next carefully examined, but found only slightly thickened and moderately distended with bile. The liver extended slightly below the costal arch. The stomach was examined, but found normal. Examination of the duodenum showed a perforation, about one-eighth of an inch in diameter, in the anterior wall, its outer portion about one and one-half inches below the pylorus. Through this opening jets of the greenish fluid came with each inspiration. The perforation was closed with three rows of silk Lembert sutures, and the peritoneal cavity was sponged out and irrigated with normal salt solution. The abdomen was closed by means of separate layers of catgut for the peritoneum and fascia, the skin being approximated with a continuous silkworm-gut suture. No drainage was used. One quart of saline solution was injected into the peritoneum just before complete closure of the abdomen, and was retained. In closure without drainage I had the support of Dr. Roswell Park and Dr. Arthur Dean Bevan, who were present at the clinic.

The notes on his condition after the operation are as follows: May 22: 10 P.M., pulse 140, temperature 101°, resting nicely. May 23: 8 A.M., pulse 110, temperature 99.2° F., quite thirsty, but no pain; 8 P.M., pulse 98, temperature 99° F., somewhat restless, but no pain. May 24: 8 A.M., pulse 74, temperature 98.6° F., some pain in abdomen, considerable tympanites; magnesii sulphas and spiritus terebinthinæ administered by high enema; patient passed considerable flatus and was much relieved; 8 P.M., patient resting well, pulse 76, temperature 99° F. May 25: 8 A.M., pulse 72, temperature 98.6°, patient had a comfortable night; 8 P.M., pulse 96, temperature 98.6°, had some pain during the day and was given an enema, passing considerable flatus afterward. May 26: 8 A.M., pulse 124, temperature 101.4°; no pain, and patient quiet; wound discharged a small quantity of foul-smelling pus; a number of stitches were removed, and an extensive infection of the cellular tissue was found; a pure culture of the bacillus coli communis was obtained from the pus, which accounted for the odor; he was quite restless during the day, with involuntary urination; slept at intervals; stools watery and brown; 8 P.M., pulse 120, temperature 101.4°. May 27: 8 A.M., pulse 124, temperature 100°, patient resting quietly, slight delirium during the day, perspiration very free, and great thirst; 8 P.M., pulse 100, temperature 99.6°, patient resting well. May 28: 8 A.M., pulse 98, temperature normal; 8 P.M., pulse and temperature same as morning, had been delirious at times during the day. May 29: 9 A.M., pulse 92, temperature 98.6°, patient feeling quite comfortable, some pain in the wound; 8 P.M., pulse 88, temperature 98.6°, very comfortable. May 30: 9 A.M., pulse 92, temperature 98.6°, resting well; 9 P.M., pulse 68, temperature 98°, resting comfortably.

From this date on patient continued to have practically normal temperature and pulse, resting quite comfortably most of the time. Wound continued to discharge, and the edges of the skin and muscles separated considerably owing to the bacillus coli communis infection of the cellular tissue. We have observed that infections with this organism produce rapid destruction of the fatty tissues, and that the best means of controlling them is with a saturated solution of bicarbonate of sodium.

The foul-smelling purulent discharge, which was abundant at first, rapidly decreased in quantity, and by June 7 had lost its odor. The wound gradually closed, and the discharge had practically ceased by June 14. On June 15 the patient developed a localized broncho-pneumonia and pleurisy on the right side, which gave rise to considerable pain, and his temperature rose to 101.2° F. This had subsided by June 20. On July 8 he had another attack of the same trouble, temperature rising to 102° on the 9th, gradually subsiding to normal on the 19th. No tubercle bacilli were found in the sputum.

July 24 patient was discharged with the wound entirely healed and feeling well. Subsequent reports showed that he progressed to complete recovery.

The following is a synopsis of the cases which we have collected. It includes all of the cases in the literature from the time of Weir's publication, May, 1900, to July 1, 1902:

CASE I.—Carter, Bolton.[11] Female, aged 20 years. Admitted to Royal Halifax Infirmary October 29, 1900. Patient presented a large, fluctuating mass in the right iliac region. Temperature 101.6° F. Appendical abscess diagnosed. Operation:

Oblique incision internal to right anterior superior spine. Large quantity of fetid pus evacuated. Abscess cavity walled off from peritoneal cavity by adhesions. Appendix not found. Cavity flushed out. Rubber drainage tube inserted. Patient improved until November 8. On the 9th blood escaped from the wound; the patient complained of severe pain over abdomen and began to vomit. Pulse reached 120 and she became collapsed. Died of general peritonitis November 10. Necropsy: General septic peritonitis; appendix sloughing, but no pus in neighborhood; blood clot in right lumbar region, which came from a perforating ulcer in anterior wall of second portion of duodenum. In this case there was no history of previous gastric trouble.

CASE II.—Clarke and Franklin.[7] Male, aged 45 years. Admitted to Leicester Infirmary November 7, 1900. Patient had passed no urine for six days. Complained of pain in right lumbar region. . On third day kidney was explored, but no stone found. Recovered from urinary suppression. Discharged January 1, 1901, well. Readmitted June 1, under Mr. Franklin. Eight days before he was suddenly seized with acute pain in abdomen, and confined to bed since. No vomiting. Some diarrhea and abdominal distension. On admission expression anxious and eyes sunken. Pulse 130 and small. Temperature normal. Abdomen distended, but not tender. No liver dulness present, and no dulness in flank; tympany all over. General peritonitis diagnosed, and abdomen opened in median line midway between pubes and ensiform. Abdominal cavity full of fecal-smelling pus. Incision extended downward and inflamed appendix removed. Peritoneal cavity flushed out and wound closed with drainage. Patient died five hours after the operation. Necropsy: Large perforating ulcer on anterior wall of first part of duodenum. Two other large non-perforating ulcers present, one opposite the perforation, involving all coats except the serous; the other a little lower down, extending through the mucous coat only. Two small superficial ulcers in stomach.

CASE III.—Fairchild, D. S.[16] Female, 50 years of age. Patient had been ill three weeks with apparently increasing obstruction of the colon near the sigmoid. Had been in poor health for several years. Operation January, 1901: Incision to the left of the umbilicus. Intestinal contents were seen escaping from beneath the transverse colon. Three perforations in the duodenum were found and sutured. Abdomen irrigated and closed with drainage. Patient died four hours later.

CASE IV.—Blum, reported by Grivot and Aguinet.[17] Male, aged 31 years. Vomiting began October 13, 1900, and this increased during the 14th and 15th. On the afternoon of the 16th patient suffered severely from pain in right hypochondriac region. The vomiting persisted, and he entered the hospital October 18. He had had no movement of the bowels for two days. Examination showed tympanites; diffuse tenderness over the abdomen, more pronounced in the right hypochondriac region, in which neighborhood there was a well-marked dulness on percussion. Temperature 37° C., pulse 120. Intestinal perforation, probably of appendical origin, was diagnosed. Operation performed by Dr. Blum. Incision same as for appendicitis; foul fluid removed from peritoneal cavity. Appendix removed. Pain disappeared after the operation, and condition temporarily improved. He soon grew rapidly worse, and died October 27. Necropsy: An abscess cavity was situated on the under surface of the liver and lined with false membrane. A brownish liquid escaped from the duodenal region. On the anterior surface of the first portion of the duodenum, about ten centimetres from the pylorus, a circular perforation was found, about one centimetre in diameter. It was evidently an old cicatrized ulcer which had ruptured during an effort at vomiting.

CASE V.—Kinnicutt, F. P. Male, aged 40 years. Admitted to hospital January 10, 1899. Patient had been drinking to excess for three days previously and had been suffering from loss of appetite, nausea, and vomiting. Had had constant epigastric pain and bowels had been constipated. Examination showed a prominence of the right epigastric region, where a mass could be felt, tender to pressure. Temperature ranged from 99.2° to 102° F. Mass increased in size, and three days after admission patient vomited blood. After several hours abdomen was opened. Stomach and liver adherent. Stomach full of blood, as was also the lesser peritoneal cavity. Circular ulcer two inches in diameter had perforated the peritoneum in the posterior wall of the duodenum, just below the pyloric ring. Patient's condition was such that it was impossible to proceed, and he died a few moments later.

CASE VI.—Labbé, Marcel.[18] Male, aged 31 years. Had been in good health, with no previous symptoms of hepatic or intestinal trouble. Was taken suddenly with severe abdominal pains one morning after breakfast. After admission to hospital pain became somewhat less severe and the next day was localized in the right side of the abdomen, with maximum intensity in the right iliac fossa. Pain soon increased; abdominal muscles became tense; there was absolute constipation; no vomiting and no fever. The diagnosis was between appendicitis and hepatic colic. On the third day condition became worse, pulse small and rapid, temperature 39° C. Tympanites became extreme, and fecaloid vomiting set in. Operation showed general peritonitis, with pus in the peritoneal cavity. Drainage established, the wound closed. Death took place that evening. Necropsy: Under the right side of the diaphragm was a localized abscess containing pus, gas, and fecal matter, and lined by a false membrane. Close to the entrance of the bile duct in the duodenum was an oval-shaped perforation one-half centimetre in diameter. This perforation connected the interior of the abscess cavity with the duodenum. In the duodenum itself an old ulcer was found on the lower portion of the anterior surface.

CASES VII., VIII., and IX.—Littlewood, H.[19]   In the transactions of the Leeds and West Riding Medico-Chirurgical Society, May 3, 1901, Mr. H. Littlewood states that he operated on three cases of acute perforating duodenal ulcer. All were in men, and the operations took place after thirty-six hours from the time of perforation. All died.

CASE X.—Lowson, D.[20]   Girl, aged 15 years. Illness began previous February with pains in the left side. Two weeks later had rigors, with depression and cyanosis. March 17, suffered profound collapse, with severe pain to the left of navel, pallor and cold sweats. March 20, began to vomit, but this ceased on the 25th, when the temperature went up and pulse increased in rapidity. April 4, the respirations were shallow, abdomen was distended, and there was a localized swelling just below the liver. The next day the swelling had disappeared and the note was tympanitic. Operation: Vertical incision through the rectus muscle showed gas in the peritoneal cavity, with shreds of food. The odor was putrid. The abscess cavity was formed by adherent intestines. A perforation which admitted a No. 6 catheter was found in the duodenum. The granulations were scraped away and the opening closed with Lembert sutures of silk. Gauze drainage was left in the wound. The ultimate result in this case is not stated in the report.

CASE XI.—Mauclaire.[21]   Male, age not stated. Had had pain between the margin of the ribs on the right side and the umbilicus, and later all over the abdomen. Pains came on suddenly

and were very severe.   Patient was seen thirty-six hours after
the onset, when the vomiting had ceased; temperature was normal, and his general condition grave.   Abdomen was tympanitic.
A diagnosis of intestinal perforation was made and laparatomy
at once performed.   Death occurred sixteen hours later, or
fifty-five hours after the onset of the attack.   Autopsy showed
general, plastic peritonitis following the perforation of an ulcer
of the duodenum two centimetres below the pylorus.

CASE XII.—Moynihan.[4]   Male, aged 44 years.   Admitted to
Leeds Infirmary April 24, 1900.   Symptoms had been present
for eighteen months, chiefly pain after taking food; vomiting
of blood, which occurred irregularly one-half to four hours after
eating.   On the 25th patient became worse and the symptoms
of peritonitis developed.   Perforation was diagnosed and laparatomy performed.   A perforating duodenal ulcer three-quarters
of an inch in diameter was found in the beginning of the second
portion.   The sutures were introduced, held imperfectly, and, as
the gut was considerably narrowed, gastroenterostomy with
Murphy button was performed.   Abdomen was cleansed and
drainage tube introduced.   Patient died May 22.

CASE XIII.—Moynihan.   Male, aged 25 years.   Admitted to
Leeds Infirmary June 18, 1901.   For four weeks had experienced
pain after taking food, and had vomited almost at once after
meals.   Had sudden, acute pain in the upper part of the abdomen, in the median line; profound collapse and persistent vomiting.   The abdomen was opened three hours and fifty minutes
after perforation.   Some gas in peritoneal cavity was found.
On examining the duodenum a perforation in the anterior wall,
one inch below the pylorus, was found.   The opening was
stitched with a continuous suture applied vertically, the abdomen
was flushed out, and a drainage tube inserted into the pelvis.   No
fluid was allowed by mouth for twenty-four hours, and saline
enemata were given every six hours.   Drainage tube taken out
in thirty-six hours and patient allowed to sit up on the nine-
teenth day.   Recovery was uneventful.

CASE XIV.—Moynihan.   Female, aged 29 years.   Admitted
to Leeds Infirmary September 29, 1900.   Had several acute attacks of pain and vomiting during last five years.   There was
blood in the vomitus the first time, and has been irregularly since
then.   Always experienced a sense of discomfort from one to
four hours after meals.   October 4, had one of these attacks,
with temperature 104° F., vomiting, tenderness in right hypo-

chondrium, and severe pain on the right of the umbilicus. October 12, laparatomy performed and many adhesions found around the duodenum, pylorus, and gall bladder. An abscess was found between the liver and the duodenum; the duodenal wall was thickened and presented a perforating ulcer at the junction of the first and second portions. Tube and gauze drainage were inserted, and the patient left the hospital November 5 with the wound entirely healed.

CASE XV.—Murphy, J. B. History of case given previously.

CASE XVI.—Pegram, J. C.[22] Male, aged 56 years; farmer. Ten years ago had stomach trouble for two years, but since then had been well. December 8, 1899, patient ate a hearty meal in the evening, and that night had dull, unlocalized pain in the abdomen. At 10 the next forenoon had violent pain in the right side of the abdomen and the bowels had not moved. Examination showed flat, rigid abdomen, with marked tenderness, especially in the right hypochondrium. Abdomen became distended, and he vomited frequently. Operation disclosed perforating ulcer in the anterior wall of the duodenum near the pylorus, with subphrenic abscess. Abscess was evacuated. No attempt was made to close the ulcer, but it was walled off with gauze. Patient died thirty-six hours later with general peritonitis.

CASE XVII.—Vince.[23] Female. Presented every symptom of intestinal obstruction. All medication being useless, an operation was performed. Upon opening the abdominal cavity gas escaped and the intestines were found to be covered with purulent, fibrinous exudate. There was no fecal matter in the peritoneal cavity. Drainage was introduced through a lumbar incision and through the cul-de-sac of Douglas. Patient died. Necropsy showed a localized abscess in a space limited by the liver, stomach, diaphragm, and transverse colon. This cavity contained the contents of the duodenum, which had escaped through the perforation in the anterior wall. The perforating ulcer was evidently a chronic one, as the edges were indurated.

CASE XVIII.—Vince.[24] Male, age not given. After lifting a heavy log, was taken with severe, acute pain in the abdomen. Upon examining the abdomen, liver dulness was found to be obliterated, and there were all the evidences of ascites. A diagnosis of intestinal perforation was made, and patient was taken to hospital and operated upon within twenty-four hours from the onset. Gas escaped from the abdominal incision, and bile flowed out. A perforation was found in the duodenum at the site of an old ulceration, about which there were numerous peritoneal adhesions. The violent effort of the patient had evidently caused the ulcer to perforate. Patient died the evening after the operation.

CASE XIX.—Wilson, A. Christy.[25] Male, aged 48 years. For several years had been troubled with indigestion. While employed at his usual labor one morning, was suddenly seized with severe pain in the epigastrium. He had all the symptoms of perforation, but refused operation until twenty hours after the onset. At that time a median incision was made, and upon opening the peritoneum a quantity of bile-stained mucus escaped. Perforation was found in the anterior wall of the duodenum one inch below the pylorus. This was closed with a double row of sutures, after which the intestines were drawn out, scrubbed, and put back. The liver, stomach, and pelvis were also cleansed thoroughly, normal saline solution being used freely. Recovery was slow but steady, and the patient is at present employed at his regular hard work.

An analysis of these cases shows: Average age in the 13 cases in which age was stated, 35 years. Of the 19 cases, 5 were females and 14 males. Of the 12 cases in which it was stated whether or not there were symptoms present previous to the perforation, in 9 cases there were symptoms (previous); in 3 cases there were no previous symptoms; in only 5 cases did the symptoms point to the stomach or duodenum; in 6 cases it was stated that the perforations were sutured—of these, 2 died, 3 recovered, in 1 the result is not stated; in 8 cases drainage only was used—of these, 7 died and 1 recovered.

CONCLUSIONS.—The diagnosis of perforating duodenal ulcer is difficult, or, better, practically impossible without an exploratory laparatomy.

In many cases there is no evidence of duodenal disease previous to the perforation. The most important physical sign, in addition to those of perforative peritonitis from perforations in other portions of the intestinal tract, is the flatness of the superficial piano percussion note in the right hypochondrium.

The leucocytosis in our case, the only one in which it was given, was pronounced, showing an inflammatory condition, in contradistinction to the usual absence of it in intestinal obstruction and fat necrosis of the pancreas. It must be borne in mind, however, that leucocytosis is not a necessary manifestation of perforation or of inflammation. It is a manifestation of the reaction of blood to infections biotic or toxic. It is often entirely absent in typhoid perforations, as we have observed in repeated blood examinations after perforation during the present epidemic in Chicago.

Collapse is absent in duodenal perforation, except where associated with severe hemorrhage. Collapse in intestinal perforation is the *manifestation of the absorption of the products of infection,* and not a manifestation of the perforation *per se.* Collapse is always secondary to abrasion or denudation of the endothelial covering of the peritoneum, which abrasion permits of rapid absorption.

Time of Operation.—In all cases of perforative peritonitis—to which duodenal perforations are no exception—operation should be performed at the earliest possible moment after perforation has taken place; and clinical experience shows that the mortality is in direct ratio to the length of time that elapses between the occurrence of perforation and the operation.

In perforation, the longer the escaping material is in contact with the peritoneum the greater the danger of destruction of its endothelial covering, and thus the greater the danger of absorption. Of 13 cases operated more than thirty hours after perforation, all terminated fatally; while in 12 cases where less than thirty hours had elapsed, 66⅔ per cent recovered (Weir). These comparisons emphasize more than words can the importance of early operation.

The operation must be complete—that is, it must be pursued to an effective suture of the perforation. Drainage is insufficient, as of 18 cases treated by drainage alone, all died (Laspèyres). The suture of the opening can be easily inserted, as in 98 per cent of the perforating ulcers into the peritoneum the opening was in the first portion of the duodenum, its most accessible portion.

Where duodenal perforation is suspected the incision should be through the right rectus muscle. It can then be carried upward to the costal arch, or downward to the symphysis pubis, without dividing any of the transverse muscles. The incision through the rectus muscle is the one which we commonly make in operating for appendicitis. It can be enlarged upward or downward without interfering with the muscle fibres.

Drainage or no drainage is a matter of personal election, influenced more or less by the pathologic condition present at the time of the operation.

The after-treatment is that commonly followed after abdominal section, except that the patient is kept elevated in bed at an angle of 35 degrees for the first forty-eight hours after the operation.

The prognosis depends: first, on the virulence of the peritonitis produced; second, on the time the material has been allowed to remain in the peritoneum; third, upon the presence or absence of blistering or abrasion of the peritoneum at the time of operation.

LITERATURE.

1. WEIR, ROBT. F.: Medical Record, May 5, 1900.

2. KINNICUTT, F. P.: Festschrift in honor of Abraham Jacobi, May, 1900.

3. ADRIANCE, VANDERPOEL: Archives of Pediatrics, April, 1901.

4. MOYNIHAN, B. G. A.: Lancet, December 4, 1901.

5. LASPÈYRES, R.: Centralblatt für die Grenzgebiete der Medicin und Chirurgie, February and March, 1902.

6. HANS: Wiener klinische Wochenschrift, 1902, p. 328.

7. CLARKE AND FRANKLIN (Leicester Infirmary): Lancet, November 2, 1901.

8. POYNTON: British Medical Journal, February 17, 1900.

9. SATTERTHWAITE, THOS. E.: Medical Record, March 24, 1900.

10. BURWINKEL, O.: Deutsche medicinische Wochenschrift, December 20, 1898.

11. CARTER, BOLTON: Lancet, November 2, 1901.

12. LADEVÈZE: Journal de Médecine et de Chirurgie Pratiques, March 25, 1901.

13. Box, C. R.: British Medical Journal, February 8, 1902.

14. ZIMNITSKI, BOLNITCH: Gaz. Botkinkina, vol. xii., No. 45. (Abstract in Philadelphia Medical Journal, June 14, 1902.)

15. LISSJANSKY, W. W.: Khirurgia, September, 1901. (Abstract in Rev. der Russ. Med. Zeitschrift, No. 2, St. Petersburg.)

16. FAIRCHILD, D. S.: Medical News, August 3, 1902.

17. GRIVOT AND AGUINET: Bull. et Mem. Soc. Anat., Paris, 1900, vol. lxxv., p. 930.

18. LABBÉ, MARCEL: Bull. et Mem. Sòc. Anat., Paris, 1901, vol. lxxvi., p. 407.

19. LITTLEWOOD, H.: Lancet, May 18, 1901.

20. LOWSON, D.: Lancet, May 11, 1901.

21. MAUCLAIRE: Journal des Praticiens, Paris, January 4, 1902. (Abstract in Philadelphia Medical Journal, April 12, 1902.)

22. PEGRAM, J. G.: Boston Medical and Surgical Journal, December 27, 1900.

23. VINCE: Cercle médical de Bruxelles, May 4, 1900. (Abstract in Gazette hebd. de Méd. et de Chir., 1900, p. 684.)

24. VINCE: Cercle médical de Bruxelles, February 11, 1901. (Abstract in Gazette hebd. de Méd. et de Chir., March 7, 1901, p. 228.)

25. WILSON, A. CHRISTY: Lancet, June 15, 1901.

CRANIOTOMY.[1]

BY

JAMES D. VOORHEES, M.D.,

Assistant Attending Physician to the Sloane Maternity Hospital,
New York.

EMBRYOTOMY literally means "a reduction in the size of the fetus by cutting or crushing any portion of the fetal body "; but the word as now used is really not so inclusive, and is applied incorrectly only to any operation mutilating the fetal trunk, as decapitation, evisceration, eventration, division, or dismemberment.

As the head most frequently presents, and as it usually offers the obstacle to delivery, some operation on the cranium, called craniotomy, is most frequently done. Craniotomy, however, strictly means a cutting into or a perforation of the skull, yet ordinarily by the term is understood any mutilation of the head. Cranioclasis, cephalotripsy, and basiotripsy all have the same definition—a crushing of the skull. These operations are generally preceded by a perforation and are designated by one of the above names, according to the kind of instrument used; for with the cranioclast itself traction on the skull alone can be applied, with the cephalotribe crushing is followed by traction, while in the basiotribe we have a compact instrument with which we can first perforate, then crush, and finally deliver.

Embryotomy is a very old operation, and its abuse led to a remonstrance on the part of the religious authorities and to the prohibition by some churches of such a measure on the living child. In the advance of the art of obstetrics, and in the improvement of the technique of cutting operations, the frequency of craniotomy has in the last few years been much lessened and the indications for its use much narrowed. Yet even to-day a child is frequently lost, either unwittingly, through ignorance, or through the fear of failure in doing a forceps or a version operation. Often after prolonged and too forcible efforts to drag the child through a pelvis relatively too small for the

[1] Read before the Society of the Alumni of the Sloane Maternity Hospital, January 24, 1902.

head, the child is born dead and autopsy shows a fracture of the skull or a cerebral hemorrhage. Sometimes it is even born alive with extensive intracranial lesions, only to die in a few hours or in a few days. In other cases we drag the head down somewhat into the pelvis and here it sticks. We have used so much traction that the fetal heart soon shows signs of cerebral compression and injury, the forceps slips (which generally means a fracture of the skull), then the child dies, and we are compelled to terminate the case by a craniotomy. Take the operation of version. By a mistake in judgment we decide a child might be born by turning. In some cases we are able to bring down a foot, but the child refuses to turn. We use so much force in pulling on this foot that we disarticulate the hip joint, or the child turns, but the head carries up with it the lower segment of the uterus and we have a uterine rupture. Again, in our manipulation the cord may prolapse and from pressure the pulsations soon stop. In another instance, after a version has been completed with ease or in the delivery of a breech presentation, we get as far as the aftercoming head and here there is a delay. Using great traction, as is often necessary, accidents will occur. The child may be born alive, but dies in a few days with symptoms of intracranial bleeding. It may be stillborn, with a fracture of the spine, fracture of the skull, or a cerebral hemorrhage. Finally, with pressure on the fundus by an assistant, with traction on the feet by another assistant, and ourselves using the Smellie-Veit method of extracting the aftercoming head, we may fail to deliver without a decapitation or a perforation of this aftercoming head.

In all of the above cases we have done a craniotomy, although it has not been a deliberate nor a premeditated undertaking with that end in view. Craniotomy remains, however, a proper procedure in certain cases, and one which, addressed to the interests of the mother only, may often serve a most useful purpose.

In the present state of obstetric surgery the operation is clearly indicated in these three conditions: (1) in a non-viable child where the mother's life is in the balance; (2) in dealing with a monstrosity; and (3) when the fetus is larger than the parturient canal and is dead when the physician first sees the patient.

1. Under the first heading we include such cases of albuminuria, eclampsia, placenta previa, chronic endocarditis, phthisis, toxemia, or any acute disease when it is all-important to deliver

quickly and to do so with as little shock as possible to the patient, already in poor condition. A tough and rigid cervix is generally the barrier in these cases, and in doing an accouchement forcé we often cannot dilate it enough for passage of the head without starting deep tears bilaterally, which will endanger the integrity of the lower uterine zone, or at any rate cause shock or a hemorrhage of sufficient degree for a fatal outcome. In such cases a simple perforation of the head will so diminish the bulk that the delivery is quickly and easily completed without unnecessary injury to the mother's soft parts.

2. In a monster, as in cases of hydrocephalus (which are the most common), no one will question for a minute the justification of doing a craniotomy. The forceps will not fit such a head, and even after a version it is senseless to try to drag such a large mass through the parturient canal with probable contusion and laceration of the maternal tissues.

3. In a dead child the indications for a craniotomy may be fairly trivial. If the mother can be saved any additional risk or suffering by the rapid delivery of a mutilated child, craniotomy is not only justifiable but advisable. In the case of a prolapsed cord, with a contracted pelvis—one of the most common conditions which call for craniotomy on the dead infant—it is far better to open the head and deliver easily by the basiotribe than to attempt version with its risks, or to apply forceps to the head at the superior strait and to subject the mother to the delay, pain, and danger of a prolonged forceps operation when nothing is to be gained by it. Esthetic conditions and regard for appearances should not be considered where the mother's safety is endangered.

Undoubtedly most of the cases which demand a craniotomy are those in which, from mistakes in judgment, from neglect, from ignorance, or by bungling work with forceps or in turning, the child dies or is killed and one is called upon to deliver. When, however, the womb contains a living child and the pelvis is too contracted to allow a normal birth *per vias naturales,* the question of sacrificing this child becomes a different matter.

To-day the knowledge of the art of obstetrics is more widespread and the need of a skilful obstetrician more and more recognized. We see our patients early in pregnancy and consequently are soon familiar with their histories, their pelves, the size of the child, its presentation, and the presence of any unusual condition obstructing the parturient canal.

To-day obstetricians are becoming surgeons, consequently more skilled in the technique of the cutting operations and less fearful of their results. So that the conclusion is now becoming established among the medical profession that a planned craniotomy or embryotomy on a living child, with mother in good condition, is not justifiable except in conditions of emergency and extreme rarity.

Pinard and others boldly hold the ground that such a procedure is never justifiable; but most modern obstetricians, although feeling it their duty to follow the rule that the child should be saved, are placed at times in circumstances where they are not free to follow the dictates of their consciences nor their best judgment. The patient herself or her friends may refuse a cutting operation. She may be in the country far away from competent assistance, or in quarters unsuitable for the major operation, consequently the accoucheur is often led to attempt an operation which, although not offering much of a chance of saving the life of the child, avoids the knife with its supposed risks. Most of such cases terminate in a stillborn baby or in a craniotomy.

A very important point to decide is whether we should recommend and perform one of the cutting operations upon the mother to save the life of the child. This decision depends upon the extra risk to which the mother is exposed by doing these operations. We all believe that the interests of the mother must take precedence during labor, and, if either must be sacrificed, it should be the child, which is an unknown quantity and has no ties to this world. If we have a case, then, of protracted labor from disproportion between size of child and pelvis, with the woman in poor condition—rapid pulse, elevated temperature, etc., and a tonic uterus—we do not hesitate for a minute to recommend a craniotomy on a living child, as by a cutting operation the mother's life would be jeopardized. Again, if the child is *in extremis* and its chance of living is very doubtful—as in cases of protracted labor or where repeated attempts have failed in the use of the forceps to deliver—then again we do not hesitate to prefer a craniotomy, unless the pelvis is so blocked that the delivery of a crushed or mangled fetus will entail more dangers to the patient than a Cesarean section. In the latter cases not only is the danger of sepsis greater, but serious injuries to the bladder and soft parts of the parturient canal may occur. But with mother and child both in good condition, and delivery by version or forceps impossible, then we have a choice between the question of Cesarean section and symphyseotomy standing over craniotomy.

Let us glance at the mortality of the above operations:

In craniotomy the combined reports of such men as Leopold, Zweifel, Fehling, Potocki, and others show a maternal mortality of 8.1 per cent, and that for the children 100 per cent, of course. A large number of these cases were done before the days of asepsis, but by skilled obstetricians. Pinard in 81 craniotomies lost 11.5 per cent of the mothers. At the Sloane Maternity Hospital, in 98 craniotomies 26 died, none, however, from the operation itself. Again, all cases of craniotomy are not reported. The statistics of the best accoucheurs alone are published. Consider the number of cases happening in the hands of the general practitioner. Among these the mortality would probably reach 35+ per cent through lack of cleanliness and unskilful work in the technique of the operation.

We argue, on the other side, that the mortality for the operation in skilful hands and selected cases ought to be *nil;* that many women *in extremis* recovered when any cutting operation would endanger their lives; and, finally, that the reason why good obstetricians and hospitals show any mortality at all is because they have to deal with cases infected, neglected, or maltreated before the case is seen by them. All of which is very true; but we must remember that with the child alive and in good condition we must institute measures to save it, if we can do so without great danger to the mother.

Even so conservative an operation as symphyseotomy, in statistics reported by F. Barnes, gives a maternal mortality of 10.8 per cent and fetal mortality of 14.5 per cent. Pinard, Ayers, Jewett, and Fry, however, give better mortality rates. For Cesarean section, an operation which showed not long ago a maternal mortality of anywhere from 50 per cent upward, the greatest reduction in the death rate has been made. Leopold. Olshausen, and others show less than 10 per cent of deaths. Barnes in collected cases gives a mortality of 7.6 per cent both for mother and child. Zweifel did 50 cases without a death, Reynolds 19 cases, and Sinclair 10 cases without a death. At the Sloane Hospital we can show 16 cases with only one death of mother and child, and that of a case moribund from extensive carcinoma of the uterus, cervix, and vagina, in which the child was already dead and beginning to macerate. In this

49

case the abdominal section was the only method of delivery without extensive lacerations and uncontrollable hemorrhage. With
such a low mortality it is now no wonder that Cesarean section
with the gain of a living baby is an operation steadily gaining
in favor. We say that this is very well for a hospital and that
these are all hospital statistics. For here we have greater
control of the patient, more favorable surroundings, plenty of
supplies on hand, many assistants in readiness who know thoroughly the entire technique of the operation. This is all very
true, and in private practice a different procedure will often be
done for the lack of the above. Yet literature to-day teems
with successful cases of Cesarean section performed in all sections of the country and by a diverse array of surgeons. The
procedure is not so difficult in technique as one ordinarily
imagines. Many much more severe operations are prepared for
and performed in private houses. Why cannot we, then, do a
Cesarean at the patient's home? Most small towns and all large
cities contain good hospitals, and in case of unfavorable surroundings at home why cannot they be transferred there for
operation?

In view of these facts we hope that craniotomy will gradually
become a very much more infrequent operation, and the day
will soon come when there will be no longer any reason to perform it on the living child.

Let us consider a few points in the technique of the operation.
Since infection is the most common and dangerous sequel, we
must be very careful in our asepsis and antisepsis. Whatever
instruments are used should be boiled. The vagina should be
thoroughly cleansed, rectum and bladder emptied, before commencing the operation. For a decapitation the best instrument
is a Ramsbotham knife-edged hook—that is, for an impacted
shoulder presentation with an arm prolapsed into the vagina.
In its use the whole hand is inserted into the vagina with palm
upward, carrying the fingers posteriorly about the neck and
placing the thumb anteriorly so that the whole neck can be controlled. Some recommend the introduction of the left hand if
the child's head is lying toward the mother's left; if the head is
directed to the right, the right hand is used. The hook can be
introduced in two ways: first, with the convexity posteriorly it
is made to encircle the neck over the fingers to reach the thumb
anteriorly, or it can be passed with the concavity backward along
the thumb and guided over the neck till it meets the fingers be-

hind. During this manipulation and in the subsequent severing of the neck we must be sure with each rocking motion that nu. thing but the neck comes in contact with the knife edge. To facilitate the cutting and to lessen the risk of injury to the mother's soft parts, traction should be made on the baby's arm to bring the neck as low in the pelvis as possible. Sometimes the neck is buttonholed by the hook, and after it comes through the head is still attached to the body by a band of skin. This can be severed by scissors. As soon as the neck is divided the body can be easily delivered by traction on the arm. The head is subse. quently extracted by forceps or basiotribe.

For evisceration we need a long, curved, blunt-pointed scis. sors and a strong volsella. We can easily open the thorax and abdomen, or cut through the spine, and break up the internal organs by means of the scissors and then remove them by the volsella. In some cases it is often necessary to twist off an extremity, so as to render the rest of the body accessible for mutilation. The operation is long and tedious, and in using the scissors we must work very carefully so as not to damage the maternal tissues.

For a craniotomy Tarnier's modern basiotribe is the best of all instruments. There are four steps in the operation:

1. Perforation.
2. Introduction and application of blades.
3. Crushing of the head.
4. Extraction of the child.

1. After the usual antiseptic preparations, the head is steadied against the cervix or brim of the pelvis by pressure above or by grasping the child's scalp with a strong volsella, which is pulled downward by an assistant. Two fingers or the whole left hand are carried into the vagina posteriorly up to the head, while with the right hand the perforator is introduced over these guide fingers to a suture or to a fontanelle which is preferably nearer the symphysis. In face presentation the perforator should be passed through the orbit, frontal bone, or through the roof of the mouth. By a boring motion the skin or scalp is perforated and the point firmly embedded in the skull. Then drawing the handle pos- teriorly almost as far as the perineum will allow, so as to be in the axis of the brim, the perforator is plunged into the cranial cavity and the brain thoroughly broken up. It is essential to be sure that the medulla and base of the brain are destroyed, for otherwise a mutilated child may be born alive, making attempts

to breathe. It is generally unnecessary to wash out the brain matter from the cranial cavity with a syringe. Ordinarily in crushing the skull this material flows out very readily.

2. The next step is often the most difficult of all—the introduction of the blades, accomplishing this without injury to the maternal soft parts. When the head is fairly movable and the cervix well dilated, this procedure is easy enough, following the rules for the introduction of the forceps either by the lateral or posterior method. The former is preferable, for in rotating the blades (using the latter method) some damage may be done to the lower uterine zone. The blades should be passed well into the uterus, so as to grasp the whole head, and the application should always be primarily with the blades to the sides of the pelvis. Before locking, the perforator should be passed well into the cranial cavity and held in place by an assistant; otherwise the vertex alone will be grasped, the crushing will only be partially accomplished, and the hold will be imperfect. When the uterus is in tonic spasm, when the pains are strong, or when the head is well wedged into the pelvis, a lateral introduction should always be done, taking the utmost care, using the least amount of force, and anesthetizing deeply to obtain as much relaxation as possible. In cases where the cervix is rigid and partially dilated we often experience the most difficulty in introducing the blades. The lack of room in the cervix will cause now and then a failure to introduce the second blade after the first is in position, or one is unable to apply the second blade, due to the fact that the absence of the ordinary pelvic and cephalic curves of the basiotribe, which curves are so essential in the forceps, renders the insertion and application of this second blade to the head almost impossible. The head is pushed over to the right when the first or left blade is in position, and seems to be in the way of the second or right blade. In just such cases as these the posterior introduction of both blades one over the other, and then rotating equally for a pelvic application, is of the highest value, remembering always to use a minimum of force in so doing.

3. The crushing of the head should not be started until we are sure of an extensive hold, for without this but little diminution of the size of the head is accomplished, the blades may slip, or we may simply pull off the cranial vault; especially is this last mentioned the result if the fetus is macerated. The crushing should be done slowly, in order to prevent the opening of the

skull from getting clogged and to allow the broken-up brain to flow out easily. Great care must be taken while crushing to keep the anterior and posterior vaginal walls, as well as the cervix, from getting pinched between the blades. It is also well to screw the windlass up to the limit, so as to reduce the head as much as possible before exerting any traction.

4. The same rules which we observe in forceps operations must be observed in extraction of the head after a cephalotripsy. Pull slowly, intermittently, and always in the axis of the parturient canal, using as little power as possible.

In flat pelves, after crushing, the head will often come through the brim more easily by first rotating the blades about a quarter of a circle. This brings the long diameter of the crushed head in the long diameter of the brim, consequently it enters the pelvis more easily. If after a few strong tractions the head does not advance, the blades can be reapplied and the head crushed again in another diameter. This procedure, however, is not often necessary if a good application is obtained in the beginning. Finally, it is well to keep the instrument on the head until the whole child is born, for the shoulders often cause delay. When such is the case and strong traction fails to deliver, or the cranial vault is pulled off, the cranioclast or strong volsella will often aid in the delivery. Sometimes even these fail, and a cleidotomy may then be necessary, or often after decapitation the arms may be brought down and then a cleidotomy done before delivery is accomplished.

For the aftercoming head, ordinarily a perforation alone is necessary. This can be readily performed with the perforator of the basiotribe. It is usually recommended to pierce through a lateral fontanelle, but with a sharp instrument any spot in the occipital region may be selected. The body of the fetus should be drawn downward and backward to bring the field of operation as low as possible and within reach of the guide finger. The perforator, guided by the fingers, is inserted as described before, brain churned up, and then the instrument removed. Simple traction, keeping the opening patent, causes the head to collapse and so it readily advances. If the obstruction is too great, the blades of the basiotribe may be applied in the manner ordinarily employed for forceps on the aftercoming head and the head crushed.

The following are the statistics for craniotomy at the Sloane Maternity Hospital from its beginning until the time of writing this article, December 28, 1901: During this period there have been 11,796 cases; among this number are recorded 91 craniotomies and 7 decapitations—in 5 of these the heads were subsequently crushed. The total, then, is 96 craniotomies—53 were primiparæ, 57 were at term.

The indications were as follows:

1. There were 3 cases of impacted brow and one of impacted face presentation, all neglected or maltreated outside the hospital; the babies were dead. In three of the cases the uterus was in tonic contraction and in two the pelves were narrowed. All four mothers recovered.

2. There were 2 cases of prolapse of the cord; the children were dead; in one the pelvis was deformed. In one forceps had been tried outside, and in the other it was attempted inside the hospital. Both mothers recovered.

3. There were 5 hydrocephalic children; 3 were alive at the time of the operation. Three heads were crushed, and in the other two the heads were only perforated after a version had been performed. All the mothers did well.

4. There were 3 cases of accidental hemorrhage. In all the cervix was rigid and the children were dead; craniotomy was considered the easiest method of delivery. One mother died of hemorrhage and shock.

5. There were 3 cases of chronic endocarditis who were almost *in extremis* with tough or immature cervices; the children were either dead or not viable. One of these cases died.

6. There was one case of a cartilaginous cervix, where forceps failed and version was performed, but the aftercoming head could not be delivered, the child dying in attempts to drag it through the cervix.

7. There was one case of pelvic tumor where the child had died through attempts to deliver outside. Patient recovered after a gangrenous sepsis.

8. There was one case of placenta previa where the aftercoming head in a non-viable child was perforated after a version, on account of the poor condition of the mother and a rigid cervix.

9. There were two cases of toxemia and albuminuria with rigid cervices and dead children. One of these mothers died.

10. There was one case of hyperemesis where the aftercoming head in a non-viable child was perforated on account of an undilatable cervix. This case died.

11. There was one case of toxic amaurosis. After a version the aftercoming head was perforated for the same reasons.

12. In 9 cases the children were very large, the gestations prolonged, with occipito-posterior positions, in most of whom previous labors had been easy. In 8 cases the children were dead, 5 on admission to hospital and 3 after attempts at forceps in the hospital. One was alive, the mother in good condition, and forceps had failed at the hospital. Two mothers of the 9 died; these two were practically moribund on admission.

13. There were 27 cases of eclampsia. In 12 of these a version was done and the aftercoming head perforated on account of a rigid cervix, in children which were already dead, macerated, or non-viable. In 2, forceps was first tried, with dead children. In 2, version was tried, with dead children. In 6, craniotomy was done at once, with dead children. In 1, craniotomy was done at once, with a live child; here a version or forceps should have been attempted. In 4, the pelves were deformed, in 2 of which forceps failed and version was done. The children in 3 cases died after the version. In 1, the child died after forceps had been tried outside. Twelve of these mothers died.

14. There were 31 cases of deformed pelves, the internal conjugate varying from 6.8 to 9.5 centimetres. In 4, labor had been induced, in one of which forceps and version both failed, and in 3 of which version was done, but delivery was impossible. In these procedures the children died. In 1, the child died after à version was done. In 4, forceps was tried and the child died after a version was done. In 2 cases the children died during attempts to deliver by forceps. In 3, the children were dead in neglected cases outside. In 11, the children were dead after forceps had failed outside the hospital, and in another case the child died after both forceps and version had failed outside the hospital. In 1, the child was alive and mother in good condition, but forceps failed. In 3, the children were alive, but the mothers or children were in poor condition. Eight mothers died in these cases of deformed pelves.

Of all the cases, 32 were neglected or mismanaged outside of the hospital, not counting the eclampsia cases. In 64 the mother's condition was such as to warrant no other procedure involving more risk.

Of the children, 1 was in very poor condition, justifying no operative procedure to save its life. Nine were alive and vigorous at the time of operation; 3 of these were hydroceph-

alic, and in 4 the mother was almost *in extremis,* so that to save
her life the child had to be sacrificed. In 26 cases the child died
after attempts to deliver by forceps and version in the hospital.
In 23, forceps had been tried outside; and in 24, forceps failed
inside the hospital. In 9, version had been attempted; and in
24, version had been completed in the hospital, in all of which
craniotomy was necessary to complete the delivery. The injuries attributable to the operation itself were merely slight or
moderate—laceration of the cervix or perineum, and in one
case a tear of the septum in a uterus septus. Twenty-four developed sepsis of different degrees of severity. Of all cases, 26
died—a mortality of 26.4 per cent.

The causes of death were as follows: Eclampsia, 10 cases;
necrosis of uterus or sepsis, 8 cases; rupture of the uterus, 5
cases; chronic endocarditis, 1 case; toxemia, 1 case; accidental
hemorrhage, 1 case.

The instruments used were in some of the early cases Smellie's
scissors or Breisky's trephine, followed by Lusk's or Scanzoni's
cephalotribe. In the large majority of the cases Tarnier's basiotribe sufficed. Occasionally Simpson's cranioclast was of service.

In 66 vertex presentations the heads were crushed. In 23, a
perforation of the aftercoming head was all that was necessary.
In 7, besides a perforation, the aftercoming head was crushed.
In 5, a decapitation of the aftercoming head was first done.
In one of the impacted shoulder cases, after decapitation the
forceps easily delivered the severed head.

In looking over these cases from our modern point of view
and with our knowledge of the success of the cutting operations,
we find at least 11 in which to-day we would not hesitate to perform either a symphyseotomy or Cesarean section, more probably
the latter operation.

From my private practice I can only cite one case of craniotomy. The patient was on the verge of eclampsia, and after
a prolonged labor, due to a rigid cervix, the indication was to
deliver. The forceps was applied to the head of a child barely
seven months along. Inasmuch as the child soon died and the
cervix started to tear, the labor was completed by a craniotomy.

Our conclusions are:

1. That craniotomy is an operation of great usefulness, but
one whose field has been narrowed to cases where the child is
dead, except on occasions of grave emergency and where the
mother's life would be jeopardized by a cutting operation.

2. That the operation of itself should be attended with prac_tically no mortality in the hands of a careful operator.

3. That the cutting operations, especially Cesarean section, should be done more frequently in proper cases, inasmuch as the maternal mortality has been reduced almost to nothing in the improvement of the technique of these operations, and inas_much as almost every baby can be saved.

Finally, I want to tender my thanks to Dr. E. B. Cragin for permission to collect the above statistics, and also wish to state that a great many of his ideas have been expressed in this article. There is no doubt that to Dr. Cragin's skill and teaching the brilliant results of our Cesarean sections at the Sloane Ma_ternity Hospital are due.

150 WEST FIFTY-NINTH STREET.

INTERPRETATION OF THE HISTOLOGY OF THE VILLI FROM EARLY INTRA- AND EXTRAUTERINE SPECIMENS; THE SYNCYTIUM.[1]

BY

FRANK A. STAHL, M.D.,
Chicago.

(With plate and seven illustrations.)

IN research work concerning the histology of the early villi and their contiguous environment, two interesting problems immediately confront the student. One is, What is the origin of the coverings of the villi; are both the syncytium and the Langhans-cell layer fetal in origin; is the one maternal and the other fetal; are they identical, of a like tissue? The second problem is, In tubal pregnancy is there a characteristic decidual development? Though both problems have been repeatedly considered by writers of recognized authority, their solutions still show so diverse opinions that the subjects are practically still open.

The interpretations are presented in sequence as they suggested themselves in the course of the work. They are from eight specimens, six intra- and two extrauterine. The intrauterine specimens are, one from an ovum estimated as being of

[1]Read before the Chicago Gynecological Society, June 25, 1902.

about the third to fourth week development; the second, of about the fourth to fifth week of development; the third, the sixth week; the fourth, three to four months; the fifth, six months; the sixth specimen is from the margin of the placenta at its union with the membranes at term. The extrauterine specimens are, one of about the second week development; the second, of about the eighth, these latter from the author's case of "Repeated Pregnancy in the Same Tube."[1] The specimens are all in splendid condition, not torn or obscured by hemorrhages.

Concerning the first problem: What is the origin of the peripheral layers of the villus?

To show the status of this question at the present time, a

[1] AMERICAN JOURNAL OF OBSTETRICS, vol. xliv., No. 4, 1901.

EXPLANATION OF PLATES.

FIG. 1.—One-third circumference of intrauterine ovum of four to five weeks. (1) Chorion, amnion not yet fused. (2) Large trunk villus to decidua reflexa (3). (4) Smaller villi. (5) Initial budding from chorion and villi well shown; syncytium always leads. (6) Little dots in intervillous field are ectoblasts surrounded by a variable-thickness layer of syncytium, like initial buds. (7) Islands of syncytium with nuclei (Langhans cells) within; previllous stage. (8) Unbroken continuity in syncytium and nuclei, and similarity in histological structure of chorion and villi well shown. (10) Empty spaces previously occupied by nuclei, probably worked out in mounting technique. In the chorion are many such empty spaces. These spaces show quite conclusively that the limiting matter of the small spaces is syncytium, not a distinct cell-limiting membrane.

FIG. 2.—Serotinal villi from same ovum as Fig. 1. (1) Large villus, longitudinal section, shows beautifully the double layer; (2) the outer nuclei in a denser, more consolidated syncytial stroma; (3) the inner nuclei surrounded by a distinct halo, this limited by a structure interpreted as undigested plasm, giving the appearance of a cell-limiting membrane. This disappears with growth, so that at maturity there is only the nucleus left. (4) Other villi in cross-section. In smaller villi observe the plasm (5) of the central body continuous into the periphery (5) without apparent change in consistence and little in color. (6) Blood vessels: corpuscles, majority non-nucleated, in the minority is seen a commencing nucleation. Most of the corpuscles appear as mere dots, nuclei. In some spots an initial encircling orange-colored plasm is observed. This gives these corpuscles the appearance of a nucleus surrounded by an orange-colored (hematinized?) plasm. In my eight-week extra- and intrauterine specimens this latter is the characteristic structural appearance of the nucleated fetal blood corpuscle. (7) Inner nuclei can be traced directly into blood vessels, demonstrating that the nuclei are concerned in furnishing corpuscles for the blood. That the nuclei should serve as a source for corpuscles for the blood seems peculiarly appropriate, for their purpose is nutrition providers and carriers. (8) A short distance from this spot, close to the inner nuclei, is a blood vessel with a nucleus touching its wall. An empty space between two nuclei just above the vessel suggests that this nucleus wandered from the empty space to enter the vessel. In places the delicate walls of the blood vessels seem to touch the border of the inner nuclei, as though to favor their entrance. This idea is conveyed at 7'. It is beautifully shown and more clearly so in a two-months specimen worked up since this case commenced. (9) Maternal blood corpuscles which have been absorbed or have penetrated the syncytium and outer row nuclei as far as the inner row nuclei, not beyond. This phenomenon is repeatedly seen in the two-months villi; just beyond the inner row nuclei the larger nucleated corpuscles of the fetal blood vessels can be seen. (8) and (9) are sketched in, since they are beyond the focus here shown.

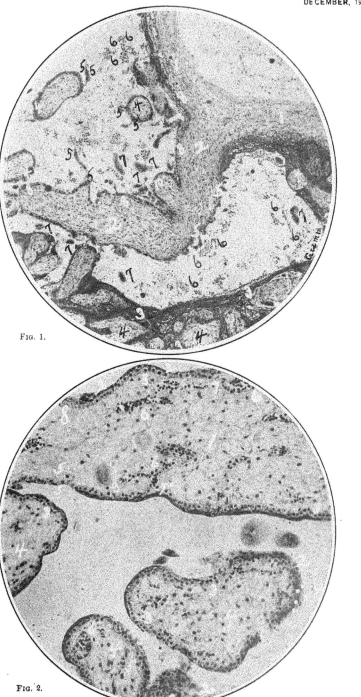

Fig. 1.

Fig. 2.

HISTOLOGY OF THE PLACENTAL VILLI.—*Stahl.*

brief citation from Ladinski's late article[1] will be *apropos*. In his paper he states that:

"The question whether this neoplasm [deciduoma malignum] takes its origin from maternal or fetal structures is still a mooted one, and will remain so until the origin of the epithelial covering of the chorionic villi is determined with some degree of accuracy.

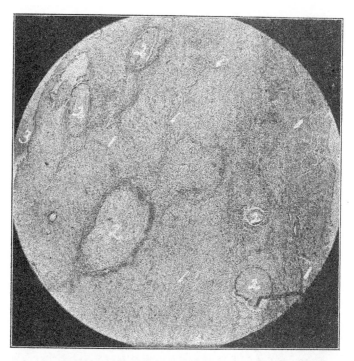

FIG. 3.—From two-weeks ampullary pregnancy. Oval desire to embed shows here a typical (tubal) mucous membrane inflammatory reaction. The intensity of this inflammation is like that characteristic of bacterial invasion, as in diphtheria. (1) Round-cell exudation. Field between round-cell margin and chorion made up of inflammatory exudate—(1') fibrin—lymphocytes, serum, and mucin. (2) Villi in cross-section. Compare with normal decidua serotina. (3) Chorion. Peripheral coverings well shown in these villi; already there is here a double row of nuclei, as in other villi. It shows conclusively a peripheral syncytial protoplasm without the intervention of the surface epithelium of the uterus (here tube), as advanced by Strahl, Merttens, Kossman, Von der Hoeven, and. J. Whitridge Williams. Another slide shows a longitudinal section of a villus, extending from the chorion to the tubal border of the inflammatory exudate, and examples the penetrating powers and length of a villus.

"All observers are now agreed, with very few exceptions, that this covering consists of a double layer of epithelium, as first pointed out by Langhans. The outer layer, that nearest the ex-

[1]Ladinski: "Deciduoma Malignum," AMERICAN JOURNAL OF OBSTETRICS, April, 1902, p. 467.

ternal wall, or syncytium, is composed of bands of protoplasm in which are very deeply staining nuclei of various shapes, arranged mostly in a single row, and not divided into definite cells. The inner layer, or Langhans-cell layer, consists of definitely marked cuboid or cylindrical epithelial cells. Beneath this is the connective-tissue stroma of the villi.

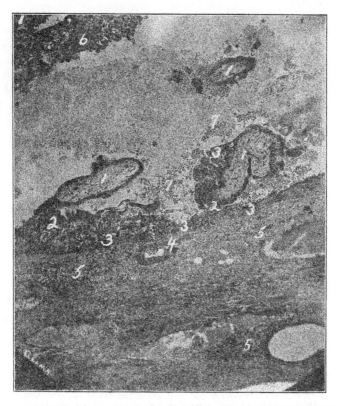

FIG. 4.—Section of tube wall, sixth to eighth week. (1) Villi with diffuse (Langhans Cell) nuClear (2) proliferation. nuClei without distinct cell wall structure, reaChing to (3) pseudo-serotina, made up of nuClear (Langhans cell) proliferatiVe tissue. (4) Eroding (malignant) effect of nuclei well shown, especially toward artery, whiCh is almost perforated. (5) ECtoblasts wandering into all the Coats of the tube. (6) InterVillous or bridging tissue made up of proliferatiVe synCytium and nuclei; for amplification see next illustration. (7) Maternal blood Corpuscles.

"There is, however, a decided difference of opinion as regards the origin of the syncytium and Langhans-cell layer. Thus we have (1) the theory of Kastschenko, Minot, Gottschall, and Albert, that the syncytium and Langhans-cell layer are both derived from the fetal ectoderm, that the syncytium is primary and the cell layer is derived from it; (2) that of **Hubrecht**, Peters, Marchand, and Aschoff, that the cell layer is primary and the syncytium derived from that; and (3) Strahl, Merttens, Kossmann, Van der Hoeven, and Williams believe that the Lang. hans-cell layer is of fetal origin and the syncytium is derived from uterine surface epithelium. The histology as well as the pathology of this disease, therefore, is far from settled and still remains a subject for controversy among pathologists.''

From my interpretations, as drawn from these studies of intra. and extrauterine specimens, I would offer the following:

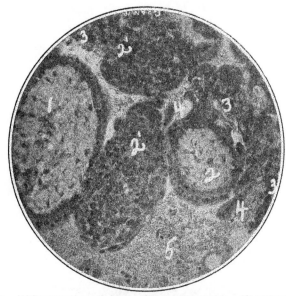

FIG. 5.—(1) Cross-section of large villus, extrauterine. (2) Oblique section of small villus. (3) Nuclear (Langhans Cell) proliferations, like tips (2') of villi. (4) Buds of syncytium with nuclei. (5) Maternal blood corpuscles. This specimen is from the proliferation tissue shown in the upper corner of Fig. 4. Both layers of nuclei in consolidated plasm. Observe nuclei here, same in general characteristics of form and size as nuclei in succeeding illustrations.

1. The syncytium with its cells, both layers, is fetal in origin.

2. The syncytium is the peripheral, muciparous stroma of the chorion or the villus as modified and added to by the ameboid activities of the nuclei (Langhans) upon their surrounding environmental tissues.

3. There is no distinct or technical cell structure presented in the so-called Langhans cell; there is only a characteristic nucleus present. In the inner layer, or Langhans layer, I find no distinct

cell structure, but a pseudo cell structure, a nucleus surrounded by a halo, and this limited by a more or less delicate filament consisting of consolidated syncytial stroma, giving the appearance of a technically considered cell-limiting membrane.

4. This is proved by (a) the appearance of the periphery of the villi in the latter half of pregnancy, after the fetal circulation has been established, where the villi show a gradual disappearance of the characteristic syncytial bordering protoplasm, with a corresponding loss of the encircling arrangement of the

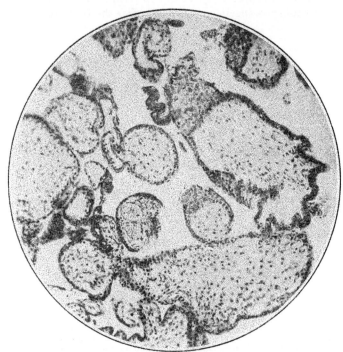

FIG. 6.—Villi in cross and partial section, intrauterine; from a three-months twin pregnancy, with single placenta, one cord—central; the second, velamentosal insertion. Double layer with inner (Langhans) cell-like appearance, again only consolidated, not yet assimilated syncytial plasm. Blood vessels with non-nucleated blood corpuscles, red and crenated appearing. Notice nuclei, especially in partially-sectioned villi, are without cell-limiting membrane. These nuclei are like those seen in extrauterine pregnancy and in malignant metastatic formations. See Figs. 5, 7, and 8.

nuclei (Langhans cells). As Minot puts it, "toward the end of pregnancy, however, the epithelium of the villi undergoes great alteration. On the larger villi a true epithelial investment has almost entirely disappeared, and instead isolated accumulations of large round nuclei are found and form protuberances *(Zell-knoten,* cell patches) on the surface of the villi.'' (*b*) By the appearance of the nuclei in the nuclear proliferation tissue con-necting the villi with the tube wall, Fig. 4 (2), where there is no cell-limiting membrane as in a technical cell. *(c)* By the appearance of the nuclei in the nuclear proliferation tissue con-necting the villi with the decidual serotina in the uterine preg-nancy. Here the contrast is definite, and shows that the nuclei

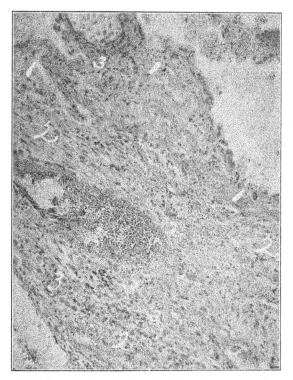

FIG. 7.—From tube wall of sixth to eighth week tubal pregnancy. (1) Sero-tinal aspect. (2) (Langhans) nuclei wandering throughout the tube wall. (3) Nuclei (in upper right corner), especially like nuclei in Fig. 6 and in Fig. 8, the latter from a deciduoma malignum.

of the proliferation tissue of the villus are without a cell-limit-ing membrane in a field of plasm, alongside the large decidual cell of the serotina, with its nucleus and characteristic cell-lim-iting membrane. (*d*) By the appearance of the nuclei in the metastatic formations of the syncytioma, where there is no cell-limiting membrane around the nuclei.

5. Syncytioma is the most correct term at the present time
descriptive of this neoplasm. Syncytioma refers to that particular structure only of the chorion or villus, and which possesses the wandering, invading, destructive, and ameboid
qualities characteristic of the syncytium and its nuclei. Further,
the term suggests a new growth, consisting of a dense protoplasm (syncytium) and nuclei (Langhans cells). Again, as
will be shown, the syncytium always leads in the sprouting
process of the chorion or villi, the nuclei follow in, this sprout-

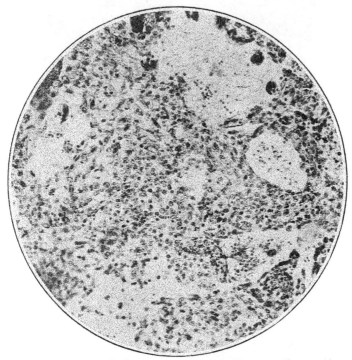

FIG. 8.—From Dr. C. S. Bacon's case of deciduoma malignum (AMERICAN
JOURNAL OF OBSTETRICS, vol. xxxi., 1895). Pulmonary metastasis. No cell
structures. Nuclei only; similarity to nuclei in Fig. 6, a normal three-months
villus; and nuclei in Fig. 7. a tube wall infiltrated with Langhans nuclei; similarity easily apparent.

ing naturally preceding the wandering of, or the possibility of,
metastatic formation of the free nuclei. As I show below, even
the free ectoblasts (nuclear division) are invested by syncytium
before they leave the mater syncytium. This term naturally,
and correctly so, excludes the thought of blood vessels and
other higher structures. Chorio-epithelioma, far more correct

than deciduoma malignum, suggests a higher order of histological merit than is present in the neoplasm. Deciduoma malignum is manifestly incorrect, for neither the decidua nor its cells give origin to the new growth.

6. Part of the nuclei in the syncytium become corpuscles of the blood. Examination of many specimens seems to confirm this thought. This seems not an untoward ultimate function for these nuclei. Control of many specimens indicates that nuclear division and growth, and naturally, therefore, of the young nuclei (ectoblasts) of the outer row, is directed outward away from the body of the villus, while the direction of disappearance

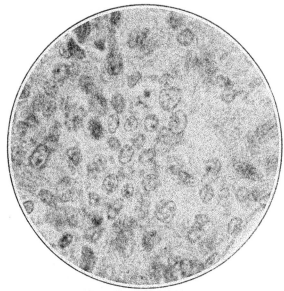

Fig. 9.—Large amplification of nuclei in Dr. C. S. Bacon's case of deciduoma malignum. Shows no Cell structure, onlY large Vesicular nuclei.

of the mature nuclei of the inner row is toward the interior of the villus. In Fig. 2 (7)· and (8) the nuclei can be traced into the blood vessels.

Again, in a two-months specimen maternal blood corpuscles are seen to penetrate through, or are absorbed by, the outer layer of the syncytium and nuclei; they extend unaltered to the inner row, but not beyond—that is, I find none. In Fig. 2 (9) I try to reproduce this effect. The penetration or absorption of these maternal blood corpuscles is not exceptional. It can be observed in many places and in many villi. I first noticed it in the extra-

50

uterine series, where I explained their appearance as material to be assimilated by the syncytium and nuclei. Another suggestion this specimen emphasizes is that the blood corpuscles (here of a two-months fetus) possess ameboid qualities—that is, they can convert outside (central and syncytial) nuclei into nucleated blood corpuscles.

Descriptive.—For the sake of clearness in description it will be convenient to speak of the early villus as presenting (1) a central body, chiefly composed of mesenchymal (mucous) tissue, in which are embedded the blood vessels, etc. (2) A peripheral border—the syncytial border—made up of syncytium, from the mesoderm, in which are several rows of nuclei (spoken of as cells—L.) from the ectoderm. This border is not a limiting membrane nor a true enveloping derm, as suggested in the term ectoderm. It is transitory in nature, disappearing as pregnancy advances, so that by maturity it exists only in the form of the isolated *Zellknoten.*

The early chorion presents externally a protoplasmic (mesenchymal) periphery, containing nuclei (double row, etc.), the so-called Langhans cells, forming the early or primal syncytium (Fig. 1). To the syncytium, with its nuclei, are given as physiologic function the properties of attacking, dissolving, and assimilating its environmental (decidua, tubal mucous membrane, peritoneum, etc.) tissues to furnish nutrition to the growing ovum. The villus is a bud, a sprout of the chorion, therefore alike in peripheral and somatic cell and stroma structure, also physiologic function. The syncytium of the villus is the same in structure and is directly continuous with the peripheral covering of the early chorion. The villi being the roots of nutrition for the ovum, in distal extremity they are unfixed, and to a certain extent need to wander as necessity of nutrition demands. Naturally, its syncytium develops a greater activity than that of the syncytium of the fixed chorion proper; therefore the greater thickness and the varying thicknesses of the syncytium in various villi of the same specimen. Both the two clearly differentiated layers of the so-called ectoderm (syncytium and nuclei) are similar in histological structure, alike both in stroma and cell. Both cell and stroma are interdependent and always associated. The stroma of the villus is a muciparous one; the villus, as a whole, in its early form and consistence might be spoken of as a highly organized gelatinous body. As has been noted, the syncytium of the villus is the peripheral muciparous stroma of the villus as modified by the activities of the nuclei, these activities corresponding to the exigencies of necessity and the resistance offered them in winning growth and nutrition for the ovum at the expense of the tissues of their environment. Hence, the syncytial protoplasm is denser than that of the central portion of the villus, for it contains in its primary stages much material, the process of nuclear and syncytial digestion of this environmental material. The outer nuclei of the early villus, with their surrounding plasm (their saliva of mastication), have a masticating and salivary function upon their environment; digestion is continued by the inner nuclei, and so on, alimentation being perfected in an inward direction. Nuclear growth occurs in an outward direction. To convert this compound granular protoplasm (villus peripheral stroma plus the absorbed broken-down particles of environmental tissues) into a clear plasm like the homogeneous plasm of the central body is also a function of the nuclei. This ameboid digestive function of the nuclei continues throughout villus expression. It is most active in the primary chorion and villi, decreasing, but not wholly disappearing, as maturity is reached. This waning of ameboid digestive function of the syncytium and nuclei is only natural, since it is consonant with the gradual lessening in the quantity of syncytium and nuclei of the villus as maturity increases. That it is not entirely lost is seen in its very slight expression (histological and physiological) in the maturer villus, for here they (syncytium and nuclei) are not so essential, since the source of nutrition now is primarily from the blood supply.

In the mature villus the perseverance of the few nuclei in the *Zellknoten* instead of the rich investment of the early villus suggests that they survive as the necessary and fitting few; that should occasion arise to demand a greater assimilative power than is possible in the more open stroma of the mature villus, then these few nuclei of the *Zellknoten* could attack the occasioning entity, break it down, and render it absorbable. As, for instance, a solid or semi-solid substance be carried by the blood current to the open stroma of the mature villus; then these few nuclei and syncytium would prove their fitness for the occasion and reason for surviving.

As budding occurs from either the chorion or villus, syncytial plasm is always projected first; then follow in its substance, and as secondary step in this budding, the nuclei. Before such a picture showing this budding process of the chorion or villus

it is .difficult to appreciate the philosophy of a maternal origin
for the syncytium. This characteristic of syncytial budding
argues against the maternal origin of the syncytium. For were
the syncytium of maternal origin, the current of initial syncytial
projection and growth should be toward the periphery of the
chorion and villi, instead of away from them toward the maternal tissues, which it does, and with so striking a malignant
effect upon those maternal tissues. The microscope always
shows an antagonistic syncytial outgrowth from the ovum
toward the uterus, not from the uterus toward the ovum.

The syncytium, both of the villus and of the chorion, in its
histological expression suggests a function similar to that seen
in the muciparous projection of other lower (reptilian, etc.) life,
viz., it halts, paralyzes, fixes, encapsulates, and assists its par-
enchymal cells, the nuclei, in the alimentation of its victims, the
tissues of its environment.

Peters' theory for the formation of the syncytium is that it
is due to the corrosive action of the maternal blood upon the
Langhans cells. In ·the early weeks of villus expression it is
easier to entertain Peters' theory as one of the causes in the
formation of the syncytium; but not as the only cause, rather
as one among several causes. But what of the corrosive action
in later villus expression, where blood activity and corrosive
possibility becomes progressively greater, and proportionately
is immensely greater? This latter thought argues against his
theory.

That the syncytium takes the stains more darkly (Figs. 1 to 7)
than the central portions of the villus stroma is due to several
causes; one, as just mentioned, the syncytium, because compound, is denser. Another factor is the greater consolidating
and hardening effects our laboratory media have upon such a
gelatinous, muciparous periphery than upon its inner central
parts. Another is the effect of the absorption and consequent
reflection of the greater amount of staining fluid taken up by the
nuclei; this effect is increased by the close arrangement of the
rows of nuclei (Langhans).

This peripheral hardening effect, due to surrounding media,
may be readily followed and seen in so simple an experiment as
a drop of the white of an egg dropped upon a slide. In a few
moments a distinct, dense, peripheral rim is observed; wipe off
the drop with a rag, a denser rim is left after the body is wiped

away. Repeat. Stain with methylene blue and observe the differences in density and shade. Control with microscope.

It is described that the ectoderm of the villi, in its earliest stages, consists of two clearly differentiated layers, a thinner outer one with smaller nuclei and without cell boundaries, and an inner one consisting of distinct cells with large nuclei (Minot). Under a low power (50, etc.) the slide on first sight seems to show a separate cell arrangement, the idea conveyed in the many illustrations of special book and article. But closer examination, even with this power, creates a doubt as to a technical cell arrangement, which is increased as the power is raised. This observation holds true, also, when applied to the slide of the syncytial neoplasm. The distinct cell picture (Fig. 2) of the inner layer, on cross-section especially, is due, I think, to several causes. One, the greater consolidating effect of the laboratory media upon the peripheral outer layer than upon the inner layer, must be taken into account. Another, the difference in the digestive-ameboid, function effect of the nuclei. The nuclei of the outer layer are more aggressive to their nutrient environmental tissues than are those of the inner layer; they have no time for assimilation of this extraneous nutrient material. This is perfected by the nuclei of the inner row; these change the denser compound granular outer protoplasm into a transparent gelatinous material similar to that of the plasm of the villus proper. *Each nucleus, having a circular influence* (Fig. 2 (3) and Fig. 6), *clears a circular space around itself, leaving, and bounded thereby, a slight intermediate margin of plasm persisting for future assimilation; thus there is given to the inner row its separate cell appearance.* Again, the separate cell appearance of the inner or Langhans layer is not always present; the consolidation persists (Figs. 4 and 5). Even in the outer layer the nuclei in some places are seen surrounded by a commencing halo, as though by a lighter protoplasm. This could be interpreted as indicative of a primitive cell formation, with commencing limiting membrane. My interpretation reads that it is due to the commencing digestive effect of the outer nuclei upon their surrounding compound plasm, giving such contiguous plasm a clearer and more transparent effect; therefore this pale halo or cell effect. Occasionally a fissure is seen in the syncytium, as though the contracting agent caused so great shrinking as to induce a fissure.

Examination of many sections shows central stroma insensibly merging into peripheral or syncytial stroma, and without apparent change in texture, often without noticeable change in color, Fig. 2 (5), suggesting an unbroken uniformity in tissue structure; at other times the syncytium is tinged with a greater eosinophilic character. In these latter cases it seems again reflexive, and due to the reflexion of the abundant staining material in the profuse cell proliferation. Again, in many sections, as oblique sections, the outer nuclei are not characteristically smaller than the inner; they vary in size; often large cells (nuclei) are externally and smaller cells (nuclei) internally. This is especially so in the extrauterine specimens. In some villi where the peripheral cells (nuclei) are almost absent, no color shades are noticeable between the peripheral and somatic stroma, similar in effect to the picture of the mature villi. This absence of syncytium and nuclei in some early villi can be explained on the theory of precocity.

From the foregoing I am led to believe that the cell bodies in the outer layer, spoken of as nuclei without cell boundaries, and the cell bodies in the inner layer, known as Langhans cells, are similar structures—nuclei only. Their surrounding plasm is without a limiting membrane, from the muciparous stroma plasm proper of the villus or of the chorion. Therefore the great deviation in size and form of the nucleus, the so-called Langhans cell, when detached from the villus. At times (Figs. 1 and 5) there is a small nucleus, with large surrounding syncytial plasm; again, a comparatively small surrounding syncytial plasm with many nuclei; again, the syncytial giant cell in its many forms and sizes; likewise the disparity in size and appearance of the nucleus in the nuclear proliferations and intervillous connecting link or bridging tissue, so well shown in the extrauterine pregnancy (Figs. 4 and 5).

Nuclear division (the Langhans cell of description) is not by mitosis; I can find none. I find only irregular cell division, in this respect resembling the pathologic karyokinesis seen in the malignant tumor. The nucleus (Langhans) viewed toward the mesoderm is of a round, polygonal, or oval form, and seems to have one, sometimes several, prominent nuclei, with traces of granules; as it nears and as it occurs in the outer syncytial periphery of the villus, the nucleus seems to have grown in activity, and now contains many nucleoli; the prominent nucleus is not apparent; the nuclear definition disappears, leaving a cell-like cluster of many separate nucleoli. Liberated into the surrounding muciparous stroma, these small bodies, ectoblasts Fig. 1 (6), are bathed, so to speak, with a muciparous (syncytial) surrounding plasm variable in thickness. These minute ectoblasts wander into surrounding tissues, directly and through the vessels, both in intra- and extrauterine pregnancy. In this aberrant structure of the nucleus (Langhans cell) lies some explanation of the difference in function between the decidual cell with its apparent distinct limiting membrane and the (Langhans) nuclear cell without such limiting membrane. The large white decidual cell is essentially a defender of maternal tissue; the syncytial nucleus, on the contrary, is a rover, a freebooter cell, which, before it consumes maternal tissue, must paralyze, hence the necessity for a free surrounding neutralizing plasm.

In the intrauterine pregnancy these infant ectoblasts are the advance posts of the villus; by their direct wandering they blaze the way into the surrounding tissues for the advancing villus by neutralizing, breaking down, and making readily absorbable the tissue structures of its environment, the decidua.

In the extrauterine pregnancy their function is a similar one, but here the picture suggests a far greater nuclear activity than in the intrauterine case. In one of the specimens from which Fig. 3 is taken a villus is seen extending all the way from the chorion down through the inflammatory exudate to its tubal margin. In the intrauterine form the nuclear activity meets with a passive resistance, as though the decidua was intended as a nutrient material for the invading but expected ovum. In the extrauterine pregnancy the nuclear activity is, and must be, greater, for here the ovum acts as an invading organism, with virulent parasitical characteristics (Fig. 3). Its every step of growth is typical of anger, like the cancer cell, as seen in its virulent active deprecatory invasion of true and various splanchnic parenchyma.

In both forms of pregnancy these ectoblasts and their maturer forms functionate like malignoblasts to the maternal tissues, more especially so in the extrauterine pregnancy.

In the intrauterine pregnancy their malignant ions are probably neutralized to a great extent by decidual function.

The picture of the early villus suggests a gelatinous tissue, expansion and rapid growth, with great nuclear activity.

The picture of the mature villus suggests a connective tissue, consolidation *(fibrosis)* and early decadence, with little nuclear activity.

In the mature villus, all stroma, the connective tissue in the trunks, and the semi-connective tissue of the buds, because of this fibrosis and consolidation, are eosinophilic, where in the earlier villus it is neutral because of its more muciparous character. In the mature villus the peripheral syncytial arrangement is not so pronounced as in the earlier villus, again because of this maturer general fibrosis. The fewer nuclei and nuclear groups of the periphery of the mature villus are the mature forms of the nuclei (the Langhans cells of description) of the early villus, now likewise showing in their denser bodies the consolidation of maturity and the waning activity of adolescence.

Embryonal growth seems essentially a nuclear one (in the usual descriptive sense). The syncytial plasmic proliferation is consonant with nuclear activity, this activity giving to the syncytial plasm virulent qualities. In the expression of the cancer juice and the cancer cell we see its analogue.

It is with pleasure that I acknowledge herewith the high technical merit and artistic enthusiasm extended me by Dr. Carl T. Gramm, Chicago, in his preparation of the photomicrographs.

RUPTURE OF THE UMBILICAL CORD.[1]

BY

HERBERT MARION STOWE, M.D.,
Demonstrator of Operative Obstetrics, Northwestern University Medical School;
Assistant Obstetrician to Provident Hospital.
Chicago.

(With illustration.)

I wish to premise my remarks by the report of two cases of traumatic partial rupture of the umbilical cord in pregnancy.

Mrs. A., aged 27, was pregnant with her second child about eight months. On June 30, 1902, while standing near her carriage, the horse suddenly kicked her in the abdomen with his hind foot. The patient was knocked down and was dazed for half an hour, but did not lose consciousness. The abdominal wall was bruised and discolored, especially in the left of the hypogastric region, where the horse's foot landed, but sustained no laceration or puncture. About thirty-five minutes after the accident the patient complained of violent fetal movements that

[1] Read before the Chicago Gynecological Society, September 19, 1902.

soon became so vigorous as to cause nausea and dizziness. The movements increased to a maximum and then gradually weakened until they were felt no more. These movements lasted fifteen minutes. When called to the case I was unable to find any heart tones or to obtain any fetal motions. The cervix was closed and there was no bleeding. The temperature was 99.6°, the pulse 100, weak and nervous. The history of the accident and the absence of any signs of fetal life led me to believe that the child was dead, and, knowing that if such were the case labor would occur spontaneously in a short time, I adopted the method of watchful expectancy. The first labor pains started in twenty-six hours after the accident. Several efforts to obtain the fetal heart sounds in the interim had failed and no life had been felt by the mother. After a normal labor of six hours the fetus (a male) was born dead. The placenta came away in

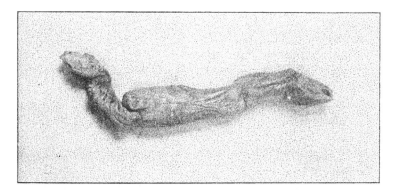

thirty minutes with slight hemorrhage. The mother made an excellent recovery.

The cord was 42 centimetres long, was inserted into the centre of the placenta, and was coiled around the child's neck twice, but not so tightly as to leave any marks. The partial rupture occurred 14 centimetres from the navel, the umbilical vein being the injured vessel. A hematoma had formed within the sheath or capsule, measuring two inches long, seven-eighths of an inch in diameter, and three inches in circumference. There was no tearing of the sheath. The cord was moderately thick and varicose in the fetal portion and contained three spirals. Between the rupture and the navel the cord was bloodless, measuring only a centimetre in width, while that portion between the rupture and the afterbirth was from two to three times as thick, was black and engorged with blood. The arteries were apparently normal. At the point of rupture the blood had been forced out into the Wharton's jelly and could be seen through the sheath as dark, ecchymotic areas irregularly distributed under the surface of the capsule.

The most reasonable theory in regard to this peculiar and rare accident seems to be that the cord at the site of the injury was lying, not around the neck, but on the child's back and next to the anterior wall of the uterus. The scarcity of liquor amnii in this instance allowed the cord to lie between two practically solid bodies, the fetal back and the uterine wall. The abdominal wall was very thin and the fetus could be readily palpated externally. The impact of the horse's hoof destroyed the integrity of the venous wall and caused an extravasation of blood into the surrounding tissues. The blood already in the fetal body was removed by way of the arteries and was found in the placenta and the proximal portion of the cord, while the fetus and the peripheral cord were left pale and bloodless. It is doubtful whether such an accident could have happened to a healthy cord, excepting when accompanied by more extensive injury to the abdominal wall. There was, however, a history of syphilis in this case, as evidenced by a former skin eruption, falling out of the hair, etc., and a stillbirth two years ago. The present fetus was poorly developed and the skin was loose and much wrinkled.

The second case is one of the more common variety of funic rupture.

Mrs. G., aged 29, IIIpara, had a rapid labor lasting two hours and thirty minutes. The pains occurred every two minutes and were violent in character. The patient was up and walking around the room, leaning on the bedpost, when the pains came on. Immediately upon my entering the room the patient gave a shriek, and while standing the fetus was forced out of the pelvis by a violent contraction and fell to the floor with a thud before I could reach her side. The cord was torn across eight centimetres from the navel, the rupture being oblique and ragged. There was no hemorrhage. The fetal end was tied and the mother quickly carried back to bed. The placenta came away in ten minutes, weighed one and a quarter pounds, and was uniformly fibrous. The cord measured 37 centimetres in length, was thin, bloodless, and, excepting a few varicosities, possessed no anomalies. The amnion and chorion were thick and fibrous. There was no perineal laceration.

It is a noteworthy fact that the strength and resistance of the umbilical cord have been greatly over-estimated. The earlier authors denied the assertion that the powers of spontaneous labor were great enough to effect a rupture either partially or totally, but increased experience and the occasional reports of cases must convince us not only as to its possibility but also as to its not infrequent occurrence.

One can no longer doubt that the majority of cord lacerations are caused by the excessive force of the expellent powers rather than any pathological condition of the cord itself, although a diseased or non-developed cord is certainly more fragile and easily ruptured than the normal and healthy one. The great rarity of rupture occurring in pregnancy before the cord has reached its full state of development precludes a positive opinion on the subject.

The fact that the powers of premature labor are weaker than those of term labor the farther the two are separated in point of time, has a great influence upon the rarity of such a rupture. In addition, the difference in the weight of the fetuses, as well as the increased elasticity of the cord in pregnancy and its increasing friableness as gestation continues, would serve to counterbalance any tendency to rupture by reason of any weakness due to non-development. The effects of torsion and consequent pressure atrophy of the umbilical vessels are equalized by the poor development of the embryo and the lack of purchase or grip the uterus would have to expel the fetus with great violence at term. Syphilis would have a similar effect, though not as marked; in fact, many of the pathological changes in the cord can be traced to this infection.

Protracted gestation theoretically would predispose to rupture on account of the increased effort of the uterus necessary to expel the over-mature head through the birth canal, especially if the pelvic floor has been torn in previous labors. The over-mature cord is weakened by fatty or calcareous change and its resistance correspondingly lessened.

Velpeau attributes rupture of the cord to some disease causing small dilatations or " small aneurysmal or varicose pouches," and states that he has seen these pouches rupture at term and communicate with a large clot which covered a large part of the placenta, which had not ruptured the amnion.

Rupture is undoubtedly favored by these varicosities or looped condition of its vessels, which prevents the operating force from being equally distributed over the entire length of the cord. We find that that part of the cord is most liable to tear that lies nearest to the central axis, that is, the funic sheath in the concavity of the loop, then generally the vessels, and finally the convex surface of the loop. The great abundance of the varicosities in the fetal portion of the cord readily explains the usual situation of the tear.

The cord ruptures either by a gradual pressure which forces the child through the pelvis, or by the sudden jerk which accompanies its exit. The first factor is rarely seen. The retracting uterus and placenta keep pace with the advancing child and the cord is always long enough in spite of its being wound about the body or neck. The great stretching the cord is capable of, from eighteen to thirty-five per cent of its length, serves to render this factor rarely operative in producing a rupture.

In the great majority of cases the rupture occurs when the fetus is nearly out of the uterus, and the head emerging from the pelvic outlet, and the cord thin or fragile and tightly wound round the child's neck. The mother at the moment of delivery is in the erect or nearly erect posture, walking about, and dropping to her knees as the child is born, or sitting in the closet and precipitating the child into the vault. Not a few cases, however, have been seen where the child has been violently forced out with the mother lying on her back in bed, and thrown, as in one case, a distance of fifty centimetres from the pelvic outlet. Budin reports two cases where the funic rupture occurred from the combined forces of the uterus and the abdominal walls while the patients were lying on their backs, and the subsequent examination of the cords showed nothing abnormal. Budin also quotes two other cases, one by Schatz and one by Duprey.

The powers of labor acting in fetal expulsion have been variously estimated. Houghton, one of the earlier writers, placed it at 512¾ pounds. Poullet gave it as 50 pounds. Duncan and Poppel measured the extremes at 5 pounds in easy and 50 pounds in difficult labor. Schatz, by means of his toco-dynamometer, finds the limits to be from 17 to 55 pounds, and this is not far from correct. These figures prove that the powers of labor are great enough to produce a rupture unaided by any outside forces.

A cord of 25 centimetres will allow of a normal delivery. If, however, its length be under 25 centimetres, one or more of four things must take place. These, in the order of frequency, are as follows, viz.: placental separation, rupture of the cord, inversion of the uterus, and ventral hernia of the child, all more or less combined with a partial lengthening of the cord. Inversion of the uterus and ventral hernia are rare. It is somewhat difficult to understand the mechanism of placental separation by gradual traction, unless we take into account the fact that during a pain when the cord is taut the fetus might strike it with his feet and thus slightly separate the placenta from the uterine wall, and then the retroplacental blood clot, aided perhaps by repeated kicks, would suffice to complete the separation. The ease with which a child kicks and moves his limbs about during a contraction depends upon the amount of liquor amnii present separating the uterine wall from the fetal body, and hence would occur more frequently in the intact bag of waters. That the fetus can and does move his limbs during a pain is a clinical fact, but his movements are certainly interfered with after the membranes have ruptured. Cazeaux in his text book states as follows: " It appears to me that such a separation can scarcely occur from a mere dragging of the cord, because during the uterine contraction the placenta is strongly pressed by the womb externally and the liquor amnii internally, and still more so, after the escape of the waters, by the body of the child. Now, these parts must react upon the fetal surfaces of the placenta with all the force of compulsion communicated by the contraction. Of course the fetus can only advance, and so the tension of the cord can only take place by the contraction, and I repeat that while it lasts the placenta is moulded on and is forcibly compressed by the parts contained within the sac and of necessity cannot be separated from the womb. I believe, therefore, that a separation of the placenta from the tension of the cord is almost impossible during the continuance of the contraction.''

Négrier was the first to investigate the resisting power of the umbilical cord. This author fastened the cord to a pulley and loaded it down with weights until it broke. In varicose cords he found it needed 3,000 grammes; in non-varicose cords, 5,250 grammes. Following him came Spaeth, of Vienna, who took twenty cords of normally-born children and weighted them

down with weights. These tests gave an average of eleven
pounds. In six cases (30 per cent) it required the weight of an
ordinary child of five to seven pounds. In four cases (20 per
cent) it necessitated a weight of more than double that of the
child, fifteen to twenty-three pounds. Carl Braun also obtained
similar results, and states that in precipitates where the full
weight of the child is brought to bear upon the cord there is
not only a great possibility but an almost certainty of rupture.
In these tests, as pointed out by Hohl, the cord was ruptured
by a gradual stretching and not by a sudden jerk as happened
in labor.

Before a complete rupture occurs a partial rupture often
takes place. This usually occurs in the capsular sheath in one or
more longitudinal rents which may connect with each other
by cross tears. Sometimes the vein tears before the arteries,
sometimes before the capsule. In one of my experiments the
arteries tore before the vein, in three the vein tore first. In
several cords I found a partial rupture of the sheath by the action of a falling weight of three to five pounds, and I believe
with Pfannkuch that small tears are more frequent than is
commonly believed, but are not looked for by the attendant.

Experiments have been made from time to time to ascertain the
relative strength of the arteries and the vein. Clifton Wintring-
ham found that the vein was to the artery as 26 was to 25. The
vena cava supported a water column of $176\frac{1}{4}$ feet, and the
aorta only 158 feet and 11 inches, or a proportion of 1,110 to
1,000. The iliac vein has been found to be greater than the
iliac artery by the ratio of 1,034 to 1,000. The portal vein of
the sheep is to the aorta as 1,414 is to 1,000. On the other hand,
Stephen Hales found that the jugular vein supported a water
column of 175 feet without breaking, while the carotid artery
broke under a pressure of 190 feet.

One of the most plausible explanations as to the prior rupture
of the vein is found in the fact that it not infrequently happens
that the vein does not lie free in the cord, but is adherent in one
or more places to the amniotic sheath, and when traction is made
the arteries are more elastic than the adherent vein. The vein
tears first and with it a portion of the adherent capsule.

The form of the rupture is largely dependent upon the manner in which the acting force is applied. The torn ends are
usually ragged and irregular, seldom transverse and even cut.

The more gradual the tension, the more the elasticity of the cord comes into play; the more numerous the spiral turns and the more irregular the course of the vessels, the more oblique and jagged is the tear, and, *vice versa,* the more sudden the jerk and the smoother the cord, the more transverse and regular is the tear.

Another factor of rupture of the cord is found in the velamentous insertion into the placenta. In many of these cases the vessels can be felt as they run in front of the presenting part of the child. The membranes are apt to rupture early in labor, tearing the vessels across and causing serious hemorrhage which will cause the child's death unless the delivery is speedily accomplished. The fetal mortality in this complication is large; according to Winckel, 18 per cent of the children die from pressure on the cord and a much larger percentage die from rupture. It is of prime importance in velamentous insertion of the cord, where the vessels can be palpated through the cervix uteri, to preserve the membranes as long as possible or until the conditions are such that immediate delivery can be effected. I believe the best instrument for this purpose is the colpeurynter, thereby opposing fluid pressure by fluid pressure.

Finally, we may rupture the cord in performing version or in the subsequent extraction. The powerful pressure of the cord between the head and the pelvis may destroy the integrity of the vessel wall and so cause obstruction and death.

The bleeding from a ruptured cord is usually very slight. In 21 of 183 cases of torn cords collected by Klein there was no hemorrhage at all. This fact accords with a general law in all the animal world, where the cord is bitten off by the mother immediately after birth. In these cases, owing to the jagged ends of the vessels and the general bruising of the parts, very few of the young die from hemorrhage. Severe hemorrhage is not likely to result, except in cases of abnormal coursing of the vessels. It is nearly always absent if the tear takes place some distance from the navel. Bleeding is very liable to occur if the cord is torn off at the navel, and especially so if torn actually within the umbilical ring.

The treatment of the more common variety of rupture of the cord may be summed up in a few words. Most important is the prophylaxis. Always aim to confine the mother on the bed in the recumbent posture, and always be on hand to control the rapidity of the delivery. If the rupture has occurred the cord should be ligated as in ordinary cases. If the cord has ruptured inside of the umbilical ring, or so close that it is impossible to tie the cord, we may transfix the navel with two steel pins at right angles to each other and then secure the vessels by passing a ligature under the pins and tying.

In the following experiments recently made, much of the material was obtained from the Chicago Lying-in Hospital through the courtesy of Dr. De Lee and the remainder from my own cases.

The first ten cords were tested to ascertain the dead weight necessary to produce a rupture. One end of the cord was fastened to a transverse beam and the other end loaded down with the weight. The cords were washed free of blood and then filled with sufficient normal salt solution to restore as closely as possible the intrapartum condition. The cords were then tied at both ends and during the test were measured to find the percentage of stretching obtained before rupture.

TABLE I

No.	Appearance of Cord.	Length.	Weight sufficient to tear, in grammes.	Percentage of stretching.
1	Thick, several nodes in fetal portion.	36	2300	19.3
2	Thin, spiral, no nodes or loops.	42	3250	22.6
3	Much twisted, full of blood.	42	2800	28.2
4	Thin, no loops, few nodes on fetal end.	50	5600	32.4
5	Moderately thick, generally spiral.	36	7650	21.6
6	Thin, no loops, no nodes.	41	6100	24.9
7	Thick, much looped.	38	4250	29.4
8	Thin three loops in fetal end.	48	3250	34.8
9	Thick, many nodes in fetal end.	38	2800	26.6
10	Thick full of blood, two loops in placental end.	40	4000	24.2

Taking the average of these tests, we find that a cord 45 centimetres long will break with a weight of 4,097 grammes, or about 8⅓ pounds, and will stretch 26.4 per cent of its length. The force applied to the cord, however, is not a dead weight, but a weight falling a distance not greater than the length of the cord itself. In fact, the fetus is shot out of the pelvis with a certain velocity much greater than that of a weight falling from a certain height.

The next ten cords were subjected to the insult of a weight falling the entire length of the cord:

TABLE II.

No.	Appearance of Cord.	Length.	Breaks at weight, in grammes.	Length of fetal end.	Description of tear
1	In fetal end badly twisted.	48	750	3 .	Uneven; oblique arteries project.
2	Medium thick, fetal end varicose.	50	500	......	Tear transverse in loop.
3	Thin, nodes and loops in fetal end.	48	1000	4.5	Ragged. oblique.
4	Thick, full of blood, three loops in fetal end.	38	500	3	Transverse; artery tears first.
5	Thick, nodes in placental end.	42	850	9	Ragged, oblique.
6	Medium thin, generally looped.	52	1000	4	As No. 3.
7	Two loops in centre, many nodes.	33	500	12	Oblique; vessels long.
8	Thin, looped in fetal end.	34	750	7.5	Ragged, oblique.
9	Thick, full of blood, nodes in placental end.	48	750	4.5	Oblique; tear of sheath.
10	Thin, no loo	48	750	4.5	Transverse; vessels torn short.

In this series only two cords were able to stand a weight of 1,000 grammes, though they may have been injured somewhat by the previous trials of 500, 750, and 850 grammes respectively. Four cords ruptured with only 500 grammes and two with 750. The cord is therefore able to stand a still weight much greater than that of a falling weight, in the two series showing an average difference of 710 and 4,097 grammes. This difference is explained by the elasticity of the cord. When subjected to a steady pull the cord stretches from 19.3 to 34.8 per cent of its length. If the test is made suddenly there is no time for stretching and the force is brought to bear at the weakest point before it can be equally distributed over the entire cord.

But the child never falls the entire length of its cord. We must subtract the distance from the fundus uteri to the pelvic outlet, and also take into account the coils that may encircle the neck and so hinder the velocity of the fall by their gradual unwinding.

The following cords were then tested by allowing the attached weight to fall one-half the entire length of the cord:

TABLE III.

No.	Appearance of Cord.	Length.	Breaks at weight, in grammes.	Length of fetal portion.	Description of tear.
1	Thin, well looped.	35	1000	15	Oblique; vein tears first.
2	Thin, two loops in fetal end.	46	1000	8	Entire cord tore transversely.
3	Thin, uniformly looped.	38	1000	16	Oblique; ragged vein tears, then arteries.
4	Thick, nodes in fetal end.	84	900	18	Long; tear of sheath, then ragged.
5	Thick (?), looped in fetal end.	49	900	12	Ragged, oblique.
6	Thin, nodes in placental portion.	56	700	14	Oblique; sheath, then vein.
7	Thick, no nodes, few loops in placental end.	42	750	26	Varix in placental end broken.

When the weight falls a distance equal to the entire length of the cord, the fetal portion is from a fifth to a seventh of the whole, whereas when the weight falls but a half of the distance the tear occurs in the 'middle. The nearer the cord tears to the acting force, the more sudden and violent that force is.

Rupture of the cord in labor is favored by one or more of the following factors:

1. The greater liability of the living cord breaking than the dead one. As shown by Casper, the experiments upon the postpartum cord do not accurately interpret the true factors which act on the living and pulsating cord. The cord whose vessels are filled with blood and whose tissues are filled with serum is shorter in length, the loops are more numerous, and its weaker spots are more exposed to external injury. Hence any difference between the living and dead cord must be taken as favoring the earlier rupture in the living one. In the experiments made by the writer the blood vessels were refilled with salt solution and ligated at both ends, except in a few cases where the test was made at the bedside with the cord filled with warm fluid blood.

Inasmuch as the child is forcibly expelled from the pelvis at the moment of birth, it is given a certain velocity which varies in different cases. The table given where the weight fell the length of the entire cord gives more accurate results than where it fell only half that distance, because at the midway point the weight has already gained a velocity similar to that possessed by the child. Where the force of gravity is added to the powers of labor the liability of rupture is of course greatly increased.

Rupture of the cord may be hindered by the loosening or separation of the placenta from the uterine wall. The traction made on the cord by the child pulls the placenta down into the lower uterine segment, and if no further resistance is offered it may be expelled with the child. If the cervix uteri should close enough to offer resistance to the afterbirth, the sudden obstruction would suffice to tear the cord, even though it lay loose in the uterine cavity. If the uterus should be in a state of relaxation at the moment of birth and the placenta adherent to it, the tug of the fetal weight would result in an inversion of the uterus. This accident, while rare, is not unknown.

If the cord is wound around the child's neck and pulled tightly, it is as liable to tear as in the other cases. Where the coils are loose the tension comes gradually into play, and the child is born in a kind of evolution and the rupture is prevented.

4433 LAKE AVENUE.

BIBLIOGRAPHY.

Archiv. f. Gynäkologie, Bd. vii., S. 28.
Lehrbuch der Geburtshülfe, S. 445.
Pract. Handbuch der gerichtl. Med., vol. i., S. 827. Casper.
Traité complet des Accouchements, 1835.
Morphologie der menschl. Nabelschnur, S. 55.
AMERICAN JOURNAL OF OBSTETRICS, February, 1899.
Progrès Médical, 1888.
American Text Book of Obstetrics.
Philadelphia Obstetrical Society, 1888.
London Lancet, 1844, p. 635.
Obstetrical Journal of Great Britain and Ireland, 1880.
Text Book of Obstetrics, Cazeaux and Tarnier.
Klinik der Geburts. u. Gynäk., 1885.
AMERICAN JOURNAL OF OBSTETRICS, May, 1901.
Text Book of Obstetrics, Spiegelberg.
Zeit. f. Geb. u. Gynäk., 1897, No. 36, S. 470.
Deutsch. med. Zeit., 1887.
Jour. de Médecine de Bordeaux.
Archiv. f. Gynäk., Bd. ix.
London Lancet, 1881, vol. ii., p. 1109.
Medical Age, January 26, 1891.
British Medical Journal, 1882, vol. ii., p. 132.

PUBERTY IN THE GIRL.[1]

BY

GEORGE WYTHE COOK, M.D.,
Washington, D. C.

THE highest and noblest function of the medical profession is the prevention of disease; and while the energizing of that function might seem to militate against the practice of medicine as a vocation in which to earn a livelihood, nevertheless it is a subject for congratulation to believe that the profession as a whole, and in its integral parts as well, has ardently striven in every possible way to eliminate the causes of disease from amongst us. I know there are those who seek to discredit these efforts and to minimize the results thus far attained, but they belong to that class which inveighs against vivisection, pooh-poohs vaccination, and trade-marks itself for the purpose of gain. In bringing to the attention of the Fellows of this Society anything that relates to the prevention of disease, even in a remote degree, I am sure of the ground upon which I stand and am confident of their interest and sympathy. Could one conceive that this race of people would eat and drink and clothe itself in such a reasonable way as is indicated by the laws of hygiene, we might expect it to be healthy, as is its natural state. But, alas! we are of those whose god is their belly, and who hitch themselves to the wheels of the chariot of fashion with such alacrity that there seems to be little hope left for an early redemption. Nevertheless I venture to offer some suggestions—which, though they are not new, should be of especial interest to a society such as this is—upon the subject of puberty in the girl. Children, male and female, are much alike up to the period of puberty. They exercise alike, romping and playing together without restraint, but as soon as sexual peculiarities are assumed a marked change is manifest. The boy separates himself from his girl companions; he becomes grosser and more self-reliant; he assumes an air of importance, but continues to

[1]President's address before the Washington Obstetrical and Gynecological Society, October 3, 1902.

engage in such sports and out-of-door exercise as tend to develop his physique in a healthy way. Not so with the girl. Her childish freedom of manners gives place to coyness and maidenly timidity. Her narrow, flat chest expands into a more capacious bust for the better accommodation of heart and lungs. The proportions of her pelvis are increased; the deposition of connective and adipose tissue transforms her angular figure into the rounded, graceful contour of the young maiden. Her eyes sparkle with a new lustre which is partially concealed by the drooping lids above them. The " mantling blood flows in her lovely cheeks '' and gives a coloring beyond the skill of painter to imitate. Her voice is soft and melodious. She is at the period when " brook and river meet,'' and is upon the eve of that which transforms her from childhood to beautiful and complete womanhood. She is ready, and awaits the great change; and when it comes she is *perfect*.

This picture but inadequately describes what woman should be in her normal state. But what do we find in consequence of the artificial conditions that surround her? Instead of the beautiful, blooming creature that she should be by nature, she is a pale, wan, and anemic weakling, poorly prepared for the great change that is to transform her into a procreating woman. Her development is far below what Nature has a right to expect, and her menstrual function is spasmodically and imperfectly performed. In a state of health, this and all functions of the body are performed without the consciousness of the individual, and unless there is departure from health there should be no so-called critical periods incident to the cycle of existence. To what is this defective development to be attributed? It lies in the fact that at the period of her existence when the girl needs much of blood and nutrition for the perfecting of her sexual peculiarities and the rounding out of her physical form, she is placed under circumstances that diminish rather than enhance her blood-making powers. Instead of being out-of-doors, exercising her young muscles and breathing the pure air of heaven and gaining the robustness that is necessary for her peculiar function to the race, the poor young thing, under the high tension of her school life, is so absorbed in the *pursuit of knowledge* and the various *fashionable accomplishments* that she has no time for such commonplace things. She is restraining the flowing spirits and joyous freedom of youth while she *studies the laws of physiology and hygiene*. I would not underrate the value of thorough education for women; but if the so-called " thorough education " is to be acquired at the expense or to the detriment of her health, there can be no question as to what course should be pursued. It is of *paramount* importance that our women should be healthy, for how can it be expected that they will be prolific and the mothers of a healthy progeny if they themselves are not vigorous? What does it advantage a woman to *attempt* to unravel the laws of physics, or to wrestle with " abstruse points in philosophy," or to solve difficult problems in mathematics, if by so doing she violates the laws of her own existence, lays the foundation for uncertain health, and renders herself unfit to be the mother of a healthy offspring? The obligation that woman owes to the race as the medium of its reproduction is far greater than any other, and just so far as that reproductive function is impaired and rendered ineffective, just so far does she fall short in her noble prerogative. I do not hesitate to say that if the choice for the girl were to lie between the road to learning and the highway to health, the latter should unquestionably be selected.

This declaration, I have no doubt, might be received by the laity with much disdain in this educational day, when in our schools all thought is turned toward investigating the laws of Nature and so little attention is paid to their practical application, especially in the case of girls. It may be said that this is in effect to assign woman to an inferior place. Such, however, is not the case, for I regard her as not only not inferior but superior to man in moral qualities and in many mental attributes. She is more liable to disease than man, but she endures pain and suffering with greater fortitude. She is not like him either anatomically, physiologically, mentally, or morally, but she is indeed his " better half." I would not abridge or hinder her *proper* education. I would have her trained in all that goes to make her a sweet and lovely woman and that fits her to become a *willing* and devoted mother. It is far more noble and far more elevated to be queen of the household, rearing lovely and healthy children, teaching them by precept and example to appreciate the true and the beautiful, and dispensing such hospitality as becomes her surroundings, than it is to be jostled in the mad rush for notoriety along the rude walks of men. Woman has been cast in a distinctive mould and she can no more escape its requirements than the planets can be turned from their courses. It is the duty of physicians, individually and collectively, to urge upon society the importance of protecting the pubescent girl from the baleful environment that endangers her health and threatens the serious impairment of her superior function. You are all perfectly aware of the truth of what I say, but are you thoroughly alive to its importance? Do you exercise the great influence of which you are capable in over-coming the pernicious mode of educating young girls? The mental excitement incident to the curriculum prescribed in our schools for girls tends to weaken their physical system and pre-vents their proper development. Such methods of education as now obtain are inefficacious. It is a conflict for blood, of which there is not enough for both, between an over-stimulated brain and an under-developed body. Instead of urging the pubescent girl to use every endeavor to " keep up with her classes, lest she fall behind and be put back in a lower grade," let her be re-stricted to a very limited amount of study. Instead of allowing her to occupy nearly all of her time with the preparation and recitation of lessons, see that she is properly clothed and let her be out-of-doors, judiciously exercising and breathing the pure air that will redden her blood so that it may adorn her cheeks with the bloom of health. See to her diet and digestion—instead of permitting her to eat sweetmeats, pickles, candies, and such " trashy stuffs," let her eat beef and lamb and poultry and some wholesome vegetables, that she may become strong and healthy and be the beautiful creature she was intended to be. Let her be clothed in suitable raiment, untrammelled by stays and trains, and she stands before us graceful and beautiful. She is indeed " God's best gift to man." If woman can acquire Latin, physics, mathematics, and political economy without dam-age to her health and her greatest function, I would not hinder her in the slightest degree; but it is of first importance to have her healthy in mind and body, and with such soundness let her have such a degree of education as will make her a cultured, sweet, and lovely mother; for

"The bearing and the training of a child
Is woman's wisdom."

LEUKEMIA IN CHILDHOOD.[1]

BY

J. R. BROMWELL, M.D.,
Washington, D. C.

LEUKEMIA—occurring generally between the ages of puberty and 50 years—belongs to general medicine; but, as the disease is not infrequent in early life, it has a legitimate place within the prescribed limits of this Society. I therefore hope you will find the report of the following case of sufficient interest to engage your attention and bring out a full discussion.

March 30, between 7 and 8 P.M., I was called to a lad of 14 years who, with his mother, arrived from a distant city the day before. His physician sent him here, hoping that this climate, where he could be more out-of-doors, would hasten a slow convalescence from grippe and malarial fever, which, some two months previous, had weakened a strong, robust constitution. His mother reported that his family history was good; that, prior to the past winter, he had been a remarkably healthy boy; that he had suffered with both grippe and malarial fever; that convalescence was retarded by chronic malarial poisoning; and that his physician had ordered change of air to a warmer climate, out-of-door life, and little if any medicine. During the day he had ridden about the city sightseeing. On returning to the hotel he complained of chilly sensations, followed by nausea and vomiting, pain over the epigastrium and abdomen, and fever. He had been unable to retain little, if anything, for the past two hours, and had slight bleeding from the nose.

He was sitting in his chair, looking tired and ill. The face was pinched and drawn, pale, but not the pearly pallor of anemia—more a muddy yellow, so often seen in cachectic conditions resulting from protracted illness and malassimilation. His appearance might have suggested an advanced but mild typhoid fever, chronic malarial poisoning, or, had he not been so young, more than all else malignant disease with sepsis.

[1]Read before the Washington Obstetrical and Gynecological Society, April 4, 1902.

The kidneys were acting freely and normally. The bowels were constipated. The respiratory sounds were normal, excepting a few bronchial râles over both lungs. The heart sounds were clear and distinct, perfectly normal. The abdomen was tympanitic, rendering it rather difficult to palpate the abdominal organs, especially as there was tenderness on pressure. The splenic region was enlarged, with increased dulness. There was also increased liver dulness and more or less diffused pain, aggravated by vomiting. The tongue was red and raw-looking from the tip to far back on the dorsum. The gums were inflamed, spongy, easily bleeding on slight irritation. The buccal membrane was inflamed, with here and there points of ulceration or lost epithelium. The breath was fetid, feverish, having the odor of fresh blood and that undergoing decomposition. There was no sordes on the teeth, and the lips were free from herpes, but dry, not cracked. His temperature was 103°, pulse 120.

I ordered him to bed, such treatment only as the exigencies of the case demanded, and liquid nourishment—when his stomach would retain it—until the following morning.

March 31: He passed a fairly good night, nausea and vomiting checked, bowels constipated, kidneys acting normally, and temperature and pulse nearly normal. There was most marked enlargement of the spleen, and the liver dulness was increased. The spleen extended about two inches below the ribs and almost to the middle line. The bulging caused by the enlarged spleen was distinctly perceptible across the room. The whole abdomen was much too large and tympanitic elsewhere. There was less pain and tenderness on pressure. The most careful search showed no lymphatic complication or involvement. There was passive bleeding from the gums and dorsum of the tongue, which annoyed and sickened him, and which he was nervously wiping away with his handkerchief. When asked how he felt, he replied, in a steady, strong voice: "Much better, and I want something to eat and plenty of it." But, notwithstanding his general condition had improved from the evening before and he was resting very comfortably, he looked more seriously ill. I ordered a purgative, followed, as soon as it acted, by full doses of muriate of quinine, turpentine stupes to the abdomen, and to continue liquid diet.

April 1, he was seemingly very much better, and, as all general conditions had decidedly improved and his temperature was normal, I yielded to his begging and allowed solid food, in small quantities, with instructions to return at once to liquid diet should nausea or pain return.

April 2, he was not so well. Nausea and vomiting returned during the night, yielding readily, however, to treatment and a return to liquid nourishment. He had fever, which was preceded by a chill or chilly sensations. The stomatitis had increased, with almost constant steady oozing of blood from gums and tongue. The blood, though mixed with the secretions of the mouth, was of normal color. The odor of the breath had improved by the use of antiseptic mouth washes, and fractional doses of carbolic acid internally. The bowels had moved sufficiently by enema. With diminished tympanites and lessened pain and tenderness on pressure, the abdominal organs were easily palpable and the margins of the very large spleen easily defined. The enlargement was unquestionably increasing, but the tenderness on pressure and pain had diminished.

April 3, there was practically little change from the day previous. The fever was running a markedly singular course, sometimes preceded, sometimes accompanied, by chilly sensations. He was comfortable and enjoyed having his mother read to him. As quinine produced no effect upon the temperature whatever and was adding to the irritability of the stomach, I ceased giving it, concluding that the cause of the trouble was much more serious than malarial poisoning; and as the symptoms pointed to the blood-making organs, especially the spleen, I requested Dr. J. B. Nichols to examine the blood for additional light. so that a correct and definite diagnosis might be made. The following report left no doubt:

The disease was acute leukemia. What type?

" Microscopic appearance: normal. Red blood corpuscles: Number of red blood corpuscles per cubic millimetre, 4,440,000; 89 per cent of normal. Hemoglobin, 85 per cent; corpuscular hemoglobin ratio, .96. Rouleau formation: normal. Leucocytes: Number of leucocytes per cubic millimetre, 85,600; proportion· of white to red corpuscles, 1 to 52. A very large number of Müller's granules in active motion. Malarial parasites: none seen."

A differential count of the leucocytes was not made, owing to a desire to have this report with no delay.

From now to April 17 the records of the daily symptoms and the clinical picture showed nothing new. The progress of the disease was singularly rapid. The fever ran its irregular course, suddenly rising from normal or thereabouts to 102° or 103°, without any appreciable cause or provocation, to fall as suddenly. There were occasional chilly sensations, but rarely well-marked chills. The bleeding from the nose was infrequent and at no time serious. There was still steady oozing of blood from the gums and dorsum of the tongue, sometimes apparently from the mucous surfaces of the mouth generally; tonsillitis and pharyngitis; slight irritable cough; nausea and digestive disturbances on the least imprudence in diet or nervous excitement. The appetite was generally ravenous, and the bowels moved only by the aid of purgatives or enema. The enlargement of the spleen increased so irregularly that there were days when there was very appreciable diminution, to be followed by rapidly increasing enlargement. The liver dulness remained stationary: and whilst there was not much pain or tenderness on pressure so long as the stupes were occasionally applied, he was rarely comfortable. There was much and increasing difficulty in breathing on the slightest exertion or nervous excitement. Nevertheless there were days when he seemed so well, and all conditions so favorable, that I hoped the little fellow would improve sufficiently to stand the journey to his home, be under the care of his physician there, and that his parents might be spared the pain and sorrow of having him die at a hotel, if not among perfect strangers. The next day, or even in an hour, all hope of anything but a speedy fatal ending would be lost. Notwithstanding he was taking sufficient nourishment and apparently digesting it, he was losing flesh daily. There was still no lymphatic involvement.

April 17, the blood examination showed as follows: Microscopic appearance: normal. Red blood corpuscles per cubic millimetre, 4,041,000; 81 per cent of normal. Hemoglobin, 65 per cent; corpuscular hemoglobin ratio, 80. Macrocytes: a few. Microcytes: a few. Polychromatophilia: not observed. Poikilocytes: few. Normoblasts: a few. Rouleau formation: normal. Leucocytes: Number of leucocytes per cubic millimetre, 529,000; proportion of white to red corpuscles, 1 to 7.6; relative proportion of leucocytes, approximately, small mononuclear 10, large mononuclear, transitional, 85, polynuclear 4.8, eosinophiles .2, myelocytes (?). Malarial parasite: none.

Dr. Nichols says: " The type is typically that of lymphatic leukemia. The clinical picture, nevertheless, is that of acute splenic leukemia, which I think is exceedinly rare. "

April 18, the spleen extended downward to within an inch and
a half or two inches of the ilium and across the middle line.
You could grasp the margins with the fingers. The edges were
thin and hard, like the rim of a dinner plate. The whole
left side, from the sixth rib to the pelvis and over the middle
line, was bulged out, producing marked deformity, and the difficulty of breathing increasing even when at rest. There was no
ascites, tenderness on pressure continued, but there was little
pain. The parotid and cervical glands were now becoming
involved. They were painful and enlarged, especially on the
left side. There was pain and difficulty in moving the head
or neck. The bleeding from the mouth steadily continued.
With moderate pressure, grasping the tongue with a napkin,
you could saturate it with what appeared pure blood. Astringent washes produced but little beneficial effect. The bleeding
from the nose, slight, occurred at irregular intervals.

The morning of April 19 Dr. M. F. Cuthbert met me in consultation. The inflammation and swelling of the glands of the
neck presented the appearance of a severe case of mumps, or
parotid infection seen in typhoid fever. There was much pain
in moving or swallowing. We examined carefully for other
lymphatic complications, finding none. Every symptom had
increased in gravity. The afternoon of April 20, between 2
and 3 o'clock, I was telephoned that he was profusely bleeding
from the nose and that the nurse failed to arrest or control it.
As I was engaged in my office, I requested Dr. Joseph Bryan to
see him—not to wait for me, but, in his capacity as a specialist,
do all possible to arrest the bleeding. He was there when I arrived, and, after an hour or more, we succeeded, by the use of
adrenalin chloride solution and plugging the nostril, in stopping
the hemorrhage. The quantity of blood lost was considerable,
but normal in appearance and readily coagulating. He was
much exhausted and resting quietly when we left.

At 10 o'clock that night, when we met again, there had been
no further bleeding; his pulse had improved; he had taken his
nourishment; and, aside from increasing weakness, there were no
marked changes. The applications were removed, rendering his
breathing easier.

April 21, 5 A.M., I was telephoned that he had waked an hour
or so before, complaining of severe pain in his head, which had
continued, and that he was then unconscious. The urinary
analysis made the day before was as follows: April 20, amount

in twenty-four hours, about 1,500 cubic centimetres (50 ounces);
amount submitted for examination, 1,445 cubic centimetres
(about two ounces lost at stool); color, medium yellow; appearance, clear; reaction, moderately acid; specific gravity, 1011;
albumin absent; nucleo-albumin absent; sugar absent; urea, 2.0
per cent, 30 grammes in twenty-four hours; hemoglobin absent;
bile pigment absent; indican diminished; uric acid, .073 per
cent, 1.1 grammes in twenty-four hours (somewhat increased);
solid undissolved matters very scanty; casts absent; epithelium,
a very few cells.

I saw him in about half an hour from receiving the message.
He was comatose, breathing slowly and irregularly, with some
stertor; the pupils were irregularly dilated, and his face was
grayish purple, enormously swollen, especially at the sides of
the neck and under the chin. His whole appearance was so
changed from only a few hours before as to be past recognition.
The pulse was slow and irregular, with partial paralysis and
inability to swallow. The picture of cerebral congestion with
hemorrhage needed no further completing touch. There were
no indications of convulsions. At 8 A.M., our next meeting,
coma was profound and paralysis seemed general. He died at
4 P.M.

Whilst the case was a very sad one, it was full of interest.
Following malarial fever and grippe, do we see cause and
effect?—the acute type of the disease; the marked difference
between the clinical and blood picture, one that of lienal or
splenic leukemia alone (a very rare disease), the other typically
that of lymphatic leukemia. The absence, or questionable existence, of myelocytes, indicating that the bone marrow was not involved, if we accept the theory that myelocytes are identical with
the marrow cells and not altered leucocytes? This can only be
answered hypothetically, as there could be no postmortem examination: that most probably, even at the last, there was no true
involvement of the lymphatic glands, the trouble there being
due to septic infection from the mouth. The very small percentage of eosinophiles, the persistent hemorrhage from the
mouth, the unsatisfied hunger, the constipation (diarrhea being
most common) and the rapid course of the disease, and the importance of thorough blood examinations in all obscure or
doubtful diagnoses, are all points of interest for discussion.

1147 CONNECTICUT AVENUE.

DIASTASIS OF THE ABDOMINAL (RECTI) MUSCLES.[1]

BY

R. P. McREYNOLDS, M.D.,
Philadelphia, Pa.

(With four illustrations.)

In the great mass of literature upon almost every conceivable disease and injury of the abdominal wall and cavity, we are surprised to find that so little has been written upon diastasis of the abdominal muscles. It is not mentioned in a number of the text books, and when it is described the author, it seems to me, fails to give it the consideration it is entitled to. The reason for this is no doubt to be attributed to the fact that it has been generally regarded as an infrequent and inoperable condition, and consequently not worthy of attention. I believe we often overlook it, for, since during the past two years I have made it a rule to examine carefully for it, I have been rewarded by finding a number of cases—some with complete and some with partial separation of the muscles.

ETIOLOGY.—In the large majority of cases it is pregnancy—frequent and rapid childbearing, improper support and protection of the abdominal wall during pregnancy and the puerperium. All of the cases I have seen have been in that class of women who do their own work. They remain in bed perhaps a week after the birth of the child, and a few days later resume their usual household duties. When the pregnant womb leaves the pelvis it begins to cause an increase in the intra-abdominal pressure. This is resisted by all of the muscles of the abdominal wall, but particularly by the recti muscles; these, as the pressure increases, gradually become flattened out and elongated. If the pressure is too great, as happens in those forms of malformations where the normal distance between the ensiform and pubis is diminished, the muscles separate and the womb is forced between them, producing what is known as a

[1] Read before the Section on Gynecology. College of Physicians of Philadelphia, October 16, 1902.

ventral hernia of the pregnant womb. This is more liable to occur in women who have poor physical development with weak and flabby abdominal muscles. The separation of the muscles, which as a rule occurs suddenly, is very extensive, and after delivery they remain so far apart that when the woman stands all of the small intestines fall in between them.

In other cases there is no marked diastasis during pregnancy, but the muscles fail to undergo the normal retrograde changes which should take place during the puerperium. The linea alba is consequently weakened and unable to withstand the pressure

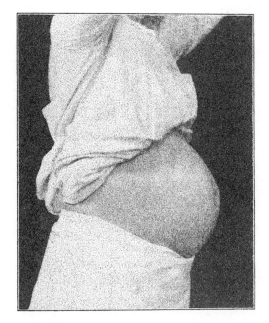

Fig. 1.—Standing posture—complete diastasis of recti muscles.

placed upon it; gradually and progressively it gives way and allows the muscles to become more or less separated.

SYMPTOMS.—There is a general upsetting of all the various functions of her body. She is nervous, anemic; suffers from headache, backache, constipation, tympanites, insomnia, anorexia, etc. She imagines she is pregnant, for she notices the increase in the size of the abdomen and mistakes the movements of the distended intestines for fetal movements, the sick stomach for the nausea and vomiting of pregnancy.

DIAGNOSIS.—When we suspect from the history and symptoms

that such a condition exists, we should have the corset removed and, if possible, examine the patient in a standing position. The intestines, in cases of complete separation of the muscles, fall in between them, giving the abdomen the shape shown in Fig. 1. If examined in the recumbent posture we can, by having her cough, get the condition of the abdomen shown in Fig. 2; if she remains passive, by gentle palpation the whole hand can easily be inserted between the muscles.

In partial diastasis of the muscles we find the shape of the abdomen is as shown in Fig. 3. In this case the woman is three and one-half months pregnant, yet the relaxed condition of the abdominal wall and the partial separation of the recti muscles

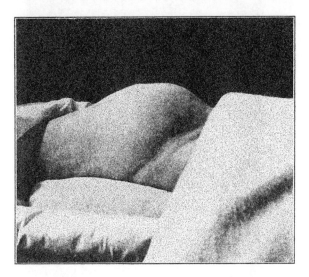

FIG. 2.—ReCumbent posture—woman straining.

give the abdomen the appearance of a seven-months pregnancy. Fig. 4 shows the same woman with properly-fitting abdominal binder; with it she is able to walk around with comparative ease and comfort; without it she can hardly walk at all.

I think a vaginal examination should always be made in these cases, for it enables us to confirm the diagnosis and to differentiate it from other diseases, such as ovarian cyst, pregnancy, phantom tumors, fat, ascites, etc. It is rather surprising how often the general practitioner mistakes the condition for ovarian cyst and sends his patient to the hospital for an operation. The absence of the wave of fluctuation, and of a central area of flatness surrounded by a ring of resonance (irrespective of the position of the patient), should exclude the diagnosis of ovarian cyst even without a vaginal examination. The subjective symptoms of pregnancy may be present, but the total absence of all of the objective signs, including, as it does, the three and only positive signs of pregnancy, should dismiss this from one of the possibilities. Phantom tumor, fat, and ascites are easily differentiated.

TREATMENT. *Prophylactic.*—If during pregnancy there are any indications of weakness of the abdominal muscles, they

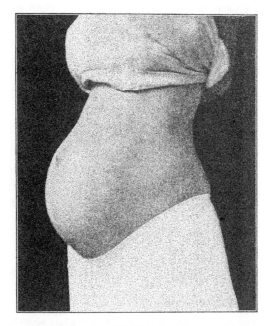

FIG. 3.—Standing posture—partial diastasis in woman three and one-half months pregnant.

should be reinforced by having the woman wear an abdominal belt which presses the abdomen upward and backward. This is (besides being a protection) a great comfort to her, for it relieves the pain in her abdomen and back and enables her to move around with facility and ease. The belt should always be removed at night and the abdominal wall massaged with cocoa butter. Every woman after her confinement should remain in bed for two weeks; during this time the abdomen should be protected by a well-fitting abdominal binder, worn both night

52

and day. She should under no circumstances be allowed to resume her household duties under six weeks.

Palliative Treatment.—This consists in the use of an abdominal belt (such as shown in Fig. 4). There can be no doubt but that a large number of women by using it are enabled to pass through a long life very comfortably. I have noticed that when wearing the belt there is a decided tendency for accumulation of abdominal fat, which may to a certain extent be overcome by systematic abdominal exercises taken morning and night, and by

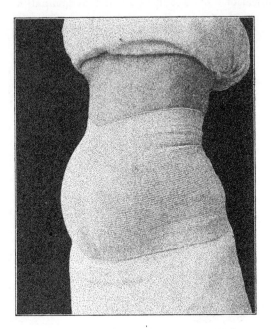

FIG. 4.—Same as Fig. 3, but with abdominal binder on.

having the muscles subjected from time to time to a course of massage and electricity.

Surgical Treatment.—I fear that the reported cases are too few to enable us to draw accurate conclusions regarding the value of the operative. treatment. Clarence Webster, in '' Progressive Medicine '' for 1901, reports a series of fifty-one cases operated upon. with what is claimed to have been satisfactory results. This is the largest number of cases that I have been able to find operated upon by one man. The operation consists in excising the connective tissue between the muscles, together with the skin and subcutaneous fat, and then suturing the recti muscles together. In well-selected cases—namely, those in which the diastasis has not been very extensive and where the muscles have not lost their tone—I believe the chances of a radical cure are sufficient to justify an operation. On the other hand, in cases where the condition has existed for a number of years and the muscles have lost their contractility and elasticity, and where there is perhaps an abnormal increase in the abdominal fat, the chances of giving permanent benefit from an operation are not brilliant and we are not warranted in recommending it.

3722 WALNUT STREET.

CARCINOMA OF THE CERVIX UTERI.[1]

SUMMARY REPORT OF THE AUTHOR'S SIXTY-TWO CASES OPERATED UPON BY HYSTERECTOMY. REMARKS.

BY

L. H. DUNNING, M.D.,
Indianapolis, Ind.

IN presenting a report of all the cases of cancer of the cervix uteri operated upon up to the date of the present writing—September 1, 1902—the author desires to state that he has excluded from this list all the cases in which a question arose in his mind as to the diagnosis of carcinoma. All but very few of the cases were examined by competent pathologists and pronounced carcinoma, and those not examined presented unmistakable signs of malignancy, such as pain, hemorrhage, and a fetid discharge with the presence of a neoplasm which was either fungoid or undergoing ulceration. There were in all 62 cases, and of these 18 are known to be alive. There were 5 deaths resulting from the operation, and one died at the end of ten years and three months.

The list has been divided into two groups, the first group including all cases operated upon previous to September 1, 1898, five years ago. In this group there are 30 cases, of which 5 (16⅔ per cent) lived longer than five years. A brief history of these 5 cases is herewith submitted. By this report it will be

[1] Read at the meeting of the American Association of Obstetricians and Gynecologists, Washington, D. C., September 16, 17, and 18, 1902.

seen that one lived ten years and three and a half months. One is alive and well at the end of six years and seven months, one at six years and eleven months, one at six years and four and a half months, and one at five years and nine months.

The second group includes those cases operated upon within the last five years. There are 32 cases in this group. Of these, 14 are still living. One is alive four years and four months after operation, one four years and three and a half months, one four years and one and a half months, two three years and ten months, one one year and ten months, one one year and seven and a half months, one one year and six months, one ten months, one nine months, one eight and a half months, one six and a half months, one five months, and one four and a half months.

All of these who have lived over three years have been examined either by myself or attending physician and found to be free from a recurrence. I cannot speak positively of several patients operated recently, other than to say that they do not present at present any symptoms leading to a fear of a recurrence.

In this report all cases are excluded in which we knew portions of the cancerous mass were left behind. In our attempts to do thorough work we sometimes jeopardized other tissues. Once a portion was cut out of the bladder and the opening was successfully sutured. Twice we caused rents in the bladder. One occurred in one of the fatal cases, and in the other case the rent was closed by a subsequent operation before the patient left the hospital. The patient died, however, of a recurrence within six months.

In three cases one ureter was severed. In two of them the corresponding kidney was extirpated. In the first, which occurred in 1893, the prognosis was unfavorable and I knew of no better way of procedure. The patient recovered from both operations, but died three months later of recurrence. In the second case I urged an abdominal section, the dissecting out of the ureter and the grafting of it into the bladder. The patient rejected this method in favor of nephrectomy. The patient is still living and seemingly well at the end of two years and eleven months. In the third case of severed ureter a rapid recurrence took place, the open end of the ureter became blocked by cancerous deposits, a hydronephrosis developed, yet the patient lived many months.

In several patients operated upon there was slight extension of the disease to the   vagina.   If the vaginal involvement is superficial and not more than one inch below the utero-vaginal junction, it is no bar to hysterectomy.

The author has several times extirpated the upper portion of the vagina, both by the lower and upper methods.   When the work is done through the vagina an incision may be made through the coats of the vagina below the growth, far enough away to enable one to seize with a forceps healthy vaginal tissue.   Now, by traction upon the forceps and finger pressure beneath the vagina, between it and the underlying structures, the vagina and neoplasm may be stripped up to the cervix.

In two or three instances I have first severed the vaginal attachment to the uterus and then stripped off portions of the vagina by forceps, traction, and finger pressure from above downward.   The former method, however, is the preferable one. The suprapubic method is certainly the preferable one when the uterus and upper portion of the vagina are to be removed.

In all five of the cases that have survived five years and longer the disease was in its incipiency.   There were two, however, in the second group—viz., the one alive at the end of four years and three and a half months and the one alive at the end of four years and one and a half months—in which the disease was so far advanced that I deemed it questionable, at the time of examination, whether the operation would be of any avail.   The first was an adenocarcinoma of the cervix and the operation a vaginal hysterectomy.   In attempting to draw the uterus down the cervix was torn off, so that the operation was greatly embarrassed.   The case proved to be one of the most satisfactory in the list.

The other case was one of a large cauliflower growth of the cervix attended by much bleeding, fetid discharges, and marked emaciation.   This patient is now enjoying good health without recurrence.   These are exceptional cases.   In the review of my experience I am greatly impressed with the necessity of early operation, if we desire to benefit the greater number of patients.

Vaginal hysterectomy was the method of operation in all but five cases.   In the five cases in which supravaginal hysterectomy was done, a technique very similar to the one proposed by Werder was employed.   The pelvic glands were removed in two cases only.   One case out of the five was fatal, and in this case the operation was most difficult and quite prolonged.   The left ureter was torn off near the bladder.[1] Fortunately the torn end of the ureter was found and transplanted into the bladder without difficulty. The result of this implantation we do not know, as the patient died at the end of two days and we were not permitted an autopsy. Only two of the remaining four patients are alive, one six and a half months and one five months after the operation. It seems to me that the question of methods is still an unsettled one.

Certainly the supravaginal operation with extensive dissection of glands and broad ligaments is attended with a larger rate of primary mortality, and the method has not been employed long enough to determine its relative merits in effecting a cure. Theoretically it appears the most promising.

"Leopold's researches show that even at a comparatively early stage of the disease too much reliance cannot be placed on this alleged immunity of dissemination, for of 127 cancerous uteri extirpated per vaginam he found dissemination in the parametrium in 68, or 54 per cent, the disease being limited to the

[1] In a recent supravaginal hysterectomy I resorted to a simple method which yielded me such admirable results that I shall employ it in the future whenever possible.

The case operated upon was one of carcinoma of the cervix in which the neoplasm extended well over toward the right lateral pelvic wall, yet it seemed just above the vaginal tissue, and the uterus and neoplasm moved freely, so I thought it possible to easily extirpate the uterus and neoplasm.

After opening the abdomen and working my way down to the neoplasm, the latter was found more extensive than we at first thought. It seemed to me the ureter was in danger. The patient was in the Trendelenburg position, and the intestines held above the pelvic brim by gauze packing. The ureter, as it came over the brim of the pelvis, was in plain view. The peritoneum lying over it was incised a distance of one-half inch. The peritoneum was dissected off the ureter, a blunt needle threaded with catgut was carried under the ureter, and a single knot was carried down to near the ureter, but not tightened.

By slight upward traction it was found to put the ureter on the stretch, so that it could be felt as a cord all the way from the thread encircling it to its entrance into the bladder.

To my satisfaction I thus demonstrated that the neoplasm in the cervix lay below the ureter, and that with a little care there was no danger of wounding it.

When the uterus was extirpated the catgut thread was cut and removed and the incised peritoneum stitched.

It seems to me this simple method could be used with marked advantage in many cases of operation upon neoplasms in the pelvis in which there is danger of wounding the ureter.

uterus in the other 59 cases." "Mackenrodt has arrived at similar conclusions."[1]

Roger Williams'[2] postmortem findings showed the largest per cent of involvement of vaginal tissue by extension, viz., 72 per cent. These findings lead us to hope for a greater number of cures when a few years more have passed and we can obtain tabulated reports of cases operated upon by the Werder method. Every supravaginal hysterectomy for cancer of the cervix should include in the procedure the removal of a portion of the upper part of the vagina, especially anteriorly, since this is the most frequent direction of the extension.

Vaginal hysterectomy for cancer of the neck of the uterus has yielded me $16\frac{2}{3}$ per cent of cures, taking the five-years time test as the standard of computation. This is a percentage corresponding to that obtained at Johns Hopkins, as recorded by Cullen in his work, "Cancer of the Uterus" (pp. 632 and 633). By consulting his table of cases of squamous-celled carcinoma of the cervix uteri, it will be seen that the whole number operated upon five years previous to the time of his report was 14. From this number two should be deducted, as they were incomplete operations. There are thus left 12 cases operated upon, and 2 of these were alive and well at the time of making the report, thus showing a percentage of recovery of $16\frac{2}{3}$ per cent.

The number of cures is not a complete index to beneficial results of operations for cancer of the uterus. The prolongation of life in many cases, and the relief of suffering, hemorrhage, and offensive discharges, must pass for much in favor of surgery. The writer's experience teaches him, however, positively the uselessness, the harmfulness of hysterectomy in cases in which there is a wide dissemination of cancerous deposits and infiltrations. He has long since abandoned all efforts in this direction. He has, however, seen much temporary benefit result from curettage and the thorough application of the thermo-cautery.

Of late there has been some discussion upon the relative merits of hysterectomy and high amputation of the cervix in incipient cancer. Several years ago the writer, following the teachings of Schröder, employed high amputation instead of hysterectomy. He abandoned this method because of the incompleteness of the operation, and because of the sufferings of the patients afterward in those operated upon before the menopause. It is probable that amputation yields a slightly less primary mortality than hys-

[1]Roger Williams: Uterine Tumors, p. 213.
[2]Ibid,. p. 224.

terectomy, but the benefits in patients surviving the hysterectomy are much greater.

It should be remembered that in a considerable percentage of cases of cancer of the cervix uteri the body of the uterus is also affected by extension through the lymphatics, and in other instances the disease spreads rapidly from below upward. Obviously amputation of the cervix is inappropriate for such cases. The ovaries and tubes are quite often invaded, even in early cases. Here also amputation is inefficient.

The painful menstruation and pelvic congestion due to stenosis following amputation of the cervix are, as a rule, very distressing and call for frequent intervention of the surgeon. Pregnancy and labor in such cases are distressing and too frequently dangerous.

We operate in cases of cancer to bring relief as well as to accomplish cures. To effect this double purpose hysterectomy is at present the best known means.

REPORT OF FIVE CASES OF CARCINOMA OF THE CERVIX UTERI ALIVE
FIVE YEARS AFTER HYSTERECTOMY.

CASE I.—Mrs. A., referred by Dr. Terrill, of Filmore, Ind., in January, 1892. The patient was 63 years old and had reached the menopause ten years previously. For several months she had had profuse uterine hemorrhages. Dr. Terrill had removed small growths from the cervix uteri several times, but new ones had quickly sprung from the site of the former ones. At the time of my examination there was a small cauliflower growth springing from the cervix and protruding into the vagina. A portion of it was examined by Dr. Ferguson and pronounced carcinoma. Vaginal hysterectomy with extirpation of the appendages was done January 4, 1892. The patient recovered. She enjoyed good health until May, 1899, when she had a slight stroke of paralysis. She made a partial recovery from this attack and died March 20, 1902, of hydrothorax. No postmortem was made. There were never any evidences of a recurrence of the carcinoma in the pelvic tissues.

CASE II.—Mrs. B., married and aged 30 years, was referred by Dr. J. R. Mauk, Cambridge City. She was emaciated as a result of uterine pain and hemorrhage. A neoplasm was found involving the cervix uteri. Dr. C. E. Ferguson examined a portion of the neoplasm and pronounced it carcinoma. A total extirpation of the uterus and appendages was effected January 30, 1896. The patient recovered from the operation and gradually regained her health. She enjoys reasonably good health and has for a number of years been employed as a stenographer. She has not been examined by me recently, but she makes no complaint indicating a recurrence.

CASE III.—Mrs. C., referred by Dr. McNutt, of Connersville, Ind. She was 45 years of age. Examined by me December 2, 1896. She gave the history of frequent and profuse hemorrhages and now has a thin, fetid discharge. Upon examination a small papillomatous growth was found upon the posterior lip of the cervix. A piece was snipped out and examined microscopically and pronounced carcinoma. Vaginal hysterectomy was done December 3, 1896. The uterine appendages were also removed. She made an excellent recovery and to-day is well. I have examined her recently and find no evidences of recurrence.

CASE IV.—Mrs. D., referred by Dr. H. Jameson. The patient was 48 years of age, mother of four children, youngest 17 years. A neoplasm involving one-half of the circumference of the cervix uteri was found upon examination. Microscopic examination showed it to be a squamous-celled carcinoma. Hysterectomy was done April 16, 1896. Patient made an excellent recovery. She reported to me by letter August 16, 1902, as being well and as having no signs of recurrence.

CASE V.—Mrs. E., about 40 years of age. Referred by Dr. E. F. Hodges. Patient married and mother of two children. Microscopical examination of cervical neoplasm was made by Dr. Hodges, who pronounced it carcinoma. A vaginal hysterectomy was done October, 1895. Patient was in ill health for some months following the operation. She has been in comparatively good health now several years. The writer examined the patient in July of this year and found a clean vagina with no signs of recurrence.

CAUSES OF RECURRENCE OF BILIARY SYMPTOMS AFTER CHOLECYSTOTOMY.[1]

BY

CHARLES S. HAMILTON, A.B., M.D.,
Columbus, O.

THE majority of surgeons who have had experience with the surgery of the biliary passages have doubtless witnessed recurrence of symptoms of biliary disease after removal of stones

[1] Read at the meeting of the American Association of Obstetricians and Gynecologists, Washington, D. C., September 16, 17, and 18, 1902.

from the gall bladder. Such recurrences may take the following forms: 1. Attacks of typical gall-stone colic, presumptively due to the passage of calculi or their temporary lodgment in the cystic duct. 2. Less painful paroxysms, apparently due to the presence of acute or subacute cholecystitis or cholangitis. 3. The recurrence of distended gall bladder with more or less pain after the thorough evacuation of stones from that viscus. 4. Disturbance (gastric or intestinal) due to adhesions involving the gall bladder and other viscera. Such apparent relapses are worthy of close investigation, as they imply occasional shortcomings in operative technique and lessen somewhat the degree of confidence with which we may recommend surgical intervention as a means of complete and permanent relief to the sufferer.

A series of causes may be regarded as responsible for such recurrences. Among them I would enumerate the following:

1. A stone may be overlooked in some part of the biliary tubes. While this does not occur so readily in the gall bladder or cystic duct, it is not infrequent in the common or hepatic duct. In fact, a stone may be felt in either of the latter two, and slip from the operator's grasp, not being again detected during the operation. As our familiarity with the disease and its operative treatment is enlarged by experience, stones will more rarely escape the hand of the surgeon.

2. There seems to be no reason why a gall stone should not occasionally re-form in the biliary tract, after even the most thorough operation, provided conditions favorable to the process are present and that a sufficient time may elapse. However this may be, there is substantial ground for believing that they may re-form if a suitable nucleus be provided. Such might be, for example, a silk suture (Kehr) which had been used in attaching the gall bladder to the peritoneum. It is hardly likely that all such sutures would find their way into the cavity of that organ; occasionally, however, they do. The propriety of using catgut for this suture is therefore self-evident, as being safer, so far as the future of the patient is concerned, than silk.

3. Stricture of the cystic, possibly of the common, duct may produce return of symptoms after a temporarily successful operation. A calculus which has lain embedded for months or years in the cystic duct may have destroyed the mucosa and have so thickened the walls of the tube that after its removal partial or total impairment of its calibre results.

4. In some instances of greatly thickened gall bladder from subacute and chronic cholecystitis, it would seem as though drainage for any reasonable period would not cure. In many such cases I believe that recurrence would be observed if the later history were known. Possibly bacteria remain embedded in the walls of the gall bladder, becoming active and producing recurrent attacks of inflammation, or the organ has been too badly damaged to perform painlessly its function of alternate expansion and contraction.

5. Adhesions which distort the biliary passages are a frequent source of pain both before and after operative procedures. That they should not form after surgical intervention implies (1) gentle handling of structures; (2) the avoidance of strong antiseptic solutions as well as absolute asepsis in operating; (3) exclusion from the field of operation, by proper padding, of all structures not directly involved.

In this connection attention may be drawn to the proper method of attaching the gall bladder to the parietes. It is very generally known that the organ should not be attached to the skin, but rather to the peritoneum and deeper muscular layers, because of the lessened tendency to persistent fistula thus secured. When the liver is greatly enlarged in a downward direction, the gall bladder should be attached to the parietes as high up as possible, the liver being even pushed upward to some extent to permit this. Otherwise, as the liver diminishes in size from removal of the cause of enlargement, the elongated gall bladder is subjected to more and more tension, together with a degree of angulation. Both of these factors are likely to produce painful symptoms.

6. Last, unrecognized pancreatitis with secondary biliary disturbance (semi-obstructions and infections) must be an occasional cause of recurrence. In some instances such conditions could be relieved only by cholecystenterostomy, if gall-bladder drainage had failed.

So far as I have been able to follow up my cases and those of my colleague, recurrence of symptoms is not infrequent. Fortunately, in the majority of instances the secondary symptoms are transitory and comparatively insignificant. That they are not always so I am sure current literature sufficiently demonstrates. Accurate knowledge of their nature, as shown by secondary operations, generally suggests the means by which they are to be avoided. It is interesting to note in this connec-

tion Kehr's statement that he is always glad to have his cases
undergo a Carlsbad cure after operation, if time and means
permit. Further, the study of these cases shows strikingly that
many of them would have been avoided by primary cholecystec-
tomy, thus justifying the growing tendency to perform that
operation more frequently.

Generally speaking, it is evident that the earlier the operation, the less complicated the surgical condition with which we
have to deal, and also the less the chance of recurrence of symptoms.

In conclusion I shall detail the history of an illustrative case.

Mrs. M. was first seen in August, 1898. She had had pain in
the right side of the abdomen when seven months pregnant three
years ago. She suffered in the same way during the puerperium,
and from that time up to the present has had a similar pain
occasionally. In connection with a miscarriage in August last
a swelling was observed in the region of the appendix. She
is a well-nourished woman of 27 years; menstruates regularly
and normally. Examination shows normal uterus and appendages; tenderness on the right side of the abdomen in the inguinal
and hypochondriac regions; no tumor can be defined. Diagnosis
uncertain.

Operation under ether. Incision through the right rectus.
Appendix and pelvic organs found normal. The gall bladder is
felt at a surprisingly low position and is much distended. The
incision is enlarged and the contents (clear mucoid, five ounces)
evacuated. Two stones of mulberry appearance are at once felt
and withdrawn. Two more stones are found in the cystic duct;
they cannot be forced bodily into the gall bladder and are therefore broken up by the curette and forceps and removed piecemeal. Directly after their removal bile escapes freely. Close
observation of the cystic duct in the region in which the stones
have been lodged shows extensive destruction of the mucous
membrane, so much so that the possibility of occlusion of the
duct at a later period was considered. Convalescence from the
operation was uneventful.

The patient returned to her home well, but within three
months began to suffer the old pain, and on examination the
gall bladder was found to be again distended; somewhat later
it discharged spontaneously through the scar. The discharge
consisted of clear mucus and was never bile-stained. It was
evidently the secretion of the mucous glands of the gall bladder.

The sinus thus established persisted until the date of the second operation, two and one-half years later. At the second operation the gall bladder was found atrophied, buried in adhesions, and terminating in a stricture of the cystic duct at the point where the stone had originally been lodged. The mucosa of the gall bladder was enucleated down to the point of stricture, the presence of adhesions rendering complete removal of the gall bladder too difficult. The recovery of the patient from operation was prompt and she has been entirely well since that time.

MANAGEMENT OF BREECH PRESENTATIONS.[1]

BY

WILLIAM D. PORTER, M.D.,
Cincinnati, O.

BREECH presentation is encountered once in about fifty cases of labor. A much higher ratio represents its pro rata agency in inflicting damage on the mother, in causing injuries to the child, and particularly in the production of fetal mortality. The mortality is variously estimated at from 10 to 35 per cent. The percentage of children that die in the twenty-four hours succeeding birth is also high. It is difficult to determine what proportion of the deaths is due to the presentation *per se.* Many of the labors are premature. A change from breech to head presentation occurs late in some pregnancies. In case of premature labor with breech presentation, dystocia incident to the presentation may cause death of the child. It may be due wholly to the premature labor, which anticipated a possible change to a vertex presentation. But it must be admitted that the presentation may cause the premature labor. The breech seldom enters the pelvis in advance of labor, which may be precipitated from lack of space. The principle is the same as that which explains the frequency of premature labors in cases of contracted pelves.

Primiparity is an important factor of fetal mortality. The abdominal wall admits of less distension, making premature labor more probable. The soft parts dilate less readily. The

[1] Read at the meeting of the American Association of Obstetricians and Gynecologists, Washington, D. C., September 16, 17, and 18, 1902.

vagina is less capacious. These conditions increase the difficulty both of labor and of manipulations, should the latter be needed.

Breech cases always require careful supervision and frequently there is urgent need of assistance. On the contrary, it is equally true that defective judgment as to whether interference is needed, and inferior skill in rendering aid, contribute in an unfortunate degree to the fetal mortality.

Breech cases are usually tedious. The position of the child is generally oblique. Its pelvis, held by the comparatively rigid portion of the spinal column, does not readily accommodate itself to the resultant of forces, as does the head under like conditions. Consequently the breech is likely to impinge against the brim near the anterior end of an oblique diameter. Much time and energy may be consumed in overcoming this obstacle.

The child's thighs are usually flexed. That the breech may engage, this flexion must be carried to an extreme degree. This is opposed by the resiliency of the tissues, reinforced doubtless by resistance on the part of the voluntary muscles. At a definite point in the labor the uterine efforts are expended in crowding the breech into the brim against this resistance. Promptly on the cessation of the pain the extension of the thighs lifts the breech out of the pelvis. The next pain is expended in doing the same work, which is as promptly undone. This seesaw will continue until finally the breech is driven so deep into the pelvis that the thighs are parallel with the body, and efforts at extension only serve to fix the breech more firmly.

The progress of the breech through the pelvis is necessarily slow. However, by the time the outlet is reached the distension of the vagina and vulva is so great that the reflexes stimulate the expulsive powers to their greatest effort. The reflexes are greater than when the head presents, owing to the greater mass within the vagina. Expulsive efforts of such power and rapidity are produced that the child is likely to be rapidly expelled, reducing its time of greatest peril to a minimum.

Serious delay in a breech case is likely to be at one of three points:

1. With the breech at the brim.
2. With the breech in the pelvis.
3. With the delivery of the head.

Delay of the breech at the brim may become a serious matter, particularly if the membranes are ruptured. The water readily escapes, and retraction of the uterine walls may occur to a degree sufficient to embarrass the utero-placental circulation. This is always a cause for apprehension, and particularly so in breech cases. For there comes a time when this circulation is suspended, owing to the compression of the cord by the chest and head as they pass through the pelvis. The ability to meet this ordeal depends largely on how well the blood is oxygenated before the ordeal begins. The principle is well exemplified in divers who give exhibitions which involve remaining under water for a comparatively long time. It is noticeable that, before undertaking such a feat, the blood is well oxygenated by a number of deep rapid respirations.

With the breech delayed at the superior strait, the usual teaching is to bring down one or both legs and make traction. This plan is excellent if the patient be a multipara and the cervix well dilated or easily dilatable. In case of a primipara, or of a multipara with the cervix imperfectly dilated and with evidence that the completion of the dilatation will require considerable force, it is a questionable procedure. With one or both legs in advance a wedge is formed whose sides taper so gradually as to form a powerful dilator. But its maximum diameter is insufficient to prepare the soft parts for the prompt passage of the head. If the resistance of the cervix is considerable, it will promptly contract when the shoulders have passed, and may cause a fatal delay of the head or a serious laceration of the cervix. Should the perineum form the chief resistance, the delivery of the head within a safe time limit will probably result in an extensive tear of the perineum and possibly of the vagina.

If greater dilatation can be safely secured before the head reaches the pelvis, there will be a manifest gain of possibly vital importance. Such a gain is inevitable if the thighs be allowed to remain flexed and the legs extended along the body of the child. If the breech is carried through the cervix and over the perineum, with the legs in this position, the dilatation is generally sufficient to permit the ready extraction of the head. Considerably more time is consumed by this plan than is needed if the legs are brought down. If interference has not been too long delayed this extra time is well spent. Minutes spent in extricating the head count for more than hours expended in bringing down the doubled breech. The cervix dilated in the slower manner, by the larger mass, is not so likely to contract about the child's neck. It would doubtless be better to do nothing in preference to bringing down the legs, though such an election would often be but the choosing of the lesser evil.

William Hunter, whose contemporary fame equalled that of his brother, the great John Hunter, was an able obstetrician and a noted teacher. At one time he advised bringing down the legs in the condition under discussion. He reasoned that by lessening the mass the dilatation would be easier and more gradual, and that the suffering of the woman would thereby be greatly lessened. In his later lectures he admitted the danger of his plan and advised strongly against it. In nearly every case in which he had brought down the legs he lost the child.

The best method of bringing down the doubled breech is to make traction over the anterior groin with a finger. In case of a multipara this is easily accomplished, particularly if only moderate traction is needed. If traction in this manner is not feasible or is inadequate, a broad tape or a handkerchief carried between the anterior thigh and the body of the child furnishes an efficient means of traction.

The objection is made that it is sometimes difficult to place the fillet in position. It is no more, or but little more, difficult than to bring down a leg. In placing the fillet the Trush forceps will be found a valuable instrument. The objection that injury has been done with the fillet is applicable to all obstetrical instruments and manipulations. If traction be made in the proper direction the force is expended largely on the pelvis rather than on the femur. Moderate traction in conjunction with the pains will, as a rule, insure gradual descent.

Delay may occur with the breech in the pelvis. Almost invariably the thighs are flexed. The mass is about as great as the pelvis can accommodate. It does not readily bend and adjust itself to the pelvic curves. This is partly due to the resistance of the inflexible thighs. Uterine inertia from exhaustion is also a possible cause of delay.

Robert Barnes taught[1] that delay, with the breech low, often gave rise to serious difficulty. He advised against direct traction on the breech in all cases, claiming that it is frequently unsuccessful, and if so does harm. His treatment was always to bring down a leg. This procedure he terms breaking up or

[1] Obstetric Operations.

decomposing the obstructing wedge. With the breech low in the pelvis it is difficult to bring down a leg. And notwithstanding the high authority, it would seem to be unnecessary.

The use of forceps on the breech is advocated by men of recognized ability. If only slight traction be needed they are doubtless safe and satisfactory. They are so poorly adapted to the shape of the pelvis that it is difficult to regard them as appropriate in cases demanding much assistance. Traction on the groin with the finger, or, if necessary, with the fillet, seldom fails to overcome the delay.

As the body of the child is delivered it should be enveloped in a warm towel. This insures a secure grasp, conserves the child's heat, and lessens the danger of premature efforts at respiration.

As the body is extracted it is well to remember that the shoulders should enter an oblique diameter of the pelvis. To keep the spinal column directly under the pubic arch, as is pictured in many of the text books, is to force the shoulders to enter the transverse diameter, with the not remote danger of fracturing a clavicle.

Among the various procedures for delivering the after-coming head, that known as the Deventer method has the sanction of good authority. With the woman in the lithotomy position, as soon as the shoulders appear traction vertically downward is made, one hand grasping the feet and the other making traction over the shoulders. The arms are undisturbed and are usually found placed along the sides of the head. The claim that by this method the head is delivered in full extension is hardly credible. The normal position of the head is that of flexion, due to the pronounced curve of the spinal column of the child *in utero*. In this position of flexion the head will in all probability enter the pelvis, unless extended by awkward efforts at suprapubic pressure. The explanation of Reynolds[1] that the chin is arrested on the pelvic floor, causing the head to become extended, is not tenable. It may be stated as an inflexible law that, *with the head in the pelvis, a change from flexion to extension or from extension to flexion is a physical impossibility.*

The so-called Prague method, but which Parvin attributes to Puzos, involves traction by the feet and shoulders, first downward and backward till the head enters the pelvis; then upward

[1] American Text Book of Obstetrics.

53

and forward, bringing the back toward the mother's abdomen as the head is delivered.

"The combined method" seeks to diminish traction on the neck and to insure flexion by pressing two fingers against the superior maxilla. This method is variously attributed to Smellie, to Veit, and to Mauriceau. Others claim to effect the same results by traction on the inferior maxilla with one or two fingers in the mouth.

Pressure over the fundus is a most valuable adjunct, whatever method be selected.

A matter of great moment is the amount of traction which can safely be exerted through the neck. This is estimated by Matthews Duncan, from experimental data, to be about 105 pounds. Goodell, from clinical experience, placed the estimate still higher. I have seen fatal injuries to the soft structures of the neck with much less traction than the estimates above given. Where such tremendous force is necessary the forceps are certainly safer and their application is a matter of seconds. For even with an obstruction at the brim, we must remember that most of the head enters the pelvis before resistance is encountered. In this condition the application of forceps is easy.

The method of delivering the head which I have found most satisfactory (though it has no original features) is as follows: After delivery of the breech, bring down the legs and grasp them, enveloped in a towel, with the left hand, making traction. Make pressure over the fundus with the right hand. The importance of this pressure cannot be overestimated. To get the best results from such pressure the woman should be anesthetized. When the shoulders appear the arms should be swept down over the face. As the head enters the pelvis it should be crowded down with the hand, keeping the pelvic curve in mind. If additional force is needed an assistant may make pressure over the fundus. Ordinarily the pressure and traction can be better timed and regulated by one person than by two. Moreover, the proper axis in which to make traction can be more accurately determined with this bimanual method. And, with all respect for the opinions of those who attribute failure to the lack of sufficient flexion, it appears more rational to explain it by traction in a wrong axis.

The possibility of a large head or of a pelvic contraction

should be anticipated by having the forceps always in readiness. If there is reason to believe that great traction will be necessary, the patient should be placed on a table of good height. The advantage of occupying a seat lower than the hips of the patient is equalled only by the satisfaction of having a firm, unyielding support for the hips. With the hips on an ordinary mattress it is necessary to vary the direction of traction with every change in the amount of traction.

To consume time in attempting to supply air to the child before delivery of the head is to forget what should be an obstetrical motto: "If in a given case it is *possible* to deliver the after-coming head, it *can* and *must* be done with promptness."

PREGNANCY AFTER THE REMOVAL OF BOTH OVARIES.

BY

J. F. BALDWIN, M.D.,

Surgeon to Grant Hospital; Fellow of the American Association of Obstetricians and Gynecologists, etc.,
Columbus, O.

IN the transactions of the Obstetrical Society of London, volume xxiv., page 231, Mr. Alban Doran reports a case of pregnancy which occurred after the removal by himself of both ovaries. In connection with his own case he has found a record of eight others in which a similar result followed. The only explanation which can be offered of such an occurrence is that ovarian tissue was left by the operator, either because he failed to remove a small bit of the ovary outside his ligature, or because ovarian tissue existed outside of the ovary itself. I desire to place on record the following two cases, the first case as adding one more to the list of pregnancies following double ovariotomy, the second as furnishing an illustration of the extraovarian existence of ovarian tissue.

CASE I.—Mrs. G. F. J., Compher, O., aged 24 years. This patient had already given birth to two living children, and was pregnant about three months at the time of the operation, which was made March 3, 1891. The operation was made at her home in the presence of her physician, Dr. E. D. Moore, of Moorefield, O., Dr. S. L. McCurdy (now of Pittsburg, Pa.), and others. She presented two ovarian tumors, each about the size of a small cocoanut. The two cysts had become adherent, but the tumors were distinct and each had quite a long and small pedicle. Owing to the known fact of her pregnancy, care was taken to avoid any manipulation of the uterus. The pedicles were ligated in the usual way and the tumors removed. Recovery was prompt, and the patient was delivered at full term September 13, 1891. A letter received from the patient under date of March 5, 1900, informed me of the later birth of two other children.

In this case, although it was supposed that both ovaries were completely removed, it is possible that a small amount of ovarian tissue may have been left upon one side or the other outside of the ligature.

CASE II.—Mrs. D. S. B., Plain City, O., patient of Dr. M. J. Jenkins; aged 32 years; mother of one child aged 9 years. Had not been well for six years following a miscarriage at two months. The patient had been affected with menorrhagia since her miscarriage. The uterus was somewhat enlarged and retroverted. She suffered a good deal with leucorrhea, and had severe pain at the menstrual periods, together with the usual constitutional symptoms. Had had a good deal of local treatment, including curetting, without benefit. Was in very poor health. She was operated upon July 15, 1893, the operation consisting in the removal of both ovaries and tubes with the intention of securing the menopause. The ovaries were not adherent, and every precaution was taken to effect their thorough removal. Recovery from the operation was entirely uneventful, but the menorrhagia and other symptoms continued as before. In June, 1894, I made a thorough curettage, but without any relief, her symptoms still continuing as bad as before. She again consulted me in November, 1894. Careful examination revealed a small mass of tissue to the left of the uterus. This was quite tender and gave her a sensation, as she described, similar to that felt by pressing upon the ovary. On the 20th of that month the abdomen was again opened, and this mass of tissue, which was between the layers of the left broad ligament and apparently just below the remains of the ovarian ligament, was easily identified and removed. It was about the size and shape of a small lima bean and presented all the characteristics of ordinary ovarian tissue. No other ovarian tissue could be found at any point, and after making a ventrofixation of the uterus the abdomen was closed. Menstruation still continued, however, showing

that some ovarian tissue still remained somewhere. Menstruation was not so profuse, however, nor painful, and her general
condition was so much better that no further operative intervention seemed desirable. At the present time she is in excellent health, but menstruation is somewhat freer than normal.

The persistence of menstruation in this case would clearly
indicate the presence of ovarian tissue outside of the ovaries,
and at the second operation the presence of such tissue was
clearly demonstrated. All writers seem to acquiesce in the
statement made by Bland-Sutton in his "Surgical Diseases of
the Ovaries," that there is no authentic instance on record of a
third ovary. Mr. Doran in his paper says that he has observed
cases in which there was present in the ovarian ligament "detached tissue containing follicles." And it is the presence of
some such tissue which offers the only explanation of the few
cases which are on record in which pregnancy has followed
double ovariotomy.

125 S. Grant Avenue.

CONDITION OF THE BLADDER AFTER HYSTEROPEXY.[1]

BY

G. KOLISCHER, M.D.,
Chicago.

While in former years attention was paid only to the different methods and the technique of the operations for displacement of the uterus, at the present time more and more study
is devoted to the changes which indicate hysteropexy and to the
conditions which follow this operation.

The intimate connection between bladder and uterus makes
it easily understood that the bladder is greatly influenced in its
circulation and function by all operations which serve to modify
the topography of both these organs. On account of the variety
of cases and the diversity in operative procedures, it is impossible at the present time to report on general types of conditions which have to be considered as sequelæ of hysteropexies;
still a certain amount of qualified observations have been accumulated which may be used as a starting point for further and
more complete researches.

To begin with the simplest operation, that of Alexander,

[1] Read before the Chicago Gynecological Society, September 19, 1902.

Bulius has already published examinations of the bladder in such cases. His demonstration and my own experience lead me to believe that this operation does not lead to any important changes in the conditions of the bladder. Neither bimanual palpation nor cystoscopic examination performed in different stages of dilatation of the bladder reveals abnormal conditions. Clinical observation also fails to show any interference with the function of the bladder; capacity, expelling force, and continence remain the same as they were before the operation was done. There is only one point, however, which could be mentioned; that is, that the impression which is made upon the fundus and vertex of the bladder by the uterine body is more pronounced, so that this bulging of the bladder wall into the viscus, which is recognized by cystoscopy, appears somewhat increased.

Abdominal hysteropexy, ventrosuspension and ventrofixation, in some cases seems to have a decided influence on the circulation and function of the bladder. I am unable to bring exact statistics, because my material, although collected from different operators, is limited, and it is not always possible to get reliable and exact information as to the conditions of the bladder and urethra previous to the operation. The following observations have been made: In some cases in which the function of the bladder previous to hysteropexy was normal the patients complained that the urinary calls became more frequent, that the resistance of the bladder against certain noxæ seemed to be reduced, so that, for instance, a slight cold would produce very disagreeable vesical sensations and an excessive increase in the number of the urinary calls. The cystoscopic examination in such cases revealed an extreme paleness of the mucosa; in some instances the epithelium appeared to be swollen and soaked. If we accept the theory that the desire for urinating is principally started by the stretching of the muscular coat of the bladder, it is easily understood that a stretching of the bladder by hanging the uterus high up will lead to this increase in the frequency of urinary calls. That by faulty abdominal hysteropexy the circulation of the bladder is interfered with seems to become apparent from the following observations:

In one case a virginal individual with normal urinary apparatus was operated on by abdominal hysteropexy in such a way that the uterus was hung up rather high. A few days after the operation, which otherwise took an absolutely normal course, the urine became cloudy and the urinary calls so frequent that even the night's rest was disturbed. This condition, with some temporary lessening of the symptoms, has continued for two years. Examination of the urine never shows anything but a few epithelial cells and detritus in the sediment. Cystoscopy demonstrates that the bladder is stretched into a sausage-shaped viscus, that the mucosa is very pale, and that many epithelial rags are floating over it. All therapeutic efforts have been of no avail. In two cases of chronic gonorrheal cystitis which existed previous to the hysteropexy, the condition of the bladder took a decided turn for the worse after ventrofixation, which, in both cases, was performed at a rather high point.

It seems that although we cannot in a general way accuse ventrosuspension of being dangerous to the bladder, in all cases where the uterus is lifted out of the pelvis, to such an extent that the bladder becomes stretched, functional disorders will set in and the soil will be prepared for pathologic changes, or already existing pathologic processes will be increased in intensity.

Vaginal hysteropexy (taking this word in a general sense, without differentiating between vaginal fixation and the different methods of shortening the round ligaments) has to be considered from two different points of view: first, as to the operative steps which may interfere with the bladder; second, as to the conditions which may arise from the dislocation of the bladder after the operation is finished and permanent conditions have been secured.

The operative step which obviously is most apt to interfere with the integrity of the viscus is the act of stripping off the bladder from the uterus. If this is done in a proper way—that is, if we sever only the connective tissue between bladder and uterus—the bladder will remain absolutely intact. But if we come too near the bladder wall, or if—which happens not so infrequently—the operator digs into the bladder wall proper. a condition will arise which I described some years ago as traumatic desquamative catarrh, a condition which has since been recognized by the gynecologists. This catarrh, a very annoying condition, is, as a rule, of a stubborn character, but always heals up in the course of time without leaving any permanent defects.

The dislocation of the bladder itself does not interfere with its function if no special complications arise. In certain cases the functional activity is even improved—a point which will be discussed later on. The tolerance of the female bladder toward dislocations and changes in form is well known. As to the topography of the viscus, if the bladder is filled up bimanual palpation will reveal the elastic tumor above and partially behind the uterus. Although some authors claim that vaginal operations which necessitate stripping the bladder from the uterus lead to prolapsus of the viscus into Douglas' pouch, I was unable to find any credible report of this kind in the literature. My personal experience is also absolutely negative in this respect.

If we have to deal with a rather enlarged bladder, we find it, as a rule, disposed to both sides of the uterus. Cystoscopic examination shows the impression of the uterus in the trigonum and the adjacent part of the fundus, instead of, as normally, in the vertex. The whole bladder appears in the shape of a saddle bag.

Quite interesting and peculiar conditions arise if vaginal fixation is performed on account of prolapse and cystocele. I have three cases on record in which the functional activity of the bladder was decidedly improved after the bladder and thus the cystocele was dislocated above and behind the uterus. While in all these cases chronic retention in the cystocele was present for years, the bladder is spontaneously and completely emptied at each micturition since the operation. I think that this phenomenon can be explained in this way:

First, the cystocele does not interfere with the complete contraction of the viscus after it is lifted up above the uterus. Second, the bladder becomes easier and more completely emptied, because under the changed conditions the part of the viscus which previously formed the cystocele comes under the influence of the abdominal pressure. The last-mentioned operation for prolapse, as private information of some operators says and as my own experience teaches, is once in a while followed by incontinence in different degrees. Two cases of my own seem to offer the following explanation:

If the uterus is stitched too low down to the vagina, it pulls the vaginal wall and consequently the posterior wall of the urethra in such a direction as to distend the urethra posteriorly. This part of the urethra is now the mainstay of continence, and, if weakened, the continence will be impaired. In both cases prompt and definite relief was furnished by the insertion of a ring pessary. In cases of this kind in which, for some reason.

the application of a pessary is not desirable, operative relief has to be looked for. Although my report is by no means a complete one, I hope that the points mentioned are interesting enough to give impulse to investigation which can only be completed by the co-operation of all gynecologists interested in this matter.

92 STATE STREET.

TRANSACTIONS OF THE
CHICAGO GYNECOLOGICAL SOCIETY.

Stated Meeting, September 19, 1902.

The Vice-President, JUNIUS C. HOAG, M.D., *in the Chair.*

DR. HERBERT M. STOWE reported a case of

TRAUMATIC RUPTURE OF A VEIN IN THE UMBILICAL CORD IN UTERO.[1]

DR. JOSEPH B. DE LEE.—I have in mind a case that occurred in the Dispensary of the Lying-in Hospital service, a normal labor, where the child was born without the aid of much expulsive force, and yet the cord was cut across as though a knife had been used. Our attention was called to the condition of the cord by the fact that the child when born was quite pale and apparently asphyxiated. It recovered very promptly. It was a case of spontaneous rupture of the cord *in utero* in a simple normal case.

DR. CHARLES S. BACON.—The first case reported is an extremely interesting one, and I agree with Dr. Stowe that the syphilitic history was undoubtedly an important element in the rupture. I fail to understand how the accident she sustained could produce the hematoma, and I believe that it is hardly necessary to take that as an explanation. Some cases of hematoma have been reported where there was no accident and where the rupture was entirely spontaneous. Of course the point of rupture may be anywhere in the cord, depending on the condition of the vessels. If section had been made of this cord, the vessel wall would no doubt have been found to be weak at the point of rupture. I believe that all cases of rupture of the umbilical vessels *in utero* have occurred in women with a syphilitic history.

DR. EFFA V. DAVIS.—I recall a case of premature delivery in which the child had several hematomata in the cord. It was a syphilitic infant and developed typical lesions in six weeks, dying three months after birth, of syphilis. Sections were made of the cord and it was found that degeneration of the blood vessels was well marked. There was no history of traumatism,

[1]See original article, p. 792.

but the labor was precipitate. The largest hematoma was about the size of a walnut, and the whole length of the cord showed more or less degeneration of its vessels.

DR. J. C. WEBSTER.—It is very interesting to have a report of Dr. Stowe's first case. Dr. Davis' case was especially interesting because the child lived. These hematomata of the cord are met with in syphilitic cases, but, apart from these, there can be little doubt that the rupture of single vessels in the cord is often associated with an abnormal arrangement of the vessels, especially in velamentous insertion or in an abnormal distribution to succenturiate portions of placenta. This variety of rupture is usually associated with some form of traumatism, especially rupture of the membranes.

It seemed to me that Dr. Stowe, in his generalization, did not differentiate sufficiently between the forms of rupture which he had in mind. There may be rupture of individual vessels, rupture of the cord as a whole, and a tearing of the cord from its placental insertion or from the umbilicus. I do not know whether he meant all of these or only one. A great deal of what he said might apply to rupture of the cord as a whole, but could not apply to rupture of individual vessels in the cord.

Albert has written a monograph on this subject in which he points out a tendency to rupture in cases in which the vein is either varicose or arranged in projections called villous knots.

I would like to call Dr. Stowe's attention to one point. When speaking of the covering of the cord he used the expression amniotic sheath. This is incorrect. The cord is not covered by the amnion. The latter stops at the placental end of the cord. The sheath is practically skin, like that of the fetus. In the earliest stage it is covered with a single layer of epithelium; in the second month there are two rows of cells; later there are several layers, the outer of which is stratified like the skin of the fetus. The old teaching was that the amnion is reflected over the cord. That view has been abandoned.

I have never paid much attention to statistics with reference to the breaking weight of the cord, because they vary so greatly. It is impossible, in my opinion, to establish an average which would be of any service from a working point of view. The size and arrangement of the vessels undoubtedly have some relationship to the strength of the cord. What is called a torsion or twisting of the cord is really not such. When we speak of torsion we mean a torsion of the vessels, especially the arteries around the vein. The former, being longer than the latter, are less likely to break when the cord is stretched.

There are also great variations in the connective tissue of the cord. The Whartonian jelly varies greatly in regard to the number of well-formed connective-tissue fibrils which may be present in late pregnancy. It is also believed that the elastic fibres in the cord determine its strength. There is no elastic coat in the vessels of the cord, but elastic fibrils can be detected in the framework of the cord. They vary considerably; in some cases they are scanty, while in others they are present in large numbers. Therefore, in view of such variations, it is not wonderful that we find so much difference in the breaking weight of the cord. I do not think that any attempt at a generalization is of very much practical value.

DR. C. S. BACON.—I would like to ask the doctor where the boundary of the amnion is on the placental side.

DR. WEBSTER.—That varies slightly, but it is usually at the junction of the cord and placenta; it may be a little above or below the junction.

DR. BACON.—Is there a union between the amnion and the allantois, as there is on the fetal side?

DR. WEBSTER.—The skin of the abdomen of the fetus is continuous with the stratified epithelium of the cord, though the junction of the two may easily be determined with the naked eye. It is different from the relationship between the covering of the cord and the amnion on the fetal surface of the placenta. The amniotic epithelium is a single layer of columnar or cubical cells; the epithelial layer of the full-time cord consists of several rows of cells.

DR. JOSEPH B. DE LEE reported a case of

ECLAMPSIA, WITH CONVULSIONS IN THE CHILD.

A primipara aged 31 entered Mercy Hospital with premonitory symptoms of eclampsia, for which she received anti-eclamptic treatment. She was put on a milk diet and was given bromides and chloral. Labor progressed normally until midnight, when suddenly, without premonition, she had a convulsion, which was followed by eight more in the course of a few hours. The coma became continuous. Labor seemed to stop and the woman's condition became serious. Her pulse was 140, and cyanosis began to show in the extremities and around the lips. I saw her about 4 in the morning, and while getting her ready for examination she had two more convulsions. Artificial respiration had to be performed after the second. It was really necessary, her breathing having stopped for a long time after the convulsions. I immediately put her under an anesthetic and dilated the cervix with two fingers, and. as is usual, tore it. I immediately applied the forceps; the child was living at the time. The head came down to the perineum without difficulty, but a large hemorrhage occurred at this time which I judged came from laceration of the vagina. The perineum began to tear and bleed profusely. I did a medio-lateral episiotomy and delivered a deeply narcotized child. It was asphyxiated and narcotized, as the woman had received chloral and morphine in large doses. The child had a faint, weak, and rare heart beat, and did not make the first gasp until after thirty minutes of active resuscitation, which consisted in clearing the trachea with a catheter and mouth-to-mouth insufflation. After thirty minutes the child made the first gasp, and after an hour of continuous insufflation the child cried and was put aside as recovered.

The mother in the meantime had an interesting history. Immediately after delivery she had another convulsion, from which she rallied without artificial respiration. I expressed the placenta at once and proceeded to sew up the lacerations. While sewing these up the hemorrhage suddenly ceased, which I ascribed to the running catgut suture. But something else was wrong, because the woman stopped breathing and her pulse almost disappeared. I waited for a pulse beat until I could not wait any longer and proceeded to resuscitate the patient. I put my thumbs under her ribs, and with the fingers over the front worked the thorax vigorously up and down. One could hear the air rushing in and out. She rallied under this treatment and I put all the sutures in the wound as fast as I could. The pulse had become uncountable. Later it came down to 144. We gave her ten drops of veratrum every hour. These doses had no effect on the pulse, and I doubled the strength of the preparation, because it was the first time in my experience that veratrum failed to slow the pulse. The woman made a slow recovery and in forty-eight hours was quite conscious.

On the first day after labor she developed a fever, but after draining the wound this disappeared, so that evidently it was due to an infection. However, on the fifth day it ran up to 105.4° and then dropped again, pursuing an irregular course until the eleventh day, when it rose high again. Although the temperature curve would suggest malaria, I do not believe that it was malaria. Temperature, morning 98°, evening 104°, for several days, beginning with chill. The plasmodium was absent from the blood and the therapeutic test failed. (Exhibited chart.)

The child immediately after resuscitation was pink and I thought would recover nicely. Toward evening, however, I noticed jaw clonus and predicted some convulsions. The next morning the child had convulsions, and had them all day and evening, having one convulsion after the other. They were typical eclamptic convulsions, and we gave the infant a grain of bromide and half a grain of chloral, which had some influence on the convulsions. When the medicine was discontinued the convulsions recommenced. After the convulsions ceased the baby had an attack of intestinal intoxication due to fermentation, which did not subside until we got mother's milk for it. A few days ago both were discharged well.

DR. CHARLES S. BACON.—The baby's history is interesting, but the fact that an infant, after a severe labor, has convulsions does not prove the nature of the convulsions. Convulsive attacks after operative delivery are not uncommon. We are generally in the habit of explaining these convulsions by assuming some brain injury. I do not know how it would be possible in this case to prove the nature of the seizures in the infant. I do not think that infants are very apt to have convulsions unless there is some brain injury. We all know the experiments that have been performed on animals, the injection of large doses of strychnine into the fetus inside the uterus, and no tetanic attacks followed, although the amount of strychnine injected was very large. I think that it is true that without some injury the child is not very apt to have convulsions. It has not as yet been proved that the eclamptic poison reacts on the child.

Dr. J. CLARENCE WEBSTER.—I remember hearing Tarnier, in a clinical lecture, raise the same objections as those raised by Dr. Bacon, stating that he had never been able to convince himself that there had been postnatal convulsions in the infant; later he had changed his mind because of several cases that had come under his observation. He pointed out that a number of cases described as convulsions were those in which forceps had been used, and also referred to the occurrence of rigor mortis in the new-born child—a condition which might be considered as eclampsia.

Kreutzmann reports a very interesting case of a woman who had marked albuminuria without eclampsia. The child was born and thirty-six hours after labor developed well-marked convulsions, which he attributed to poison sucked from the breasts. There was no instrumental delivery in this case.

There is no reason to disbelieve in fetal eclampsia. It is very probably the death of the fetus *in utero* in some cases is preceded by marked movements which are of the nature of convulsions. It is also likely that postnatal eclamptic phenomena might occasionally occur.

Dr. G. KOLISCHER.—I think Dr. De Lee is correct in his diagnosis. There is no doubt that we have to deal here with a case of eclampsia in both mother and child. The differential diagnosis between eclamptic and other convulsions is made by the presence of temperature. As I understand it, the child had fever, so that there is no doubt that the convulsions were eclamptic. I think that these cases support the theory that eclampsia is due to saturation of the maternal system with the products of the metabolism of the fetus.

Dr. EMIL RIES.—I think the question of fetal eclampsia is satisfactorily settled since Schmorl reported postmortems of cases where the child had convulsions and which showed the typical lesions of the eclampsia as found in the mother, who died also.

Dr. EFFA V. DAVIS.—The case Dr. Webster mentioned recalls to my mind a case I had some time ago where the mother had premonitory symptoms of eclampsia but no eclampsia. It was a twin pregnancy and the labor was exceedingly tedious; a case of inertia uteri. The babies were well developed, weighing eight and one-quarter pounds each. The second child was born seven hours after the first, being delivered by forceps. There was no pressure on the head, as the delivery was easy, everything having been prepared by the first birth. Within thirty-six hours after its birth this child began to develop a high temperature (103° to 104° F.) and some opisthotonos, but no convulsions. Both children were affected, the second most severely. The mother had marked albuminuria, a very severe postpartum hemorrhage, but no convulsions. The second child died at the end of a week. At the postmortem examination nothing could be found to account for its death. The first child lived for six or eight months and died in convulsions. I do not know whether this had anything to do with the previous condition, but it never recovered from the peculiar rigidity. The condition of these children seemed very peculiar to me, and I called in several of my friends to see these cases, thinking that it was a poisoning from the maternal condition.

DR. CHARLES S. BACON.—It would be interesting if Dr. Ries would tell us what the typical postmortem findings of eclampsia are. In regard to the proof that Dr. Kolischer gives of the presence of eclampsia, if every infant that has a temperature a day or two after birth suffers from eclamptic poisoning, eclampsia is very common.

DR. EMIL RIES.—The postmortem findings typical of eclampsia are especially the focal necroses in the liver and the changes in the kidneys. These focal necroses have been found by Schmorl so regularly in eclamptic women that he considers them quite typical, especially as he does not find them in any other condition. As to their origin, that is doubtful, because we do not know whether it is due to syncytial masses carried into the liver or whether it is simply a toxemia. I know that these findings have not been considered typical by all men, but Schmorl has carried on his investigations for some years, and, as he finds them so regularly, I think considerable importance should be attributed to them.

DR. FRANK A. STAHL.—Though the history is very suggestive of malaria, I would ask whether any thrombi were found in the pelvic vessels. I remember a case of abortion which behaved very much like the case cited. So much has been said of infection that it occurred to me that possibly there were thrombi which disintegrated, and that the disintegration and absorption of the products were marked by rise in temperature.

DR. DE LEE (closing the discussion).—I purposely left open the question as to whether or not the convulsions were eclamptic. I am inclined to think that they were toxemic. A careful examination of the infant after birth showed a highly nervous condition, as was evidenced by the jaw clonus. No external head injuries of any kind could be found. When the first convulsion occurred I examined the baby very carefully for paralyses, but found none. Then I investigated to see if the convulsions began at any particular point constantly, thinking that perhaps the child had a cerebral hemorrhage or a fracture of the skull. The baby would have convulsions beginning on one side, then on the other, then in the legs, and then in the face, without any degree of regularity. I examined the skull to determine increase of intracranial tension. The fontanelle was not prominent, but depressed. In cases of hemorrhage in the brain the fontanelle is always prominent or flat and tense, but there cannot be much hemorrhage without producing bulging of the fontanelle.

The child passed very little urine and not often. On one occasion it went twenty-four hours without urinating. I catheterized and found a tiny trace of albumin. The child did not have sufficient kidney action, in spite of the large amount of water given it. The child had fever, which came on long after the convulsions, so that it could not be meningitis. In order to confirm my position in the matter, I got Dr. Walls and Dr. Abt, both of whom have had considerable experience with infants, to see the baby, and they leaned toward my diagnosis; and that is the position in which I would leave it.

Regarding the delivery producing head injuries, I agree with Dr. Bacon that most cases of convulsions occurring after operative deliveries are due to injury. The temperature is probably due to infection. Examination a few days ago showed a little thickening on the right side and parametritis. I would like Dr. Watkins to express his opinion, as he saw the case with me.

DR. THOMAS J. WATKINS.—I examined the patient a few days ago and was unable to account for the temperature.

DR. EMERSON M. SUTTON, of Peoria, read a paper entitled

CANCER OF THE POSTERIOR VAGINAL WALL INVOLVING THE RECTUM.

Dr. Sutton reported a case of cancer of the posterior vaginal wall which penetrated to the submucosa of the rectum, with fibrous but non-malignant infiltration around the rectum, producing a stricture. He operated by the sacral route, using the Von Volkmann-Rose incision. He resected the vagina, rectum, and one-half of the cervix, anchoring the healthy end of the sigmoid to the gluteal incision side of the wound. He cited several cases collected from the literature of the subject, and gave his reasons for attempting operations for extensive cancerous growths situated in the pelvis.

DR. GUSTAV KOLISCHER.—The history of this case and the specimen itself impress me with the idea that we have to deal with a rectal and not a vaginal carcinoma. So far as the method of operating is concerned, the idea of attacking malignant vaginal growths, or so-called inoperable carcinoma of the cervix and uterus, by sacral operations was proposed in 1888 by Hochenegg and Herzfeld and taken up by our surgeons later. It has since been abandoned: first, because results have been poor; second, because the operation is very dangerous and leaves the patient in a pitiful condition; third, because all this extensive resecting is absolutely unnecessary in females. and Senn claims it is unnecessary even in male patients. We can make accessible per vaginam the whole pelvis, and reach all the lymphatics which can be reached through the sacral route. By Schuchart's or Rehn's incision it is unnecessary to perform this mutilating incision. I would like to ask the doctor why he did not follow out Hochenegg's method and pull down the large intestine and fix it to the anus, which was indicated. Hochenegg advocates this method and uses it in every case where there is a chance of preserving the anus. All pads and supports do not help to keep the patient from being excluded from human society if he has a sacral anus. In order to reach all the lymphatics of the pelvis the abdominal route is the best. It is important to reach the primary cancer, and not only the secondarily infected areas, if we have to deal with these cases. If, in case of carcinoma, the lymphatics are once infected, the patient in most cases is lost, and the result of very extensive operations is absolutely temporary. I cannot see that anybody is justified, with the methods at hand, in resecting a part of the sacrum when operating on a supposed vaginal carcinoma.

Dr. Carl Wagner.—By studying the topography of this specimen I am inclined to believe that the fibrous induration existed prior to the development of the carcinoma. It reminds me a great deal of two cases reported by Zahn (some seven or eight years ago), which were described as round ulcers of the vagina (ulcus rotundum vaginæ) and represent the only two cases existing in literature. I am of the opinion that for a long while this rare condition, called round ulcer of the vagina (ulcus rotundum vaginæ), existed and caused an inflammatory infiltration of the tissue surrounding it, which reactive wall later on organized represents this fibrous mass encircling the rectum so heavily. The carcinoma itself developed only secondarily upon the ground of the primarily existing round ulcer of the vagina, quite analogous to a similar process in the stomach.

Dr. Emil Ries.—What interests me particularly in this case, aside from the pathology of the organs removed, would be the question which lymphatics would have to be considered as involved. Dr. Evans, in his pathological report, mentioned two routes and two groups of lymphatics which might be involved, the anterior and the posterior. Perhaps it might be advisable to take into consideration also the lateral group. In a case like this, where the carcinoma is inside the vagina, the lymphatics involved would most probably be the deep inguinal. In malignant neoplasm of the external organs the superficial inguinal would probably be involved; in carcinoma of the upper two-thirds of the vagina, the deep inguinal and the iliac; in carcinoma of the cervix itself, the iliac and lumbar; in carcinoma of the rectum, the glands along the mesentery. For the removal of the glands possibly involved in a case like this the sacral route offers distinct disadvantages. These can be removed thoroughly either by an abdominal incision or by the hypogastric method of Mackenrodt.

As there was no carcinoma in this rectum, neither the lumbar nor mesenteric lymphatics would be involved. Examination of the deep inguinal glands would probably have shown carcinoma, or the patient may show it in the future by recurrence in these glands.

DR. SUTTON (closing the discussion).—It seemed to me that drainage was much better with the wound open than closed. The sacral route is a matter of individual preference. There are carcinomas of the rectum, vagina, and cervix that no one will do much for except to give momentary benefit. When the sacrum is out of the way the results in inoperable carcinoma of the cervix will be much better. It leaves a healthy wound, provided the surgeon's technique is such as to prevent contamination of the wound by feces. This can be prevented to a large extent by the use of a Paquelin cautery.

In regard to the question whether it was a round ulcer, I left that to the pathologists. As three pathologists gave exactly the same report, I am satisfied with their findings.

The inguinal glands were not involved and I hope they never will be. With the modern treatment for recurrent carcinoma I still have hopes for the patient.

DR. GUSTAV KOLISCHER read a paper entitled

CONDITION OF THE BLADDER AFTER HYSTEROPEXY.[1]

TRANSACTIONS OF THE SECTION ON GYNECOLOGY OF THE COLLEGE OF PHYSICIANS OF PHILADELPHIA.

Meeting of October 16, 1902.

CHARLES P. NOBLE, M.D., *in the Chair.*

DR. R. P. MCREYNOLDS read an essay on

DIASTASIS OF THE ABDOMINAL (RECTI) MUSCLES.[2]

DR. CHARLES P. NOBLE.—This is a subject in which I have been interested for a good many years. I have operated repeatedly and with very satisfactory results. The operation for the cure of the condition is a simple one, and whenever the symptoms are distressing I think the condition should be operated on and cured. The method which I have used has been to make an incision usually to the right of the median line. That, of course, opens into the sheath of the right rectus, always up as far as the umbilicus, and in some cases almost to the ensiform cartilage. Then the sheath of the left rectus is split open, and when the incision goes above the umbilicus the umbilicus is excised and the peritoneum sewed up with a running suture. Then the muscle and the fascia aponeurosis are dealt with as they are

[1] See original article, p. 837.   [2] See original article, p. 814.

always dealt with in closing an abdominal wound. The under surface of the aponeurosis on the right side is bared by detaching it from the muscle, and the upper side of the aponeurosis on the left side of the wound is bared and the right aponeurosis sewed on top of the left, so that we have a double thickness of aponeurosis. The lapping should extend only about three-quarters of an inch; sometimes as much as an inch. I have used a double row of continuous sutures to accomplish that. In that way there is no difficulty in bringing the recti muscles together and getting a good, strong abdominal wall. I am sure the number operated on has run into the dozens, and so far I have never had these cases come back with any trouble. I have, therefore, no question but that they can be cured by that method.

In connection with the so-called Glenard's disease, where we have the kidneys, uterus, stomach, and intestines all prolapsed, there is no doubt whatever that anatomically the patients are imperfectly cured if we simply stitch up the uterus and kidneys, if there is also diastasis of the abdominal muscles, because the abdominal muscles no longer support the intestinal contents.

Dr. J. M. Baldy exhibited

SPECIMENS OF MYOMA OF THE OVARY.

Peterson reports a series of 82 cases of fibroma of the ovary that he had found in the literature (and reported two at the meeting of the American Gynecological Society last spring), only taking those cases in which the diagnosis had been verified by microscopical examination. He made no effort to distinguish between fibroma and myoma, only dealing with the clinical aspect. Pfannenstiel has reported a case of true myoma as distinguished from fibroma of the ovary, and has noted in his paper having seen four other cases. Dornan reports a myoma of the ovary, and says that at one time he questioned whether myoma of the ovary could exist. Myoma presupposes the presence of muscular tissue, and it has not been believed that muscular tissue existed in the ovary. Gessner reported fibromyoma from the ovarian ligament, and states there are not only muscular fibres in the ovarian ligament itself, but that there are muscle cells in the cortex of the ovary; and Dornan,, in commenting on his own case, which is an unquestionable one, says that Gessner has stated in connection with his tumor, which was the size of a bean and located in the ovarian ligament half-way between the uterus and ovary, that he believed a myoma may spring from that point and spread over to and involve the ovary and convert it into a myomatous growth. Dornan says that his own specimen goes a great way to prove this point and that he has been of the opinion that such a condition could exist.

The specimen I have to show to-night is one of such a character. It would be a pure matter of speculation at present, from the size of this growth, to say where it began to grow, whether in the ligament or the ovary or at the junction of the two, because the ovary and ligament have completely disappeared and are involved in the tumor.

I operated on the patient for uterine fibroma, and you will see that there is a large fibromyoma of the uterus which is split open and that the walls of the uterus contain a number of nodules of the fibroma. On the left side the ovary and the tube are plainly seen. The tube is in a condition of distension, containing a gelatinous fluid. On the right side there is no trace of ovary. The relations of this tumor are that it extends from the side of the uterus as an ordinary nodule or subperitoneal fibroid nodule, with this difference, that after it passes away from the uterus it lies under the broad ligament on its posterior surface in the position of the ovary. It has all the relations and attachments to the broad ligament, Fallopian tube, and round ligament above that an ovary has, and hangs free like the ovary. A subperitoneal fibroid can grow from the uterus in two ways and can take two courses. It may be a pedunculated fibroid hanging in the peritoneal cavity. A mere glance will show this is not such a one. The tumor might have sprung from the uterus at the junction of the broad ligament and grow extraperitoneally, in which case it would always be extraperitoneal in all its parts. Even then you would not have the relations to the Fallopian tube and broad ligament, etc., that this specimen has. I take it that the relations demonstrate perfectly that this tumor cannot be either of those. As far as anatomical relations are concerned, we can exclude fibromata of the uterus. The uterine tumors here are fibromyomata, the one of the ovary is pure myoma. This is a difference which exists in this case sufficiently to add just a bit of corroborative evidence to the theory of its growth. Any other solid tumor of the broad ligament we would have to consider and exclude, and this is readily done in this case. We come down to the possibility, as suggested by Gessner and Dornan, of a myoma developing in either the ovarian ligament or developing at the cortex of the ovary. Granting that that should happen, we would have in the resulting tumors exactly such attachments as we have here: subperitoneal at one point (against the uterus), and from that point out perfectly free on its under, anterior, and lateral surfaces. It should have also, if it grew into and involved the ovary, all the anatomical relations that the ovary has in health. This theory explains every relation anatomically this tumor has, and is the only possible one that does so.

As a bit of corroborative evidence, we find a point of ovarian tissue toward the fimbriated end of the tube from which I have been able to secure two sections, which show under the microscope the normal ovarian tissue. The slide shows from above downward ovarian tissue, connective tissue, and then the underlying myomatous tissue, that is, the underlying tumor tissue. We have a tumor which is microscopically a myoma, and it has been proved absolutely by Dornan that a pure myoma of the ovary does and can exist. It has all the anatomical relations that such a growth could have. No other growth I can think of in this region can produce these same anatomical relations. This specimen is spoiled by much handling to a great extent, but the essential points are still easily seen. I think it undoubtedly is a pure myoma of the ovary. I am unable to find a single evidence of proof to the contrary. The pathologist has mentioned that in the microscope slide, between the ovarian tissue and tumor tissue, there is a layer of connective tissue which they say indicates pathologically a capsule, and there is the probability of the ovarian tissue simply overlying the tumor. This point, however, seems to me still further corroborative proof of the true condition; that the portion of the ovary remaining and the tumor are one and the same thing, with the ordinary connection that any circumscribed tumor would have with a remnant of any organ from which it developed, in a connective-tissue connection.

Dr. John B. Shober.—It seems to me the manner of development of this tumor is unusual. I have seen only three cases of fibroma of the ovary. One of these occurred in my practice three years ago in an old woman past 60 years of age. We diagnosed the condition ovarian tumor. Upon opening the abdomen we found that there was some ascites. This led us to suppose that possibly it was a malignant growth, but the tumor did not present appearances of malignancy. It was about the size of a large cocoanut, weighed five to six pounds, and had a long pedicle. The pathologist reported that the tumor was composed entirely of fibrous tissue. He was unable to find any muscular tissue in his examination, though he did not examine it everywhere. The interesting point was the accompanying ascites, in the presence of which we rather expect malignant disease. It is also of special interest to find pure fibroma of the ovary of some considerable size. The specimens of these cases are extremely rare.

Dr. Wilmer Krusen.—I think undoubtedly that Dr. Baldy has presented one of the most unique specimens recently exhibited before this Section. After hearing Dr. Peterson's paper on "Fibroma of the Ovary" at Atlantic City, I had, in a few weeks, a case of fibroma of the ovary accompanied by ascites. The patient was a woman of 36. The tumor was posterior to the uterus, adherent to it, and I made the diagnosis of subperitoneal fibroid tumor. Upon opening the abdomen and breaking up the adhesions I found that the tumor was a part of the ovary. I am now having a microscopical report made on it. The most curious part is the ascitic accumulation so often associated. It is curious also that fibroma of the ovary will produce irritation and cause serum, while a movable pedunculated fibroid will not do so. Dr. Baldy says there was no ascitic accumulation about the growth itself. There must be some other condition producing the effusion in the peritoneal cavity. I have no doubt we have all heard of a number of cases in Philadelphia since Dr.

Peterson read his paper. It shows that these growths have probably been overlooked, and that very frequently, in cases of multilocular ovarian cyst, possibly fibrous tissue would be found if a more careful examination of the growth were made.

DR. CHARLES P. NOBLE.—I have had several cases of fibroma of the ovary, but never one in which the pathologist reported myoma. I am sure that I have had quite a number of fibromas of the ovary years ago when under the current teaching we supposed them to be sarcomas, and unless a microscopic examination were made they were set down as being sarcomas. I am sure I have had five or six such cases. It seems to me that, as a rule, the ascites comes because there are degenerative changes in the veins and the return circulation of the tumor is interfered with, whereas the arterial circulation is maintained. I think we should emphasize the fact that the mere presence of ascites does not indicate, as formerly taught, that the tumor is malignant.

DR. JOHN B. SHOBER.—The presence of ascites is rare in cases of pedunculated fibroids of the uterus, because these tumors are covered by a smooth, non-irritating serous membrane; whereas a fibroid tumor of the ovary has no such capsule, and its surface is usually rough and gives rise to ascites by mechanical irritation of the general peritoneum.

DR. BALDY (closing).—I think that Dr. Peterson's examinations showed that about 25 or 30 per cent of cases of fibroma of the ovary had ascites. I do not know whether Dr. Shober's explanation would hold good or not in considering the cases. In fibroma of the ovary, some have been very small, not larger than some hypertrophied ovaries. The hypertrophied ovary would have the rough cortex as well as would the neoplasm, and be coarser than the peritoneum covering the uterus, and still of the character Nature has put into the peritoneal cavity. The cavity is therefore used to friction from such surfaces. In the hypertrophied ovary, however, we never find ascites. Many of the large cases of fibroma had no ascites. Some were very small and were accompanied by ascites. The mere size, therefore, would rather indicate that that was not a factor either. Like Dr. Noble, in the past I have had a number of cases which were probably fibromas. The specimens were never examined.

TRANSACTIONS OF THE
NEW YORK OBSTETRICAL SOCIETY.

Meeting of October 14, 1902.

The President, MALCOLM McLEAN, M.D., *in the Chair.*

SUPRAVAGINAL HYSTERECTOMY FOR MYOFIBROMA.

DR. HERMAN J. BOLDT.—This specimen was removed from Mrs. S. H., æt. 43 years, married twenty-three years, who has had four children, the last eleven years ago. For the last four years she has had atypical hemorrhages, very profuse in character, passing many clots with the flow. She has had backache and pains radiating down the right thigh. The pelvis and lower abdomen were filled by a fluctuating tumor which was but slightly mobile in its upper aspect. The appearance of the patient was very anemic, in fact cachectic—so much so that maligant degeneration of the tumor was considered probable. The hemoglobin was reduced 38 per cent; erythrocytes, 2,800,000.

Bimanual examination was painful. The operation was performed this morning. At the beginning intravenous infusion of saline solution was begun by an assistant and 1,500 cubic centimetres introduced. The difficulty in raising the fibromyomatous uterus so as to clamp the broad ligament was considerable. The omentum was adherent all around its base.

This specimen is presented to bring up the question of the desirability of using the angiotribe throughout as a hemostatic. I have done four hysterectomies with the angiotribe, have used four modifications of the instrument, and have come to the conclusion that the original Tuffier's angiotribe is the most satisfactory, if one desires to use such instruments at all. So far as the saving of time is concerned, I have been unable to find them superior to ligatures. Further, the Tuffier angiotribe is so heavy and clumsy that it requires an additional assistant to hold the instrument in place while one is continuing the operation. Modifications of Tuffier's angiotribe have in my hands not given sufficient pressure to completely obliterate the vessels, so that it became necessary to use ligatures, bleeding beginning a few minutes after removal of the instruments. It is my opinion that if we could get angiotribes which exert as much pressure as the Tuffier without possessing the same clumsiness, and somewhat longer in the jaws, then the use of such an instrument may be more desirable than ligatures, first, by the saving of time, and, second, by not requiring the use of foreign material on the vessels and to close over the peritoneal folds of the broad ligaments.

Dr. J. Riddle Goffe.—I have been using the angiotribe during the past five years, and with me it is a routine custom. I always have it with me whether I operate from above or below, and I make constant use of it. I began with the Tuffier instrument and I never have had occasion to regret its use. But it is rather clumsy, and, after it is once applied, it requires support from an assistant to keep it from dragging while waiting for the two minutes to expire during its application. I have experimented with several varieties of these instruments, and in operating upon one case for carcinoma I used three instruments in succession, to see if one was more desirable than another. All acted equally well. Since then Dr. Child has modified the instrument by making it lighter and more easy to handle; his instrument I have used several times, and he has used it. The Tuffier instrument gives a pressure of 3,000 pounds; Dr. Child's,

1,600. It certainly simplifies the operation of vaginal hysterectomy in those cases where it is difficult to drag the uterus down within reach of the ligature. Often we find firm adhesions holding the appendages high up in the pelvis; I can clamp the lower half of the broad ligament and set the uterus free, making room to drag down the appendages in cases in which it would have been impossible to apply the ligatures. And even in cases in which the appendages cannot be brought down, this instrument can be slid up into the pelvis and the broad ligaments pinched off beyond the appendages. The angiotribe greatly facilitates vaginal hysterectomies in either simple or complicated cases.

DR. CHILD.—In using the Tuffier instrument we find serious objections. First, its great weight, which causes a dragging down of the tissues and makes it very clumsy to handle. Secondly, by the scissors action of the jaws the tissues are squeezed out at the end of the blades. To obviate these features I devised an instrument in which the blades come together in a parallel direction; they remain parallel until the completion of the action. I also believe that a pressure of 3,000 pounds in the Tuffier instrument is more than is needed. My instrument will exert a pressure of 1,600 pounds, and I believe that to be sufficient to control hemorrhage from the uterine or ovarian arteries and even larger vessels. I have found that it acts very satisfactorily as a hemostatic. It is about one-third the weight of the Tuffier instrument.

DR. JOSEPH E. JANVRIN.—I should like to reinforce the remarks of Dr. Goffe regarding the use of the angiotribe. I have used the instrument, particularly in doing vaginal hysterectomies, during the past five years, ever since its first introduction into this country. It works admirably and always does its work. As Dr. Goffe has stated, it shortens the time of operation very much. I have never had any trouble from pressing out the tissues from the end of the blade, as mentioned by Dr. Child. I always make it a point, after the two minutes are up after its application, to sever the tissues nearly up to the point of the blade and there stop. I never quite cut up to the points of the blades and consequently never have any hemorrhage. I have always used the Tuffier instrument.

HYDATIDIFORM DEGENERATION OF THE CHORION.

DR. HOWARD C. TAYLOR.—The patient from whom the specimen was obtained was admitted to the Roosevelt Hospital in April, 1902, with this history: She is 27 years old, married nine years; has had three children, eight years, four years, and three years ago respectively. She has also had six miscarriages, the first four at six weeks, the last two at ten weeks, and in order were seven years, six years, four years, three and one-half years, two years, and six months ago. That is, in nine years she has been pregnant nine times and has given birth to only three living children and has had six early miscarriages. No history of syphilis.

For two months previous to her admission to the hospital she had a discharge, watery in character, and at times brown or bloody. At one time the bloody discharge was so profuse that she was obliged to remain in bed for three weeks. There had been moderate pain in back and some increase in size of the abdomen. Labor-like pains began the day before her admission, and shortly after entering the hospital the mole was passed.

Under ether the uterus was found enlarged and appendages normal. The uterus was curetted and washed with normal saline solution. The patient left the hospital one month later. I examined the case again on October 13, 1902. The uterus was not enlarged, retroverted but movable, the appendages normal. In general health the patient had been well since her operation, had gained fifteen pounds in weight. She has no pain. Since the curetting she has flowed but once (for two days) about two weeks after the curetting. She is not pregnant.

Dr. H. N. VINEBERG.—I have had a case under observation for a year in which there is no malignancy; this case was curetted. In two other cases that I saw some years ago no malignancy followed.

Dr. W. S. STONE.—I had such a case last winter in my service at the Lying-in Hospital, and it proved to be very interesting, because she entered the hospital as a case of ordinary pregnancy with a dead fetus and a chronic diffuse nephritis. Under anesthesia, in dilating the cervix I found the uterus entirely filled with a mass of soft, cystic material. I removed it all with the hand and washed out the uterus. When dilating the cervix I noted that it was rather friable and tore quite deeply upon the left side. She did well and soon left the hospital. In about six or seven weeks she returned to the hospital and complained of a considerable bloody discharge from the vagina. She had lost some flesh. The physical examination revealed a rather large uterus, and upon the left side was a tumor that felt, very much like a fibroid; it was situated near the horn of the uterus. She had a temperature of 99.5° F. She was kept under observation for a few days. The bloody discharge persisted. I did a laparatomy and found, much to my surprise, that the tumor was an ovarian abscess and its hardness resulted from an adherent and thickened omentum. I also removed the uterus for surgical reasons. The interior of that organ was found to be simply the seat of an endometritis. The cystic material had been examined previously, and there had been some question as to whether a deciduoma had not already begun to grow.

Dr. R. A. MURRAY.—I have carefully observed for some years half a dozen cases. None have shown any evidences of malignancy at the time of operation or since.

VAGINAL COUNTERPRESSURE DIRECTOR.

DR. H. N. VINEBERG.—This instrument is to facilitate an incision into the vagina from above through Douglas' cul-de-sac where drainage or packing is indicated. The usual method of thrusting a blunt instrument through Douglas' cul-de-sac into the vagina is not always as easy as it is said to be. With the aid of this instrument a free incision can be made in a very short space of time, and, by clamping the edges of the incision with a clamp until a suture is applied, the patient can be saved from the slightest loss of blood. I have used the instrument in several cases and have found it very valuable.

DR. JOSEPH E. JANVRIN.—For many years I have occasionally used a somewhat similar method, lifting the posterior cul-de-sac with a big cork attached to a staff. This answers the same purpose as the instrument presented by Dr. Vineberg. It is very rare, however, that any instrument is absolutely necessary for the purpose of lifting up the cul-de-sac, as ordinarily the opening can be easily made from below upward by the scissors and easily enlarged by tearing with the fingers.

DR. J. RIDDLE GOFFE.—I do not believe in much instrumentation in opening through the posterior fornix, for we are very apt to have hemorrhage. The less cutting the better. It is better to make a wide incision in the vaginal mucous membrane and a small incision through the peritoneum, and then tear and stretch the tissues. In this way we rarely risk a hemorrhage or do mischief.

DR. GEORGE T. HARRISON.—It is rarely necessary, if we operate as we should operate, to use drainage. In case drainage *is* necessary I wish to make an emphatic protest against the method of drainage through the cul-de-sac. You should drain from above. Why make a new wound which adds a complication and increases the danger of infection? I am assuming that the method of operation is by the abdominal route.

DR. H. N. VINEBERG.—The method mentioned by Dr. Goffe is the one I have been using in the past, and it struck me as not being satisfactory because it never gave an opening large enough; if we are to drain at all we should have a good-sized opening both for the purpose of drainage and for the easy removal of the gauze. With this instrument a good-sized opening from one and a half to two inches in length can be made, and it has the further advantage that with it the incision can be made in the most dependent part of Douglas' cul-de-sac where the opening into the vagina is made just behind the cervix; as is usually the case it is at a higher level than the bottom of the cul-de-sac, and in consequence the drainage cannot be as good as when the opening is made at the most dependent part.

A FEW DISPUTED POINTS IN THE TREATMENT OF PYOSALPINX.

DR. RALPH WALDO.—When called to the bedside of a woman suffering from acute pelvic inflammation, the first question that presents itself is, what is the exact-pathological condition present, and is operative interference indicated or not? If there are secundines in the uterus they should be removed; or if there is a fluctuating point indicating the presence of pus, this should be evacuated by free incision by the most direct course. There are some who in such instances advocate radical operation, arguing that it will have to be done sooner or later; which statement is true in a few instances, while the large majority may be cured, so far as disagreeable symptoms are concerned, and subsequent normal labor may take place. When in a puerperal woman you have a septic endometritis and salpingitis on one or both sides and the early stages of peritoneal infection in Douglas' pouch, I believe that free incision and drainage of Douglas' pouch with gauze will not only very materially shorten the duration of the inflammatory disease, but will in many instances prevent irreparable disease of the tubes.

There is another large class of patients who have an old pyosalpinx, which is usually confined to the tubes, but occasionally extends to the neighboring structures, especially the pelvic peritoneum, when the patient states that she has had a number of similar attacks, which she attributes to various causes, as indiscretion of diet, fatigue, constipation, etc. Examination usually shows a localized process in one or both tubes and involving very little else. More frequently a large part of the pelvic peritoneum is involved and no special stricture can be satisfactorily palpated. In rare instances a general peritonitis will be found. In the first and second classes of cases, where you are convinced that the disease has its origin in the tubes and involves them principally, the question that most forcibly presents itself is, shall an operation be immediately performed or not? Excepting where there is a very rapidly extending virulent peritonitis, I want to say all I can in opposition to operative interference of any kind during the acute stage of the disease, and especially when you are first called to see the patient when the acute stage has passed. There are many instances where competent gynecologists have made a diagnosis of acute pyosalpinx and strongly urged immediate operation, and, this being refused, 'the patient has not only recovered from the acute attack, but has gone years without discomfort or subsequent attack.

After the acute process has entirely subsided and you can palpate one or both tubes, enlarged and more or less tender, an operation is indicated, and I believe that the abdomen should be opened from above and, as far as possible, the diseased structure removed.

Where it is impossible to separate adhesions without allowing the escape of pus into the field of operation, which in every instance should be separated from the remainder of the peritoneal cavity by sterile gauze sponges and towels, the escaping pus must be removed as rapidly as possible from the wound.

After removal of the diseased tube, and possibly ovary, peroxide of hydrogen is thoroughly applied to the region. The entire field is wiped clean with sterile sponges, which are frequently wet with sterile water. In rare instances the field of operation, never the general peritoneal cavity, is thoroughly irrigated with hot normal saline solution. A sterile gauze sponge is placed over the surface from which the tube has been removed, the superficial layer of sponges is removed, the hands of the operator and assistants are thoroughly cleansed, and the other side investigated, and, if found to contain pus, treated as the first.

In every instance where pus has escaped, the peritoneal cavity is drained from the deepest portion of the wounded area—which is usually Douglas' pouch—anteriorly through the lower angle of the abdominal wound by means of a Mikulicz drain, the outer portion of which is composed of sterile gauze, and usually the inner portion of iodoform gauze. Iodoform gauze is never allowed to come in contact with living tissue. The upper portion of the wound is closed, taking great care not to constrict the drain as it passes through the abdominal wall. Externally a moist bichloride dressing is applied. which is changed as often as it is soiled by the discharges. On the third day the central portion of the drain is partially removed, and on the fifth day it is entirely removed. Usually on the seventh or eighth day the outer portion of the drain is found to have separated from the surrounding structures, and is removed, and a small strip of gauze is placed in the wound. Primary union almost invariably takes place above the drain, and it is seldom that any pus discharges from the drained portion. In no case is the drain introduced so as to make marked pressure against any of its neighboring structures, but is so applied that it is a drain, never a packing. The drain should be left in as long as indicated, because during the first three or four days there is a free discharge of material, and after this the drain is adherent to the neighboring structures, and its removal will cause severe pain and leave a bleeding surface, and a rise of temperature will ensue, which is not the case when the drain is removed at the end of a week when it is not adherent. A few months after the operation the scar will show very little evidence of a drain having been used, which is not the case when it is removed soon after the operation. When the drain is removed within a few days after the operation, it is not uncommon for the intestine or omentum to be drawn into the wound and so have a condition that later results in hernia.

DR. HERMAN J. BOLDT.—I was under the impression that although drainage was a method in vogue and extensively used by abdominal surgeons years ago, it had now been dispensed with, except under exceptional circumstances. There are a large number of instances in which operations have been performed for the removal of a pyosalpinx when the tubes have ruptured during enucleation and the patients have done equally well when the pus was wiped out of the pelvis with gauze and the abdomen closed. The only instance in which a gauze drain would be applicable, in my opinion, is where there has been a large, torn adhesion surface; then it is used only for the purpose of stopping the oozing and of giving exit for twenty-four or thirty-six hours to the sero-bloody oozing which takes place from that site. The virulent secretion in gonorrheal suppurative salpingitis is, as a rule, at the time when such patients are operated upon, sterile; therefore the uselessness of draining in that class of cases. (Personally I consider drainage, if used at all, from below preferable.) So far as the question of hernia is concerned, I can conceive how that is possible when we leave in the gauze drain for a number of days; such an abdominal scar will yield more readily to intra-abdominal pressure than when the drain gauze is removed early.

Dr. E. H. Grandin.—I presume that we are all here for a free interchange of opinion, and therefore I trust that the reader of the paper will pardon me if I take issue with regard to the manner of drainage. His description carried me back to the days when I began the study of, and taught, gynecology; then it was the custom to place in glass tubes from above down in the cul-de-sac and expect the pus and blood to flow uphill. I have seen Bantock in London, and Lister in 1878 and 1879, introduce these glass tubes with fenestræ and expect fluids to flow uphill. I can recall some cases of intestinal obstruction the result of using these fenestrated glass tubes. I have been taught by some who are present here to-night, and by others who are dead, to place gauze in from above; but it did not take me a long time to make up my mind that that was a false method for trying to secure drainage. If we wish to drain well we should endeavor to imitate Nature's method; water finds it impossible to flow uphill and so will serum, blood, or pus which gravitates down to Douglas' cul-de-sac. The point that I really wish to make is this: If I should look over my statistics I could tell you that I have had many successful cases drain downward into the vagina which equal in number the cases reported by the reader of the paper which drained upward. The logical conclusion to be drawn is this: that I can see no indication for draining at all with gauze or anything else. If we have performed a clean operation and if we insert gauze it is for the purpose Dr. Boldt has already mentioned, of covering over the raw surface to prevent the intestinal adhesions. I am still deluded enough to carry gauze into the vagina after total hysterectomies for fibroids when there is no pus present. When pus is present I believe in packing gauze over the raw surface, and I carry it into the vagina and not upward. Within twenty-four hours after an abdominal section, gauze, no matter where it is placed, will not drain the general peritoneal cavity; therefore why place it in for drainage? I have reached the conclusion that after a clean abdominal operation drainage is not necessary. If it is used to protect raw surfaces against adhesions of intestines, that is right; if not introduced, the gut will adhere. After a pyosalpinx where pus, contrary to expectations or wishes, has oozed into the lower pelvis, and where we have cleaned the lower pelvis, I question very much, if it is an old pyosalpinx, if it is necessary to insert gauze. If it should be necessary to insert gauze we should imitate Nature and allow the fluids to flow downhill, and not try to work against Nature's method by carrying the gauze upward. Much of the so-called drainage, by the way, is not drainage at all, but is simply oozing from raw surfaces, the necessary outcome of placing gauze (or any foreign body) against them.

DR. A. F. CURRIER.—I suppose that almost all of us have reached a point in our experience when we have definite views upon the question of drainage. With regard to the question of hemorrhage, it is certain that, in cases of very difficult removal of pus tubes, it is a serious question to decide whether it is prudent to allow the continuance of hemorrhage from surfaces denuded of peritoneum, which sometimes even requires subsequent reopening of the abdomen. I should like to refer to an experience that I have had lately. By the use of Cargile's membrane, or sterilized peritoneum, in cases where the denudation has been quite extensive, very satisfactory results have been obtained. After the surface has been carefully dried this substance adheres to it at once. As an additional security a large rubber tube is introduced to the bottom of the cul-de-sac, and if, at the end of twenty-four hours, the hemorrhage is insignificant, the tube is withdrawn. It is a tentative measure and in my experience thus far has been satisfactory. I cannot say absolutely, of course, that the substance has remained where it was applied, because no mishaps have been observed where it has been used, but whether *post hoc* or *propter hoc* I am unable to say.

DR. H. N. VINEBERG.—It seems to me that the value of this discussion does not rest upon whether a drain should be introduced or not, but whether in cases of pyosalpinx a waiting policy should be pursued—*i.e.*, waiting until the pus has become sterile. I think, gentlemen, that is a step backward and gynecologists have not kept pace with surgeons in this branch of surgery. It is not good surgery to wait four or five weeks when we have to deal with suppurating tubes or ovaries, in the hope that the pus may become sterile. I think that in the future gynecologists will take a different stand in the treatment of these cases and attack from below, evacuating the pus first and then completing this operation from above, if necessary. I wish to make mention of one case which I think is rather instructive in connection with this class of cases. During the summer a patient came into the hospital; she had been curetted outside by a physician, and in consequence she had a large suppurating mass on the right side. The woman was in very poor condition and I was loath to operate upon her, hoping that rest in bed would cause a subsidence of the temperature and time would elapse for the pus to become sterile. In spite of that her temperature ranged from 103° to 104° F. at night and from 99° to 100° in the morning. The mass was getting larger and the patient was losing ground. Believing that if I attempted to operate from above the patient would die, I determined to evacuate the pus from below, and so I entered the mass, which was high up, and with considerable difficulty evacuated a large quantity of pus. However, before she left the operating room she had a profuse hemorrhage, and in spite of our efforts the hemorrhage persisted, and the only thing left for me to do was to open the abdomen and enucleate this pus sac. This patient made a slow but good recovery. This illustrates what can be done in similar cases. I think it would have been better to have had an operation sooner. It is only a question of being able to remove pus sacs without infecting the general peritoneal cavity; that, I think, is the main question, and not the question that Dr. Waldo raises, that, in some cases diagnosed as such, the patients get well. The cases he refers to I believe to have been cases in which there were inflammatory exudates and collections of serum, which are so frequently found in pelvic inflammations; I do not believe they were true cases of pyosalpinx, such as we understand by that term—tubes distended with a considerable amount of pus.

Dr. C. A. Von Ramdohr.—I wish to call attention to the fact that there has not been enough stress laid upon the difference between pyosalpinx depending upon gonorrheal or puerperal or septic origin resulting from an operation. In the first instance you can wait; in the others you are occasionally obliged to operate on account of the danger of rupture of the tube. We can never wait in puerperal pyosalpinx without being well aware that rupture into the peritoneum will mean quick death to the patient. I remember one particular case that Dr. Boldt saw with me, in which a puerperal pyosalpinx was not diagnosed and which ruptured three hours later, too late to save the patient. In puerperal pyosalpinx it takes a good deal of ripe experience to exactly balance the time when to operate. In all cases of course it is always good surgery to empty the pus tubes or else remove them from the body at the earliest possible moment.

So far as drainage is concerned, I urge absolutely against the employment of rubber tubes in the abdomen, even for twenty-four hours. Drainage is not necessary, if we have a clean field of operation; here the fluid left is sterile. Drainage, so-called, chiefly serves to keep the intestines away from the wound, thus preventing adhesions, and to stop hemorrhage uncontrollable by other methods.

Dr. A. P. Dudley.—The subject of the paper was interesting enough to draw me out to-night, because I thought this subject was long since settled.

With regard to this question of drainage it should be borne in mind that it is the care of the drain which makes it effective. In twenty-four hours the gauze is stuck in the cul-de-sac and all the secretions or excretions will be confined within the pelvis. The gauze should be moved daily. The presence of a tube in the pelvis is a greater menace than damming up the secretions for a short time. The poor drainage comes from a lack of knowledge in handling the drain properly. Another good point is that we should not remove the gauze too early. I would not place in a drain from above. The Mikulicz drain is bad. If we could confine the suppuration to the pelvis, drainage from below will be proper and will not produce any fistula, will be sufficient, and you will be doing what you know to be right. Another advantage in using the gauze is that you do not permit the admission of air into the abdominal cavity, as you would if drainage was instituted from above. No matter what you use, the rubber, gauze, or Mikulicz drain, you will get air in. Gauze is really used to protect the raw surfaces and to remove the secretions that have accumulated.

Dr. George T. Harrison.—I do not think that drainage should be used at all in these cases, nor do I think that the majority of men put in Mikulicz's tampon for the purpose of drainage. As Dr. Boldt has stated, you may sometimes have a large raw surface, and the Mikulicz dressing is then used for the purpose of preventing intestinal adhesions. In some cases in which there is an extensive hemorrhage, the Mikulicz tampon can be used for the purpose of preventing more hemorrhage by the compression which it exerts. I wish to call attention to a force in Nature called capillary attraction, which Dr. Grandin seems to have ignored.

Dr. G. W. Jarman.—I wish to refer to one point that has not been spoken of in reference to drainage from below, which I have found to be of great advantage. I refer to posture. I believe in drainage was used. Those are the cases I drain. If septic, or been stated, that if you pull little by little upon the gauze a gush of fluid will appear; this certainly does occur, and I have had better results in cases of sepsis or possible sepsis when such drainage was used. Those are the cases I drain; if septic, or possibly septic, I drain from below and raise the head of the bed, lifting it from twelve to sixteen inches. At first I feared there would be too much strain on the weakened heart, but no evil results have ever followed. I have not seen a case where the least risk was run by reason of this posture, and I have seen cases recover which I believe would not have been saved otherwise. By gravity everything goes to the lower part of the pelvis. Follow a case in such a posture for a few days and see how much discharge comes away, provided a few inches of gauze are removed each day.

DR. J. RIDDLE GOFFE.—I believe in evacuating pus as soon as it is discovered.

With regard to the method of attack, I believe that the cases described by the reader can be operated on from below—*i.e.*, through the vagina. I also believe in drainage in all cases. I draw out a little day by day, beginning on the fourth day. The gauze is kept moist and the adhesions dissolved with vaginal douches of boric acid solution. These are continued daily and a few inches of the gauze packing removed daily also. If Dr. Jarman will add this practice of giving boric acid douches to the system of handling gauze drains which he has described, I think he will find it a distinct advantage. A gauze packing, in order to drain, must be kept moist at its outer end.

DR. RALPH WALDO.—The object of my paper was to elicit discussion, and it has succeeded. Among the many things mentioned in the paper was drainage. Dr. Goffe and I agree equally on the question of drainage. The question is whether we should drain from above or below. In regard to its removal, I agree with what he has stated, and pull out the gauze little by little, beginning on the third day, and remove it all by the end of the week. I use the Mikulicz drain. I drain for the removal of discharge and prevention of adhesions; I do not want to leave a raw bleeding surface by tearing off the drain, but wait until it separates and then remove it.

If gauze does not drain, where does the large amount of bloody serum and other discharges that saturate the dressings as late as the third or fourth day after the operation come from? I have heard of the diagnosis of pyosalpinx having been made and no pus found. You may have remembered that I stated that there was no question as to the propriety of opening when we felt a fluctuating point. I wish it to be understood that I am not discussing pelvic abscesses.

There is another class of cases I referred to to-night, where there is inflammatory disease in the tube and the tube contains from one drachm to three or four ounces of pus, and the neighboring structures are thick and hard, and there is no fluctuating point. You say, " I think there is pus present," but you do not know positively. I have seen many such patients get well without operation.

Regarding the etiology of pyosalpinx, a great many are caused by extension into the tubes from septic endometritis, usually following an abortion, or less frequently labor. Pyosalpinx may occur, but it is not frequent, from gonorrhea. I did not speak of that class of cases of marked inflammatory disease of the tubes where there was some pus in the tubes, not in a cavity, but as an infiltration. I did not speak of the cases in which we operate and take out so-called catarrhal tubes.

I had more interest in the absolute impropriety of removing

normal tissue from a human being intentionally than in any other part of the paper. I admit that one will take out a uterus thinking that there is malignant disease there; but when I am dealing with pus tubes I leave everything that is normal. This is a point that I was more interested in than the one of drainage.

TRANSACTIONS OF THE WASHINGTON OBSTETRICAL AND GYNECOLOGICAL SOCIETY.

Meeting of April 4, 1902.

The President, G. W. Cook, M.D., *in the Chair.*

Dr. J. R. Bromwell read the report of a case of

LEUKEMIA IN CHILDHOOD.[1]

Dr. J. B. Nichols said that, according to the accepted statements in the manuals of medicine, the division of cases of leukemia into two distinct types, splenic (or spleno-medullary) and lymphatic, would appear to be clearly and finally settled. The splenic type is ordinarily held to exhibit the characteristic enlargement of the spleen with a large proportion of myelocytes in the circulating blood; while the lymphatic type is supposed uniformly to present primary enlargement of the lymph glands with great increase of the lymphocytes or mononuclear leucocytes in the blood. Recent findings, however, will apparently unsettle these views and necessitate a revision of the current classification of the varieties of leukemia. Cases of splenic enlargement, for instance, occur without an increase of lymphocytes; exhibiting, that is, the splenic type of the disease with the blood picture supposedly belonging to lymphatic leukemia. Three distinct varieties of blood changes are now recognized: (1) that in which the myelocytes are increased, forming 40 per cent or more of all the leucocytes (myelocythemia); (2) that in which the small mononuclears are increased, up to 90 per cent or more; and (3) that in which the large mononuclears are enormously increased. Any one of these blood varieties may be associated with either the splenic or the lymphatic changes. Usually, but not always, splenic leukemia and myelocythemia go together, and lymphatic enlargement is usually associated with increase of the lymphocytes. The cases exhibiting increase in the large mononuclears seem usually to be acute.

The case reported by Dr. Bromwell is one of those in which the blood picture and the organic changes are reversed from the association ordinarily laid down in the works on medicine: that

[1]See original article, p. 808.

is, there was typical and enormous enlargement of the spleen, practically without involvement of the lymph glands, with enormous increase of the large lymphocytes in the blood, but without myelocytes. The case further departs from the types of acute leukemia as recently laid down by Cabot, in that the splenic hypertrophy was enormous, and the number of leucocytes reached as high a figure as ordinarily characterizes the chronic forms of leukemia.

Possibly the question may ultimately be settled somewhat after these lines. When the bone marrow is primarily involved myelocytes will appear in the blood in large numbers; the spleen or lymph glands, or both, are also involved, especially the spleen. When either the spleen or the glands are primarily involved, the leucocytes increased in the blood will be of the mononuclear variety—small mononuclear in the more chronic cases, large mononuclear in the more acute cases.

Dr. Bromwell's case was acute, with increase of the large mononuclear leucocytes, and (so far as can be judged without autopsy findings) practically of purely splenic form, without involvement of lymph glands or bone marrow.

The retiring President, DR. COOK, read an address on

PUBERTY IN THE GIRL.[1]

TRANSACTIONS OF THE OBSTETRICAL SOCIETY OF LONDON.

Meeting of October 8, 1902.

The President, PETER HORROCKS, M.D., *in the Chair.*

COMPLETE INVERSION OF UTERUS OF SEVEN MONTHS' DURATION ; FAILURE OF ELASTIC PRESSURE WITH REPOSITORS; OPERATION OF ANTERIOR VAGINAL CELIOTOMY, ANTERIOR UTEROTOMY AND REPLACEMENT; RECOVERY.

MR. JOHN TAYLOR described a case of complete inversion of the uterus causing dangerous hemorrhage and obstinate vomiting, the treatment adopted for the alleviation of the symptoms, and the operation finally carried out for the reduction of the inversion. He remarked on the rarity of complete inversion, on its clinical character, and on the operative difficulties which may be met with during treatment.

MR. BUTLER SMYTHE congratulated Mr. Taylor on the success attending his operation. He wished, however, to ask why Aveling's repositor had not been tried in this case as well as Tait's instrument. So far as his knowledge went, Aveling's repositor was almost always successful, and a well-known author even

[1] See original article, p. 804.

went so far as to say "he had never known it to fail." Mr. Butler Smythe asked his question because he looked upon Aveling's repositor as a simpler and more reliable instrument than that introduced by Tait. The former, being without any spring. was less liable to slip during the attempts at replacement.

DR. VICTOR BONNEY was much interested to learn that in Dr. Taylor's case complete obliteration of the junction between cervix and vagina had occurred. This entirely bore out the deductions he had made on the specimen he had just exhibited, and he thought there could be no doubt but that the mechanism by which this was brought about was the same in the two cases.

DR. HEYWOOD SMITH considered that in cases of chronic inversion of the uterus sufficient consideration had not been given to direct manipulation of the uterine body. His experience went to prove that intermittent squeezing of the inverted fundus. though it might prove a tedious process, yet in many cases was very effectual, pressure tending to empty the blood vessels and causing the muscular tissue to relax; then, if pressure is made with the thumb at the orifice of one of the oviducts where the uterine tissue is thinner, it would be comparatively easy to reduce the inversion.

DR. HANDFIELD-JONES regretted that he could not agree with the line of treatment adopted in this case. He had had a similar case under his care, in which the inversion was so acute that no line of definition between vagina and end of cervix could be made out. The uterus hung as a pear-shaped mass from the vaginal roof, and the finger passed from the vaginal mucous membrane on to the cervical mucous membrane without the possibility of distinction. The same difficulty had arisen as in Mr. Taylor's case, viz., that the womb was so movable that it was extremely difficult to keep the cup of the Aveling's repositor on the uterine body. However, by packing swabs round the womb in the upper vagina and patient watching, reposition had been effectually secured. He could not help thinking that a similar good result might have been obtained in the present instance.

There were two other points worthy of notice. In the first place, the result of the operation in Mr. Taylor's case was to leave a long, weak scar in the anterior uterine wall, and this might be a source of danger if the patient became gravid again. In the second place, if a patient was so collapsed and in such a critical state as had been described by Mr. Taylor, would not removal of the womb per vaginam be an operation shorter, simpler, and attended by less shock?

DR. HERBERT SPENCER thought we were much indebted to Mr. Taylor for pointing out the peculiar absence of any groove between the cervix and body. He alluded to the great value of Aveling's repositor in these cases—an instrument which, as Dr. Cullingworth said, appeared to be almost unknown on the Continent, and was even, he believed, spoken of somewhat contemptuously by a foreign gynecologist. His own opinion was that

there was no method of reducing an inverted uterus to be compared with reposition with Aveling's instrument, and that the
cases must be very rare in which the instrument would fail. The
difficulty of slipping of the cup off the fundus was present
in many cases. In one case of the kind he had held the
instrument in place and had then rapidly reduced an .inver-
sion which was previously very obstinate. He was interested
in the case of manual reposition mentioned by Dr. Heywood
Smith, because it seemed to support an opinion he had always
held, that, with patience, continuous pressure (with Aveling's
instrument) would overcome the resistance of the uterine muscle
and restore the organ in nearly every case. He would like to
know if Mr. Taylor had persevered with the taxis and had
ascertained that the cup had not slipped off the fundus.

DR. DUNCAN agreed with Dr. Cullingworth that the Society
was indebted to Mr. Taylor for bringing forward another method
of reducing a completely inverted uterus. At the same time he
could not help feeling that if Aveling's repositor had been applied to the inversion and kept there by packing the vagina carefully all around, the inversion would have been reduced. Dr.
Duncan mentioned a case which he reported many years ago in
the *Lancet,* in which by this method he reduced a complete inversion which had existed for nine years.

DR. BLACKER asked why Mr. Taylor had incised the uterus anteriorly, instead of first opening Douglas' pouch and attempting reduction after separation of the adhesions, as recommended
by Küstner.[1] He thought the objection raised by Dr. Handfield-
Jones one of great importance. In a recent case of his own,
where he had reduced a chronic inversion of some four months'
standing by Aveling's repositor, the patient became pregnant
and had recently been delivered of a full-term child. As these
cases usually occurred in young women who might subsequently
become pregnant, the danger of rupture of the uterus was considerable, more especially when it was necessary, as in Mr. Taylor's case, to carry the incision from the fundus uteri to the
external os.

EPITHELIOMA OF THE CERVIX.

DR. LOCKYER read a short communication of a case in which
the uterus showed rapidly growing epithelioma of the cervix.
Death from recurrence of the disease had occurred five months
after removal of the womb.

DR. VICTOR BONNEY showed a specimen of

UTERUS AND CHILD IN THE SECOND STAGE OF LABOR.

DR. HERBERT SPENCER exhibited a

MEDAL

which had been struck to commemorate the twenty-fifth anni-

[1]Centralb. f. Gynäk., 1893, No. 4.

versary of the first Porro operation, and also presented to the Society a copy of the work which had been published in connection with that event.

REVIEWS.

THE MEDICAL RECORD VISITING LIST, or Physicians' Diary for 1903. New Revised Edition. New York: William Wood & Company.

This well-known visiting list contains the usual pages for cash accounts, engagements, records, and addresses, preceded by useful information in compact form. The latter consists of a calendar, tables for the conversion of weights and measures into the common or metric system, tables of maximum doses of drugs and of other facts relating to them, directions for the care of emergeney cases, and hints on the writing of wills. The List is compact, well bound and well printed, but is chiefly commendable for the omission of much of the useless information which too often adds to the weight of a visiting list.

A MANUAL OF SURGERY. For Students and Practitioners. By WILLIAM ROSE, M.B., B.S. Lond., F.R.C.S., Professor of Clinical Surgery in Kings College, London, Senior Surgeon to Kings College Hospital, etc.; and ALFRED CARLESS, M.S. Lond., F.R.C.S., Surgeon to Kings College Hospital and Teacher of Operative Surgery in Kings College, London, etc. Fifth Edition. Pp. 1212. New York: William Wood & Company, 1902.

Each of the rapidly succeeding editions of this popular work has been a marked improvement over its predecessors, and the present volume is no exception to the rule.

It continues to present the facts of surgical science in a succinct and clear form, so that a vast amount of material is compressed into a small space. The authors have abandoned the idea that a knowledge of inflammation and its treatment is the first and most important element in surgical practice, and have given the foremost place to bacteriology and the principles of aseptic and antiseptic surgery. Many little changes and additions are apparent. A number of new plates have been added throughout the text, notably a series of very beautiful X-ray pictures showing fractures and other surgical affections of bone.

PHYSICIANS' VISITING LIST FOR 1903. Philadelphia: P. Blakiston, Sons & Co.

This well-known list contains, besides the blank leaves for visits, memoranda, etc., tables of incompatibility, antidotes, metric weights and measures, doses, calculation of date of labor, and treatment of asphyxia and apnea.

BRIEF OF CURRENT LITERATURE.

OBSTETRICS.

Management of the Third Stage of Labor.—R. W. Holmes (*Phil. Med. Jour.*, Aug. 9), directly after cutting the cord, or even before, turns the woman on her back, if the second stage has been conducted on the side. The buttocks and vulva are cleaned, fresh linen placed under her, and a sterile pad applied to the vulva. The thighs should be closely apposed. The hand resting lightly upon the uterus will determine the condition of the organ, but no massage should be practised. In from ten to thirty minutes the placenta will pass into the vagina. Now the placenta may be expressed. Credé's method should have a small place in the treatment of the third stage; if there be some uterine relaxation with hemorrhage after a contraction, Credé may be appropriately carried out.

First Stage of Labor.—E. H. Tweedy (*Jour. Obst. and Gyn. Br. Emp.*, Oct.) believes: 1. The first stage of labor begins when the polarity of the uterus is established. 2. Uterine polarity results from an over-stretched condition of the nerves which course through the lower uterine segment and are distributed to the circular muscular fibres of the cervix. The painless contractions and retractions of pregnancy thin out and stretch the segment, and thus ultimately induce polarity. 3. The cervix being fully dilated does not necessarily imply a sufficiently open os to permit of the passage of the fetus. 4. The anterior cervical lip is not easily nipped or incarcerated between the pubes and the descending fetus. The cause of its elongation is due rather to the retraction of the posterior cervical lip and the consequent dragging upward of the os, which cannot sufficiently dilate to permit of the passage of the fetus through it. 5. Such an os will, in the case of primiparæ, rupture almost certainly in order to permit of the commencement of the second stage of labor, an expansion sufficiently large to permit the passage of the greatest diameter of the presenting portion of the fetus. 6. Such a laceration cannot be treated by immediate suture, not alone because of the great edema of the anterior lip, but chiefly for the reason that the posterior lip is taken up and there is therefore nothing to which to stitch it. 7. A multiparous cervix is not always the weakest portion of the uterus. When this is so, a uterine rupture occurring as a consequence of rigid os will be preceded by none of the usual premonitory symptoms, and the tear will be most likely to involve the vagina.

Indications for Cesarean Section.—A. L. Galabin (*Br. Med. Jour.*, Oct. 11) advises Cesarean section in the place of embryotomy, provided that the decision can be made before labor cr early in labor, that the patient has not been exposed to sepsis, and that an operator skilled in abdominal section is available. When the patient is exhausted by prolonged labor, and in houses where perfect asepsis cannot be obtained, embryotomy is preferable. It is advisable to let the patient decide whether she shall be rendered sterile at the time of delivery or left so that she may bear other children. If sterilization is decided upon, the best operation is likely to prove to be supravaginal hysterectomy, one or both ovaries being left. Where cancer of the cervix exists, Cesarean section is called for if any considerable part of the circuit of the os is involved; but the risk of sepsis renders the prognosis much less favorable than in cases of contracted pelvis.

In cases where extraction by forceps is likely to be difficult, an operator successful in Cesarean section may advise operation with the prospect of diminishing the risk to the child and little if any increase of risk to the mother. For placenta previa the operation is only advisable for those skilled in Cesarean section.

Murdock Cameron *(Br. Med. Jour.*, Oct. 11) states that the operators who advise Cesarean section for placenta previa are surgeons of little or no experience in obstetric practice. A skilled obstetrician would never think of such a procedure. With a diameter under two and one-half inches, where engagement of the head is impossible, no one would hesitate to advise Cesarean section, although there will always remain cases—such as where the child is dead or a subject of hydrocephalus—in which craniotomy may be resorted to. Experience alone will enable one to avoid extreme measures in cases with a conjugate diameter measuring more than three inches, and where the skilled practitioner will weigh the chances between premature induction of labor and symphyseotomy.

Fritsch's Fundal Incision.—J. M. Munro Kerr *(Br. Med. Jour.*, Oct. 11) finds (1) that the only advantage of Fritsch's fundal incision is that the child can be more easily extracted; (2) the only proved objection to the incision is that the uterus becomes attached higher up to the abdominal wall and remains larger; (3) weighing the one against the other, an anterior longitudinal incision, if made high, is the best for routine practice; but when the uterus has also to be removed subsequently to the extraction of the child, Fritsch's fundal incision is the better.

Potassium Chlorate in Pregnancy.—Robert Jardine *(Br. Med. Jour.*, Oct. 11) uses potassium chlorate in the treatment of cases of habitual death of the fetus in the latter months of pregnancy. He uses it in ten-grain doses three times a day, beginning about the end of the third month. He reports several cases in which he used it successfully.

Puerperal Eclampsia.—H. O. Nicholson *(Br. Med. Jour.*, Oct. 11) finds that thyroid extract is a very valuable remedy in some cases of eclampsia, if only for the purpose of re-establishing the flow of urine. It may be advantageously used in all cases of eclampsia, but when convulsions are frequent and severe at least one large dose of morphine should be given. Besides these measures, saline infusions may accelerate diuresis. In cases with coma and high fever a cold or tepid bath seems to afford the best chance of recovery. In the comatose type one would not use morphine. Thyroid extract should be tried in some of those rare cases of suppression of urine occurring after labor. ·

GYNECOLOGY AND ABDOMINAL SURGERY.

Abdominal Hysterectomy for Fibromyoma Uteri.—Herbert R. Spencer *(Br. Med. Jour.,* Oct. 11) concludes that in fibromyoma uteri total abdominal hysterectomy is preferable to supravaginal amputation, and Doyen's is the best method of performing the operation.

The Knee-Chest Posture in Some Operations upon the Vesical End of the Ureters.—The advantages claimed by Howard Kelly *(Jour. A. M. A.,* Aug. 9) for the knee-chest posture are as follows: 1. The opening into the bladder is made in a few seconds, and can be extended from cervix to urethra so as to include the entire base of the bladder. 2. In some cases, after catheterizing the ureters so as to mark their location, a wide lateral incision, or two incisions, can be made to secure a still wider exposure and render the remoter parts of the bladder more accessible. 3. The opening into the bladder is made more accessible by a strong retraction of the perineum with a Simon's speculum pulling in the direction of the sacrum. 4. The anterior vesical wall can be reached best by inserting a retractor, 2.5 to 3 centimetres in width, into the bladder through the incision, and then using it to draw the incision down to the vaginal orifice, producing a displacement of 4 to 5 centimetres. 5. A beautiful means of inspection of all parts of the bladder is afforded by means of a large cylindrical speculum, about 12 centimetres in length and about 3 in diameter, with a large handle similar to a proctoscope. 6. For operations on the vertex and lateral vesical walls, the assistant's hand may be of the utmost service in pushing the bladder up into the vaginal wound; in this way a tumor or an area of ulceration at the top of the bladder can often be removed with as much ease as a growth in the anterior vaginal wall.

Myomectomy versus Hysterectomy.—Andrew McCosh *(Med. News,* Sept. 27) finds that in young women with uterine fibroids demanding removal myomectomy should always be the operation of choice. Myomectomy is possible and advisable in the great majority of cases of fibroids in young women. For the safe performance of myomectomy the strictest asepsis is needed, otherwise it becomes a most dangerous operation. In the operation of myomectomy fear of hemorrhage should be cast aside and bold and rapid methods should be adopted. The operation is attended by the same danger to life as is hysterectomy. The ultimate results as regards menstruation, pain, and pregnancy are satisfactory.

Retrodisplacements of the Uterus.—F. H. Davenport *(Ann. of Gyn. and Ped.,* Aug.) finds the pessary of value in simple cases of retroverted uterus without complication which have lasted only a short time; retroversion following childbirth; and cases complicating neurasthenia where operation is inadvisable until the patient's health is built up. The pessary treatment is not applicable to cases in young girls where local treatment of any kind is inadvisable, to cases complicated with lacerations, or to cases of long standing where secondary changes in the circulation of the uterus have followed.

DISEASES OF CHILDREN.

Arthrodesis of the Ankle for Infantile Paralysis.—John Dane *(Amer. Med.,* Aug. 16, 1902) urges an early operation, and gives the following points in its favor: 1. It avoids the use of costly apparatus for a period of years, thus saving money and trouble. 2. At an early stage in the trouble the bones are relatively normal, both as regards their shapes and their mutual articulations; nor are there marked malpositions of the foot as a whole, which so often have to be overcome in operations at a later stage. 3. The tissues are then in a period of great plastic activity, when repair is both quicker and more perfect than in the older child. Cartilage is being changed into bone all through the foot, and we have less fear of a failure to secure bony union at the site of operation. 4. When at an early age the foot is secured in a relatively normal position, the statics of the lower limb are not so much disturbed, and growth goes on under more nearly normal conditions than can be possible when there is a constantly increasing tendency to the transmission of weight along abnormal lines. 5. By avoiding mechanical support the unaffected and partially paralyzed muscles are not subjected to the injury inseparable from the use of constricting bands and straps. They have in consequence a freer blood supply and develop more rapidly. Against the early operation two strong objections have been urged. They are: (1) the fear of an insecure cartilaginous union, which will make the use of retaining apparatus as necessary as it was before; (2) the danger of injury to the lower tibio-fibular epiphysis, causing interference with the growth of the limb and a consequent shortening. X-ray pictures of cases show the spicules of new bone forming between the tibia and the astragalus. In order to secure this union the author would lay special stress on the necessity of an accurate approximation of the opposing denuded surfaces. It is not enough to scrape away most of the cartilage and bring the bones "fairly well together." The joint must be thoroughly exposed and then an attempt be made to secure as square a line of contact between the bones as in a "typical" excision of the knee. As to the second objection, of injury to the growing epiphysis, destruction could only arise by the grossest carelessness on the part of the operator. As to irritation, even should this occur, which is problematical, it is a well-recognized fact that a moderate amount of irritation of a growing epiphysis acts as a stimulus, and causes, not a retardation, but an increase of growth, and it has been suggested in Germany that use should be made of this fact in operations on paralyzed joints.

Chondrodystrophy Fetalis.—John Lovett Morse *(Arch. of Ped.,* Aug., 1902) reports a case belonging to the class which has been variously described as fetal rickets, osteogenesis imperfecta, achondroplasia, and chondrodystrophy fetalis. In a general way, in these cases the trunk is normal, the extremities short and deformed, the head large, and the bridge of the nose flattened. Although a considerable number of cases has been thoroughly worked up, both macroscopically and microscopically, by competent observers, no scientific classification on pathological lines is at present possible. While the pathological lesions in the different specimens resemble each other in a general way, no two cases show exactly the same changes. Certain points, however, seem pretty well established. The most important pathological process is a disturbance of the normal process of ossification of the primary cartilage. It takes place early in fetal life, probably most often between the third and sixth months, and has ceased before birth. Hence chondrodystrophy fetalis seems the most suitable and comprehensive name to apply to it. There is nothing in common between it and rickets except the macroscopical appearances. Microscopically, the changes which produce such similar appearances are seen to be radically different. Some authors consider chondrodystrophy and cretinism to be intimately related, but shortening of the base of the skull may be due to failure of development as well as to synostosis (which is pathognomonic of cretinism). The pathological changes in the long bones are dissimilar in the two diseases, and in chondrodystrophy other signs of cretinism are lacking. In no case have the parents been cretinistic; no case has as yet been reported in regions where cretinism occurs; in cretinism the intelligence is subnormal, in chondrodystrophy it is normal. As the disease affects general nutrition as well as the osseous system, the fetus usually dies *in utero* or a few days after birth. Milder cases may reach adult life. But few cases of this condition have been reported in this country.

Diphtheria.—J. W. Pearce *(Amer. Pract. and News,* July 15, 1902) relates as follows the way he treats diphtheria, and he has never lost a case. If he can get perfectly fresh antitoxin he gives it, but if it cannot be had perfectly fresh he does not. Whether antitoxin is given or not, he gives ecthol, in full doses appropriate for the age of the patient, every three hours, administered by the mouth. The entire fauces, larynx, and pharynx are sprayed with a mixture of ecthol and peroxide of hydrogen, three parts of the former to one of the latter, every fifteen to thirty minutes. Calomel in small doses is administered every hour until the bowels are thoroughly moved. Nourishing and supporting diet is given at short, regular intervals, and plenty of fresh air admitted. In a series of 24 cases treated in this manner, seven received antitoxin and seventeen did not. The seventeen did as well as the seven. All recovered, and the author attributes most of the remedial effects to the ecthol, which was used in all cases throughout the entire attack.

A Fatal Case of Staphylococcus Pyogenes Aureus Infection of the Throat Resembling Diphtheria.—John Girdwood *(Maryland Med. Jour.,* Sept., 1902) reports a case in which the chief points of interest were the following: Infection by a pure culture of staphylococcus pyogenes aureus. The impossibility of distinguishing the condition from diphtheria without bacteriological examination of the exudate. The large amount of antitoxin administered, being in all six injections of 12,500 units, which the author thinks was the strongest clinical evidence against the diagnosis of true diphtheria. Large amounts of strychnia sulphate administered without evidence of physiological effects. The absence of metastatic abscesses or other clinical complications.

Infant Feeding.—Alexander McAlister *(Jour. Am. M. A.,* Aug. 2, 1902) says that it is universally admitted that such diseases as gastroenteritis, scurvy, rickets, etc., are peculiar to artificially-fed infants and children; but these are merely extreme manifestations of malnutrition. One need not observe very closely a general infant mortality table to see that the percentage of deaths is larger among the artificially-fed than among the breast-nursed. The former are always inferior physically to the latter. They may appear in robust health, and to the casual observer stronger than the average breast-nursed child of the same age, but they succumb first to the acute maladies of childhood. This fact is practically unknown among the common people, and, it is to be feared, does not receive proper consideration by physicians. An infant ruthlessly deprived of mother's milk succumbs to an attack of measles or whooping cough in childhood. Blame is never placed on the mode of early feeding, while it is likely that if the child had received the benefits of normal breast-nursing it would in all probability have survived the attack.

Lobar Pneumonia in Young Children.—J. A. Coutts *(Edin. Med. Jour.,* Sept., 1902) says that it may be safely asserted that no treatment yet devised has in any way shortened the natural course of this disease. The principal points in the active treatment of croupous pneumonia in children are comprised in the efforts to control the temperature when excessive, to alleviate pain, to procure sleep, and to relieve the strain upon the right heart. Very often the means used for the successful accomplishment of one of these purposes are effective in dealing with one or more of the others. As to reduction of the fever, the author believes that a high temperature is dangerous *per se,* in the direction of producing temporary degenerative changes in the heart and other viscera. Tepid sponging has the advantages of being easily performed and of being generally efficacious and sufficient. If this is so temporary in its relief as to have to be too often repeated, to the distress of the patient, there is no valid objection to the occasional use of a guarded dose of antipyrin. Its depressing effects can be mitigated by administering alcohol at the same time. Quinine in large doses, such as three grains for a child a year old and five grains for a child 2 years old, produces a much more lasting reduction of temperature, but requires so long a time to act that it is well to combine the antipyrin with the quinine. A single dose of opium is very valuable for the relief of pain associated with hyperpyrexia and insomnia in the first "shock" of the complaint. Pain arising from pleural inflammation may call for the application of one or two leeches to the affected side. Insomnia, if not cured by the measures used for the relief of hyperpyrexia and pain, is sometimes overcome by a copious warm enema. For cardiac failure, strychnine, with the exception of alcohol, is the only drug on which any reliance can be placed. Should these two remedies fail, bleeding may save the cases in which the urgency of the symptoms has been of comparatively gradual onset, when the cyanosis and heart extension to the right are more marked, and when the distended veins in the neck when depleted by the finger have filled the more readily up from below.

Pyloric Stenosis in Infants.—E. W. Saunders (*Med. Times and Register,* July, 1902) says that in the treatment of this disease the indications are: First, the administration of some medicinal agent which shall overcome to a greater or less extent the violent contraction of the pylorus. Among the drugs to be recommended are belladonna, bromides, and chloral. Second, the treatment of the secondary gastric irritation. This results from the stagnation of food, and should be treated by washing out the stomach and by giving it rest; rectal feeding should therefore be resorted to from time to time, and for twenty-four hours nothing but water given by the mouth; when food by the mouth is again allowed, the stomach should be washed out occasionally to remove a possible residuum of undigested food. Third, the diet of the child should consist of food which forms no coagulum in the stomach. Milk or any food containing undigested casein will not answer, consequently the mother's milk is usually unsuitable, while the milk of a wet-nurse in advanced lactation will succeed. Whey or peptonized milk, or a mixture of both, is usually the best food. The deficiency in fat should be supplied by cod-liver-oil. A very small percentage of cream can be gradually added. To aid the motor power of the stomach by gravity, the infant should be placed on its right side after nursing. The end to be accomplished is hypertrophy of the gastric wall without dilatation, hence the quantity of food should not be large. Gaseous distension of the stomach should by all means be prevented. When the infant fails in spite of rational treatment, surgical intervention must be advised.

INDEX.

A

C

G

H

I

TO CONTRIBUTORS AND SUBSCRIBERS.

ALL COMMUNICATIONS TO THIS JOURNAL, OF ANY NATURE WHATSOEVER. M
ONTRIBUTED TO IT EXCLUSIVELY. THE EDITOR RELIES ON ALL CONTRIBUTOR
ORMING STRICTLY TO THIS RULE.

The JOURNAL will be pleased to receive, and to translate at its own expens
ributions by Continental authors written in French, German, Swedish, or Ital
n examination they prove desirable.

The Editor is not responsible for the views of contributors.

LITHOGRAPHIC PLATES OR ILLUSTRATIONS on wood are prepared FREE wh
equired.

ALTERATIONS in the proof involving an excessive amount of work will be c
authors at the rate of 50 cents an hour.

REPRINTS.—Contributors desiring *extra copies* of their articles can
hem at reasonable rates by *application to the printers*, STETTINER BROS., Nos.
6, 58 Duane Street, New York, *immediately after the acceptance of the article
ditor.*

Twenty reprints, of articles published among "ORIGINAL COMMUNICATION
urnished *free, provided the request is distinctly stated on the manuscript* whe
ent to the Editor. ☞ Neither Editor nor Publishers take orders for reprints c
ind.

CONTRIBUTIONS, LETTERS, and all other communications relating solely 1
ditorial management of the JOURNAL should be sent DIRECTLY and EXCLUSIV
Dr. BROOKS H. WELLS. No. 34 West 45th Street, New York.

SUBSCRIPTIONS, EXCHANGES, BOOKS FOR REVIEW, and all business communic
hould be addressed to the publishers, 51 Fifth Avenue, New York.

PUBLISHERS and AUTHORS are informed that the space of the JOURNAL is s
occupied by matter pertaining solely to the branches to which it is devoted, tha
works treating of these subjects can be reviewed or noticed. Books and monog
native and foreign, on *Obstetrical. Gynecological, and Pediatrical* topics will
riewed without fail, according to their merits and the space at disposal.

WILLIAM WOOD & COMPANY, PUBLISHERS,
51 FIFTH AVENUE, NEW YORK.

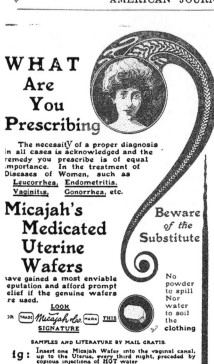
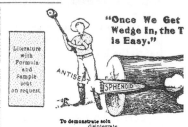